Core Curriculum *for* Progressive Care Nursing

AMERICAN
ASSOCIATION
of CRITICAL-CARE
NURSES

CORE CURRICULUM *for* PROGRESSIVE CARE NURSING

SAUNDERS

ELSEVIER

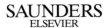

11830 Westline Industrial Drive
St. Louis, Missouri 63146

Core Curriculum for Progressive Care Nursing　　　　　　　ISBN: 978-1-4160-9987-1

Notice

Knowledge and best practice in this field are constantly changing. As new research and experience broaden our knowledge, changes in practice, treatment and drug therapy may become necessary or appropriate. Readers are advised to check the most current information provided (i) on procedures featured or (ii) by the manufacturer of each product to be administered, to verify the recommended dose or formula, the method and duration of administration, and contraindications. It is the responsibility of the practitioner, relying on their own experience and knowledge of the patient, to make diagnoses, to determine dosages and the best treatment for each individual patient, and to take all appropriate safety precautions. To the fullest extent of the law, neither the Publisher nor the Author assumes any liability for any injury and/or damage to persons or property arising out of or related to any use of the material contained in this book.

The Publisher

Library of Congress Cataloging-in-Publication Data

Core curriculum for progressive care nursing / American Association of Critical-Care Nurses. – 1st ed.
　　p. ; cm.
　Includes bibliographical references and index.
　ISBN 978-1-4160-9987-1 (pbk. : alk. paper)
　1. Progressive patient care. 2. Nursing. I. American Association of Critical-Care Nurses.
　[DNLM: 1. Critical Illness–nursing–Outlines. 2. Critical Care–methods–Outlines.
3. Progressive Patient Care–methods–Outlines. WY 18.2 C79727 2010]
　RT120.P76.C67 2010
　610.73–dc22

　　　　　　　　　　　　　　　　　　　　　　　　　　　　　　2008047438

Managing Editor: Maureen Iannuzzi
Senior Developmental Editor: Jennifer Ehlers
Book Production Manager: Gayle May
Project Manager: Tracey Schriefer
Book Designer: Amy Buxton

Printed in Canada

Last digit is the print number:　9　8　7　6　5　4　3　2　1

Working together to grow
libraries in developing countries

www.elsevier.com | www.bookaid.org | www.sabre.org

ELSEVIER　　BOOK AID International　　Sabre Foundation

Expert Panel

Kathleen M. Stacy, RN, MS, CNS, CCRN, PCCN, CCNS
Clinical Nurse Specialist–Intermediate Care Unit
Palomar Medical Center
Escondido, California
Adjunct Faculty Member
School of Nursing, College of Health and Human Services
San Diego State University
San Diego, California

Susan V. Helms, RN, MSN, CCRN, PCCN
Director of Professional Practice
   and Critical Care
Community Memorial Healthcenter
South Hill, Virginia

Sheryl E. Leary, RN, MS, CNS, CCNS,
   CCRN, PCCN
Clinical Nurse Specialist, Direct Observation
   Unit
Clinical Instructor, VA Nursing Academy
San Diego VA Healthcare System
San Diego State University
San Diego, California

Ellen Peller, RN, MSN, CNS, PCCN, CCRN
Staff Nurse
Cardiac Intensive Care Unit
Deaconess Medical Center
Spokane, Washington

Laura Savage, RN, MSN, PCCN
Cardiothoracic Clinical Nurse Specialist
Virginia Commonwealth University
Richmond, Virginia

Preface

As early as the 1970s, journals advertised for nurses to care for cardiac patients who needed heart rhythm monitoring but did not require intensive nursing care and continuous observation. Some were medical cardiology patients; others were recovering from cardiac surgery. The nurses worked in areas designated as step-down, telemetry, or intermediate care units.

Since then, the acuity of patients admitted to hospitals has steadily increased and with it the demand for a higher level of care. To accommodate the increased demand, stabilized patients are transferred out of critical care units while they continue to require an increased level of nursing care and vigilance. The units to which they are transferred have collectively become known as progressive care units, although they continue to carry other names that now include transitional care and direct observation, along with the familiar step-down, telemetry, and intermediate care units.

In 2001, the American Association of Critical-Care Nurses (AACN) recognized the need to define and identify the distinct needs of progressive care nurses, to define the progressive care environment, and to delineate the core competencies and basic knowledge and skill requirements of progressive care nursing. The AACN Certification Corporation developed the first progressive care certification examination in 2003, following completion of a national study of practice and using the AACN Synergy Model for Patient Care as the framework for matching patient needs with nurse competencies to achieve optimal patient outcomes. The Synergy Model identifies patients on the basis of the characteristics and needs they present rather than the beds they occupy. A second study of progressive care practice was completed in 2007. Its data were used to revise the PCCN certification examination.

AACN recognizes progressive care as part of the continuum of critical care. Progressive care nursing is delivered to patients whose needs fall along the less acute end of the continuum. Progressive care patients are moderately stable with less complexity. They require moderate resources and intermittent nursing vigilance. Or they may be stable with a high potential for becoming unstable, requiring increased intensity of care and vigilance. Characteristics of progressive care patients include decreased risk of a life-threatening event, decreased need for invasive monitoring, increased stability, and increased ability to participate in care decisions. Progressive care can be generalized, as in the care of patients with multisystem problems, or specialized, as in cardiac care.

The geographic domain of progressive care continues to expand with designated progressive care units, by any name, found in an ever-growing number of hospitals. Progressive care patients can now receive care based on the needs and nursing interventions they require, not the location where the care is provided. Where designated progressive care units do not exist, patients requiring this level of care are located throughout the hospital.

Critical care represents a continuum of complexity and acuity, so the competencies, knowledge, and skill requirements for progressive care logically derive from those used in intensive care units. This book presents the core curriculum necessary for learning how to provide progressive care and fills a much needed gap.

Caryl Goodyear-Bruch, RN, PhD, CCRN
AACN President 2008-2009

Acknowledgments

The American Association of Critical-Care Nurses gratefully acknowledges the work of the editor, JoAnn Grif Alspach, RN, MSN, EdD, and the contributors of *Core Curriculum for Critical Care Nursing,* 6th edition, which formed the basis for *Core Curriculum for Progressive Care Nursing:*

Jan Marie Belden, MSN, APRN, BC, FNP
Nancy Blake, RN, MN, CCRN, CNAA
Pamela J. Bolton, RN, MS, ACNP, CCNS, CCRN, PCCN
Dennis J. Cheek, RN, PhD, FAHA
Kathleen Ellstrom, RN, PhD, APRN, BC
Susan Gallagher, RN, MSN, CNS, PhD
Mary A. Hall, RN, MSN
Elizabeth A. Henneman, RN, PhD, CCNS, FAAN
Reneé Holleran, RN, PhD, CEN, CCRN, CFRN, FAEN
M. Lindsay Lessig, BSN, MSEd, MBA
Kim Litwack, RN, PhD, CFNP, FAAN
Karen A. McQuillan, RN, MS, CCRN, CNRN
Nancy C. Molter, RN, MN, PhD
Amy A. Nichols, RN, CNS, EdD
Jan Odom-Forren, RN, MS, CPAN, FAAN
Ginette A. Pepper, RN, PhD, FAAN
Patricia Radovich, RN, MSN, CNS, FCCM
Marilyn Sawyer Sommers, RN, PhD, FAAN
June L. Stark, RN, BSN, MEd

Thanks to Laura Savage, RN, MSN, PCCN, who consulted on initial content development and to the nurses who participated in the content survey that informed the editorial direction for *Core Curriculum for Progressive Care Nursing:*

Christie Artuso, RN, MA, CCRN, PCCN
Katie Brick, RN, MSN, CCNS, CCRN, PCCN
Beverly Clayton, RN, MSN, CCRN, CRT, LMT
Jo Ellen Craghead, RN, MSN, CCRN, PCCN
Joanna Entrekin-Callahan, RN, CCRN-CSC-CMC, PCCN

Don Everly, RN, MSN, CCRN-CMC, PCCN, CCNS
Allynda Hammond, RNC, MS, CCRN, PCCN, CMC
Patti Henry, RN, MSN, FNP, CNS, CCNS, CCRN, PCCN
Mary Ann House-Fancher, ACNP, MSN, CCRN-CSC, PCCN
Stephanie Maillie, RN, MSN, PCCN, CCRN, CCNS
Shirley Sebastian, RN, CCRN, PCCN
Nancy Rowley, RN, CCRN, PCCN
Jackie Myers, RN, CCRN, PCCN, CSC, CNP
Kathleen M. Stacy, RN, MS, CNS, CCRN, PCCN, CCNS
Dawn M. Specht, RN, MSN, CEN, CCRN, PCCN, CCNS
Carol A. Rauen, RN, MS, CCNS, CCRN, PCCN
Ann M. Peterson, RN, MS, CNS, PCCN
Jeanette Meyer, RN, MSN, CCRN, CCNS, PCCN
Jennifer M. McCord, RN, MSN, CCRN, PCCN, CCNS
Jane Lindblad, RN, BSN, CCRN, PCCN
Susan V. Helms, RN, MSN, CCRN, PCCN
Judy Giovannelli, RN, CCRN, PCCN
Lisa Thomas Barile, RN, MSN, CCRN, PCCN

AACN gives special thanks to the progressive care subject matter experts who reviewed and revised the manuscript for *Core Curriculum for Progressive Care Nursing,* whose significant contributions made this edition possible: Kathleen M. Stacy, RN, MS, CNS, CCRN, PCCN, CCNS; Susan V. Helms, RN, MSN, CCRN, PCCN; Sheryl E. Leary, RN, MS, CCNS, CCRN, PCCN, CNS; Ellen Peller, RN, MSN, CCRN, PCCN, CNS; and Laura Savage, RN, MSN, PCCN.

Thanks also to the clinical practice specialists on the AACN national office staff who provided expert consultation and review: Linda Bell, RN, MSN; Mary Pat Aust, RN, MS; Pamela Shellner, RN, MA; Laura McNamara, RN, MSN, CCRN, CCNS; RoseMarie Faber,

RN, MSN/ED, CCRN; and to Carol Hartigan, RN, MA, and Karen Harvey, RN, MSN, of the AACN Certification Corporation national office staff for consultation on the PCCN certification examination test plan.

To the team at Elsevier: thanks to Maureen Iannuzzi, Jennifer Ehlers, Julia Curcio, Tracey Schriefer, Amy Buxton, and their colleagues for bringing this book to progressive care nurses.

Introduction

The evolution of progressive care nursing practice has paralleled historical changes and demands for additional environments in which high-acuity, overflow critical care patients and patients requiring specialized surveillance could be safely cared for. Such areas have a variety of names including transitional care unit, stepdown unit, progressive care unit, intermediate care unit, and telemetry unit. The formation of these new patient care units created new challenges in the development of standards of practice, guidelines for care, and admission and discharge criteria. In 2001 the American Association of Critical-Care Nurses (AACN) created a task force and advisory panel who defined this emerging new patient care environment and provided some guidance on competency requirements for nurses practicing in progressive care. *Progressive care* is the term AACN uses to collectively represent the variety of high-acuity units described previously. AACN envisions progressive care as part of the critical care continuum where patients are in less critical condition than those in traditional critical care units. Progressive care is a place where highly skilled nurses combine skills of assessment, surveillance, communication, patient teaching, and coaching into what is called progressive care nursing.

Definition

AACN recognizes progressive care as part of the continuum of critical care. AACN's vision is dedicated to creating a health care system driven by the needs of patients and families in which critical care nurses make their optimal contribution. The AACN Synergy Model for Patient Care is the conceptual framework that actualizes the vision. It defines nursing practice according to the needs of the patient and the characteristics of the nurse so that optimal patient outcomes can be achieved.

Progressive care defines the care that is delivered to patients whose needs fall along the less-acute end of the continuum. Progressive care patients are in moderately stable condition with less complexity, require moderate resources, and require intermittent nursing vigilance or are in stable condition with a high potential for becoming unstable and require increased intensity of care and vigilance. Characteristics of progressive care patients include decreased risk for life-threatening events, decreased need for invasive monitoring, increased stability, and increased ability to participate in their care.

Location of Progressive Care Patients

Using the AACN Synergy Model for Patient Care will assist in defining the progressive care patient. The Synergy Model identifies patients according to the characteristics and needs they present rather than the location of the bed they occupy. As in critical care, the geographic domain of progressive care is expanding. Care provided to progressive care patients is not limited by geography but is based on the needs and required interventions of the patient. Although specific progressive care units can be identified, patients requiring progressive care nursing can be located throughout the hospital.

Progressive care can be very specialized, with care focused on a specific system such as cardiac, or more generalized, as in the care of patients with multisystem problems.

Educational Requirements

Progressive care nursing has expanded beyond the basic cardiac telemetry that marked its beginning and now encompasses many of the same technologies and therapies that were once synonymous with critical care units. To meet the changing needs of the patient, nurses caring for progressive care patients must demonstrate competencies that are influenced by ever-changing technology. Progressive care nurses must demonstrate the following core competencies:

- Dysrhythmia monitoring techniques
- Basic and advanced life support
- Basic dysrhythmia interpretation and treatment
- Drug dosage calculation, continuous medication infusion administration, and patient monitoring for medication effects (e.g., nontitrated vasoactive agents, platelet inhibitors, antiarrhythmic agents, insulin)
- Patient monitoring using standardized procedures for preoperative, intraoperative, and postoperative procedures (e.g., cardioversion, transesophageal echocardiography, cardiac catheterization with percutaneous coronary intervention, bronchoscopy, esophagogastroduodenoscopy, percutaneous endoscopic gastrostomy tube placement, chest tube insertion)
- Hemodynamic monitoring including equipment setup and troubleshooting, monitoring, and recognition of signs and symptoms of patient instability
- Recognition of the signs and symptoms of cardiopulmonary emergencies and initiation of standardized interventions to stabilize the patient awaiting transfer to critical care
- Interpretation of arterial blood gas analysis and communication of findings
- Recognition of indications for and management of patients requiring noninvasive oxygen delivery systems including oral airways, bilevel positive airway pressure, and continuous positive airway pressure
- Assessment of the patient receiving mechanical ventilation to monitor patient response and ensure delivery of the prescribed treatment
- Assessment and understanding of long-term mechanical ventilation and weaning
- Recognition of the indications for and complications of enteral and parenteral nutrition
- Assessment, monitoring, and management of patients requiring renal therapeutic interventions (e.g., hemodialysis, peritoneal dialysis, stents, continuous bladder irrigation, urostomies)
- Recognition of and evaluation of the family's need for enhanced involvement in care to facilitate the transition from hospital to home

The Synergy Model describes patient function according to these characteristics: stability, complexity, vulnerability, resiliency, predictability, resource availability, participation in care, and participation in decision making. Characteristics of the nurse that typically represent comprehensive nursing practice include clinical judgment, advocacy, caring practices, collaboration, systems thinking, response to diversity, clinical inquiry, and facilitator of learning. The model therefore takes into account the unpredictability of the progressive care patient and the competencies of the progressive care nurse on the basis of the patient's and family's needs.

Competency development for progressive care nurses has historically been based on the essential components of critical care education. However, progressive care nurses may have the opportunity to enhance and further develop certain areas of practice. Some of the most common patient presentations that progressive care nurses experience are patients who have less technology available for assessment and intervention than what is typically found in the critical care environment. The progressive care nurse's greatest tool in providing patient care is personal clinical assessment skill development. The development of keen assessment skills using such techniques as palpation, auscultation, observation, and percussion becomes the progressive care nurse's greatest asset. Progressive care nurses care for patients who have experienced a critical illness and have progressed to a state of recovery. The needs of patients and families at this stage along the care continuum require consideration for increasing independence and self-care; patient education becomes an important competency. Some patients are admitted to the progressive care area for heightened surveillance and specialized care and may require transfer to the critical care unit. The progressive care nurse's ability to identify subtle changes in the patient's condition, communicate those changes in a meaningful way, and prepare the patient and family for the transfer is an essential lifesaving skill.

Evidence-Based Practice

Some progressive care units may require nurses to obtain additional training such as ventilator management, transplant care, and specialized surgical interventions. Such units may be institution specific and have specific competency requirements for the nursing staff. We acknowledge that there are challenges in consistent standards of care and nursing practice in progressive care units as this new environment is emergent. At the Mayo Clinic clinical nurse specialists created a progressive care practice committee that standardized practice and promoted utilization of evidence-based practice across seven progressive care units. A major accomplishment for this progressive care practice committee was establishment of guidelines for intravenous drug infusion including types and frequency of monitoring required based on the pharmacologic action and potential side effects of each drug. These practice standards were implemented across all progressive care units. The many similarities of progressive care nursing are being described in various practice venues and provide opportunities for progressive care nurses to explore ways of improving patient care using evidence-based knowledge.

Staffing

Staffing in progressive care units has been challenging. Few resources are available for staffing progressive care using the standard hours per patient day calculations and conventional staffing standards. St. Mary's Hospital Medical Center in Madison, Wisconsin, completed an extensive analysis of hours per patient day delivered in various nursing care units from 1992 to 2005, during which time hours per patient day in the intermediate and progressive care units increased by approximately 23%. The National Database of Nursing Quality Indicators provides benchmarks to participating hospitals for comparison with like units and like hospitals. As progressive care units become more and more prevalent within acute care hospitals, research is needed to further define the staffing requirements for units that fit the progressive care definition.

Progressive Care Job Analysis

AACN Certification Corporation completed the second study of practice and job analysis for adult progressive care nursing in 2007. The study of practice defines the scope of progressive care practice and provides clarification on the commonalties in progressive care nursing practice. A panel of experts developed a survey using the AACN Synergy Model as the framework for a practice analysis for the progressive care practice environment. In the study, nurses across the United States were surveyed to ascertain the frequency and significance of the various elements of progressive care practice. The job analysis underwent an extensive review process to ascertain content validity to provide a foundation for revising the progressive care certification examination on the basis of the study of practice. The findings were used in the revision of the progressive care test plan for the progressive care certification examination.

PCCN Certification Credential

PCCN is a registered service mark of the AACN Certification Corporation and is the credential granted to nurses who meet the eligibility criteria and successfully pass the PCCN certification examination. The PCCN examination, which is approved by the National Commission for Certifying Agencies, requires 2.5 hours and comprises 125 multiple-choice items derived from a progressive care study of practice completed in 2007. The certification examination and recertification process are based on the AACN Synergy Model for Patient Care, the established model of care whose hallmark is matching patient needs with nurse competencies.

We hope this text will assist nurses who practice in a variety of clinical settings to increase their skills, knowledge, and confidence in the care of high-acuity patients. It is intended to serve as a guide for core competency development and support preparation for the PCCN progressive care certification examination. We hope it will be helpful in preparing nurses to deliver the highest quality of patient care in the progressive care environment.

About the Text

Core Curriculum for Progressive Care Nursing provides the fundamental knowledge required to care for the patient in the progressive care unit. This book is designed to meet the needs of the nurse new to the specialty of progressive care nursing and the nurse studying for the PCCN exam. Classic references are identified in each chapter with a star icon. Information required for the PCCN exam is identified in a colored font for ease of identification. Given the extremely diverse nature of progressive care, additional content is provided to meet the needs of the nurse going into the specialty of progressive care regardless of the type of unit. Therefore, if the focus of the progressive care unit is pulmonary and the nurse is expected to care for patients on ventilators, additional content on mechanical ventilation has been provided even though it is not on the PCCN exam. Thus it is the intent of *Core Curriculum for Progressive Care Nursing* to

- Present the essential information required for the nurse studying for the PCCN exam
- Provide the foundational knowledge needed for the nurse new to the specialty of progressive care

■ Serve as a resource for the nurse already working in the progressive care unit

With the exception of the first chapter, the book is segregated into chapters by body systems using an embellished outline formation for presentation. Each chapter contains subsections related to physiologic anatomy, patient assessment, patient problems, and disorders. Chapter 1, Professional Caring and Ethical Practice, provides a comprehensive description of AACN's perspective on progressive care nursing; the Synergy Model of Patient Care; and AACN's mission, vision, and values statements. In addition, information regarding healthy work environments, patient safety, ethical practice, and legal aspects of progressive care nursing are presented.

REFERENCES

American Association of Critical-Care Nurses. *AACN Scope and Standards for Acute and Critical Care Nursing Practice*. Aliso Viejo, CA: AACN; 2008.

American Association of Critical-Care Nurses. Progressive Care Fact Sheet. http://www.aacn.org/WD/Practice/Content/progressivecarefactsheet.pcms?menu=Practice. Accessed July 22, 2008.

Beglinger JE. Quantifying patient care intensity: an evidence-based approach to determining staffing requirements. *Nurs Adm Q.* 2006;30(3):193-202.

McCabe PJ, Kalpin P. Bold voices in progressive care: using shared decision making to implement evidence-based practice in progressive care. *Crit Care Nurse.* 2005;25(2):76-87.

Nasraway SA, Cohen IL, Dennis RC, et al. American College of Critical Care Medicine of the Society of Critical Care Medicine: Guidelines on admission and discharge for adult intermediate care units. *Crit Care Med.* 1998;26(3):607-610.

Contents

Professional Caring and Ethical Practice

AMERICAN ASSOCIATION OF CRITICAL-CARE NURSES: MISSION, VISION, AND VALUES

Mission

Patients and their families rely on nurses at the most vulnerable times of their lives. Acute and critical care nurses rely on the American Association of Critical-Care Nurses (AACN) for expert knowledge and the influence to fulfill their promise to patients and their families. AACN drives excellence because nothing less is acceptable (AACN, 2008).

Vision

A health care system driven by the needs of patients and families in which nurses can make their optimal contribution.

Values

As AACN works to promote its mission and vision, it is guided by values that are rooted in, and arise from, the association's history, traditions, and culture. Therefore, AACN and its members, volunteers, and staff will:
1. Be accountable to uphold and consistently act in concert with ethical values and principles.
2. Advocate for organizational decisions that are driven by the needs of patients and their families.
3. Act with integrity by communicating openly and honestly, keeping promises, honoring commitments, and promoting loyalty in all relationships.
4. Collaborate with all essential stakeholders by creating synergistic relationships to promote common interest and shared values.
5. Provide leadership to transform thinking, structures, and processes to address opportunities and challenges.
6. Demonstrate stewardship through fair and responsible management of resources.
7. Embrace lifelong learning, inquiry, and critical thinking to enable each to make optimal contributions.
8. Commit to quality and excellence at all levels of the organization, meeting and exceeding standards and expectations.
9. Promote innovation through creativity and calculated risk taking.
10. Generate commitment to and passion for the organization's causes and work.

SYNERGY OF CARING

What Nurses Do

1. Attend to the full range of human experiences of and responses to health and illness.
2. Integrate objective data with knowledge of the patient as a person and understanding of the patient's subjective experience.
3. Apply scientific knowledge to the process of diagnosis and treatment of the responses to health and illness.
4. Establish a caring relationship that facilitates healing (ANA, 2003).

What Progressive Care Nurses Do

In 2007, the AACN Certification Corporation Progressive Care Practice Analysis Task Force developed a survey tool that asked the following questions:
■ What do you mean by progressive care nursing?
■ What are the characteristics of acutely ill patients?
■ How are they different from critically ill patients?
■ What special knowledge, skill, and abilities are necessary for nurses to work in progressive care areas, caring for high-acuity patients?

Nurses from all across the nation responded with the answers that provide the job analysis of progressive care nurses. The findings of this analysis were used to develop the test blueprint for the PCCN examination and are available online at http://www.aacn.org/WD/Certifications/content/pccnexamblueprint.pcms.

1. Progressive care nurses deal with human responses to life-threatening problems.
2. The Scope of Practice includes all ages and involves a dynamic interaction between the critically ill patient, the patient's family, the progressive care nurse, and the environment.
3. The framework of practice includes the scientific body of specialized knowledge, an ethical model for decision making, a commitment to interdisciplinary collaboration, and the AACN Synergy Model for Patient Care. Progressive care nurses rely on this framework to do the following (Bell, 2008):
   a. Restore, support, promote, and maintain the physiologic stability of vulnerable patients across the lifespan.
   b. Assimilate and prioritize information sources to take immediate and decisive patient-focused action.
   c. Anticipate, respond with confidence and adapt to rapidly changing patient conditions.
   d. Respond to the unique needs of patients and families coping with unanticipated treatment, quality of life, and end-of-life decisions.
   e. Manage appropriately the interface between the patient and technology that may be threatening, invasive, and complex so that human needs for a safe, respectful, healing, humane, and caring environment are established and maintained.
   f. Monitor and allocate progressive care services, recognizing the fiduciary role of nurses working in a resource-intensive environment.
   g. Use healthcare interventions designed to restore, rehabilitate, cure, maintain, or palliate for patients across the lifespan.

The Environment of Progressive Care

1. Progressive care patients require moderate to complex assessment and therapies, surveillance and specialized monitoring, vigilance, education, and rehabilitation.
2. Organizational model for a humane, caring, and healing environment
   a. The progressive care nurse works with an interdisciplinary team to create a humane, caring, and healing environment. There are five elements of an organizational model for health and healing (Malloch, 2000; Molter, 2003):
      i. Common values of health as a function of mind-body-spirit interrelationships
      ii. Patient and family–centered philosophy
      iii. Physical environment that supports healing
      iv. Use of complementary and alternative therapies, as well as conventional therapies
      v. Organizational culture that promotes personal growth

    b. The progressive care nurse is a constant in the environment and works to develop an organizational culture that supports the following (Bell, 2008):

        i. Providers acting as advocates on behalf of patients, families, and communities

        ii. Patient's and family's values and preferences driving care decisions

        iii. Practice based on research and best evidence

        iv. The expectation and promotion of ethical decision making

        v. Collaboration and collegiality

        vi. The fostering of leadership at all levels

        vii. Lifelong learning for professional growth

        viii. Optimization of existing talents and resources

        ix. The rewarding of innovation, creativity, and clinical inquiry through meaningful recognition

        x. Valuing and incorporating diversity in healthcare delivery

        xi. The expectation of effective communication at all levels

        xii. A professional practice model that drives the delivery of nursing care

3. Patient safety

    a. The Institute of Medicine in its 2004 report *Keeping Patients Safe: Transforming the Work Environment for Nurses* describes the essential elements and interplay of an effective safety culture in organizations where low levels of errors and accidents occurred:

        i. Environmental structures and processes within the organization that promote safety

        ii. Strong attitudes and perceptions of safety of the workers

        iii. Strong safety behaviors exhibited by individuals in the organization

    b. The creation of a culture of safety requires changing attitudes and behaviors to a new paradigm of continuous consciousness of safety. *AACN Standards for Establishing and Sustaining Healthy Work Environments* (Barden, 2005) provides progressive care nurses with standards that can be implemented to create a culture of safety:

        i. Skilled communication

        ii. True collaboration

        iii. Effective decision making

        iv. Appropriate staffing

        v. Meaningful recognition

        vi. Authentic leadership

    c. The progressive care work environment's location on the patient care trajectory provides a great opportunity for progressive care nurses to demonstrate the effectiveness of healthy work environments. Lewis and Vickers (2008), in their poster presentation "Unit Based Shared Governance Leads the Journey of Creating a Healthy Work Environment," demonstrated how a progressive care unit (PCU) base council using the Healthy Work Environment Standards could increase the involvement of bedside nurses in practice decisions, quality improvement, research, recruitment, and retention and improve collaboration and communication between nursing and all disciplines. Measuring the success of implementing the standards can be accomplished by using available tools. Kramer and Schmalenberg (2008) provide a comparison of the Essentials of Magnetism and the Healthy Work Environment Standards. The Essentials of Magnetism tool can be used to assess the extent to which the healthy work environment strategies are in place in PCUs.

    d. The Joint Commission's National Patient Safety Goals (2009)* include the following:

        i. Improve the accuracy of patient identification by using at least two patient identifiers when providing care, treatment, and services, including collection specimens, medication administration, transfusion, and treatment. The care provider must involve the patient in the process of accurate identification whenever possible. The patient's room number or physician is not used as a method of identifying the patient.

        ii. Improve the effectiveness of communication among caregivers by reading back verbal or telephone orders and critical laboratory results; standardizing abbreviations, acronyms, and symbols not to be used in the organization; improving the timeliness of receiving and reporting critical test results and values; and standardizing the "hand-off" of communications.

iii. Improve the safety of using medications by standardizing and limiting the number of drug concentrations available in the organization; identifying and reviewing a list of look-alike/sound-alike drugs; taking action to prevent errors involving the interchange of these drugs; labeling all medications, medication containers, or other solutions in perioperative and other procedural settings; implementing a defined anticoagulation management program; and individualizing the care of patients receiving this therapy.

iv. Reduce the risk of health care–associated infections by complying with current World Health Organization (WHO) and Centers for Disease Control and Prevention (CDC) hand hygiene guidelines and managing as sentinel events all identified cases of unanticipated death or major permanent loss of function associated with a health care–associated infection. Implement evidence-based practices that prevent multiple drug–resistant organisms and implement best practice guidelines that prevent central line–associated bloodstream infections and surgical site infections.

v. Accurately and completely reconcile medications across the continuum of care by implementing a process to obtain and document a complete list of the patient's current medications on the patient's admission to the organization, by comparing the medications on the list with those available in the organization, and by communicating the list to the next provider of service and documenting the communication when a patient is referred or transferred within the hospital. Provide a complete list of reconciled medications to the patient's known primary care provider or next health care provider on discharge.

vi. Reduce the risk of patient harm resulting from falls by implementing a fall-reduction program and evaluating its effectiveness.

vii. Implement strategies that allow patients to participate in their own care, including mechanisms for patients and families to report safety concerns.

viii. Implement strategies that identify safety risks in emotional and behavioral disorders present in the patient population by implementing a risk assessment of population.

ix. Improve recognition of changes in the patient's condition by implementing a system for calling additional expert help for the assessment and treatment of changes in the patient's condition. This system allows patients and families to access this help when the patient's condition worsens.

e. Patient safety practices have significant implications in the progressive care environment where patient are at a moderate to high acuity level. Patient safety goals that have a significant impact on the delivery in progressive care include the following:

i. Patient Safety Goal 2 focuses on safety in communication. PCUs are known for the high number of patients that are handed off through transfers and for tests. Skilled handoff communication using techniques such as Situation, Background, Assessment, and Recommendation (SBAR) is paramount to successful interaction and safe patient care delivery (Haig, Sutton, & Whittington, 2006).

ii. Patient Safety Goal 3 addresses the procedural time-out requirement. This safety goal applies only to surgical suites and to preoperative and postoperative care. It applies to procedures that are commonly done in progressive care, including chest tube insertions, elective cardioversions, and complex dressing changes. The standardization and limiting of drug concentrations in the organization has implications for PCUs. Progressive care patient populations vary from institution to institution, and standardization of patient care medication delivery is an important patient safety consideration.

iii. Patient Safety Goal 5 identifies the need to reconcile medications across the continuum of care. The reconciliation of progressive patients' medications can be a challenge for patients who have been transferred from PCUs. These patients enter a phase of rehabilitation and may be discharged from the PCU. Attention to the details during medication reconciliation on transfer and discharge becomes an important consideration of the progressive care nurse.

The "Synergy" of the AACN Synergy Model for Patient Care

1. Synergistic practice and patient and family safety: The AACN Synergy Model for Patient Care (Curley, 1998) describes nursing practice in terms of the needs and characteristics of patients. The model's premise is that the needs of the patient and family system drive the competencies required by the nurse. When this occurs, synergy is produced, and optimal outcomes can be achieved. Buckminster Fuller stated that "synergy is the only word in our language that means behavior of whole systems unpredicted by the separately observed behaviors of any of the system's separate parts or any subassembly of the system's parts" (Carlson, 1996). The synergy created by practice based on the Synergy Model helps the patient-family unit safely navigate the health care system.
2. The Synergy Model and ethical practice: The Synergy Model provides a foundation for addressing ethical concerns related to progressive care nursing practice (McGaffic, 2001). The model focuses on the characteristics of patients, the competencies needed by the progressive care nurse to meet the patient's needs on the basis of these characteristics, and the outcomes that can be achieved through the synergy that develops when nursing competencies are driven by the patient's needs. AACN is committed to helping members deal with ethical issues through education (Glassford, 1999).

AACN SYNERGY MODEL FOR PATIENT CARE

Origin of the Synergy Model for Patient Care

In 1992, AACN developed a vision of a health care system driven by the needs of patients and their families in which progressive care nurses can make their optimal contribution. AACN Certification Corporation in tandem was rethinking the contributions of certification to the care of patients. Patient needs and outcomes must be the central focus of certification. A think tank was convened in 1992 to reconceptualize certified practice (Caterinicchio, 1995; Villaire, 1996).

Purpose

Before development of the Synergy Model, the certification process conceptualized nursing practice according to the dimensions of the nurse's role, the clinical setting, and the patient's diagnosis. The Synergy Model reconceptualized certified practice to recognize that the needs and characteristics of patients and families influence and drive the competencies of nurses.

Overview of the Synergy Model

1. Description of the Synergy Model (Figure 1-1): Synergy results when the needs and characteristics of a patient, clinical unit, or system are matched with a nurse's competencies. All patients have similar needs and experience these needs across wide ranges or continuums from health to illness. Logically, the more compromised patients are, the more severe or complex are their needs. The dimensions of a nurse's practice are driven by the needs of a patient and family.

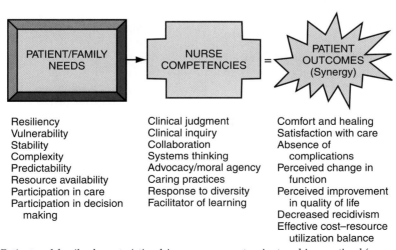

FIGURE 1-1 ■ Patient and family characteristics drive nurse competencies to achieve optimal (synergistic) outcomes.

This requires nurses to be proficient in the multiple dimensions of the nursing continuums. When nurse competencies stem from patient needs and the characteristics of the nurse and patient synergize, optimal patient outcomes can result (AACN, 2003).

2. Assumptions guiding the AACN Synergy Model for Patient Care (AACN, 2003): These characteristics must be viewed in the context of various assumptions regarding nurses, patients, and families that guide the Synergy Model:
   a. Patients are biological, psychological, social, and spiritual entities who present at a particular developmental stage. The whole patient (body, mind, and spirit) must be considered.
   b. The patient, family, and community all contribute to providing a context for the nurse-patient relationship.
   c. Patients can be described by a number of characteristics. All characteristics are connected and contribute to each other. Characteristics cannot be looked at in isolation.
   d. Similarly, nurses can be described on a number of dimensions. The interrelated dimensions paint a profile of the nurse.
   e. A goal of nursing is to restore a patient to an optimal level of wellness as defined by the patient. Death can be an acceptable outcome, in which the goal of nursing care is to move a patient toward a peaceful death.
3. Patient characteristics: Characteristics unique to each patient and family span the continua of health and illness. The first five are intrinsic to the patient, and the last three are extrinsic. Each characteristic is described in terms of a range of levels from 1 to 5 in Table 1-1.
   a. Resiliency: The capacity to return to a restorative level of functioning using compensatory and coping mechanisms; the ability to bounce back quickly after an insult
   b. Vulnerability: Susceptibility to actual or potential stressors that may adversely affect patient outcomes
   c. Stability: The ability to maintain a steady-state equilibrium
   d. Complexity: The intricate entanglement of two or more systems (e.g., body, family, therapies)
   e. Predictability: A characteristic that allows one to expect a certain course of events or course of illness
   f. Resource availability: Extent of resources (e.g., technical, fiscal, personal, psychologic, social) the patient, family, and community bring to the situation
   g. Participation in care: Extent to which the patient and/or family engages in aspects of care
   h. Participation in decision making: Extent to which the patient and/or family engages in decision making
4. Nurse characteristics: Nursing care is an integration of knowledge, skills, experience, and individual attitudes. The continua of nurse characteristics needed are derived from the patient's needs and range from a competent to an expert level as outlined in Table 1-2.
   a. Clinical judgment: Clinical reasoning, which includes clinical decision making, critical thinking, and a global grasp of the situation, coupled with nursing skills acquired through a process of integrating education, experiential knowledge, and evidence-based guidelines
   b. Advocacy/moral agency: Working on another's behalf and representing the concerns of the patient/family and nursing staff; serving as a moral agent in identifying and helping to resolve ethical and clinical concerns within and outside the clinical setting
   c. Caring practices: Nursing activities that create a compassionate, supportive, and therapeutic environment for patients and staff, with the aim of promoting comfort and healing and preventing unnecessary suffering. These caring behaviors include but are not limited to vigilance, engagement, and responsiveness. Caregivers include family and health care personnel.
   d. Collaboration: Working with others (e.g., patients and families, health care providers) in a way that promotes each person's contributions toward achieving optimal and realistic patient and family goals. Collaboration involves intradisciplinary and interdisciplinary work with colleagues and community.
   e. Systems thinking: The body of knowledge and tools that allow the nurse to manage whatever environmental and system resources exist for the patient, family, and staff within or across health care and non–health care systems
   f. Response to diversity: The sensitivity to recognize, appreciate, and incorporate differences into the provision of care. Differences may include, but are not limited to, cultural, spiritual, gender, race, ethnicity, lifestyle, socioeconomic, age, and values.

■ **TABLE 1-1**
■ ■ **The Synergy Model—Patient Characteristics**

Characteristic and Description	Continua of Health and Illness*
INTRINSIC CHARACTERISTICS	
RESILIENCY The capacity to return to a restorative level of functioning using compensatory and coping mechanisms; the ability to bounce back quickly after an insult	*Level 1: Minimally resilient* • Unable to mount a response • Failure of compensatory/coping mechanisms • Minimal reserves • Brittle *Level 3: Moderately resilient* • Able to mount a moderate response • Able to initiate some degree of compensation • Moderate reserves *Level 5: Highly resilient* • Able to mount and maintain a response • Intact compensatory/coping mechanisms • Strong reserves • Endurance
VULNERABILITY Susceptibility to actual or potential stressors that may adversely affect patient outcomes	*Level 1: Highly vulnerable* • Susceptible • Unprotected, fragile *Level 3: Moderately vulnerable* • Somewhat susceptible • Somewhat protected *Level 5: Minimally vulnerable* • Safe; out of the woods • Protected, not fragile
STABILITY The ability to maintain a steady-state equilibrium	*Level 1: Minimally stable* • Labile; unstable • Unresponsive to therapies • High risk of death *Level 3: Moderately stable* • Able to maintain steady state for limited period of time • Some responsiveness to therapies *Level 5: Highly stable* • Constant • Responsive to therapies • Low risk of death
COMPLEXITY The intricate entanglement of two or more systems (e.g., body, family, therapies)	*Level 1: Highly complex* • Intricate • Complex patient/family dynamics • Ambiguous/vague • Atypical presentation *Level 3: Moderately complex* • Moderately involved patient/family dynamics *Level 5: Minimally complex* • Straightforward • Routine patient/family dynamics • Simple/clear-cut • Typical presentation
PREDICTABILITY A characteristic that allows one to expect a certain course of events or course of illness	*Level 1: Not predictable* • Uncertain • Uncommon patient population or illness

Continued

■ TABLE 1-1
■ ■ The Synergy Model—Patient Characteristics—Cont'd

Characteristic and Description	Continua of Health and Illness*
PREDICTABILITY—CONT'D	• Unusual or unexpected course
	• Does not follow critical pathway, or no critical pathway developed
	Level 3: Moderately predictable
	• Wavering
	• Occasionally noted patient population or illness
	Level 5: Highly predictable
	• Certain
	• Common patient population or illness
	• Usual and expected course
	• Follows critical pathway
EXTRINSIC CHARACTERISTICS	
RESOURCE AVAILABILITY	*Level 1: Few resources*
Extent of resources (e.g., technical, fiscal, personal, psychologic, and social) the patient, family, and community bring to the situation	• Necessary knowledge and skills not available
	• Necessary financial support not available
	• Minimal personal/psychologic supportive resources
	• Few social systems resources
	Level 3: Moderate resources
	• Limited knowledge and skills available
	• Limited financial support available
	• Limited personal/psychologic supportive resources
	• Limited social systems resources
	Level 5: Many resources
	• Extensive knowledge and skills available and accessible
	• Financial resources readily available
	• Strong personal/psychologic supportive resources
	• Strong social systems resources
PARTICIPATION IN CARE	*Level 1: No participation*
Extent to which patient and/or family engages in aspects of care	• Patient and/or family unable or unwilling to participate in care
	Level 3: Moderate participation
	• Patient and/or family need assistance in care
	Level 5: Full participation
	• Patient and/or family fully able and willing to participate in care
PARTICIPATION IN DECISION MAKING	*Level 1: No participation*
Extent to which patient and/or family engages in decision making	• Patient and/or family have no capacity for decision making; require surrogacy
	Level 3: Moderate participation
	• Patient and/or family have limited capacity; seek input/advice from others in decision making
	Level 5: Full participation
	• Patient and/or family have capacity, and make decisions themselves

From AACN Certification Corporation.
*Note that the continua of health and illness levels vary in order of rating based on the characteristic.

   g. Clinical inquiry or innovation and evaluation: The ongoing process of questioning and evaluating practice and providing informed practice; creating changes through evidence-based practice, research utilization, and experiential knowledge

   h. Facilitator of learning: The ability to facilitate learning for patients and families, nursing staff, other members of the health care team, and community; includes both formal and informal facilitation of learning

▓ TABLE 1-2
▓ ▓ The Synergy Model—Nurse Characteristics

Characteristic and Description	Continua of Level of Expertise (Levels 1-5 Range from Competent to Expert)
CLINICAL JUDGMENT Clinical reasoning, which includes clinical decision making, critical thinking, and a global grasp of the situation, coupled with nursing skills acquired through a process of integrating education, experiential knowledge, and evidence-based guidelines	*Level 1* • Collects and interprets basic-level data • Follows algorithms, protocols, and pathways with all populations and is uncomfortable deviating from them • Matches formal knowledge and clinical events to make basic care decisions • Questions the limits of one's ability to make clinical decisions and defers the decision making to other clinicians • Recognizes expected outcomes • Often focuses on extraneous details *Level 3* • Collects and interprets complex patient data focusing on key elements of case; able to sort out extraneous detail • Follows algorithms, protocols, and pathways and is comfortable deviating from them with common or routine patient population • Recognizes patterns and trends that may predict the direction of illness • Recognizes limits and utilizes appropriate help • Reacts to and limits unexpected outcomes *Level 5* • Synthesizes and interprets multiple, sometimes conflicting, sources of data • Makes judgments based on an immediate grasp of the "big picture," unless working with new patient populations; uses past experiences to anticipate problems (applies principles from old situations to new situations) • Helps patient and family see the "big picture" • Recognizes the limits of clinical judgment and seeks multidisciplinary collaboration and consultation with comfort • Recognizes and responds to the dynamic situation (following patient/family lead) • Anticipates unexpected outcomes • Acts on and directs others to act on identified clinical problems • Assists nursing staff in identifying daily goals for patients
ADVOCACY/MORAL AGENCY Working on another's behalf and representing the concerns of the patient/family and nursing staff; serving as a moral agent in identifying and helping to resolve ethical and clinical concerns within and outside the clinical setting	*Level 1* • Works on behalf of the patient and self • Begins to self-assess personal values • Aware of ethical conflicts/issues that may surface in clinical setting • Makes ethical/moral decisions based on rules/guiding principles and on own personal values • Represents patient if consistent with own framework • Aware of patient rights • Acknowledges death as an outcome

Continued

■ **TABLE 1-2**
■ ■ **The Synergy Model—Nurse Characteristics—Cont'd**

Characteristic and Description	Continua of Level of Expertise (Levels 1-5 Range from Competent to Expert)
ADVOCACY/MORAL AGENCY—Cont'd	*Level 3* • Works on behalf of patient and family • Considers patient values and incorporates in care, even when differing from personal values • Supports patients, families, and colleagues in ethical and clinical issues, identifying internal resources • Moral decision making can deviate from rules • Demonstrates give and take with patients/family, allowing them to speak/represent themselves when possible • Aware of and acknowledges patient and family rights • Recognizes that death may be an acceptable outcome • Facilitates patient/family comfort in the death and dying process *Level 5* • Works on behalf of patient, family, and community • Advocates from patient/family perspective, whether similar to or different from personal values • Advocates for resolution of ethical conflict and issues from patient's, family's, or colleague's perspective; utilizes and participates in internal and external resources • Recognizes rights of patient/family to drive moral decision making • Empowers the patient and family to speak for/represent themselves • Achieves mutuality within patient/family/professional relationships
CARING PRACTICES Nursing activities that create a compassionate, supportive, and therapeutic environment for patients and staff, with the aim of promoting comfort and healing and preventing unnecessary suffering. These caring behaviors include but are not limited to vigilance, engagement, and responsiveness. Caregivers include family and health care personnel.	*Level 1* • Focuses on basic and routine needs of the patient • Bases care on standards and protocols • Maintains a safe physical environment *Level 3* • Responds to subtle patient and family changes • Engages with the patient to provide individualized care • Employs caring and comfort practices to provide individualized care for patient/family • Optimizes patient/family environment *Level 5* • Has astute awareness and anticipates patient/family changes and needs • Fully engaged with and senses how to stand alongside the patient/family and community • Patient/family needs determine caring practices • Anticipates hazards and promotes safety, care, and comfort throughout transitions along the health care continuum • Initiates the establishment of an environment that promotes caring • Provides patient/family the skills to navigate transitions along the health care continuum (i.e., facilitates safe passage)

■ **TABLE 1-2**
■ ■ **The Synergy Model—Nurse Characteristics—Cont'd**

Characteristic and Description	Continua of Level of Expertise (Levels 1-5 Range from Competent to Expert)
COLLABORATION Working with others (e.g., patients, families, health care providers) in a way that promotes each person's contributions toward achieving optimal and realistic patient/family goals. Collaboration involves intradisciplinary and interdisciplinary work with colleagues and community.	*Level 1* • Willing to be taught, coached, and/or mentored • Participates in team meetings and discussions regarding patient care and/or practice issues • Open to various team members' contributions *Level 3* • Willing to be taught/mentored • Participates in preceptoring and teaching • Initiates and participates in team meetings and discussions regarding patient care and/or practice issues • Recognizes and critiques multidisciplinary participation in care decisions *Level 5* • Seeks opportunities to role model, teach, mentor, and be mentored • Facilitates active involvement and contributions of others in team meetings and discussions regarding patient care and/or practice issues • Involves/recruits multidisciplinary resources to optimize patient outcomes • Role models, teaches, and/or mentors professional leadership and accountability for nursing's role within the health care team and community
SYSTEMS THINKING Body of knowledge and tools that allow the nurse to manage whatever environmental and system resources exist for the patient/family and staff, within or across health care and non–health care systems	*Level 1* • Utilizes previously learned strategies or standardized processes • Identifies problems but unclear of health care systems to resolve problems • Sees patient and family within the isolated environment of the unit • Sees self as key resource for patient/family • Applies personal experiences to identify patient/family needs *Level 3* • Develops processes/strategies based on needs and strengths of patient/family • Able to make connections within pieces or components of the health care system • Sees and begins to use negotiation as a tool for practice-based decisions • Recognizes and reacts to needs of patient/family as they move through health care systems • Recognizes how to obtain and utilize resources within the health care system *Level 5* • Develops, integrates, and applies a variety of strategies that are driven by the needs and strengths of the patient/family • Recognizes global or holistic interrelationships that exist within and across both health care and non–health care systems

Continued

■ TABLE 1-2
■ ■ The Synergy Model—Nurse Characteristics—Cont'd

Characteristic and Description	Continua of Level of Expertise (Levels 1-5 Range from Competent to Expert)
SYSTEMS THINKING—Cont'd	• Knows when and how to negotiate and navigate through the system on behalf of patients and families • Develops core plans based on anticipated needs of patients/families • Utilizes a variety of resources as necessary to optimize patient/family outcomes
RESPONSE TO DIVERSITY The sensitivity to recognize, appreciate, and incorporate differences into the provision of care. Differences may include, but are not limited to, cultural, spiritual, gender, race, ethnicity, lifestyle, socioeconomic status, age, and values.	*Level 1* • Assesses diversity and acknowledges differences but uses standardized plans of care • Provides care based on own belief system • Practices within the culture of the health care environment • Recognizes barriers • Recognizes practices based on diversity that have potential negative outcomes *Level 3* • Inquires about cultural differences and considers their impact on care • Accommodates personal and professional differences in plans of care • Helps patient/family understand the culture of the health care system • Recognizes barriers and seeks strategies for resolution • Identifies and utilizes resources that promote and support diversity *Level 5* • Anticipates needs of patient/family based on identified diversities and develops plans accordingly • Acknowledges and incorporates differences • Adapts health care culture, to the extent possible, to meet the diverse needs and strengths of the patient/family • Anticipates and intervenes to reduce/eliminate barriers • Incorporates patient/family values with evidence-based practice for optimal outcomes
CLINICAL INQUIRY The ongoing process of questioning and evaluating practice and providing informed practice; creating changes through evidence-based practice, research utilization, and experiential knowledge	*Level 1* • Follows policies, procedures, standards, and guidelines without deviation • Uses research-based practices as directed by others • Recognizes the need for further learning to improve patient care • Recognizes obvious changing patient situation (e.g., deterioration, crisis) and seeks assistance to identify patient problems and solutions • Participates in data collection (e.g., research, continuous quality improvement [CQI], quality improvement [QI]) *Level 3* • Utilizes policies, procedures, standards, and guidelines, adapting to patient needs • Applies research findings when not in conflict with current clinical practice

Characteristic and Description	Continua of Level of Expertise (Levels 1-5 Range from Competent to Expert)
CLINICAL INQUIRY—Cont'd	• Accepts advice or information to improve patient care • Recognizes subtle changes in patient condition and begins to compare and contrast possible care alternatives • Participates on team (e.g., CQI, survey, research) *Level 5* • Improves, modifies, or individualizes policies, procedures, standards, and guidelines for particular patient situations or populations on the basis of experiential or published data • Questions and/or evaluates current practice based on patient/family's responses, review of the literature, research, and education/learning • Seeks to validate whether research answers clinical questions • Embraces lifelong learning and acquires knowledge and skills needed to address questions arising in practice to improve patient care • Evaluates outcomes of studies and implements changes (converging of clinical inquiring and clinical judgment allows for anticipation of patient needs)
FACILITATOR OF LEARNING The ability to facilitate learning for patients and families, nursing staff, other members of the health care team, and community; includes both formal and informal facilitation of learning	*Level 1* • Follows planned educational programs using standardized educational materials • Sees patient/family education as a separate task from delivery of care • Provides information without seeking to assess learner's readiness or understanding • Has basic knowledge and/or understanding of the patient/family's educational needs • Focuses educational plan on nurse-identified patient/family needs • Sees the patient/family as a passive recipient *Level 3* • Adapts planned educational programs to meet individual patient's needs • Begins to recognize and integrate different ways of implementing education into delivery of care • Assesses patient's/family's readiness to learn, develops education plan based on identified needs, and evaluates learner understanding • Recognizes the benefits of educational plans from different health care providers' perspectives • Sees the patient/family as having input into educational goals • Incorporates patient's/family's perspective into individualized education plan *Level 5* • Creatively modifies or develops patient/family education programs

Continued

■ **TABLE 1-2**
■ ■ **The Synergy Model—Nurse Characteristics—Cont'd**

Characteristic and Description	Continua of Level of Expertise (Levels 1-5 Range from Competent to Expert)
FACILITATOR OF LEARNING—Cont'd	• Integrates patient/family education throughout delivery of care • Evaluates patient/family readiness to learn and provides comprehensive individualized education evaluating behavior changes related to learning, adjusting to meet the educational goal • Collaborates and incorporates all health care providers' ideas into ongoing educational plans for the patient/family • Sees patient/family as having choices and consequences that are negotiated in relation to education

From AACN Certification Corporation and PES. *Final Report of a Comprehensive Study of Critical Care Nursing Practice.* Aliso Viejo, CA: The Corporation; 2004.

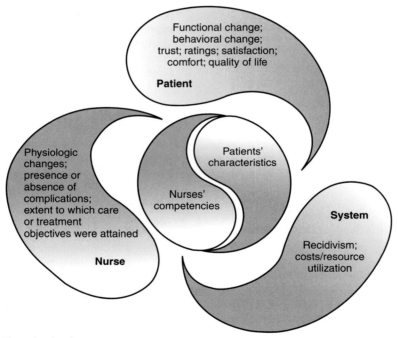

FIGURE 1-2 ■ Three levels of outcomes delineated by the AACN Synergy Model for Patient Care: those derived from the patient, those derived from the nurse, and those derived from the health care system. (From Curley M. Patient-nurse synergy: optimizing patients' outcomes. *Am J Crit Care.* 1998;7:69.)

5. Outcomes of patient-nurse synergy (Figure 1-2) (Curley, 1998)
   a. Patient-derived outcomes
      i. Behavior change: Based on the dispensing and receiving of information. Requires caregiver trust. Patients and families grow in their knowledge about health and take greater responsibility for their own health.
         (a) Functional change and quality of life: Multidisciplinary measures that can be used across all populations of patients but provide specific information to a population of patients when analyzed separately

(b) Satisfaction ratings: Subjective measures of individual health and quality of health services. Satisfaction measures query about expectations (technical care provided, trusting relationships, and education experiences) and the extent to which they are met. Often linked with functional change and quality-of-life perceptions.

(c) Comfort ratings and perceptions: Quality-of-care outcomes based on caring practices with the aim of promoting comfort and alleviating suffering

   b. Nurse-derived outcomes

   i. Physiologic changes: Require monitoring and managing instantaneous therapies and noting changes. The nurse expects a specific trajectory of changes when he or she "knows" the patient (Tanner, Benner, & Chesla, 1993).

   ii. The presence or absence of preventable complications: Through vigilance and clinical judgment, the nurse creates a safe and healing environment

   iii. Extent to which care and treatment objectives were attained: Reflects the nurse's role as an integrator of care that requires a high degree of collaboration

   c. System-derived outcomes

   i. Recidivism: Decrease in rehospitalization or readmission, which adds to the personal and financial burden of care

   ii. Cost and resource utilization: Organizations usually evaluate financial cost based on an episode of care. Achieving cost-effective care requires knowing the patient and providing continuity of care. Resource utilization can affect patient outcomes when there is not enough care given by competent nurses (Aiken et al, 2001). When nurses cannot provide care at an appropriate level to meet patient needs, they are dissatisfied and turnover is high, which results in increased costs for the organization (Cornerstone Communication Group, 2001).

Application of the Synergy Model

There are many applications for the model in clinical operations, clinical practice, education, and research.*

1. **Clinical operations**

   a. Leadership: Use of the model for achieving organizational objectives of nursing excellence and building an organizational structure to achieve magnet status (Kaplow & Reed, 2008)

   b. Development of standards: Use of the model to develop practice standards and align patient needs with new technologic advancements (Reilly & Humbrecht, 2007)

   c. Development of a staff mentoring tool with use of the Synergy Model (Kanaskie, 2006)

   d. Use of the model to study providing spiritual nursing care to patients (Smith, 2006)

2. **Clinical practice**

   a. Providing care to acute and progressive care patients in the military setting (Freyling, Kesten, & Heath, 2008)

   b. Use of the Synergy Model to study spirituality in progressive care (Smith, 2006)

   c. Use of the model in the delivery of care to progressive care patient populations (Helms & Ennis, 2005)

3. **Education**

   a. Use of the model to develop a preceptor program that addresses the needs of the preceptee to provide an optimal orientation experience (Alspach, 2006)

   b. Use of the model to develop online education and simulation of progressive care courses (Brady et al, 2006)

4. **Research**

   a. Validation in the AACN Certification Corporation Progressive Care Study of Practice (Muenzen, Greenberg, & Pirro, 2004)

   b. Validation study of patient characteristics along the continuum of care

   c. Further research needed related to consumer perspective, staffing, and productivity implications for nursing, patient outcomes measurement, and development of a quantitative tool based on the model for rapidly assessing patients and determining the nursing characteristics needed

---

*Refer to the AACN Certification Corporation website (http://www.certcorp.org) for up-to-date applications.

GENERAL LEGAL CONSIDERATIONS RELEVANT TO PROGRESSIVE CARE NURSING PRACTICE

State Nurse Practice Acts

1. Purpose: To protect the public
2. Statutory laws: Written by the individual states
3. Usual authorization: Board of nursing to oversee nursing (by use of regulations or administrative law)
4. Content: Define scope of practice for nurses

Scope of Practice

Provides guidance for acceptable nursing roles and practices, which vary from state to state

1. Nurses are expected to follow the nurse practice act and not deviate from usual nursing activities.
2. Advanced nursing practice: Expanded roles for nurses include nurse practitioner, clinical nurse specialist (CNS), certified registered nurse anesthetist (CRNA), certified nurse-midwife (CNM), and doctorate of nursing practice. These roles require education beyond the basic nurse education and usually involve a master's or doctorate degree (Advanced Practice Registered Nurses [APRN] Consensus Work Group and the National Council of State Boards of Nursing APRN Advisory Committee, 2008). An APRN model of regulation has been proposed. In this model there are four roles: CRNA, CNM, CNS, and certified nurse practitioner (CNP). These four roles are given the title of APRN.
3. A scope of practice and standards for the acute and critical care CNS (Bell, 2002) and the acute care nurse practitioner (Bell, 2006) were published by the AACN.

Standards of Care

1. A standard of care is any established measure of extent, quality, quantity, or value; an agreed-on level of performance or a degree of excellence of care that is established.
2. Standards are established by usual and customary practice, institutional guidelines, association guidelines, and legal precedent.
3. Standards of care, standards of practice, policies, procedures, and performance criteria all establish an agreed-on level of performance or degree of excellence:
   a. *AACN Scope and Standards for Acute and Critical Care Nursing Practice* (Bell, 2008)
   b. ANA standards: Generic and also specialty standards (e.g., for medical-surgical nursing)
   c. *Scope and Standards of Practice for the Acute Care Nurse Practitioner* (Bell, 2006).
   d. *Scope of Practice and Standards of Professional Performance for the Acute and Critical Care Clinical Nurse Specialist* (Bell, 2002)
4. National facility standards: Include those published by The Joint Commission, the National Committee for Quality Assurance (NCQA),* the Institute for Healthcare Improvement (IHI), and the National Quality Forum (NQF)
5. Community and regional standards: Standards prevalent in certain areas of the country or in specific communities
6. Hospital and medical center standards: Standards developed by institutions for their staff and patients
7. Unit practice standards, policies, and protocols: specific standards of care for specific groups or types of patients or specific procedures (e.g., insulin or massive blood transfusion protocols)
8. Precedent court cases: Standard of a "reasonable, prudent nurse" (i.e., what a reasonable, prudent nurse would have done in the given situation)

---

*The NCQA website contains the various standards the committee endorses and/or publishes (http://www.ncqa.org/index.asp).

9. Other nursing and interdisciplinary specialty organization standards (such as the American Heart Association, Society of Critical Care Medicine, and Association of Perioperative Registered Nurses)

Certification in a Specialty Area

1. Certification is a process by which a nongovernmental agency, using predetermined standards, validates an individual nurse's qualification and knowledge for practice in a defined functional or clinical area of nursing.
2. A common goal of specialty certification programs is to promote consumer protection and to promote high standards of practice.
3. The certified nurse may be held to a higher standard of practice in the specialty than the non-certified nurse; certification validates the nurse's knowledge and experience in a specialty area.
4. Certifications are awarded by AACN Certification Corporation. AACN Certification Corporation is accredited by the National Commission for Certifying Agencies, the accreditation arm of the National Organization for Competency Assurance.
   a. PCCN: Separate certification process for nurses in progressive care
   b. CCRN: Separate certification processes for critical care nurses practicing with neonatal, pediatric, or adult populations
   c. CCNS: Advanced practice certification for clinical nurse specialists who practice in acute, progressive, and critical care.
   d. ACNP: Advanced practice certification for acute care nurse practitioners who practice in acute, progressive, and critical care

Professional Liability

1. Professional negligence: An unintentional act or omission; the failure to do what the reasonable, prudent nurse would do under similar circumstances, or an act or failure to act that leads to an injury of another. Six specific elements are necessary for professional negligence action and must be established by a person bringing a suit against a nurse (plaintiff) (Giordano, 2003; Guido, 2006):
   a. Duty: To protect the patient from an unreasonable risk of harm
   b. Breach of duty: Failure by a nurse to do what a reasonable, prudent nurse would do under the same or similar circumstances. The breach of duty is a failure to perform within the given standard of care. The standard defines the nurse's duty to the patient.
   c. Proximate cause: Proof that the harm caused was foreseeable and that the person injured was foreseeably a victim. This element can determine the extent of damages for which a nurse may be held liable.
   d. Injury: The harm done
   e. Direct cause of injury: Proof that the nurse's conduct was the cause of or contributed to the injury to the patient
   f. Damages: Proof of actual loss, damage, pain, or suffering caused by the nurse's conduct
2. Malpractice: A specific type of negligence that takes account of the status of the caregiver, as well as the standard of care (Giordano, 2003; Guido, 2006). Professional negligence is malpractice. It is differentiated from ordinary negligence (e.g., failure to clean up water from the floor).
   a. Malpractice includes professional misconduct, improper discharge of professional duties, or a failure by a professional to meet the standard of care that results in harm to another person.
   b. Malpractice is the failure of a professional person to act in accordance with prevailing professional standards or a failure to foresee consequences that a professional person who has the necessary skills and education would foresee.
   c. Most common types of malpractice or negligence in progressive care settings include medication errors, failure to prevent patient falls, failure to assess changes in clinical status, and failure to notify the primary provider of changes in patient status.
3. Delegation and supervision:
   a. Definitions (National Council of State Boards of Nursing, 1995)
      i. Delegation: Transferring to a competent individual the authority to perform a selected nursing task in a selected situation; the nurse retains accountability for the delegation

      ii. Accountability: Being responsible and answerable for actions or inactions of self or others in the context of delegation

      iii. Authority: Deemed present when a registered nurse (RN) has been given the right to delegate based on the state nurse practice act and also has the official power from an agency to delegate

      iv. Unlicensed assistive personnel (UAP): Any unlicensed personnel, regardless of title, to whom nursing tasks are delegated

      v. Delegator: The person making the delegation

      vi. Delegatee: The person receiving the delegation

      vii. Competent: Demonstrating the knowledge and skill, through education and experience, to perform the delegated task

  b. The five "rights" of delegation

      i. Right task: The RN ensures that the task to be delegated is appropriate to be delegated for that specific patient. Example: Delegating suctioning of secretions in a tracheostomy in a stable patient to a licensed practical nurse is appropriate. If the patient has a head injury and becomes bradycardic and hypotensive during suctioning, then delegation of this task for this patient may not be appropriate.

      ii. Right circumstances: The RN ensures that the setting is appropriate and that resources are available for successful completion of the delegated task.

      iii. Right person: The RN delegates the right task to the right person to be performed on the right person.

      iv. Right direction and communication: The delegating nurse provides a clear explanation of the task and expected outcomes; the RN sets limits and expectations for performance of the task.

      v. Right supervision: The RN does appropriate monitoring and evaluation and intervenes as needed; the RN provides feedback to the delegatee and establishes parameters for receiving feedback about the outcome of the task.

  c. Model of the delegation decision-making process: The nurse must ensure that delegation of nursing tasks is based on appropriate assessment, planning, implementation, and evaluation. Box 1-1 describes the model for delegation established by the National Council of State Boards of Nursing.

  d. Nurse executives must ensure the following:

      i. Policies and procedures concerning supervision and delegation are in place and are consistent with state nurse practice acts.

      ii. Job descriptions for UAPs do not include responsibilities for whose performance a license is required.

      iii. Adequate training and consistent orientation for UAPs are provided.

      iv. A mechanism for regular evaluation of UAPs is in place.

  e. In the progressive care environment, many of the concepts for delegation to UAPs can also be applied to delegation of care to other professional nurses and licensed practical or vocational nurses (through assignments made by charge nurses or nurse managers).

      i. The job descriptions and scope of practice for personnel with various levels of expertise and for various roles must be clearly defined.

      ii. When assignments are made, the patient's characteristics (as defined by the Synergy Model) and required care procedures guide the decision regarding the competency level of the nurse who should provide the care.

      iii. Nurse executives and nurse managers must ensure that nurses have demonstrated and documented levels of expertise necessary to provide the care required by specific patients.

      iv. Additional training and experience are required for performance of many of the complex therapies needed by vulnerable critically ill patients.

4. Adequate staffing

  a. Staffing is a process and an outcome. The term can refer to the process by which human resources are used within a nursing care unit or to the number of staff members required to provide care. The individuals managing health care services have ethical responsibilities to ensure that policies and processes are in place to ensure the safety of the patients

▓ **BOX 1-1**
▓ **NATIONAL COUNCIL OF STATE BOARDS OF NURSING MODEL FOR DELEGATION DECISION-MAKING PROCESS**

I.   Delegation criteria
   A. Nursing Practice Act
     1. Permits delegation
     2. Authorizes task(s) to be delegated or authorizes the nurse to decide to delegate
   B. Delegator qualifications
     1. Within scope of authority to delegate
     2. Appropriate education, skills, and experience
     3. Documented or demonstrated evidence of current competency
   C. Delegatee qualifications
     1. Appropriate education, training, skills, and experience
     2. Documented or demonstrated evidence of current competency
   Provided that this foundation is in place, the licensed nurse may enter the continuous process of delegation decision making.
II. Assess the situation.
   A. Identify the needs of the patient, consulting the plan of care.
   B. Consider the circumstances and setting.
   C. Ensure the availability of adequate resources, including supervision.
   If patient needs, circumstances, and available resources (including supervisor and delegatee) indicate that patient safety will be maintained with delegated care, proceed to step III.
III. Plan for the specific task(s) to be delegated.
   A. Specify the nature of each task and the knowledge and skills required to perform it.
   B. Require documentation or demonstration of current competence by the delegatee for each task.
   C. Determine the implications for the patient, other patients, and significant others.
   If the nature of the task, competence of the delegatee, and patient implications indicate that patient safety will be maintained with delegated care, proceed to step IV.
IV. Ensure appropriate accountability.
   A. As delegator, accept accountability for performance of the task(s).
   B. Verify that delegatee accepts the delegation and the accountability for carrying out the task correctly.
   If delegator and delegatee accept the accountability for their respective roles in the delegated patient care, proceed to steps V-VII.
V. Supervise the performance of the task.
   A. Provide directions and clear expectations of how the task(s) is (are) to be performed.
   B. Monitor performance of the task(s) to assure compliance with established standards of practice, policies, and procedures.
   C. Intervene if necessary.
   D. Ensure appropriate documentation of the task(s).
VI. Evaluate the entire delegation process.
   A. Evaluate the patient.
   B. Evaluate the performance of the task(s).
   C. Obtain and provide feedback.
VII. Reassess and adjust the overall plan of care as needed.

From National Council of State Boards of Nursing. Delegation: concepts and decision-making process. National Council position paper. http://www.ncsbn.org/regulation/uap_delegation_documents_delegation.asp. Accessed May 4, 2005. Used with permission of the National Council of State Boards of Nursing, Chicago, IL, copyright 1995.

and the staff (Box 1-2) (Curtin, 2002a, 2002b). The 42 Code of Federal Regulations (42CFR 482.23[b]) requires hospitals certified to participate in Medicare to "have adequate numbers of licensed registered nurses, licensed practical (vocational) nurses, and other personnel to provide nursing care to all patients as needed."

b. The ANA launched the "Safe Staffing Saves Lives" campaign in 2008 (http://www. safestaffingsaveslives.org), which promotes safe staffing legislation. The ANA advocates for staffing ratios mandated by legislation with the actual number of nurses set at the unit level

■ **BOX 1-2**
■ **ETHICAL RESPONSIBILITIES OF HEALTH CARE DELIVERY MANAGERS**

In order of priority, the following are the ethical responsibilities of those managing health service delivery systems:
1. Ensuring the safety of the services delivered
2. Ensuring a safe environment for those receiving and those delivering the health care services
3. Ensuring the responsible use, care, and distribution of the materials needed for safe delivery of services
4. Carefully developing and implementing a budget
5. Developing responsible institutional policies
6. Intelligently interpreting and implementing institutional policies
7. Knowing and adhering to all applicable laws governing practice and personnel management

Adapted from Curtin L. The ethics of staffing—part 1. *J Clin Syst Manage.* 2002;4(3):6-7.

with RN input. The ANA's proposal is not a "one size fits all" approach to staffing. The ANA staffing proposal is congruent with the AACN Synergy Model, matching patient acuity with the right skill mix and experience of the nursing staff.
  c. The AACN Health Work Environment Standards are an AACN priority and provide standards and critical elements that are achievable and that create a work environment that promotes quality patient and family care.
  d. The gap between the supply and demands of nurses continues to grow (Welton, 2007). Higher-acuity patients are in the hospital for shorter periods of time. They are quickly discharged, and hospital beds are then filled with sicker patients with greater needs. Progressive care unit (PCU) nurses care for patients with higher-acuity needs and require additional surveillance for those with the potential to become unstable. Staffing PCUs by matching the patient's needs with the competencies and experience of the PCU nurse is a crucial consideration today.
  e. Patient and family–focused care requires matching the right caregiver to each patient, identifying systems that provide the right support in delivering care, incorporating legal and regulatory considerations, and measuring the outcomes of care.
  f. AACN *Standards for Establishing and Sustaining Healthy Work Environments* (Barden, 2005), Standard No. 4, Adequate Staffing, provides critical elements that must be in place to address critical staffing shortages:
    i. The health care organization has staffing policies in place that are solidly grounded in ethical principles and support the professional obligation of nurses to provide high-quality care.
    ii. Nurses participate in all organizational phases of the staffing process from education and planning—including matching nurses' competencies with patients' assessed needs—through evaluation.
    iii. The health care organization has formal processes in place to evaluate the effect of staffing decisions on patient and system outcomes. This evaluation includes analysis of when patient needs and nurse competencies are mismatched and how often contingency plans are implemented.
    iv. The health care organization has a system in place that facilitates team members' use of staffing and outcomes data to develop more effective staffing models.
    v. The health care organization provides support services at every level of activity to ensure nurses can optimally focus on the priorities and requirements of patient and family care.
    vi. The health care organization adopts technologies that increase the effectiveness of nursing care delivery. Nurses are engaged in the selection, adaptation, and evaluation of these technologies.

Documentation

1. Mandates of regulatory agencies
  a. Federal requirements: Related to narcotics, controlled substances, organ transplantation

      b. National voluntary requirements: The Joint Commission requirements related to quality improvement activities

      c. State requirements: May exist in specific situations (e.g., in relation to minors)

      d. Community (regional or local) standards: May include enhanced documentation in specific areas of practice (e.g., epidural medication)

      e. Hospital, medical center, or health maintenance organization requirements

2. Purposes of nursing care documentation in the patient record

      a. To provide clear and concise communication between providers

      b. To facilitate planning and evaluation of care and demonstrate use of the nursing process

      c. To show progress of patient treatment, changes in condition, and continuity of care and to record patient status, appearance, and behavior

      d. To protect the patient; the medical record may be used in litigation

      e. To protect health care professionals and institutions and reduce risk for possible litigation

3. Documentation requirements

      a. General requirements regarding patient records

            i. Should contain accurate, factual observations

            ii. Should include times, dates, and signatures for notations and events entered

            iii. Reflect patient status and unusual events

            iv. Should reflect documentation of the nursing process on a continuing basis throughout the hospitalization

            v. Should note omissions of care and rationale

            vi. Should show that the physician was informed of unusual or adverse situations and record the nature of the physician's response

            vii. Should note deviations from standard hospital practice and the rationale for such deviations

            viii. Should be legible

            ix. Should carefully document method of the patient's admission, condition on admission, discharge planning, and condition on discharge

      b. Specific Joint Commission requirements regarding patient records

            i. Patient's name, address, date of birth, and name of any legally authorized representative

            ii. Legal status of patient receiving mental health services

            iii. Emergency care, if any, provided to the patient before arrival

            iv. Findings of the patient assessment, including assessment of pain status, learning needs and barriers to learning, and cultural or religious needs that may affect care

            v. Conclusions or impressions drawn from the medical history and physical examination

            vi. Diagnosis or diagnostic impression

            vii. Reasons for admission or treatment

            viii. Goals of treatment and the treatment plan; evidence of interdisciplinary plan of care

            ix. Evidence of known advance directives or documentation that information about advance directives was offered

            x. Evidence of informed consent, when required by hospital policy

            xi. Diagnostic and therapeutic orders, if any

            xii. Records of all diagnostic and therapeutic procedures and all test results

            xiii. Records of all operative and other invasive procedures performed, with acceptable disease and operative terminology that includes etiology, as appropriate

            xiv. Progress notes made by the medical staff and other authorized persons

            xv. All reassessments and any revisions of the treatment plan

            xvi. Clinical observations and reports of patient's response to care

            xvii. Evidence of patient education

            xviii. Consultation reports

            xix. Records of every medication ordered or prescribed for an inpatient

            xx. Records of every medication dispensed to an ambulatory patient or an inpatient on discharge

            xxi. Records of every dose of medication administered and any adverse drug reaction

            xxii. All relevant diagnoses established during the course of care

    xxiii. Any referrals and communications made to external or internal care providers and to community agencies

    xxiv. Conclusions at termination of hospitalization

    xxv. Discharge instructions to the patient and family

    xxvi. Clinical discharge summaries, or a final progress note or transfer summary. Discharge summary contains reason for hospitalization, significant findings, procedures performed and treatment rendered, patient's condition at discharge, and instructions to the patient and family, if any, including pain management plan.

Good Samaritan Laws

1. Various states have enacted laws to allow health care personnel and citizens trained in first aid to deliver needed emergency care without fear of incurring criminal and civil liability (Guido, 2006).
2. Laws vary among states; thus, nurses should be familiar with the relevant state law. Look for these elements when evaluating the state's law:
   a. Who is covered under the law?
   b. Where does the coverage extend?
   c. What is covered?
3. Most laws require that care be given in good faith and that it be gratuitous.
4. There is no legal duty to render care to strangers in distress.

ETHICAL CLINICAL PRACTICE

Foundation of Ethical Nursing Practice

1. ANA Code of Ethics with Interpretive Statement
   a. The foundation of ethical practice for nursing is the ANA Code of Ethics (Box 1-3). The ANA code is a statement of the ethical obligations and duties of every nurse, a nonnegotiable ethical standard for the profession, and an expression of the nursing profession's commitment to society.
   b. The preface to the ANA Code of Ethics states: "Ethics is an integral part of the foundation of nursing. Nursing has a distinguished history of concern for the welfare of the sick,

▓ **BOX 1-3**
▓ **PROVISIONS OF THE AMERICAN NURSES ASSOCIATION CODE OF ETHICS**

> The nurse, in all professional relationships, practices with compassion and respect for the inherent dignity, worth, and uniqueness of every individual, unrestricted by considerations of social or economic status, personal attributes, or the nature of health problems.
>
> The nurse's primary commitment is to the patient, whether an individual, family, group, or community.
>
> The nurse promotes, advocates for, and strives to protect the health, safety, and rights of the patient.
>
> The nurse is responsible and accountable for individual nursing practice and determines the appropriate delegation of tasks consistent with the nurse's obligation to provide optimum care.
>
> The nurse owes the same duties to self as to others, including the responsibility to preserve integrity and safety, to maintain competence, and to continue personal and professional growth.
>
> The nurse participates in establishing, maintaining, and improving health care environments and conditions of employment conducive to the provision of quality health care and consistent with the values of the profession through individual and collective action.
>
> The nurse participates in the advancement of the profession through contributions to practice, education, administration, and knowledge development.
>
> The nurse collaborates with other health professionals and the public in promoting community, national, and international efforts to meet health needs.
>
> The profession of nursing, as represented by associations and their members, is responsible for articulating nursing values, for maintaining the integrity of the profession and its practice, and for shaping social policy.

injured, and vulnerable and for social justice. This concern is embodied in the provision of nursing care to individuals and the community. Nursing encompasses the prevention of illness, the alleviation of suffering, and the protection, promotion, and restoration of health in the care of individuals, families, groups, and communities. Nurses act to change those aspects of social structures that detract from health and well-being. Individuals who become nurses are expected not only to adhere to the ideals and moral norms of the profession but also to embrace them as a part of what it means to be a nurse. The ethical tradition of nursing is self-reflective, enduring, and distinctive. A code of ethics makes explicit the primary goals, values, and obligations of the profession" (ANA, 2005).

2. AACN Standards of Care for Acute and Critical Care Nursing (Bell, 2008), Standard V: AACN's mission, vision, and values are framed within an ethic of care and ethical principles. An ethic of care is a moral orientation that acknowledges the interrelatedness and interdependence of individuals, systems, and society. An ethic of care respects individual uniqueness, personal relationships, and the dynamic nature of life. Essential to an ethic of care are compassion, collaboration, accountability, and trust. Within the context of interrelationships of individuals and circumstances, traditional ethical principles provide a basis for deliberation and decision making. These ethical principles include the following:
   a. Respect for persons: A moral obligation to honor the intrinsic worth and uniqueness of each person; to respect self-determination, diversity, and privacy
   b. Beneficence: A moral obligation to promote good and prevent or remove harm; to promote the welfare, health, and safety of society and individuals in accordance with beliefs, values, preferences, and life goals
   c. Justice: A moral obligation to be fair and promote equity, nondiscrimination, and the distribution of benefits and burdens based on needs and resources available; to advocate on another's behalf when necessary

Emergence of Clinical Ethics

1. Definition of clinical ethics: "The systematic identification, analysis, and resolution of ethical problems associated with the care of particular patients" (Ahronheim, Moreno, & Zuckerman, 2005)
2. Goals:
   a. Promote patient-centered decision making that honors the rights and interests of the patient
   b. Facilitate the involvement of all clinicians (e.g., physicians, nurses, social workers, and other health care professionals) who require assistance in this complex field
   c. Promote organizational commitment, as well as cooperation among all involved parties, to implement plans on behalf of the patient
3. "Rethinking the Conceptual and Empirical Foundations of Clinical Ethics" (McCullough, 2008)
   a. Phillips (2006) describes how the use of a ethical model is helpful in resolving issues of noncompliance during the rehabilitative stages of a patient's illness.
   b. A qualitative study by Hough (2008) provides evidence of the importance of direct experience, a reflective process, and educational programs that teach ethical decision making.
   c. A book review by Grossenbacher (2007) on *The Case of Terri Schiavo: Ethics at the End of Life* by Caplan et al speaks to the importance of talking with families and documenting wishes to avert moral dilemmas at the end of life.
   d. Fowler (2004) describes the use of reflection to evaluate the ethics of truth telling.
   e. Mathes (2005) describes the two orientations of ethical decision making and their effect on nursing frameworks.
4. Religion and clinical ethics (Ahronheim et al, 2005)
   a. "Clinical ethics" now refers to secular bioethics.
   b. Religious leaders continue to play a role in the deliberation of moral and ethical dilemmas; often provide wisdom to secular community.
   c. Religious convictions of competent adults should be honored and respected (Brett & Jersild, 2003). This can be difficult for health care providers when it involves decision making by parents for dependent children.
   d. Pesut (2008) describes the importance of using self in understanding the spiritual state of individuals in the delivery of spiritual care.

5. Cultural competence and clinical ethics: Cultural competence is the ability to identify the effects of a patient's culture on the health of the patient (Ahronheim et al, 2005). The health care provider should use a framework of ethical decision making that factors in the patient's culture while avoiding cultural stereotyping.
6. Five modes of ethical leadership and interventions (Johnson, 2005); the modes of ethical leadership intervention depend on the culture of the organization.
   a. Inspiration: the setting of an example for others to follow in achieving organizational goals (lowest degree of intervention)
   b. Facilitation: supporting and guiding members of an organization
   c. Persuasion: appealing to reason and convincing members of the organization to achieve goals
   d. Manipulation: the process of offering extrinsic incentives to members for achieving goals
   e. Coercion: the process of forcing members who are not committed to achieve the organizational goals (highest degree of intervention)
7. Ethics across the life span: Issues include the following (Ahronheim et al, 2005):
   a. Before pregnancy: Carrier screening for genetic disorders, testing for human immunodeficiency virus, in vitro fertilization and related technologies, potential for human cloning, stem cell research, and surrogacy
   b. During pregnancy: Manipulation of embryos, substance abuse during pregnancy, abortion, prenatal genetic diagnosis, implications of multiple births due to reproductive technologies
   c. Infants: Treatment of infants born with severe impairments
   d. Children and adolescents: Role in decision making
   e. Elderly: Issues related to truth telling and confidentiality have shifted for this generation; planning with patient for potential lapses in decision making; emphasis on advance directives for this age group; end-of-life care issues
   f. Caring for the family: Although the rights of the individual patient are still presumed to outweigh those of the family, this is being challenged in many situations and often leads to significant ethical conflicts. Conflicts center on autonomy and confidentiality. A philosophy of family-centered care has the potential to prevent such conflicts or reduce their effects on the care provided to patients (Clarke et al, 2003; Curtis et al, 2001; Henneman & Cardin, 2002; Levine & Zuckerman, 1999; Levy & Carlet, 2002).

Standard Ethical Theory

1. **Deontology** (Ahronheim et al, 2005)
   a. Duty-based ethics; health care providers have special duties of care to their patients
   b. Associated with German philosopher Immanuel Kant
2. **Utilitarianism** (Ahronheim et al, 2005)
   a. Belief that actions are morally evaluated on the basis of the extent to which they facilitate or promote happiness or well-being; health care providers' actions often based on achieving a desired outcome or preoccupation with consequences of an intervention
   b. Associated with English philosophers John Locke and John Stuart Mill

Ethical Principles

1. **Patient autonomy and self-determination** (Ahronheim et al, 2005)
   a. Principle that a competent adult patient has the right to make his or her own health care decisions
   b. Autonomy: the potential to be self-determining; clinically supported through the informed consent process, which facilitates decision making that is individualized on the basis of the patient's own values
   c. Paternalism: the term used when health care providers make the decisions for the patient based on the rationale that it is in the patient's best interest. This practice denies the patient the autonomy to make his or her own decisions.
2. **Beneficence** (Ahronheim et al, 2005)
   a. Principle that the competent patient or appropriate surrogate is the best judge of the patient's best interests

    b. Source of common ethical conflicts when there are disagreements between physician and patient or surrogate. Conflict may arise between the physician's perceived obligation to do good and obligation to respect the patient's expressed wishes.

3. Nonmaleficence (Ahronheim et al, 2005)

    a. Principle to "do no harm"

    b. Often considered same principle as beneficence

4. Justice (Ahronheim et al, 2005)

    a. Principle that everyone fundamentally deserves equal respect

    b. Point of reference for social policy related to access to health care

    c. Distributive justice in health care usually involves how resources are allocated (e.g., scarcity of organs for donation, availability of intensive care unit [ICU] beds or health care staff, futility of care versus patient autonomy, cost-benefit ratio of treatments, and limiting of access to expensive treatments)

        i. Macroallocation decisions (e.g., public health policy)

        ii. Microallocation decisions (e.g., triage during wartime); area of distributive justice involving the clinician role

Common Ethical Distinctions

Should common ethical distinctions be used in clinical ethics assessments? According to Ahronheim et al (2005), there are four common distinctions used in clinical ethics discussions. These authors believe it is important to determine whether these distinctions are logically valid (i.e., capable of sorting actions into two different groups without ambiguity) and morally relevant (i.e., one of the actions identified is morally justifiable whereas the other is not).

1. Active versus passive means to an end (or commission versus omission)

    a. Often associated with euthanasia

    b. Validity questioned because the decision to omit medical interventions to bring about a certain end often involves active behaviors (such as calling a meeting)

    c. Involves serious moral issues similar to those in the distinction between "killing" and "letting die." (For instance, it can be argued that it is justifiable to actively hasten a death if the alternative is to passively stand by while a patient suffers a prolonged death.)

    d. Recommended not to use this distinction in clinical ethics assessments

2. Ordinary versus extraordinary means

    a. Attempts to identify interventions on the basis of whether or not they are standard of practice

    b. Practice standards: a reflection of what is being done, not necessarily what should or should not be done on the basis of scientific principles. Should a patient be required to accept any kind of standard means of extending life even if properly grounded in science?

    c. Not recommended as part of a clinical ethics assessment unless a patient adheres to a particular faith that prohibits a specific intervention(s)

3. Killing versus letting die

    a. "Killing" infers a deliberate and physically active process such as giving a lethal injection; "letting die" refers to letting the disease process take its course. No one has a moral obligation to rescue a person if the attempt would not prolong life or the attempt would put the rescuer at risk for significant harm.

    b. The distinction appears to be valid and morally relevant but creates significant ethical dilemmas, especially in relation to assisted suicide.

4. Withholding versus withdrawing

    a. "Withholding" means never starting a given treatment; "withdrawing" means removing or stopping a treatment already started.

    b. Logical validity is questionable because there are only a few situations in which the distinction between the two actions is clear. There is no legal basis for the distinction.

    c. There is no clear distinction in terms of moral relevance. Is it more justifiable not to intubate a patient than to extubate a patient when the end point is similar in both situations?

    d. Despite the lack of logical validity and moral relevance, this distinction is commonly applied in clinical ethics.

Informed Consent and Patient Self-Determination

1. Informed consent for clinical care: Physicians or independent licensed practitioners have a separate duty to provide needed facts to a patient so that the patient can make an informed health care decision. The right to treat a patient is based on a contractual relationship grounded in mutual consent of the parties (Guido, 2006).

   a. Types of consent (Guido, 2006)
      i. Expressed consent: Given directly by written or verbal words
      ii. Implied consent: Presumed in emergency situations or implied by the patient's behavior (such as presenting an arm to the practitioner to have blood drawn)
      iii. Partial or complete consent: May be given by patient for only part of a proposed therapy, for example, consenting to a breast biopsy but not to a mastectomy should it be needed

   b. Elements of informed consent for clinical treatment (Guido, 2006)
      i. Explanation of treatment or procedure
      ii. Name and qualifications of the person to perform the procedure and those of any assistants
      iii. Explanation of significant risks (those that may lead to serious harm, including death)
      iv. Explanation of alternative therapies to the procedure or treatment, including the risk of doing nothing at all
      v. Explanation that the patient can refuse the treatment or procedure without having alternative care or support discontinued
      vi. Explanation that the patient can still refuse the treatment or procedure even after it has started

   c. Standards of informed consent disclosure (Guido, 2006)
      i. Medical community standard (reasonable medical practitioner standard): Disclosure of facts related to the treatment or procedure that a reasonable medical practitioner in a similar community would disclose
      ii. Objective patient standard (prudent patient standard): Disclosure of risks and benefits based on what a prudent person in the given patient's situation would deem material
      iii. Subject patient standard (individual patient standard): Disclosure of facts relevant to a particular patient's situation and what he or she would deem important to know to make an informed decision
      iv. Medical disclosure laws: Requirement by some states that certain risks and consequences be printed on a consent form
      v. Evolving standard proposed by Piper (1994): Patient and physician determine together what informed consent means to them; patient must communicate his or her values and expectations of the procedure or treatment to the physician, ask questions and seek clarification of the physician-patient discussion, evaluate symptoms and report impressions of how well the treatment or procedure is working or worked, and make good-faith efforts to participate in the treatment.

   d. Exceptions to informed consent (Guido, 2006)
      i. Emergency situations: Consent is implied if there is no time for disclosure and informed consent.
      ii. Therapeutic privilege: Primary health care providers are allowed to withhold information that they feel would be detrimental to the patient's health (i.e., likely to hinder or complicate necessary treatment, cause severe psychological harm, or cause enough anxiety to make a rational decision by the patient impossible).
      iii. Patient waiver: The patient may waive full disclosure while consenting to the procedure, but this cannot be suggested by the health care provider; the waiver must be initiated by the patient.
      iv. Prior patient knowledge: If the patient has had the same procedure previously and knows the risks and benefits as explained for the first procedure, then consent can be waived.

   e. Accountability for obtaining informed consent (Guido, 2006)
      i. The physician or independent practitioner has full accountability for obtaining informed consent.

      ii. A hospital is responsible for informed consent only if those obtaining the consent are employed by the hospital or if the hospital fails to take appropriate actions when informed consent was not obtained and the hospital is aware it was not obtained.

      iii. The nurse's role in obtaining informed consent varies with the situation, institution, and state law.

          (a) Nurses should explain all nursing care procedures to patients and families. Such procedures rely on orally expressed consent or implied consent. If a patient refuses a procedure or care, this must be honored.

          (b) Physicians can delegate the obtaining of informed consent to nurses. They do so at their own risk, but the nurse must ensure that all aspects of an informed consent are disclosed. Some hospitals do not allow nurses to obtain informed consent to limit the hospital's liability.

          (c) If a nurse has knowledge that an already signed consent form does not meet the criteria for informed consent or the patient revokes the consent, the nurse must notify the supervisor and/or physician.

      iv. To obtain blood at the request of law enforcement personnel without consent, five conditions must be present and documented:

          (a) The suspect is under arrest.

          (b) The likelihood exists that the blood drawn will produce evidence for criminal prosecution.

          (c) A delay in drawing blood would lead to destruction of evidence.

          (d) The test is reasonable and not medically contraindicated.

          (e) The test is performed in a reasonable manner.

2. Consent forms (Guido, 2006)

  a. Blanket consent: Required before admission and covers routine and customary care

  b. Specific consent forms: Often mandated by states; a detailed consent form with the following elements:

      i. Signature of a competent patient or legally authorized representative; "competent" means that the patient has not been declared incompetent by a court of law and the person is able to understand the consequences of his or her actions

          (a) The signature cannot be coerced.

          (b) The patient cannot be impaired because of medications previously received.

      ii. Name and description of procedure in lay language

      iii. Description of risks and alternatives to treatment (including nontreatment)

      iv. Description of probable consequences of proposed procedure

      v. Signatures of one or two witnesses as mandated by state law; the witness is attesting that the patient actually signed the form

3. Informed consent in human research (Guido, 2006)

  a. Since 1974, the U.S. Department of Health and Human Services has required an institutional review board to approve protocols for human research.*

  b. Special precautions are in place to protect vulnerable patient populations such as minors, mentally disabled persons, children, and prisoners

  c. Informed consent must include the following basic elements:

      i. A description of the purpose of the research, procedures that are experimental and those that are part of regular care, and expected duration of the subject's participation

      ii. Description of foreseeable risks or discomforts

      iii. Benefits, if any, to the subject

      iv. Disclosure of alternative courses of treatment available

      v. Description of how confidentiality of information will be maintained

      vi. Explanation of any compensation that will be provided and explanation of medical care that will be provided if injury occurs

---

*For comprehensive resources related to the protection of human research subjects, see the website for the Office for Human Research Protections, Department of Health and Human Services (http://www.hhs.gov/ohrp/).

      vii. Contact information for further questions about the research and the subject's rights as a research volunteer

      viii. A clear statement that the subject understands that he or she is a volunteer and has not been coerced into participating; also a statement that the subject may withdraw consent to participate any time during the procedure without loss of benefits or penalties to which the subject is entitled

      ix. Language that is easy to understand and includes no exculpatory wording (such as that the researcher has no liability for the patient's outcome). Participants should be advised of:

        (a) Any additional cost they may incur

        (b) Potential risk

        (c) Rights to withdraw at will without question

        (d) The consequences of withdrawal before the completion of the study

        (e) A statement that informs subject that new finds will be disclosed to them

        (f) The number of participating subjects in the study

4. Advance directive: A document in which a person gives directions in advance about medical care or designates who should make medical decisions if he or she should lose decision-making capacity

    a. Living will: Generic term for an advance directive; some states do not recognize these

      i. Not binding for medical practitioners

      ii. Does not protect practitioner from criminal or civil liability

    b. Natural death acts: Enacted by many states to protect practitioners from civil and criminal lawsuits and to ensure that the patient's wishes are followed if the patient is not competent to make his or her own health care decisions.

      i. A legally recognized living will

        (a) Must be developed by a competent adult 18 years of age or older

        (b) Must be witnessed by two persons; some states put restrictions on who can witness

        (c) May be revoked by physically destroying, revoking in writing, or verbally rescinding

        (d) Remains valid until revoked

        (e) Becomes effective only when the person becomes qualified (i.e., is terminally ill or has an irreversible condition with loss of decision-making capacity). Usually two physicians must certify that procedures or treatments will not prevent death but merely prolong it.

        (f) Does not apply to medications and therapies given to prevent suffering and to provide comfort

    c. Durable power of attorney for health care: Allows competent adults to designate someone to make their health care decisions for them if they become unable to make their own decisions

    d. Medical or physician directive: Allowed in some states; lists a variety of treatments and procedures that the patient may want depending on the patient's condition at the time he or she cannot make his or her own decisions; similar to a living will and with equal legal worth

    e. Uniform Rights of the Terminally Ill Act: Adopted in 1980 and revised in 1989

      i. Act is similar to natural death acts.

      ii. Scope is narrow and limited to treatment that is life prolonging in patients with a terminal or irreversible condition.

      iii. Patients who are in a persistent vegetative state are not qualified to use the provisions of this act

    f. Patient Self-Determination Act of 1990

      i. Mandates patient education about advance directives and provides assistance in executing such directives

      ii. States that providers may not discriminate against a patient on the basis of the presence or absence of an advance directive

    g. Do-not-resuscitate (DNR) directives: Institution-based policies that allow patients and physicians to make a decision not to resuscitate in the event of cardiopulmonary arrest

  i.   Some states have out-of-hospital DNR laws that allow an individual to request not to be resuscitated by emergency personnel. These orders are still in effect for outpatient treatment, including emergency department care, unless revoked.

  ii.   Some hospitals do not recognize DNR orders during surgery. Others believe that the decision to resuscitate or not to resuscitate should be made together by the patient, the physician, and the anesthesiologist. Whatever decision is made should be clearly documented in the medical record before surgery.

5. Declaration of death

  a. World Medical Association Declaration on Death*

  b. Uniform Determination of Death Act (UDDA): Guidelines developed by the President's Commission for the Study of Ethical Problems in Medicine and in Biomedical and Behavioral Research, which state that "any individual who has sustained either irreversible cessation of circulatory and respiratory functions, or irreversible cessation of all functions of the entire brain, including the brainstem, is dead" (http://www.ascensionhealth.org/ethics/public/issues/udda.asp)

  c. Continued existence of confusion and controversy over the term brain death and the relation of such death to donorship for organ transplantation (Capron, 2001; Truog, 2003)

  d. Procedural guidelines for the declaration of death

   i.   Triggering of a neurologic evaluation: As soon as the responsible physician has a reasonable suspicion that an irreversible loss of all brain functions has occurred, he or she should perform the appropriate tests and procedures to determine the patient's neurologic status.

   ii.   Obligation to declare a patient dead

    (a)   Cardiopulmonary criteria for determining death are recognized in all states. When the physician determines that the patient has experienced an irreversible cessation of cardiopulmonary functions, he or she declares the patient dead. Consent of the surrogate, family, or concerned friends is not required.

    (b)   Sensitivity to family or surrogate needs is required in declaring brain death. Family members have the option to obtain a second opinion about brain death.

   iii.   cessation of treatment after a declaration of death: Once the declaration of death has been made, all treatment of the patient ordinarily should cease; exceptions to this might be when efforts are made to use the body or body parts for purposes stated in the Uniform Anatomical Gift Act (UAGA) (education, research, advancement of medical or dental science, therapy, transplantation) or when the patient is pregnant and efforts are being made to save the life of the fetus.

   iv.   In cases involving organ donation, health care professionals who make the declaration of death

    (a)   Should not be members of the organ transplantation team

    (b)   Should not be a member of the patient's family

    (c)   Should not have malpractice charges pending against them that are related to the case

    (d)   Should not have any other special interest in declaration of the patient's death (i.e., stand to inherit anything according to patient's will)

6. Organ donation

  a. World Medical Association Statement on Human Organ and Tissue Donation and Transplantation (World Medical Association, 2006)†

  b. Types of organ donors

   i.   Tissue donor or living organ donor: Donor may be alive (e.g., bone marrow, kidney donor) or deceased (e.g., eye donor); organ donation by living donors poses special concerns because of the increased risk to donors' lives (Benner, 2002).

---

*For the text of the declaration, go to http://www.wma.net/e/policy/d2.htm.

†Adopted in 2000 to address the professional obligations of physicians and hospitals related to organ donation and transplantation. The complete statement can be found at http://www.wma.net/e/policy/wma.htm.

      ii. Heart-beating donor: Donor is brain dead but respiratory function is supported mechanically while cardiac function continues spontaneously.

      iii. Non–heart-beating donor: Organs are procured immediately after cessation of cardio-respiratory function

  c. A recent study (Exley, White, & Martin, 2002) indicated that the following characteristics significantly influence the likelihood that families will make a decision to donate tissues or organs:

      i. Anglo-American ethnicity

      ii. Any religious affiliation

      iii. Discussion of donation initiated by someone: This person could be family member, physician, or organ procurement organization coordinator, but it is helpful to include the organ procurement organization coordinator early in the process.

      iv. Death caused by gunshot or suicide

      v. Issuing of request before or during declaration of brain death

      vi. Presence of signed donor card

7. Emergency Medical Treatment and Labor Act (EMTALA)

  a. This 1986 law requires hospitals participating in Medicare to screen patients for emergency medical conditions and stabilize them or provide protected transfers for medical reasons (Centers for Medicare and Medicaid Services, 2004; Frank, 2001).

  b. Failure to adhere to the law results in large fines or loss of Medicare funding.

  c. Patients may sue hospitals in federal or state court for damages under EMTALA's private right of action provision.

  d. First case was decided by the U.S. Supreme Court in 1998.

  e. In 2006, the National Conference of Commissioners on Uniform State Law introduced revisions to the UAGA. This act replaced the previous 1968 and 1987 versions of the Act. The 2006 revision was prepared with the active participation of the whole range of stakeholders. The Act was designed to provide uniformity and facilitate organ donations where minutes are too precious to permit wasting time deciphering divergence in state laws. By June 2008, 29 states had adopted the UAGA Act (http://www.anatomicalgifttact.org). Improvements to the Act provide clear definitions and enhance the rights of individuals (including minors) to donate gifts.

8. Futile care

  a. Concept is an evolving standard (Ahronheim et al, 2005).

  b. Definitions of futility lack consensus and are value laden, but futile care involves interventions that sustain life for prolonged periods even when there is no hope of improvement or achieving the goals of therapy (American Medical Association Council on Ethical and Judicial Affairs, 1999). Many questions remain unresolved and lead to ethical dilemmas and conflict.

      i. Who establishes the goals of therapy? Is it the physician, the patient, the family, or all of them?

      ii. What does the physician or hospital do if the medical decision is in conflict with that of the patient and family, who may have an unrealistic expectation for improvement (Curtis & Burt, 2003; Lofmark & Nilstun, 2002)?

  c. The American Medical Association Council on Ethical and Judicial Affairs (1999) recommends resolution of futility conflicts using a process-based framework.

  d. There is some evidence that bioethics consultation resulting in cessation of therapy shortens the length of therapy significantly (Rivera et al, 2001; Schneiderman, Gilmer, & Teetzel, 2000; Schneiderman et al, 2003).

9. Legal barriers to end-of-life care (Meisel et al, 2000)

  a. The legal context of care affects interventions and outcomes.

  b. Legal myths and counteracting reality include the following:

      i. *Myth:* Forgoing life-sustaining treatment for a patient without decision-making capacity requires evidence that this is the patient's wish.
        Reality: Only a few states require "clear and convincing evidence." Most states will allow forgoing life-sustaining treatment on the basis of a surrogate's word that it was the patient's wish. Some states even allow termination of such treatment if no one knows the patient's wishes and it is deemed in the patient's "best interest."

    ii. *Myth:* Withholding or withdrawing artificial nutrition or hydration from terminally ill or permanently unconscious patients is illegal.
    Reality: Just like any other therapy, fluids and nutrition may be withheld if it is the patient's or surrogate's wish.

    iii. *Myth:* Risk management personnel must be consulted before life-sustaining medical treatment can be stopped.
    Reality: This may be a hospital policy, but there is no legal requirement to notify risk management personnel.

    iv. *Myth:* Advance directives must be developed with use of specific forms, are not transferable to other states, and govern all future decisions. Advance directives given orally are not enforceable.
    Reality: Oral statements made by the patients may be legally valid directives. The patient does not have to be competent to revoke an advance directive but does have to be competent to make one. There are no specific forms required by any law to be used to document advance directives. Most states honor directives developed in other states.

    v. *Myth:* Physicians will be criminally prosecuted if they prescribe high dosages of medication for palliative care (to relieve pain or discomfort symptoms) that result in death.
    Reality: In 1997 the U.S. Supreme Court ruled on the constitutionality of laws making physician-assisted suicide a crime. The physician has not committed assisted suicide or homicide if the pain medications were ordered to relieve pain. The doctrine of "double effect" states that if an intervention is used for its intended purpose (such as pain relief) but has an unintended effect that would be illegitimate if it were intended (such as the death of the patient), then the physician is not morally responsible for the unintended effect. In reality the application of this doctrine can be ambiguous, and acting under the double-effect doctrine does not eliminate the risk of prosecution. Although a good defense can be made under the doctrine, such defense takes a toll on the physician. As a result, undertreatment of pain at the end of life often occurs.

    vi. *Myth:* There are no legal options for easing suffering in a terminally ill patient whose suffering is overwhelming despite palliative care.
    Reality: Terminal sedation is an option to treat otherwise intractable symptoms in patients imminently dying. Only Oregon gives physicians the right to prescribe oral medication to competent patients who intend to commit suicide with the medication. The patient must take his or her own medication. The physician can only prescribe the drugs. The 1997 U.S. Supreme Court decision on assisted suicide leaves other states free to legalize or prohibit the practice.

Clinical Ethics Assessment

1. Identification of ethical issues and ethical decision-making models
    a. Distinction between ethical and nonethical problems and dilemmas: Three characteristics must be present for a problem to be deemed an ethical one (Curtin as cited in Stanton, 2003):
        i. The problem cannot be resolved with just empirical data.
        ii. The problem is inherently perplexing.
        iii. The result of the decision making will affect several areas of human concern.
    b. Elements of ethical decision-making models (Ahronheim et al, 2005; Stanton, 2003): There are many decision-making models. Common elements include the following actions:
        i. Gather all data (including information from all the stakeholders) related to the issue.
        ii. Analyze and interpret the data: Is it an ethical issue versus a legal or policy issue? What ethical principles are involved? What ethical conflicts are present? What are the capabilities of the stakeholders involved?
        iii. Identify courses of action and analyze the benefits and burdens of each course; project the consequences of the action.
        iv. Choose a plan of action and implement the plan; provide support to the stakeholders as needed.
        v. Evaluate the consequences of the actions taken.
        vi. Evaluate the ethical decision-making process.

2. Ethical conflicts
   a. Conflicts between moral principles
   b. Conflicts between interpretations of a patient's best interest
   c. Conflicts between moral principles and institutional policy or the law
3. Institutional ethics committees
   a. Multidisciplinary team resource for patients and families, clinicians, and the institution
      i. Assist with clarifying issues.
      ii. Assist with the development of institutional policies and procedures related to clinical ethical issues.
   b. Goals including promoting the rights of patients, fostering shared decision making between patients and clinicians, promoting fair policies and procedures that maximize the likelihood of good patient-centered outcomes, and enhancing the ethical practice of health care professionals and health care institutions
   c. Education of staff and the community to achieve goals
   d. Ethics consultation: The most common situations triggering consultations by physicians include the following (DuVal et al, 2001):
      i. End-of-life care
      ii. Patient autonomy
      iii. Conflicts among persons involved
   e. Composition: Should include representatives of all disciplines and of the institution administration, and community-at-large members
4. Ethics consultation: Process elements
   a. Who has access to the process (all clinicians, patients, and/or families) should be delineated.
   b. Patients (or surrogates), if appropriate, and attending physicians should be notified (providing reason for the consultation, describing the process, and inviting participation).
   c. Documentation should be in patient record or some other permanent record.
   d. Case review or process evaluation should be done to promote accountability.
5. Core skills and knowledge required for effective ethics consultations (Society for Health and Human Values, 1998)
   a. Core skills (Table 1-3)
      i. Ethical assessment skills required to identify the nature of the ethical dilemma or conflict
      ii. Process skills required to focus on efforts to resolve the ethical dilemma or conflict
      iii. Interpersonal skills critical to the consultation process
   b. Core knowledge areas
      i. Moral reasoning and ethical theory as it relates to consultation
      ii. Bioethical issues and concepts that typically emerge in ethical consultations
      iii. Health care systems as they relate to ethics consultation
      iv. Clinical knowledge as related to the ethics consultation
      v. Knowledge of the health care institution and institution policies in the context of the ethical consultation
      vi. Beliefs and perspectives of the patient and staff populations served by the ethics consultation
      vii. Relevant code of ethics, standards of professional conduct, and guidelines of accrediting organizations as they relate to ethics consultation
      viii. Health law relevant to ethics consultation

Nurse's Role as Patient Advocate and Moral Agent

1. Organizational ethics and the nurse as patient advocate: AACN takes the position that the role of the progressive care nurse includes being a patient advocate (AACN, 2006). The health care institution is instrumental in providing an environment in which patient advocacy is expected and supported. Patient advocacy is a fundamental nursing characteristic in the Synergy Model (Hayes, 2000). As a patient advocate, the acute/critical care nurse does the following:
   a. Respects and supports the right of the patient or the patient's designated surrogate to autonomous, informed decision making

▓ **TABLE 1-3**
▓ ▓ **Core Skills for Ethics Consultation**

Skill Category	Specific Skills
Ethical assessment skills	***Ability to:*** Discern and gather relevant data Assess social and interpersonal dynamics Distinguish ethical dimensions of case from other dimensions (i.e., legal, medical, psychiatric) Identify the assumptions that stakeholders bring to the situation Identify values held by the various stakeholders (requires knowledge to access and analyze the relevant laws, policies, and bioethical knowledge needed) Use relevant moral considerations in case analysis Identify and justify a range of morally acceptable options and their consequences Evaluate evidence for and against the options presented for action Recognize and acknowledge personal limitations and potential areas of conflict between personal views and role as ethics consultant (may involve accepting group decisions that are morally acceptable but in conflict with personal viewpoint)
Process skills	***Ability to:*** Identify key stakeholders and involve them in the process Set ground rules for formal meetings Stay within the limits of the consultant's role Create an atmosphere of trust that respects privacy and confidentiality and promotes honest discussion of issues Build moral consensus by helping individuals analyze the values underlying their assumptions and decisions, negotiating and resolving conflicts, and engaging in creative problem solving Use institutional structure and resources to facilitate the implementation of the selected course of action Document the consultation and elicit feedback about the process for evaluation
Interpersonal skills	***Ability to:*** Listen well and communicate respect, support, and empathy to stakeholders Educate about the ethical dimensions of the case Elicit the moral views of stakeholders Represent the views of all involved parties to the others Enable involved parties to communicate effectively and be heard by others Recognize and attend to communication barriers

Adapted from Society for Health and Human Values–Society for Bioethics Consultation Task Force on Standards for Bioethics Consultation. *Core Competencies for Health Care Ethics Consultation.* Glenview, IL: American Society for Bioethics and Humanities; 1998:12-14.

    b. Intervenes when the best interest of the patient is in question
    c. Helps the patient obtain necessary care
    d. Respects the values, beliefs, and rights of the patient
    e. Provides education and support to help the patient or the patient's designated surrogate make decisions
    f. Represents the patient in accordance with the patient's choices
    g. Supports the decisions of the patient or the patient's designated surrogate or transfers care to an equally qualified acute/progressive care nurse
    h. Intercedes for a patient who cannot speak for himself or herself in situations that require immediate action
    i. Monitors and safeguards the quality of care the patient receives
    j. Acts as liaison among the patient, the patient's family, and health care professionals
  2. Patient rights
    a. American Hospital Association (AHA) Patient Bill of Rights (AHA, 1992); first published in 1973, revised in 1992; posted in all hospitals in the United States

  b. Ethics of restraints: The use of restraints in acute/critical care has the potential to violate several ethical principles (Reigle, 1996) and thus should be undertaken with caution.
   i. Nonmaleficence, or preventing harm; and beneficence, or doing good. Restraints are often used to prevent harm, but unintended consequences may violate this principle. The patient's autonomy is breached, and restraints often cause significant physical harm. In many cases use of restraint does not prevent the disruption of medical therapy.
   ii. Informed consent should be obtained from the patient and/or family before use of restraints. A discussion of alternative treatments should be included. A patient with decision-making capacity should be able to choose to forgo restraint. Paternalism is involved in situations in which one overrides another's decision to prevent harm to the person or maximize the benefits of treatment. There may be justifications for such actions in the progressive care environment. If the patient lacks decision-making capacity and no surrogate decision maker is available, the nurse is obligated to use restraints to prevent significant or irreversible harm.
   iii. Trust is important to the patient and family members. They trust nurses, and thus ongoing communication about restraint decisions is crucial. Family members become upset when the patient is restrained without their knowledge.
  c. Ethics of pain management (American Pain Society, 2006; McCaffery & Pasero, 1999)
   i. Patients have the right to have their reports of pain believed.
   ii. Patients have the right to have pain addressed appropriately.
   iii. Clinicians, patients, and families must be educated about pain treatment.
   iv. Pain and pain management must be made visible and emphasized in organizations.
   v. Policies on reimbursement for the services of health professionals, medications, and other palliative treatments must be designed so that they do not create barriers to symptom treatment.
   vi. Development of policies to ensure adequate treatment of symptoms should take precedence over legalization of physician-assisted suicide and euthanasia.
 3. Family-centered care versus patient-centered care
  a. Family members are not visitors (Molter, 2003).
  b. The family has a vital role in supporting the patient through a critical illness (Simpson, 1991). When family members' needs are not attended to or met, significant conflict occurs (Chesla & Stannard, 1997; Levine & Zuckerman, 1999).
  c. Family-centered care focuses on the whole patient as a member of a family unit. It incorporates the family as a team member in the healing process. Improving family communications at the end of life can be cost-effective for the family and institution (Ahrens et al, 2003).
  d. The family-centered care philosophy was developed by pediatric practitioners (Edelman, 1995). Box 1-4 summarizes the key tenets of the family-centered care philosophy. It is a collaborative approach to care and not a unilateral approach on the part of the clinicians or the family. It can be practically established in PCUs (Henneman & Cardin, 2002).
 4. End-of-life care
  a. AACN organized a consortium to develop an agenda for the nursing profession on end-of-life care (EOLC) (Nursing Leadership Consortium on End-of-Life Care, 1999). Nine priorities were identified:
   i. Education: Integrate EOLC into all curricula and develop interdisciplinary education on palliative care.
   ii. Professionalism: Create an environment for collaboration among health care systems, educational institutions, associations, and government agencies to meet the needs of EOLC.
   iii. Clinical and patient care: Establish practice guidelines that incorporate supportive strategies to prevent pain and suffering and promote comfort and well-being.
   iv. Research: Provide health care staff with research-based information on EOLC.
   v. Patient and family advocacy: Educate and empower the consumer of health care services about EOLC.
   vi. Decision making: Develop a dynamic process for making decisions about EOLC.
   vii. Culture: Create a national environment in which EOLC is freely discussed.

▓ **BOX 1-4**
▓ **EIGHT ELEMENTS OF FAMILY-CENTERED CARE**

1. Incorporating into policy and practice the recognition that the family is the constant in a person's life, while the service systems and support personnel within those systems fluctuate
2. Facilitating family/professional collaboration at all levels of hospital, home, and community care
3. Exchanging complete and unbiased information between families and professionals in a supportive manner at all times
4. Incorporating into policy and practice the recognition and honoring of cultural diversity, strengths, and individuality within and across all families
5. Recognizing and respecting different methods of coping and implementing comprehensive policies and programs that provide developmental, educational, emotional, environmental, and financial supports to meet the diverse needs of families
6. Encouraging and facilitating family-to-family support and networking
7. Ensuring that hospital, home, and community service and support systems for individuals and their families needing specialized health and development care are flexible, accessible, and comprehensive in responding to diverse family-identified needs
8. Appreciating families as families and individuals as individuals, recognizing that they possess a wide range of strengths, concerns, emotions, and aspirations beyond their need for specialized health services and support

From Edelman L, ed. *Getting on Board: Training Activities to Promote the Practice of Family-Centered Care.* 2nd ed. Bethesda, MD: Association for the Care of Children's Health; 1995:4-5.

    viii. Systems of care: Structure a health care system that allows all dying patients and their families access to pain management and hospice care.
    ix. Resource allocation policy: Enact legislation that provides comprehensive financing for palliative care that is not limited to skilled nursing episodes or hospice care.
  b. Quality indicators for EOLC have been described (Clarke et al, 2003). Consensus was established by the Robert Wood Johnson Foundation Critical Care End-of-Life Peer Workgroup. Seven domains were identified with specific indicators:
    i. Patient and family–centered decision making
      (a) Recognize the patient and family as the unit of care.
      (b) Assess the patient's and family's decision-making style and preferences.
      (c) Address conflicts in decision making within the family.
      (d) Assess, together with appropriate clinical consultants, the patient's capacity to participate in decision making about treatment and document this assessment.
      (e) Initiate advance care planning with the patient and family.
      (f) Clarify and document the status of the patient's advance directive.
      (g) Identify the health care proxy or surrogate decision maker.
      (h) Clarify and document resuscitation orders.
      (i) Assure the patient and family that decision making by the health care team will incorporate their preferences (Heyland et al, 2003).
      (j) Follow ethical and legal guidelines for patients who lack both capacity and a surrogate decision maker.
      (k) Establish and document clear, realistic, and appropriate goals of care in consultation with the patient and family.
      (l) Help the patient and family assess the benefits and burdens of alternative treatment choices as the patient's condition changes.
      (m) Forgo life-sustaining treatments in a way that ensures that patient and family preferences are elicited and respected.
    ii. Communication within the team and with patients and families
      (a) Meet as an interdisciplinary team to discuss the patient's condition, clarify goals of treatment, and identify the patient's and family's needs and preferences (Curtis et al, 2001).

    (b) Address conflicts among the clinical team before meeting with the patient and/or family.

    (c) Use expert clinical, ethical, and spiritual consultants when appropriate.

    (d) Recognize the adaptations in communication strategy required for the patient and family depending on the chronic versus acute nature of illness, cultural and spiritual differences, and other influences.

    (e) Meet with the patient and/or family on a regular basis to review the patient's status and to answer questions.

    (f) Communicate all information to the patient and family, including distressing news, in a clear, sensitive, unhurried manner and in an appropriate setting.

    (g) Clarify the patient's and family's understanding of the patient's condition and goals of care at the beginning and end of each meeting.

    (h) Designate a primary clinical liaison(s) who will communicate with the family daily.

    (i) When indicated, prepare the patient and family for the dying process.

  iii. Continuity of care

    (a) Maximize continuity of care across clinicians, consultants, and settings.

    (b) Orient new clinicians regarding the patient and family status.

    (c) Prepare the patient and/or family for a change of clinician(s) and introduce new clinicians.

  iv. Emotional and practical support

    (a) Elicit and attend to the needs of the dying person and his or her family.

    (b) Distribute written material for families that includes orientation to the progressive care environment and open visitation guidelines, logistical information (nearby hotels, banks, restaurants; directions), listings of financial consultation services, and bereavement programs and resources.

    (c) Facilitate strengthening of patient-family relationships and communication.

    (d) Maximize privacy for the patient and family.

    (e) Value and support the patient's and family's cultural traditions.

    (f) Arrange for social support for a patient without family or friends.

    (g) Support the family through the patient's death and their bereavement.

  v. Symptom management

    (a) Emphasize the comprehensive comfort care that will be provided to the patient.

    (b) Institute and use uniform quantitative symptom assessment scales appropriate for communicative and noncommunicative patients on a routine basis.

    (c) Standardize and follow best clinical practices for symptom management.

    (d) Use nonpharmacologic, as well as pharmacologic, measures to maximize comfort as appropriate and desired by the patient and family.

    (e) Reassess and document symptoms after interventions.

    (f) Eliminate unnecessary tests and procedures (laboratory work, weighing, routine monitoring of vital signs) and maintain intravenous catheters only for symptom management in situations in which life support is being withdrawn.

    (g) Attend to the patient's appearance and hygiene.

    (h) Ensure the family's and/or clinician's presence so the patient is not dying alone.

  vi. Spiritual support

    (a) Assess and document spiritual needs of the patient and family on an ongoing basis.

    (b) Encourage access to spiritual resources.

    (c) Elicit and facilitate spiritual and cultural practices that the patient and family find comforting.

  vii. Emotional and organizational support for progressive care clinicians

    (a) Support health care team colleagues caring for dying patients.

    (b) Adjust nursing staff and medical rotation schedules to maximize continuity of care providers for dying patients.

    (c) Communicate regularly with the interdisciplinary team regarding the goals of care.

(d) Establish a staff support group, based on the input and needs of the staff and experienced group facilitators, and integrate meeting times into the routine of the PCU.

(e) Enlist palliative care experts, pastoral care representatives, and other consultants to teach and model aspects of EOLC.

(f) Facilitate the establishment of rituals for the staff to mark the death of patients.

5. Good palliative care practice (Kirchhoff, 2002)

   a. Goals to enable the patient to achieve a peaceful end of life (Ruland and Moore, 1998)

      i. The patient will be pain free.

      ii. The patient will feel comfortable.

      iii. The patient will experience dignity and respect.

      iv. The patient will be at peace.

      v. The patient will be close to significant others.

   b. Precepts of palliative care*

      i. Respect patient goals, preferences, and choices.

      ii. Provide comprehensive care.

      iii. Utilize the strengths of interdisciplinary resources.

      iv. Acknowledge and address caregiver concerns.

      v. Build systems and mechanisms of support.

   c. Development of the competencies needed to provide care to patients at the end of life†

REFERENCES AND BIBLIOGRAPHY

AACN Certification Corporation. *PCCN Test Plan* (date unknown). http://www.aacn.org/WD/Certifications/content/pccnexamblueprint.pcms?menu=Certification;2008. Accessed October 20, 2008.

AACN Certification Corporation. *Safeguarding the patient and the profession: The value of critical care certification*, 2002. http://www.aacn.org/WD/PressRoom/Docs/exesum02.pdf; 2008.Accessed October 21, 2008.

APRN Consensus Work Group and the National Council of State Boards of Nursing APRN Advisory Committee. *Consensus Model for APRN Regulation: Licensure, Accreditation, Certification & Education*, 2008. http://www.aacn.nche.edu/Education/pdf/APRNReport.pdf; 2008. Accessed October 14, 2008.

Agich GJ, Arroliga AC. Appropriate use of DNR orders: a practical approach. *Cleve Clin J Med*. 2000;67:392, 395, 399–400.

Ahrens T, Yancey V, Kollef M. Improving family communications at the end of life: implications for length of stay in the intensive care unit and resource use. *Am J Crit Care*. 2003;12:317–324.

Aiken LH, Clarke SP, Sloane DM, et al. Nurses' reports on hospital care in five countries. *Health Affairs*. 2001;20:43–53. http://www.healthaffairs.org. Accessed October 15, 2008.

Alspach G. Extending the Synergy Model to preceptorship. *Crit Care Nurse*. 2006;26(2):10-13.

American Association of Critical-Care Nurses. *Mission, Vision and Values*, 2008. http://www.aacn.org/WD/Memberships/Content/Mission_vision_values_ethics.pcms?menu=AboutUs. Accessed October 15, 2008.

American Association of Critical-Care Nurses. *The AACN Synergy Model for Patient Care*, 2003. http://www.aacn.org/WD/Certifications/content/synmodel.pcms?pid=1&&menu=. Accessed October 16, 2008.

American Association of Critical-Care Nurses. *Role of the Critical Care Nurse*, 2006. http://classic.aacn.org/AACN/pubpolcy.nsf/64c71bdeda6f392a882567310071cbf2/4b9dd3eb98c7a273882566090004b13f?OpenDocument. Accessed October 15, 2008.

★ American Nurses Association. *Nursing's Social Policy Statement*. 2nd ed. Washington, DC: The Association; 2003.

Annis TD. The interdisciplinary team across the continuum of care. *Crit Care Nurse*. 2002;22:76-79.

Barden C, ed. *Standards for Establishing and Sustaining Healthy Work Environments*. Aliso Viejo, CA: American Association of Critical-Care Nurses; 2005.

Bell L, ed. *AACN Scope and Standards for Acute and Critical Care Nursing Practice*. 4th ed. Aliso Viejo, CA: American Association of Critical-Care Nurses; 2008.

---

*The actual document developed by the Last Acts Task Force on Palliative Care in 1997 can be found at https://www.aacn.org/AACN/practice.nsf/Files/ep/$file/2001Precep.pdf.

†Competencies recommended by the American Association of Colleges of Nursing are found at http://www.aacn.nche.edu/Publications/deathfin.htm.

Bell L, ed. *Scope and Standards of Practice for the Acute Care Nurse Practitioner*. Aliso Viejo, CA: American Association of Critical-Care Nurses; 2006.

Bell L, ed. *Scope of Practice and Standards of Professional Performance for the Acute and Critical Care Clinical Nurse Specialist*. Aliso Viejo, CA: American Association of Critical-Care Nurses; 2002.

Brady D, Molzen S, Graham S, O'Neil V. Using the synergy of online education and simulation to inspire a new model for a community critical care course. *Crit Care Nurs Q*. 2006;29(3):231-236.

Brewer BB, Wojner-Alexandrov AW, Triola N, et al. AACN Synergy Model's characteristics of patients: psychometric analyses in a tertiary care health system. *Am J Crit Care*. 2007;158-167.

Carlson MB. Engaging synergy: kindred spirits on the edge. *J Humanistic Psychol*. 1996;36(3):85-102.

★ Caterinicchio MJ. Redefining nursing according to patients' and families' needs: an evolving concept. The AACN Certification Corporation. *AACN Clin Issues*. 1995;6:153-156.

Chesla CA, Stannard D. Breakdown in the nursing care of families in the ICU. *Am J Crit Care*. 1997;6:64-71.

Cohen SS, Crego N, Cuming RG, et al. The Synergy Model and the role of clinical nurse specialists in a multihospital system. *Am J Crit Care*. 2002;11:436-445.

Collopy KS. Advance practice nurses guiding families through systems. *Crit Care Nurse*. 1999;19:80-85.

Cornerstone Communications Group. *Analysis of American Nurses Association Staffing Survey*. Washington, DC: American Nurses Association; 2001.

Curley MAQ. Patient-nurse synergy: optimizing patients' outcomes. *Am J Crit Care*. 1998;7:64-72.

Curtis JR, Patrick DL, Shannon SE, et al. The family conference as a focus to improve communication about end-of-life care in the ICU: opportunities for improvement. *Crit Care Med*. 2001;29(suppl 2):N40-N45.

Czerwinski S, Blastic L, Rice B. The Synergy Model: building a clinical advancement program. *Crit Care Nurse*. 1999;19:72-77.

Doble RK, Curley MAQ, Hession-Leband E, et al. Using the Synergy Model to link nursing care to diagnosis-related groups. *Crit Care Nurse*. 2000;20:86-92.

Ecklund MM, Stamps DC. Promoting synergy in progressive care. *Crit Care Nurse*. 2002;22:60-66.

Edelman L, ed. *Getting on Board: Training Activities to Promote the Practice of Family-Centered Care*. 2nd ed. Bethesda, MD: Association for the Care of Children's Health; 1995.

Edwards DF. The Synergy Model: linking patient needs to nurse competencies. *Crit Care Nurse*. 1999;19:97-99.

Exley M, White N, Martin JH. Transplantation: why families say no to organ donation. *Crit Care Nurse*. 2002;6:44-51.

Fowler E. An ethical dilemma. Is it ever acceptable to lie to a patient? *Br J Perioper Nurs*. 2004;14:448-451.

Freyling M, Kesten K, Heath J. The Synergy Model at work in a military ICU in Iraq. *Crit Care Nurs Clin North Am*. 2008;20(1):23-29.

Glassford BA. Goals aimed at helping to integrate ethics into practice. *AACN News*. 1999;16(11).

Grossenbacher J. The case of Terri Schiavo: ethics at the end of life. *J Leg Med*. 2007;28:419-427.

Haig KM, Sutton S, Whittington, J. SBAR: a shared mental model for improving communication between clinicians. *J Comm J Qual Patient Safe*. 2006;32(3):167-175.

Hardin S, Hussey L. AACN Synergy Model for patient care: case study of CHF patient. *Crit Care Nurse*. 2003;23:73-76.

Hartigan RC. Establishing criteria for 1:1 staffing ratios. *Crit Care Nurse*. 2000;20:114-116.

Hayes C. Strengthening nurses' moral agency. *Crit Care Nurse*. 2000;20:90-94.

Helms S, Ennis R. *Synergizing Your Progressive Care Environment* [CD-ROM]. Aliso Viejo, CA: American Association of Critical-Care Nurses; 2005.

Henneman EA, Cardin S. Family-centered critical care: a practical approach to making it happen. *Crit Care Nurse*. 2002;22:12-16, 18-19.

Hough C. Learning, decisions, and transformation in critical care nursing practice. *Nursing Ethics*. 2008;15:322-331.

Institute of Medicine. *Keeping Patients Safe: Transforming the Work Environment for Nurses*. Washington, DC: The National Academies Press; 2006.

Johnson KW. *The role of leadership in organizational integrity and five modes of ethical leadership*, 2005. http://www.ethicaledge.com/Components%20of%20Ethical%20Leadership%20July%2001.pdf. Accessed October 14, 2008.

Kanaskie M. Mentoring—a staff retention tool. *Crit Care Nurs Q*. 2006;29:248-252.

Kaplow R. Applying the Synergy Model to nursing education. *Crit Care Nurse*. 2002;22:77-81.

Kaplow R, Reed K. The AACN Synergy Model for patient care: a nursing model as a force of magnetism. *Nurs Econ*. 2008;1(11):11-20.

Kerfoot K. The Synergy Model in practice: the leader as synergist. *Nurs Econ*. 2001;19:29-30.

Kirchhoff KT. Promoting a peaceful death in the ICU. *Crit Care Nurs Clin North Am*. 2002;14:201-206.

Schmalenberg C, Kramer M. Clinical units with the healthiest work environments. *Crit Care Nurse*. 2008:28(3):65-77.

Levy MM, Carlet J. Compassionate end-of-life care in the intensive care unit. *Crit Care Med*. 2002;29(suppl 2):N1.

Lewis L, Vickers A. *Unit based shared governance leads the journey of creating a healthy work environment*, 2008. http://classic.aacn.org/AACN/NTIPoster.nsf/vwdoc/2008CSLLewis. Accessed October 14, 2008.

Malloch K. Healing models for organizations: description, measurement, outcomes. *J Healthc Manag* 2000;45:332-345.

Markey DW. Applying the Synergy Model: clinical strategies. *Crit Care Nurse*. 2001;21:72-76.

Mathes M. Ethical decision making and nursing. *Medsurg Nurs* 2005;13:429-431.

McCaffery M, Pasero C. *Pain: Clinical Manual*. 2nd ed. St Louis, MO: Mosby; 1999.

McCullough L. Rethinking the conceptual and empirical foundations of clinical ethics. *J Med Philos*. 2008;33(1):1-5.

McGahey PR. Family presence during pediatric resuscitation: a focus on staff. *Crit Care Nurse*. 2002;22:29-34.

Moloney-Harmon P. The Synergy Model: contemporary practice of the clinical nurse specialist. *Crit Care Nurse*. 1999;19:101-104.

Molter NC. Creating a healing environment for critical care. *Crit Care Nurs Clin North Am*. 2003; 15:295-304.

★ Molter NC. The Synergy Model: creating safe passage in healthcare. In: Biel M, ed. *Reconceptualizing Certified Practice: Envisioning Critical Care Practice of the Future*. Aliso Viejo, CA: American Association of Critical-Care Nurses Certification Corporation; 1997.

Muenzen PM, Greenberg S, Pirro KA. *Final Report of a Comprehensive Study of Critical Care Practice*, 2004. http://www.aacn.org/WD/Certifications/Docs/executivesummaryjobanalysis03.pdf. Accessed October 21, 2008.

National Conference of Commissioners on Uniform State Law. *Revised Uniform Anatomical Gift Act, 2007*. http://www.anatomicalgiftact.org/DesktopDefault.aspx?tabindex=1&tabid=63. Accessed October 14, 2008.

National Council of State Boards of Nursing. *Delegation: Concepts and Decision-Making Process*, 1995. https://www.ncsbn.org/323.htm#Introduction. Accessed October 22, 2008.

National Council of State Boards of Nursing. *Working with Others: A Position Paper*, 2005. https://www.ncsbn.org/Working_with_Others.pdf. Accessed October 15, 2008.

Nursing Leadership Consortium on End-of-Life Care. *Designing an Agenda for the Nursing Profession on End-of-life Care*, 1999. http://classic.aacn.org/AACN/practice.nsf/Files/da/$file/Designing%20Agenda.pdf. Accessed October 14, 2008.

Pesut B. Spirituality and spiritual care in nursing fundamentals textbooks. *J Nurs Educ*. 2008;47:167-173.

Phillips S. Ethical decision-making when caring for noncompliant patient. *J Infus Nurs*. 2006;29:266-277.

Reilly T, Humbrecht D. Fostering synergy: a nurse-managed remote telemetry model. *Crit Care Nurse*. 2007;27(3):22-33.

Ruland CM, Moore SM. Theory construction based on standards of care: a proposed theory of the peaceful end of life. *Nurs Outlook*. 1998;46:169-175.

Sechrist KR, Berlin LE, Biel M. Overview of the theoretical review process. *Crit Care Nurse*. 2000;20:85-86.

Simpson T. The family as a source of support for the critically ill adult. *AACN Clin Issues Crit Care Nurs*. 1991;2:229-235.

Smith AR. Using the Synergy Model to provide spiritual nursing care in critical care setting. *Crit Care Nurse*. 2006;26(4):41-47.

★ Stannard D. Being a good dance partner. *Crit Care Nurse*. 1999;19:86-87.

Tanner CA, Benner P, Chesla C, et al. The phenomenology of knowing the patient. *Image*. 1993;25:273-280.

Task Force on Palliative Care. *Last Acts. Precepts of Palliative Care*, 1997. http://www.aacn.org/WD/Palliative/Docs/2001Precep.pdf. Accessed October 19, 2008.

van Walraven C, Forster AJ, Stiell IG. Derivation of a clinical decision rule for the discontinuation of in-hospital cardiac arrest resuscitation. *Arch Intern Med*. 1999;159:129-134.

Villaire M. The Synergy Model of certified practice: creating safe passage for patients. *Crit Care Nurse*. 1996;16:95-99.

Welton J. Mandatory hospital nurse to patient staffing ratios: time to take a different approach. *Online J Issues Nurs*. 2007;12:1-16.

Legal Aspects of Care

Benner P. Living organ donors: respecting the risks involved in the "gift of life." *Am J Crit Care*. 2002;11:266-268.

Capron AM. Brain death—well settled yet still unresolved. *N Engl J Med*. 2001;344:1244-1246.

Centers for Medicare and Medicaid Services. *Interpretive Guidelines-Responsibilities of Medicare Participating Hospitals in Emergency Cases*, 2004. http://www.cms.hhs.gov/manuals/Downloads/som107ap_v_emerg.pdf. Accessed October 20, 2008.

Frank G. EMTALA: an expert tells us what it's all about. *J Emerg Nurs*. 2001;27:65-67.

Giordano K. Legal counsel: examining nursing malpractice: a defense attorney's perspective. *Crit Care Nurse*. 2003;23:104-106, 108.

Guido GW. *Legal and Ethical Issues in Nursing*. 4th ed. Stamford, CT: Appleton & Lange; 2006.

Meisel A, Snyder L, Quill T, et al. Seven legal barriers to end-of-life care: myths, realities, and grains of truth. *JAMA*. 2000;284:2495-2501.

Piper A Jr. Truce in the battlefield: a proposal for a different approach to medical informed consent. *J Law Med Ethics*. 1994;22:301-313.

Truog RD. Role of brain death and the dead donor rule in the ethics of organ transplantation. *Crit Care Med*. 2003;31:2391-2396.

World Medical Association. *World Medical Association Declaration on Death*, 1983. http://www.wma.net/e/policy/d2.htm. Accessed October 24, 2008.

World Medical Association. *World Medical Association Statement on Human Organ and Tissue Donation and Transplantation*, 2006. http://www.wma.net/e/policy/wma.htm. Accessed October 24, 2008.

Ethical Aspects of Care

Ahronheim JC, Moreno JD, Zuckerman C. *Ethics in Clinical Practice.* 2nd ed. Sudbury, MA: Jones & Barlett; 2005.

★ Alexander S. They decide who lives, who dies. *Life.* November 9, 1962;11:102.

★ American Hospital Association. *Patient Bill of Rights.* Chicago, IL: The Association; 1992.

American Association of Colleges of Nursing. *Peaceful death: Recommended competencies and curricular guidelines for end-of-life nursing care,* 2004. http://www.aacn.nche.edu/Publications/death-fin.htm. Accessed October 14, 2008.

American Medical Association, Council on Ethical and Judicial Affairs. Medical futility in end-of-life care: report of the Council on Ethical and Judicial Affairs: 1999. *JAMA.* 1999;281:937-941.

American Nurses Association. *Code of Ethics for Nurses with Interpretive Statements,* 2005. http://www.nursingworld.org/ethics/code/protected_nwcoe303.htm. Accessed October 22, 2008.

American Pain Society. *Treatment of Pain at the End of Life,* 2006. http://www.ampainsoc.org/advocacy/treatment.htm. Accessed October 10, 2008.

Beauchamp TL, Childress JF. *Principles of Biomedical Ethics.* 5th ed. New York, NY: Oxford University Press; 2001.

Brett AS, Jersild P. "Inappropriate" treatment near the end of life: conflict between religious convictions and clinical judgment. *Arch Intern Med.* 2003;163:1645-1649.

Burns JP, Edwards J, Johnson J, et al. Do-not-resuscitate order after 25 years. *Crit Care Med.* 2003;31:1543-1550.

Clarke EB, Curtis JR, Luce JM, et al. Quality indicators for end-of-life care in the intensive care unit. *Crit Care Med.* 2003;31:2255-2262.

Curtin L. The ethics of staffing—part 1. *J Clin Syst Manage.* 2002a;4:6-7, back cover.

Curtin L. The ethics of staffing—part 2. *J Clin Syst Manage.* 2002b;4:13, 18.

Curtis JR, Burt RA. Why are critical care clinicians so powerfully distressed by family demands for futile care? *J Crit Care.* 2003;18:22-24.

DePalo V, Iacobucci R, Crausman RS. Do-not-resuscitate and stratification-of-care forms in Rhode Island. *Am J Crit Care.* 2003;12:239-241.

★ Duff R, Campbell AGM. Ethical dilemmas in the special care nursery. *N Engl J Med.* 1973;289:890-894.

DuVal G, Sartorius L, Clarridge B, et al. What triggers requests for ethics consultations? *J Med Ethics.* 2001;27(Suppl 1):i24-29.

Heyland DK, Tranmer J, O'Callaghan CJ, et al. The seriously ill hospitalized patient: preferred role in end-of-life decision-making. *J Crit Care.* 2003;18:3-10.

In re *Quinlan,* 429 US (1992), *cert denied,* 355 A2d 647 (NJ 1976).

Khalafi K, Ravakhah K, West BC. Avoiding the futility of resuscitation. *Resuscitation.* 2001;50:161-166.

Levine C, Zuckerman C. The trouble with families: toward an ethic of accommodation. *Ann Intern Med.* 1999;130:148-152.

Lofmark R, Nilstun T. Conditions and consequences of medical futility—from a literature review to a clinical model. *J Med Ethics.* 2002;28:115-119.

★ Lynn J, Harrold J. *Handbook for Mortals: Guidance for People Facing Serious Illness.* New York, NY: Oxford University Press; 1999.

MacLean SL, Guzzetta ce, White C, et al. Family presence during cardiopulmonary resuscitation and invasive procedures: practices of critical care and emergency nurses. *Am J Crit Care.* 2003;12:246-257.

McGaffic C. Family care giving: the Synergy Model as a foundation of ethical practice. *AACN News.* 2001;18(10). http://classic.aacn.org/AACN/aacnnews.nsf/GetArticle/ArticleThree1810#family. Accessed October 14, 2008.

★ Reigle J. The ethics of physical restraints in critical care. *AACN Clin Issues.*1996;7:585-591.

Rivera S, Kim D, Morgenstern L, et al. Motivating factors in futile clinical intervention. *Chest.* 2001;119:1944-1947.

Scanlon C. Ethical concerns in end-of-life care: when questions about advance directives and the withdrawal of life-sustaining interventions arise, how should decisions be made? *Am J Nurs.* 2003;103:48-55.

Schneiderman LJ, Gilmer T, Teetzel HD. Impact of ethics consultations in the intensive care setting: a randomized controlled trial. *Crit Care Med.* 2000;28:3920-3924.

Schneiderman LJ, Gilmer T, Teetzel HD, et al. Effects of ethics consultations on nonbeneficial life-sustaining treatments in the intensive care setting: a randomized controlled trial. *JAMA.* 2003;290:1166-1172.

Singer PA, Pellegrino ED, Siegler M. Clinical ethics revisited. *BMC Med Ethics.* 2001;2:1. http://biomedcentral.com/1472-6939/2/1. Accessed October 17, 2008.

Society for Health and Human Values–Society for Bioethics Consultation Task Force on Standards for Bioethics Consultation. *Core Competencies for Health Care Ethics Consultation.* Glenview, IL: American Society for Bioethics and Humanities; 1998.

Spencer EM, Mills A, Rorty MV, et al. *Organization Ethics for Healthcare Organizations.* New York, NY: Oxford University Press; 1999.

Stanton K. Nursing management of end-of-life issues: ethical and decision-making principles. *AACN News.* 2003;20(4):12-13, 15.

2 The Pulmonary System

SYSTEMWIDE ELEMENTS

Physiologic Anatomy

1. **Respiratory circuit**
   a. The pulmonary system exists for the purpose of gas exchange. Oxygen (O_2) and carbon dioxide (CO_2) are exchanged between the atmosphere and the alveoli, between the alveoli and pulmonary capillary blood, and between the systemic capillary blood and all body cells.
   b. Atmospheric O_2 is consumed by the body through cellular aerobic metabolism, which supplies the energy for life.
   c. CO_2, a byproduct of aerobic metabolism, is eliminated primarily through lung ventilation.
   d. The respiratory circuit includes all structures and processes involved in the transfer of O_2 between room air and the individual cell and the transfer of CO_2 between the cell and room air.
   e. Cellular respiration cannot be directly measured but is estimated by the amount of CO_2 produced ($\dot{V}_{CO_2}$) and the amount of O_2 consumed ($\dot{V}_{O_2}$). Ratio of these two values is called the respiratory quotient. Respiratory quotient is normally about 0.8 but changes according to the nutritional substrate being burned (i.e., protein, fats, or carbohydrates). Patients fully maintained on intravenous (IV) glucose alone will have a respiratory quotient approaching 1.0 as a result of the metabolic end product, CO_2.
   f. Exchange of O_2 and CO_2 at the alveolar-capillary level (external respiration) is called the *respiratory exchange ratio* (R). This is the ratio of the CO_2 produced to the O_2 taken up per minute. In homeostasis, the respiratory exchange ratio is the same as the respiratory quotient, 0.8.
   g. Proper functioning of the respiratory circuit requires efficient interaction of the respiratory, circulatory, and neuromuscular systems.
   h. In addition to its primary function of O_2 and CO_2 exchange, the lung also carries out metabolic and endocrine functions as a source of hormones and a site of hormone metabolism. In addition, the lung is a target of hormonal actions by other endocrine organs.
2. **Steps in the gas exchange process**
   a. *Step 1—Ventilation:* Volume change, or the process of moving air between the atmosphere and the alveoli and distributing air within the lungs to maintain appropriate concentrations of O_2 and CO_2 in the alveoli
      i. Structural components involved in ventilation

(a) Lung
    (1) Anatomic divisions: Right lung (three lobes—upper, middle, lower); left lung (two lobes—upper, lower). Lobes are divided into bronchopulmonary segments (10 right, nine left). Bronchopulmonary segments are subdivided into secondary lobules.
    (2) Lobule: Smallest gross anatomic units of lung tissue; contain the primary functional units of the lung (terminal bronchioles, alveolar ducts and sacs, pulmonary circulation). Lymphatics surround the lobule, keep the lung free of excess fluid, and remove inhaled particles from distal areas of the lung.
    (3) Bronchial artery circulation: Systemic source of circulation for the tracheobronchial tree and lung tissue down to the level of the terminal bronchiole. Alveoli receive their blood supply from the pulmonary circulation.

(b) Conducting airways: Entire area from the nose to the terminal bronchioles where gas flows, but is not exchanged, is called anatomic dead space ($\dot{V}Danat$). Amount is approximately 150 ml but varies with patient size and position. Airways are a series of rapidly branching tubes of ever-diminishing diameter that eventually terminate in the alveoli.
    (1) Nose
        a) Serves as a passageway for air movement into the lungs
        b) Preconditions air by the action of the cilia, mucosal cells, and turbinate bones
            1) Warms air to within 2° to 3° F of body temperature; humidifies it to full saturation before it reaches the lower trachea
            2) Filters by trapping particles larger than 6 mcg in diameter
        c) Has voice resonance, olfaction, sneeze reflex functions
    (2) Pharynx: Posterior to nasal cavities and mouth
        a) Separation of food from air is controlled by local nerve reflexes.
        b) Opening of eustachian tube regulates middle ear pressure.
        c) Lymphatic tissues control infection.
    (3) Larynx: Complex structure consisting of incomplete rings of cartilage and numerous muscles and ligaments
        a) Vocal cords: Speech function
            1) Vocal cords are the narrowest part of the conducting airways in adults.
            2) Contraction of muscles of the larynx causes the vocal cords to change shape.
            3) Vibration of the vocal cords produces sound. Speech is a joint function of the vocal cords, lips, tongue, soft palate, and respiration, with control by temporal and parietal lobes of the cerebral cortex.
            4) The rima glottis is the opening between the vocal cords.
        b) Valve action by the epiglottis: Helps to prevent aspiration
        c) Cough reflex: Occurs when cords close and intrathoracic pressure increases to permit coughing or Valsalva maneuver
        d) Cricoid cartilage
            1) Only complete rigid ring
            2) Narrowest part of the child's airway
            3) Inner diameter sets the limit for the size of an endotracheal tube (ETT) passed through the larynx.
    (4) Trachea: Tubular structure consisting of 16 to 20 incomplete, or C-shaped, cartilaginous rings that stabilize the airway and prevent complete collapse with coughing
        a) Begins the conducting system, or tracheobronchial tree
        b) Warms and humidifies air
        c) Has mucosal cells that trap foreign material
        d) Has cilia that propel mucus upward through the airway
        e) Cough reflex present, especially at the point of tracheal bifurcation (carina)
        f) Smooth muscle innervated by the parasympathetic branch of the autonomic nervous system

(5) Major bronchi and bronchioles
(6) Terminal bronchioles
    a) Smooth muscle walls (no cartilage); bronchospasm may narrow the lumen and increase airway resistance
    b) Ciliated mucosal cells: These become flattened, with progressive loss of cilia toward the alveoli
    c) Sensitive to CO_2 levels: Increased levels induce bronchiolar dilation, decreased levels induce constriction
(c) Gas exchange airways: Semipermeable membrane permits the movement of gases according to pressure gradients. These airways are not major contributors to airflow resistance but do contribute to the distensibility of the lung. The acinus (terminal respiratory unit) is composed of the respiratory bronchiole and its subdivisions (Figure 2-1).
    (1) Respiratory bronchioles and alveolar ducts
        a) Terminal branching of airways
        b) Distribution of inspired air
        c) Smooth muscle layer diminishes
    (2) Alveoli and alveolar bud
        a) Most important structures in gas exchange
        b) Alveolar surface area: Large, depends on body size. Total surface area is about $70\,m^2$ in a normal adult. Thickness of the respiratory membrane is about $0.6\,\mu m$. This fulfills the need to distribute a large quantity of perfused blood into a very thin film to ensure near equalization of O_2 and CO_2.
        c) Alveolar cells
            1) Type I: Squamous epithelium, adapted for gas exchange, sensitive to injury by inhaled agents, structured to prevent fluid transudation into the alveoli
            2) Type II: Large secretory, highly active metabolically; origin of surfactant synthesis and type I cell genesis

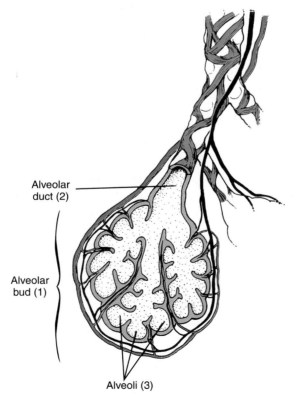

FIGURE 2-1 ■ Components of the acinus. (From Eubanks DH, Bone RC. *Comprehensive Respiratory Care: A Learning System*. 2nd ed. St Louis, MO: Mosby; 1990:168.)

      3) Alveolar macrophages: Phagocytize foreign materials

  d) Pulmonary surfactant

      1) Phospholipid monolayer at the alveolar air-liquid interface; able to vary surface tension with alveolar volume

      2) Enables surface tension to decrease as alveolar volume decreases during expiration, which prevents alveolar collapse

      3) Decreases the work of breathing, permits the alveoli to remain inflated at low distending pressures, reduces net forces causing tissue fluid accumulation

      4) Reduction of surfactant makes lung expansion more difficult; the greater the surface tension, the greater the pressure needed to overcome it.

      5) Surfactant also detoxifies inhaled gases and traps inhaled and deposited particles.

  e) Alveolar-capillary membrane (alveolar epithelium, interstitial space, capillary endothelium)

      1) Bathed by interstitial fluid; lines the respiratory bronchioles, alveolar ducts, and alveolar sacs; forms the walls of the alveoli

      2) About 1 mcg or less thick (less than one red blood cell); permits rapid diffusion of gases; any increase in thickness diminishes gas diffusion

      3) Total surface area of about 70 m² in an adult in contact with about 60 to 140 ml of pulmonary capillary blood at any one time

  f) Gas exchange pathway (Figure 2-2): Alveolar epithelium → alveolar basement membrane → interstitial space → capillary basement membrane → capillary endothelium → plasma → erythrocyte membrane → erythrocyte cytoplasm

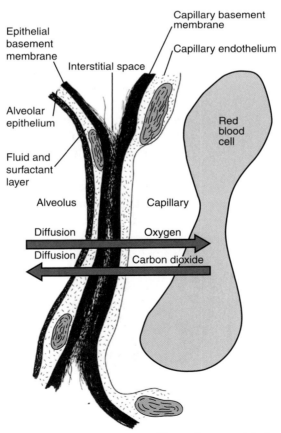

FIGURE 2-2 ■ Ultrastructure of the respiratory membrane. (From Guyton AC, Hall JE. *Textbook of Medical Physiology*. 9th ed. Philadelphia, PA: Saunders; 1996:508.)

ii. Alveolar ventilation ($\dot{V}_A$): That part of total ventilation taking part in gas exchange and, therefore, the only part useful to the body
   (a) Alveolar ventilation is one component of minute ventilation.
      (1) Minute ventilation (($\dot{V}_E$): Amount of air exchanged in 1 minute.
         a) Equal to exhaled tidal volume (V_T) multiplied by respiratory rate (RR or f):

$$V_T \times RR = \dot{V}_E$$

         b) Normal resting minute ventilation in an adult is about 6 L/min:

$$500\,ml \times 12 = 6000\,ml$$

      (2) Minute ventilation is composed of both alveolar ventilation ($\dot{V}_A$) and physiologic dead space ventilation ($\dot{V}_D$):

$$\dot{V}_E = \dot{V}_D + \dot{V}_A$$

         a) Physiologic dead space ventilation is that volume of gas in the airways that does not participate in gas exchange. It is composed of both anatomic dead space ventilation ($\dot{V}D_{anat}$) and alveolar dead space ventilation ($\dot{V}D_A$).
      (3) Ratio of dead space to tidal volume (V_D/V_T) is measured to determine how much of each breath is wasted (i.e., does not contribute to gas exchange). Normal values for spontaneously breathing patients range from 0.2 to 0.4 (20% to 40%).
   (b) Alveolar ventilation cannot be measured directly; it is inversely related to arterial CO_2 pressure (Pa_{CO_2}) in a steady state by the following formula:

$$\dot{V}_A = \frac{\dot{V}_{CO_2} \times 0.863}{Pa_{CO_2}}$$

   where 0.863 = correction factor for differences in measurement units and conversion to standard temperature (0° C) and pressure (760 mm Hg), dry (STPD)
   (c) Because $\dot{V}_{CO_2}$ remains the same in a steady state, measurement of the patient's Pa_{CO_2} reveals the status of the alveolar ventilation.
   (d) Pa_{CO_2} is the only adequate indicator of effective matching of alveolar ventilation to metabolic demand. To assess ventilation, Pa_{CO_2} must be measured.
   (e) If Pa_{CO_2} is low, alveolar ventilation is high; hyperventilation is present:

$$\downarrow Pa_{CO_2} = \uparrow \dot{V}_A$$

   (f) If Pa_{CO_2} is within normal limits, alveolar ventilation is adequate:

$$\text{Normal } Pa_{CO_2} = \text{Normal } \dot{V}_A$$

   (g) If Pa_{CO_2} is high, alveolar ventilation is low and hypoventilation is present:

$$\uparrow Pa_{CO_2} = \downarrow \dot{V}_A$$

iii. Defense mechanisms of the lung
   (a) Although an internal organ, the lung is unique in that it has continuous contact with particulate and gaseous materials inhaled from the external environment. In the healthy lung, defense mechanisms successfully defend against these natural materials by the following means:
      (1) Structural architecture of the upper respiratory tract, which reduces deposited and inhaled materials
      (2) Processing system, including respiratory tract fluid alteration and phagocytic activity
      (3) Transport system, which removes material from the lung
      (4) Humoral and cell-mediated immune responses, which may be the most important bronchopulmonary defense mechanisms
   (b) Loss of normal defense mechanisms may be precipitated by disease, injury, surgery, insertion of an ETT, or smoking.
   (c) Upper respiratory tract warms and humidifies inspired air, absorbs selected inhaled gases, and filters out particulate matter. Soluble gases and particles larger than 10 μm are aerodynamically filtered out. Normally, no bacteria are present below the larynx.

(d) Inhaled and deposited particles reaching the alveoli are coated by surface fluids (surfactant and other lipoproteins) and are rapidly phagocytized by pulmonary alveolar macrophages.

(e) Macrophages and particles are transported in mucus by bronchial cilia, which beat toward the glottis and move materials in a mucus-fluid layer, eventually to be expectorated or swallowed. This process is referred to as the mucociliary escalator. Pulmonary lymphatics also drain and transport some cells and particles from the lung.

(f) Antigens activate the humoral and cell-mediated immune systems, which add immunoglobulins to the surface fluid of the alveoli and activate alveolar macrophages.

(g) Disruption of or injury to these defense mechanisms predisposes to acute or chronic pulmonary disease.

iv. Lung mechanics

(a) Muscles of respiration: Act of breathing is accomplished through muscular actions that alter intrapleural and pulmonary pressures and thus change intrapulmonary volumes

   (1) Muscles of inspiration: During inspiration, the chest cavity enlarges. This enlargement is an active process brought about by the contraction of the following:

      a) Diaphragm: Major inspiratory muscle
         1) Normal quiet breathing is accomplished almost entirely by this dome-shaped muscle, which divides the chest from the abdomen.
         2) Diaphragm is divided into two "leaves"—the right and left hemidiaphragms.
         3) Downward contraction increases the superior-inferior diameter of the chest and elevates the lower ribs.
         4) Innervation is from the C3 to C5 level through the phrenic nerve.
         5) Normally, diaphragm accounts for 75% of tidal volume during quiet inspiration.
         6) Diaphragm facilitates vomiting, coughing and sneezing, defecation, and parturition.

      b) External intercostal muscles
         1) These increase the anterior-posterior (A-P) diameter of the thorax by elevating the ribs.
         2) A-P diameter is about 20% greater during inspiration than during expiration.
         3) Innervation is from T1 to T11.

      c) Accessory muscles in the neck: Scalene and sternocleidomastoid
         1) Lift upward on the sternum and ribs and increase A-P diameter
         2) Are not used in normal, quiet ventilation

   (2) Muscles of expiration: During expiration, the chest cavity decreases in size. This is a passive act unless forced, and the driving force is derived from lung recoil. Muscles used when increased levels of ventilation are needed are the following:

      a) Abdominals: Force abdominal contents upward to elevate the diaphragm
      b) Internal intercostals: Decrease A-P diameter by contracting and pulling the ribs inward

(b) Pressures within the chest: Movement of air into the lungs requires a pressure difference between the airway opening and alveoli sufficient to overcome the resistance to airflow of the tracheobronchial tree (Table 2-1)

   (1) Air flows into the lungs when intrapulmonary air pressure falls below atmospheric pressure.
   (2) Air flows out of the lungs when intrapulmonary air pressure exceeds atmospheric pressure.
   (3) Intrapleural pressure is normally negative with respect to atmospheric pressure as a result of the elastic recoil of the lungs, which tend to pull away from the chest wall. This "negative" pressure prevents the collapse of the lungs.
   (4) Increased effort (forced inspiration or expiration) may produce much greater changes in intrapulmonary and intrapleural pressures during inspiration and expiration.

TABLE 2-1
Example of Changes in Pressures Throughout the Ventilatory Cycle

Pressure	At Rest (No Airflow) (mm Hg)	Inspiration (mm Hg)	Expiration (mm Hg)
Atmospheric (P_B)	760	760	760
Intrapulmonary or intra-alveolar (P_{alv})	760	757	763
Intrapleural (P_{pl}) or intrathoracic	756	750	756

(c) Structural components of the thorax
  (1) For protection: Sternum, spine, ribs
  (2) Pleura
    a) Visceral layer next to the lungs; parietal layer next to the chest wall
    b) Pleural fluid between layers: Allows smooth movement of the visceral layer over the parietal layer
    c) Adherence: Pleural space is normally a potential space (vacuum); because of a constant negative pressure (less than atmospheric pressure by 4 to 8 mm Hg), any change in the volume of the thoracic cage is reflected by a similar change in the volume of the lungs
    d) Nerve supply: Parietal pleura has fibers for pain transmission, but visceral pleura does not
(d) Resistances
  (1) Elastic resistance (static properties)
    a) Lung, if removed from the chest, collapses to a smaller volume because of lung elastic recoil. This tendency of the lungs to collapse is normally counteracted by the chest wall tendency to expand. Volume of air in the lungs depends on the equal and opposite balance of these forces.
    b) Compliance (C_L) is an expression of the elastic properties of the lung and is the change in volume (ΔV) accomplished by a change in pressure (ΔP):

$$C_L = \frac{\Delta V}{\Delta P}$$

    If compliance is high, the lung is more easily distended; if compliance is low, the lung is stiff and more difficult to distend.
  (2) Flow resistance (dynamic properties)
    a) Airway resistance must be overcome to generate flow through the airways.
    b) Changes in airway caliber affect airway resistance. Examples are changes caused by bronchospasm or secretions.
    c) Flow through the airway depends on pressure differences between the two ends of the tube, as well as resistance. Driving pressure for flow in airways is the difference between atmospheric and alveolar pressures.
(e) Work of breathing
  (1) To minimize the work required to maintain a given level of ventilation, the body automatically changes the respiratory pattern.
  (2) Work performed must be sufficient to overcome the elastic resistance and the flow resistance.
  (3) In diseased states, the workload increases.
  v. Control of ventilation: Although the process of breathing is a normal rhythmic activity that occurs without conscious effort, it involves an intricate controlling mechanism within the central nervous system (CNS). Basic organization of the respiratory control system is outlined in Figure 2-3.
    (a) Respiratory generator: Located in the medulla and composed of two groups of neurons

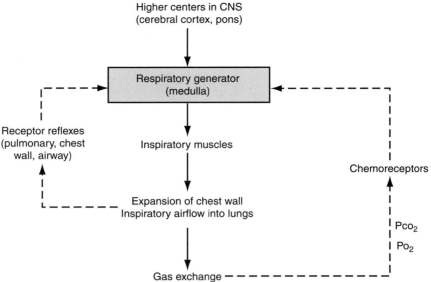

FIGURE 2-3 ■ Schematic diagram depicting the organization of the respiratory control system. The dashed lines show feedback loops affecting the respiratory generator. P_{CO_2}, Partial pressure of carbon dioxide; P_{O_2}, partial pressure of oxygen. (From Weinberger SE. *Principles of Pulmonary Medicine.* 2nd ed. Philadelphia, PA: Saunders; 1992:206.)

      (1) One group initiates respiration and regulates its rate.
      (2) One group controls the "switching off" of inspiration and thus the onset of expiration.
    (b) Input from other regions of the CNS
      (1) Pons: Input is necessary for normal, coordinated breathing
      (2) Cerebral cortex: Exerts a conscious or voluntary control over ventilation
    (c) Chemoreceptors: Contribute to a feedback loop that adjusts respiratory center output if blood gas levels are not maintained within the normal range
      (1) Central chemoreceptors: Located near the ventrolateral surface of the medulla (but are separate from the medullary respiratory center)
        a) Central chemoreceptors respond not directly to blood partial pressure of carbon dioxide (P_{CO_2}) but, rather, to the pH of the extracellular fluid (ECF) surrounding the chemoreceptor.
        b) Feedback loop for CO_2 can be summarized as follows: Increased arterial P_{CO_2} → increased brain ECF P_{CO_2} → decreased brain ECF pH → decreased pH at chemoreceptor → stimulation of central chemoreceptor → stimulation of medullary respiratory center → increased ventilation → decreased arterial P_{CO_2}.
      (2) Peripheral chemoreceptors: Located in the carotid body and aortic body
        a) Sensitive to changes in the partial pressure of oxygen (P_{O_2}), with hypoxemia stimulating chemoreceptor discharge
        b) Minor role in sensing P_{CO_2}
    (d) Other receptors
      (1) Stretch receptors in the bronchial wall respond to changes in lung inflation (Hering-Breuer reflex).
        a) As the lung inflates, receptor discharge increases.
        b) Receptors contribute to the start of expiration.
      (2) Irritant receptors in the lining of the airways respond to noxious stimuli, such as irritating dust and chemicals.
      (3) "J" (juxtacapillary) receptors in the alveolar interstitial space have the following functions:

a) They cause rapid shallow breathing in response to deformation from increased interstitial volume because of high pulmonary capillary pressures (such as in heart failure or inflammation).

b) Stimulation can also cause bradycardia, hypotension, and expiratory constriction of the glottis.

(4) Receptors in the chest wall (in the intercostal muscles)

a) Involved in the fine tuning of ventilation

b) Adjust the output of the respiratory muscles for the degree of muscular work required

b. *Step 2—Diffusion:* Process by which alveolar air gases are moved across the alveolar-capillary membrane to the pulmonary capillary bed and vice versa. Diffusion occurs down a concentration gradient from a higher to a lower concentration. No active metabolic work is required for the diffusion of gases to occur. Work of breathing is accomplished by the respiratory muscles and the heart, which produce a gradient across the alveolar-capillary membrane.

i. Ability of the lung to transfer gases is called the diffusing capacity of the lung (D_L). Diffusing capacity measures the amount of gas (O_2, CO_2, carbon monoxide) diffusing between the alveoli and pulmonary capillary blood per minute per millimeter Hg mean gas pressure difference.

ii. CO_2 is 20 times more diffusible across the alveolar-capillary membrane than O_2. If the membrane is damaged, its decreased capacity for transporting O_2 into the blood is usually more of a problem than its decreased capacity for transporting CO_2 out of the body. Thus, the diffusing capacity of the lungs for O_2 is of primary importance.

iii. Diffusion is determined by several variables:

(a) Surface area available for gas exchange

(b) Integrity of the alveolar-capillary membrane

(c) Amount of hemoglobin (Hb) in the blood

(d) Diffusion coefficient of gas, as well as contact time

(e) Driving pressure: Difference between alveolar gas tensions and pulmonary capillary gas tensions (Table 2-2). This is the force that causes gases to diffuse across membranes.

(1) During the breathing of 100% O_2, the alveolar O_2 tension (PAO_2) becomes so large that the difference between PAO_2 and PvO_2 (mixed venous O_2 tension) significantly increases, proportionately increasing the driving pressure.

(2) Therefore, hypoxemia due solely to diffusion defects is usually improved by breathing 100% O_2.

c. *Step 3—Transport of gases in the circulation*

i. Approximately 97% of O_2 is transported in chemical combination with Hb in the erythrocyte, and 3% is carried dissolved in the plasma. PaO_2 is a measurement of the O_2 tension in the plasma and is a reflection of the driving pressure that causes O_2 to dissolve in the plasma and combine with Hb. Thus, O_2 content is related to PaO_2.

ii. Oxyhemoglobin dissociation curve is described as follows (Figure 2-4):

(a) Relationship between O_2 saturation (and content) and PaO_2 is expressed in an S-shaped curve that has great physiologic significance. It describes the ability of Hb to bind O_2 at normal PaO_2 levels and release it at lower PO_2 levels.

(b) Relationship between the content and pressure of O_2 in the blood is not linear.

■ **TABLE 2-2**
■ ■ **Driving Pressures**

Alveolar Gas	Alveolar-Capillary Membranes	Pulmonary Capillaries
PAO_2 104 mm Hg	Diffusion →	PvO_2 40 mm Hg
$PaCO_2$ 40 mm Hg	Diffusion →	$PvCO_2$ 45 mm Hg

$PaCO_2$, Arterial partial pressure of carbon dioxide; *PAO_2*, alveolar partial pressure of oxygen; *$PvCO_2$*, mixed venous partial pressure of carbon dioxide; *PvO_2*, mixed venous partial pressure of oxygen.

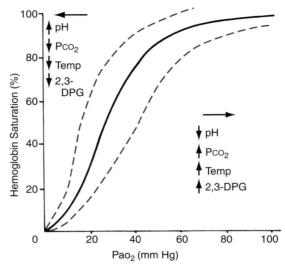

FIGURE 2-4 ■ The oxyhemoglobin dissociation curve, relating percent hemoglobin saturation and arterial partial pressure of oxygen (Pao_2). The normal curve is depicted by the solid line; the curves shifted to the right or left (along with the conditions leading to them), by the dashed lines. *2,3-DPG*, 2,3-Diphosphoglycerate; *Pco_2*, partial pressure of carbon dioxide; *Temp*, temperature. (From Weinberger SE. *Principles of Pulmonary Medicine*. 2nd ed. Philadelphia, PA: Saunders; 1992:10.)

     (1) Upper flat portion of the curve is the arterial association portion. Dissociation relationship in this range protects the body by enabling Hb to retain high saturation with O_2 despite large decreases (down to 60 mm Hg) in Pao_2.

     (2) Lower steep portion of the curve is the venous dissociation portion. Dissociation relationship in this range protects the body by enabling the tissues to withdraw large amounts of O_2 with small decreases in Pao_2.

  (c) Hb O_2 binding is sensitive to O_2 tension. The binding is reversible; the affinity of Hb for O_2 changes as Po_2 changes.

     (1) When Po_2 is increased (as in pulmonary capillaries), O_2 binds readily with Hb.

     (2) When Po_2 is decreased (as in tissues), O_2 unloads from Hb.

  (d) Increase in the rate of O_2 utilization by tissues causes an automatic increase in the rate of O_2 release from Hb.

  (e) Shifts of the oxyhemoglobin curve are as follows:

     (1) Shifts to the right: More O_2 is unloaded for a given Po_2, which thus increases O_2 delivery to the tissues. These shifts are caused by the following:

       a) pH decrease (acidosis), the Bohr effect

       b) Pco_2 increase

       c) Increase in body temperature

       d) Increased levels of 2,3-diphosphoglycerate (2,3-DPG)

     (2) Shifts to the left: O_2 is not dissociated from Hb until tissue and capillary O_2 are very low, which thus decreases O_2 delivery to the tissues. These shifts are caused by the following:

       a) pH increase (alkalosis), the Bohr effect

       b) Pco_2 decrease

       c) Temperature decrease

       d) Decreased levels of 2,3-DPG

       e) Carbon monoxide poisoning

     (3) 2,3-DPG is an intermediate metabolite of glucose that facilitates the dissociation of O_2 from Hb at the tissues. Decreased levels of 2,3-DPG impair O_2 release to the tissues. This may occur with massive transfusions of 2,3-DPG–depleted blood and anything that decreases phosphate levels.

iii. Ability of Hb to release O_2 to the tissues is commonly assessed by evaluating the P_{50}.
   (a) P_{50} = The partial pressure of O_2 at which the Hb is 50% saturated, standardized to a pH of 7.40.
   (b) Normal P_{50} is about 26.6 mm Hg; varies with the disease process.
iv. Each gram of normal Hb can maximally combine with 1.34 ml of O_2 when fully saturated (values of 1.36 or 1.39 ml are sometimes used).
v. Amount of O_2 transported per minute in the circulation is a factor of both the arterial O_2 concentration (Cao_2) and cardiac output. This amount reflects how much O_2 is delivered to tissues per minute and is dependent on the interaction of the circulatory system (delivery of arterial blood), erythropoietic system (Hb in red blood cells), and respiratory system (gas exchange) according to the following equations:
   (a) O_2 content (Cao_2) is calculated from O_2 saturation, O_2 capacity, and dissolved O_2.
      (1) O_2 capacity is the maximal amount of O_2 the blood can carry. It is expressed in milliliters of O_2 per deciliter (100 ml) of blood (ml/dl) and is calculated by multiplying Hb in grams by 1.34.
      (2) O_2 saturation is the percentage of Hb actually saturated with O_2 (Sao_2 or Svo_2) and is usually measured directly.
      (3) O_2 content is the actual amount of O_2 the blood is carrying (oxyhemoglobin plus dissolved O_2):

$$O_2 \text{ content} = (O_2 \text{ capacity} \times O_2 \text{ saturation}) (0.0031 \times Pao_2)$$

   (b) Systemic O_2 transport:

$$\text{ml/min} = \text{Arterial } O_2 \text{ content (ml/dl)} \times \text{Cardiac output (L/min)} \times 10 \text{ (conversion factor)}$$

      (1) Normal cardiac output = approximately 5 to 6 L/min (range, 4 to 8 L/min).
      (2) Normal arterial O_2 content = approximately 20 ml/dl.
      (3) Therefore, systemic O_2 transport averages about 1000 to 1200 ml/min.
vi. Focusing only on the O_2 tension of the blood is unwise because an underestimation of the severity of hypoxemia may result. O_2 content and transport are more reliable parameters because they take into account the Hb concentration and cardiac output.
vii. In CO_2 transport, CO_2 is carried in the blood in three forms, as follows:
   (a) Physically dissolved ($Paco_2$), which accounts for 7% to 10% of CO_2 transported in the blood
   (b) Chemically combined with Hb as carbaminohemoglobin. This reaction occurs rapidly, and reduced Hb can bind more CO_2 than oxyhemoglobin. Thus, unloading of O_2 facilitates loading of CO_2 (Haldane effect) and accounts for about 30% of CO_2 transport.
   (c) As bicarbonate (HCO_3^-) through a conversion reaction:

$$CO_2 + H_2O \overset{CA}{\leftrightarrow} H_2CO_3 \leftrightarrow H^+ + \text{(Hb buffer)} + HCO_3^-$$

   where CA = carbonic anhydrase
      (1) Reaction accounts for 60% to 70% of CO_2 in the body.
      (2) Reaction is slow in plasma and fast in red blood cells because of the CA enzyme.
      (3) When the concentration of these ions increases in red blood cells, HCO_3^- diffuses but H^+ remains.
      (4) To maintain electrical neutrality, chloride diffuses from the plasma (the "chloride shift").
viii. Pulmonary circulation (pulmonary artery, arterioles, capillary network, venules, and veins) has the following functions:
   (a) Pulmonary vessels are peculiarly suited to maintaining a delicate balance of flow and pressure distribution that optimizes gas exchange. They are richly innervated by the sympathetic branch of the autonomic nervous system.
   (b) In contrast to the systemic circulation, the pulmonary circulation is a low-resistance system. Pulmonary arteries have far thinner walls than systemic arteries do, and vessels distend to allow for increases in volume from systemic circulation. Intrapulmonary blood volume increases or decreases of approximately 50% occur with changes in the relationship between intrathoracic and extrathoracic pressure.

    (c) Pulmonary arteries accompany the bronchi within the lung and give rise to a rich capillary network within the alveolar walls. Pulmonary veins are not contiguous with the bronchial tree.

    (d) Primary function of the pulmonary circulation is to act as a transport system.

        (1) Transport of blood through the lung

            a) Flow resistance through vessels (R) is defined by Ohm's law:

$$R = \frac{\Delta P}{F}$$

            where ΔP = the pressure difference between the two ends of the vessel (upstream and downstream pressures) and F = flow

              Driving pressure for flow in the pulmonary circulation is the difference between the inflow pressure in the pulmonary artery and the outflow pressure in the left atrium.

            b) In the lung, measurement of flow resistance is pulmonary vascular resistance (PVR):

PVR = [Mean pulmonary artery pressure – Mean left atrial (or pulmonary wedge) pressure]/Cardiac output

            c) About 12% of the total blood volume of the body is in the pulmonary circulation at any given time.

            d) Normal pressures in the pulmonary vasculature are as follows:

                1) Mean pulmonary artery pressure: 10 to 15 mm Hg

                2) Mean pulmonary venous pressure: 4 to 12 mm Hg

                 3) Mean pressure gradient: Approximately 10 mm Hg (considerably less than the systemic gradient)

                4) Pressures higher at the base of the lung than at the apex

                5) Perfusion better in the dependent areas of the lung

            e) Unique characteristic of the pulmonary arterial bed is that it constricts in response to hypoxia. Diffuse alveolar hypoxia causes generalized vasoconstriction, which results in pulmonary hypertension. Localized hypoxia causes localized vasoconstriction that does not increase pulmonary hypertension. This localized vasoconstriction directs blood away from poorly ventilated alveoli and thus improves overall gas exchange.

            f) Chronic pulmonary hypertension (increased PVR) can result in right ventricular hypertrophy (cor pulmonale).

                1) Transvascular transport of fluids and solutes

                    a) Transvascular fluid filtration in the lung (and all other organs) is described by the Starling equation. This means that fluid and solutes move because of increases or decreases in hydrostatic or osmotic filtration pressures or because of changes in the permeability of vessel walls to fluids or proteins.

                    b) Thus, excess fluid in the lung (pulmonary edema) can result from either a net increase in hydrostatic pressure forces (favoring filtration) or a decreased resistance to filtration.

                2) Metabolic transport

                    a) All cardiac output passes through the lung before reaching systemic circulation. Therefore, pulmonary circulation can influence the composition of the blood supplying all organs.

                    b) Several humoral substances are added, extracted, or metabolized in the lung. Examples are inactivation of vasoactive prostaglandins, conversion of angiotensin I to angiotensin II, and inactivation of bradykinin.

  d. *Step 4—Diffusion between the systemic capillary bed and body tissue cells*

    i. Pressure gradients allow for the diffusion of O_2 and CO_2 among systemic capillaries, interstitial fluid, and cells (Figures 2-5 and 2-6).

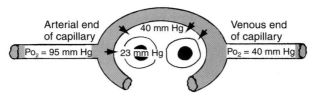

FIGURE 2-5 ■ Diffusion of oxygen from a tissue capillary to the cells. P_{O_2}, Partial pressure of oxygen. (From Guyton AC, Hall JE. *Textbook of Medical Physiology*. 9th ed. Philadelphia, PA: Saunders; 1996:514.)

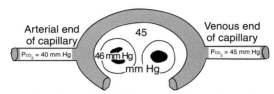

FIGURE 2-6 ■ Uptake of carbon dioxide by the blood in the capillaries. P_{CO_2}, Partial pressure of carbon dioxide. (From Guyton AC, Hall JE. *Textbook of Medical Physiology*. 9th ed. Philadelphia, PA: Saunders; 1996:515.)

    ii. Within the mitochondria of each individual cell, O_2 is consumed through aerobic metabolism. This process produces the energy bonds of adenosine triphosphate and the waste products of CO_2 and water.

3. Hypoxemia: Hypoxemia is a state in which the O_2 pressure or saturation of O_2 in arterial blood, or both, is lower than normal. Hypoxemia is generally defined as Pa_{O_2} less than 55 mm Hg or Sa_{O_2} below 88% at sea level in an adult breathing room air. Disorders that lead to hypoxemia do so through one or more of the following processes.

  a. Alveolar hypoventilation (increased Pa_{CO_2})

    i. Alveolar hypoventilation is a decrease in alveolar ventilation from disorders of the respiratory center, peripheral nerves that supply the muscles of respiration, the respiratory muscles of the chest wall, or the lungs; medications that diminish ventilation.

    ii. This causes an increase in Pa_{CO_2}, which results in a fall in PA_{O_2} according to the alveolar air equation.

    iii. Hypoxemia will improve with ventilation.

  b. $\dot{V}/\dot{Q}$ mismatch

    i. $\dot{V}/\dot{Q}$ mismatch is the most common cause of hypoxemia.

    ii. Ideally, ventilation of each alveolus is accompanied by a comparable amount of perfusion, which yields a $\dot{V}/\dot{Q}$ ratio of 1.00. Usually, however, there is relatively more perfusion than ventilation, which yields a normal $\dot{V}/\dot{Q}$ ratio of 0.8. Normal amount of blood perfusing the alveoli ($\dot{Q}$) is 5 L/min, and normal amount of air ventilating the alveoli ($\dot{V}$) is 4 L/min. Figure 2-7 presents in simplified form the possible relationships between ventilation and perfusion in the lung.

    iii. When $\dot{V}/\dot{Q}$ is decreased (<0.8), a decrease of ventilation in relation to perfusion has occurred. This is similar to a right-to-left shunt because more deoxygenated blood is returning to the left side of the heart. Low $\dot{V}/\dot{Q}$ ratios and hypoxemia occur together, because good areas of the lung cannot be overventilated to compensate for the underventilated areas. (Hb cannot be saturated to more than 100%.) Atelectasis, pneumonia, and pulmonary edema are clinical examples of intrapulmonary shunt.

    iv. When $\dot{V}/\dot{Q}$ is increased (>0.8), a decreased perfusion relative to ventilation exists, the equivalent of dead space or wasted ventilation. Examples of cases in which this occurs are pulmonary emboli and cardiogenic shock.

    v. Hypoxemia that is thought to be due to $\dot{V}/\dot{Q}$ mismatch can be corrected by giving the patient a simple incremental fraction of inspired oxygen (F_{IO_2}) test. For example, if the Pa_{O_2} increases significantly in response to an F_{IO_2} change from 0.30 to 0.60, the primary problem is low $\dot{V}/\dot{Q}$. If the Pa_{O_2} does not increase significantly, a right-to-left shunt exists.

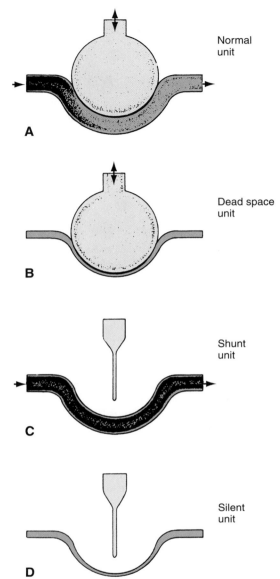

FIGURE 2-7 ■ The theoretical respiratory unit. **A,** Normal ventilation, normal perfusion. **B,** Normal ventilation, no perfusion. **C,** No ventilation, normal perfusion. **D,** No ventilation, no perfusion. (From Shapiro BA, Peruzzi WT, Templin R, et al. *Clinical Application of Blood Gases*. 5th ed. St Louis, MO: Mosby; 1994:22.)

c. Shunting
   i. Shunting occurs when a portion of venous blood does not participate in gas exchange. An anatomic shunt may occur (a portion of right ventricular blood does not pass through the pulmonary capillaries) or a portion of pulmonary capillary blood may pass by airless alveoli.
   ii. Normal physiologic shunting amounts to 2% to 5% of cardiac output (this is bronchial and thebesian vein blood).
   iii. Shunting occurs in arteriovenous malformations, acute lung injury (ALI), atelectasis, pneumonia, pulmonary edema, pulmonary embolus, vascular lung tumors, and intracardiac right-to-left shunts.
   iv. Breathing at an increased F_{IO_2} level does not correct shunting because not all blood comes into contact with open alveoli and shunted blood passes directly from pulmonary veins to arterial blood (venous admixture). Lack of improvement of hypoxemia with O_2 therapy is a hallmark of shunting.

4. Acid-base physiology and blood gases
    a. Terminology
        i. *Acid:* Donor of hydrogen ions (H^+); substance with a pH below 7.0
        ii. *Acidemia:* Condition in which the blood pH is below 7.35
        iii. *Acidosis:* Process (metabolic or respiratory) that causes acidemia
        iv. *Base:* Acceptor of H^+ ions; any substance with a pH above 7.0
        v. *Alkalemia:* Condition in which the blood pH is above 7.45
        vi. *Alkalosis:* Process (metabolic or respiratory) that causes alkalemia
        vii. *pH:* Negative logarithm of the H^+ ion concentration
            (a) Increase in $[H^+]$ = lower pH, more acidic
            (b) Decrease in $[H^+]$ = higher pH, more alkaline
    b. Buffering: Normal body mechanism that occurs rapidly in response to acid-base disturbances to prevent changes in $[H^+]$
        i. Bicarbonate (HCO_3^-) buffer system:

$$[H^+] + HCO_3^- \leftrightarrow H_2CO_3 \leftrightarrow CO_2 + H_2O$$

        This system is very important because HCO_3^- can be regulated by the kidneys and CO_2 can be regulated by the lungs.
        ii. Phosphate system
        iii. Hb and other proteins
    c. Henderson-Hasselbalch equation: Defines the relationship between pH, P_{CO_2}, and bicarbonate. Arterial pH is determined by the logarithm of the ratio of bicarbonate concentration to arterial P_{CO_2}. Bicarbonate is regulated primarily by the kidney and P_{CO_2} is regulated by alveolar ventilation:

$$pH = pK + \log\frac{\left[HCO_3^-\right]}{Pa_{CO_2}}$$

    where pK = a constant (6.1)
        i. As long as the ratio of HCO_3^- to CO_2 is about 20:1, the pH of the blood will be normal. It is this ratio, rather than the absolute values of each, that determines blood pH.
        ii. pH must be maintained within a narrow range of normal because the functioning of most enzymatic systems in the body depends on the H^+ concentration (Figure 2-8).
    d. Normal adult blood gas values (at sea level): See Table 2-3. Note: Knowledge of blood gas values neither supersedes nor replaces sound clinical judgment.
    e. Effect of altitude on blood gas values
        i. Pa_{O_2} and Sa_{O_2} are lower at high altitudes because of a lower ambient O_2 tension.
        ii. Normal for 5280 feet (Denver) = Pa_{O_2} of 65 to 75 mm Hg, Sa_{O_2} of 94% to 95%.

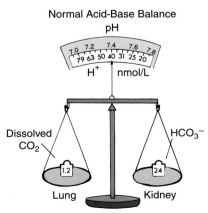

FIGURE 2-8 ■ The balance between bicarbonate (HCO_3^-) (24) and dissolved carbon dioxide (CO_2) (1.2 of arterial partial pressure of CO_2 [Pa_{CO_2}] = 40) is normally 20:1, and this is usually associated with a pH of about 7.40 and an H^+ concentration of about 40 nmol/L. (From Cherniack RM, Cherniack L. *Respiration in Health and Disease.* 3rd ed. Philadelphia, PA: Saunders; 1983:85.)

■ **TABLE 2-3**
■ ■ **Normal Adult Blood Gas Values (at Sea Level)**

	Arterial	Mixed Venous
pH	7.40 (7.35-7.45)	7.36 (7.31-7.41)
P_{O_2}	80-100 mm Hg	35-40 mm Hg
Sa_{O_2}	≥95%	70%-75%
P_{CO_2}	35-45 mm Hg	41-51 mm Hg
HCO_3^-	22-26 mEq/L	22-26 mEq/L
Base excess	−2 to +2	−2 to +2

Hco_3^-, Bicarbonate; Pco_2, partial pressure of carbon dioxide; Po_2, partial pressure of oxygen; Sao_2, arterial oxygen saturation.

f. Respiratory parameter (Pa_{CO_2}): If the primary disturbance is in the Pa_{CO_2}, the patient is said to have a respiratory disturbance
  i. Pa_{CO_2} is a reflection of alveolar ventilation.
    (a) If increased, hypoventilation is present.
    (b) If decreased, hyperventilation is present.
    (c) If normal, adequate ventilation is present.
    (d) To assess relationships, measurements of both Pa_{CO_2} and minute ventilation are needed.
  ii. Respiratory acidosis (elevated Pa_{CO_2}) may be caused by hypoventilation of any etiology and may be acute or chronic. Treatment generally consists of improving alveolar ventilation.
    (a) Obstructive lung disease, sleep apnea, and other lung diseases resulting in inadequate excretion of CO_2
    (b) Oversedation, head trauma, anesthesia, and drug overdose
    (c) Neuromuscular disorders: Guillain-Barré syndrome
    (d) Pneumothorax, flail chest, or other types of chest wall trauma that interfere with breathing mechanics
    (e) Inappropriate mechanical ventilator settings
  iii. Respiratory alkalosis (low Pa_{CO_2}) may be caused by hyperventilation of any etiology. Treatment consists of correcting the underlying cause.
    (a) Nervousness and anxiety
    (b) Hypoxemia, interstitial lung disease
    (c) Excessive ventilation with mechanical ventilator, as a response to metabolic acidosis (diabetic ketoacidosis) or from respiratory stimulant drugs, such as salicylates, theophylline, catecholamines
    (d) Pregnancy
    (e) Pulmonary embolus, pulmonary edema
    (f) Bacteremia (sepsis), liver disease, or fever
    (g) CNS disturbances, such as brainstem tumors and infections
g. Nonrespiratory (renal) parameters (HCO_3^-): If the primary disturbance is in the bicarbonate level, the patient has a metabolic disturbance
  i. Concentration is influenced by metabolic processes.
    (a) When HCO_3^- is elevated, metabolic alkalosis results.
      (1) Loss of nonvolatile acid
      (2) Gain of HCO_3^-
    (b) When HCO_3^- is decreased, metabolic acidosis results.
      (1) H^+ is added in excess of the capacity of the kidney to excrete it.
      (2) HCO_3^- is lost at a rate exceeding the capacity of the kidney to regenerate it.
  ii. Causes of metabolic alkalosis (elevated HCO_3^-)
    (a) Chloride depletion (vomiting, prolonged nasogastric suctioning, diuretic therapy)

      (b) Cushing's syndrome, hyperaldosteronism, potassium deficiency, renal artery stenosis, licorice ingestion

      (c) Exogenous administration of alkali (massive blood transfusions containing citrate, bicarbonate administration, ingestion of antacids)

  iii. Causes of metabolic acidosis (decreased HCO_3^-)

      (a) Increase in unmeasurable anions (acids that accumulate in certain diseases and poisonings); high anion gap

        (1) Diabetic ketoacidosis, starvation

        (2) Drugs: Salicylates, ethylene glycol, methanol alcohol, paraldehyde

        (3) Lactic acidosis resulting from tissue hypoperfusion and subsequent anaerobic metabolism (shock, sepsis)

        (4) Renal failure, uremia

        (5) Easy mnemonic is MULEPAK—methanol, uremia, lactic acidosis, ethylene glycol, paraldehyde, aspirin (salicylates), and ketoacidosis

      (b) No increase in unmeasurable anions, normal anion gap

        (1) Diarrhea, ureterosigmoidostomy (long or obstructed ileal conduit)

        (2) Drainage of pancreatic juices

        (3) Rapid IV infusion of non–bicarbonate-containing solutions causing a dilutional acidosis

        (4) Certain drugs, renal tubular acidosis

        (5) Hyperalimentation (causes hyperchloremic acidosis)

h. Compensation for acid-base abnormalities: Physiologic response to minimize pH changes by maintaining a normal bicarbonate to Pco_2 ratio

  i. pH is returned to near normal by changing component that is not primarily affected.

  ii. Respiratory disturbances result in kidney compensation, which may take several days to become maximal.

      (a) Compensation for respiratory acidosis

        (1) Kidneys excrete more acid.

        (2) Kidneys increase HCO_3^- reabsorption.

        (3) Compensation is slow (days).

      (b) Compensation for respiratory alkalosis

        (1) Kidneys excrete HCO_3^-.

        (2) Compensation is slow (days).

  iii. Metabolic disturbances result in pulmonary compensation, which begins rapidly but takes a variable amount of time to reach maximal levels.

      (a) Compensation for metabolic acidosis

        (1) Hyperventilation to decrease $Paco_2$

        (2) Rapid compensation (begins in 1 to 2 hours and reaches maximum in 12 to 24 hours)

      (b) Compensation for metabolic alkalosis

        (1) Hypoventilation (limited by the degree of the rise in $Paco_2$)

        (2) Rapid compensation (minutes to hours)

  iv. Body does not overcompensate. Therefore, the acidity or alkalinity of the pH identifies the primary abnormality if there is only one. Abnormalities may be multiple; each is not a discrete entity. Mixed acid-base disturbances often occur.

i. Correction of acid-base abnormalities: Caused by a physiologic or therapeutic response

  i. pH returned to normal by altering the component primarily affected; blood gas values are returned to normal

  ii. Correction for respiratory acidosis: Increased ventilation, treatment of cause

  iii. Correction for respiratory alkalosis: Decreased ventilation, treatment of cause

  iv. Correction for metabolic acidosis

      (a) Treatment of underlying cause

      (b) Administration of bicarbonate intravenously or orally (given only under specific circumstances)

  v. Correction for metabolic alkalosis

       (a) Treatment of underlying cause

       (b) Direct reduction by isotonic hydrochloric acid solution (cautious IV administration required) via a central line at a rate no higher than 0.2 mEq/kg/hr)

       (c) Acetazolamide (carbonic anhydrase inhibitor–diuretic) used in certain situations

j. Arterial blood gas (ABG) analysis

  i. Purpose

       (a) Shows end result of what occurs in the lung

       (b) Confirms the presence of respiratory failure and indicates acid-base status

       (c) Absolutely necessary in monitoring patients in acute respiratory failure (ARF) and patients on ventilators

  ii. Main components: Pa_{O_2}, Pa_{CO_2}, pH, base excess, HCO_3^-, Sa_{O_2}, O_2 content, Hb. Both FI_{O_2} and body temperature must be measured for proper interpretation. It is also essential to know whether HCO_3^- and Sa_{O_2} are directly measured or are calculated.

k. Guidelines for interpretation of ABG levels and acid-base balance

  i. Examine pH first (Table 2-4).

       (a) If pH is reduced (<7.35), the patient is acidemic.

          (1) If Pa_{CO_2} is elevated, the patient has respiratory acidosis.

          (2) If HCO_3^- is reduced, the patient has metabolic acidosis.

          (3) If Pa_{CO_2} is elevated and HCO_3^- is reduced, the patient has combined respiratory and metabolic acidosis.

       (b) If pH is elevated (>7.45), the patient is alkalemic.

          (1) If Pa_{CO_2} is decreased, the patient has respiratory alkalosis.

          (2) If HCO_3^- is elevated, the patient has metabolic alkalosis.

          (3) If Pa_{CO_2} is decreased and HCO_3^- is elevated, the patient has combined metabolic and respiratory alkalosis.

       (c) Expected change in pH for changes in Pa_{CO_2}: Commonly used rule is that the pH rises or falls 0.08 (or 0.1) in the appropriate direction for each change of 10 mm Hg in the Pa_{CO_2}

       (d) If the pH is normal (7.35 to 7.45), alkalosis or acidosis may still be present as a mixed disorder (Box 2-1).

  ii. Assess the hypoxemic state and tissue oxygenation state (Box 2-2).

       (a) Arterial oxygenation is considered compromised when Hb saturation is less than 88% (Pa_{O_2} is <60 mm Hg). If the Pa_{O_2} is below 55 mm Hg, hypoxemia is present.

       (b) If the patient is receiving supplemental O_2 therapy, Pa_{O_2} values must be interpreted in relation to the FI_{O_2} delivered. One way involves examination of the two as a ratio (Pa_{O_2}/FI_{O_2}). Normal Pa_{O_2}/FI_{O_2} ratio is 286 to 350, although levels as low as 200 may be clinically acceptable. Another way to assess oxygenation is to use the following formula to calculate the A-a arterial P_{O_2} gradient ($PA_{O_2} - Pa_{O_2}$):

$$PA_{O_2} = [FI_{O_2} (P_B - 47) - Pa_{CO_2}]/R$$

where 47 = vapor pressure of water at 37° C (in mm Hg) and R = respiratory quotient, the ratio of CO_2 production to O_2 consumption ($\dot{V}_{CO_2}/\dot{V}_{O_2}$); assumed to be 0.8

■ **TABLE 2-4**
■ ■ **Analysis of the Acid-Base Balance of an Arterial Blood Gas**

pH	↑	Alkalemia
	↓	Acidemia
Pa_{CO_2}	↑	Acidemia: pH should be ↓
	↓	Alkalemia: pH should be ↑
HCO_3^-	↑	Alkalemia: pH should be ↑
	↓	Acidemia: pH should be ↓

pH and Pa_{CO_2} go in opposite directions; pH and HCO_3^- go in the same direction.
HCO_3^-, Bicarbonate; Pa_{CO_2}, arterial partial pressure of carbon dioxide.

■ **BOX 2-1**
■ **ARTERIAL BLOOD GAS ANALYSIS: ACID-BASE EXAMPLE**

MEASUREMENTS
pH: 7.38
$Paco_2$: 70 mm Hg
HCO_3^-: 32 mEq/L
Pao_2: 65 mm Hg
Sao_2: 92%

ANALYSIS
pH: Normal, but on acidic side
$Paco_2$: Elevated—acidotic
HCO_3^-: Elevated—alkalotic
  Primary disorder is respiratory acidosis (pH is on the acidic side and $Paco_2$ is elevated). Secondary disorder is metabolic alkalosis (HCO_3^- is elevated) as compensation.

INTERPRETATION
Compensated respiratory acidosis (e.g., patient with stable chronic obstructive pulmonary disease)

Hco_3^-, Bicarbonate; *$Paco_2$*, arterial partial pressure of carbon dioxide; *Pao_2*, arterial partial pressure of oxygen; *Sao_2*, arterial oxygen saturation.

■ **BOX 2-2**
■ **ARTERIAL BLOOD GAS ANALYSIS: OXYGENATION EXAMPLE**

MEASUREMENTS
pH: 7.38
$Paco_2$: 70 mm Hg
HCO_3^-: 32 mEq/L
Pao_2: 65 mm Hg
Sao_2: 92%
Cao_2: 19.0 g/dl
Hb: 18 g/dl
Hct: 54%
On 2 L/min O_2 by nasal cannula, at sea level

ANALYSIS
pH: Normal, not in lactic acidosis from hypoxia
Pao_2: Low but adequate
Sao_2: Low but adequate
Cao_2: Within normal limits
Hb: Elevated
Hct: Elevated

INTERPRETATION
Adequate oxygenation on 2 L/min O_2. Hb/Hct elevated as compensatory mechanism to increase O_2-carrying capacity and compensate for underlying lung disease (chronic obstructive pulmonary disease) producing hypoxemia.

Cao_2, Arterial oxygen concentration; *Hb*, hemoglobin level; *Hco_3^-*, bicarbonate; *Hct*, hematocrit; *$Paco_2$*, arterial partial pressure of carbon dioxide; *Pao_2*, arterial partial pressure of oxygen; *Sao_2*, arterial oxygen saturation.

Normal $PA_{O_2} - Pa_{O_2}$ difference is less than 10 to 15 mm Hg. Although it provides an estimate of oxygenation, the gradient does not take into account the normal increasing gradient as a function of increasing F_{IO_2} levels. The higher the F_{IO_2}, the larger the increase in the A-a gradient can be without changing the level of intrapulmonary shunt or oxygenation. (Note: Primarily used for patients on a ventilator when the F_{IO_2} is known. F_{IO_2} is unknown [and its value therefore unreliable] with other O_2 delivery methods, but it can be estimated.)

(c) Excessively high Pa_{O_2} (>100 mm Hg) is generally not necessary, and in such cases F_{IO_2} should be reduced

(d) Assessment of cardiac output and O_2 transport determines tissue oxygenation. Pv_{O_2} and Sv_{O_2} may be useful guides in evaluating the adequacy of overall tissue oxygenation.

(e) Effectiveness of O_2 transport may be judged clinically by examining the patient carefully for mental status, skin color, urine output, and heart rate. Tests that measure end-organ function are also important clinical assessment tools.

Patient Assessment

1. **Nursing history: Nursing history follows the sequence and length of the standard history-taking process and is modified as needed for acutely ill patients**
   a. Patient health history: Patient's interpretation of his or her signs and symptoms and the emotional response to them play a significant role in the development or exacerbation of symptoms, especially as related to dyspnea
   i. Common symptoms
      (a) Dyspnea: Subjective feeling of shortness of breath or breathlessness
         (1) Quantifying objectively is difficult.
            a) Count the average number of words the patient is able to speak between breaths, or whether the patient can speak in full sentences.
            b) Ask the patient to rate breathing comfort on a visual analogue or dyspnea scale from 1 to 10.
         (2) Emotional problems may cause an increased awareness of respirations and complaints of inability to get enough air, despite normal blood gas values.
         (3) Dyspnea caused by increased work of breathing accompanies both obstructive and restrictive lung diseases, as well as the dysfunction of nerves, respiratory muscles, or thoracic cage.
         (4) Question the patient regarding exercise tolerance; some dyspnea is normal with exercise but is abnormal if exercise tolerance is decreased.
         (5) Assess whether the patient's dyspnea is acute or chronic, and whether it has recently increased or decreased.
         (6) Determine all circumstances under which dyspnea occurs (walking, stair climbing, eating) and how long the patient has experienced dyspnea with those activities.
         (7) Assess orthopnea or dyspnea when the patient is lying flat; ask how many pillows the patient generally uses for sleep and whether for comfort or shortness of breath.
         (8) Assess for paroxysmal nocturnal dyspnea by asking whether dyspnea ever awakens the patient from sleep.
         (9) Determine whether dyspnea is accompanied by other symptoms, such as cough, wheezing, or chest pain.
         (10) In some patients, it is difficult to differentiate cardiac from pulmonary dyspnea.
      (b) Cough: Normal when it occurs as a lung defense mechanism
         (1) Determine whether cough is acute and self-limiting or chronic (lasting more than 6 weeks) and persistent.
         (2) Note any change in character and frequency.
         (3) Determine what the timing is (both daily and seasonal) and whether the cough is accompanied by sputum production, hemoptysis, wheezing, chest pain, blackouts or falls, or dyspnea.

(4) Most common etiologic mechanisms are as follows:
    a) Inhaled irritants or airway diseases (asthma, bronchitis)
    b) Aspiration or lung diseases (pneumonia, lung abscess, tumor)
    c) Left ventricular failure (pulmonary edema)
    d) Side effect of medications (some angiotensin-converting enzyme inhibitors)
(c) Sputum production
    (1) Quantify amount by asking how many teaspoons, cups, or shot glasses of sputum are coughed up daily.
    (2) Determine aggravating and alleviating factors.
    (3) Assess the character of the sputum (color, odor, consistency).
    (4) Determine whether current sputum characteristics (quantity and quality) are changed from usual.
(d) Hemoptysis: Expectoration of blood from the lungs or airways
    (1) Determine whether the material coughed up is grossly bloody, blood streaked, or blood tinged (pinkish).
    (2) Try to differentiate from hematemesis. Product of hemoptysis is often frothy, alkaline, and accompanied by sputum; product of hematemesis is nonfrothy, acidic, and dark red or brown, with food particles.
    (3) Determine the approximate amount of blood produced in hemoptysis using a reasonable measurement guideline, such as the number of teaspoons or shot glasses per day. Assess whether all expectorated specimens contain blood or whether this is an isolated event.
    (4) Blood may originate from the nasopharynx, airways, or lung parenchyma; blood from these sites remains red because of the contact with atmospheric O_2.
    (5) Etiologic mechanisms of hemoptysis fall into three categories by location: airways, pulmonary parenchyma, and vasculature.
        a) Airways disease: Most common; bronchitis, bronchiectasis, and bronchogenic carcinoma
        b) Parenchymal causes: Often infectious—tuberculosis (TB), lung abscess, pneumonia
        c) Cardiovascular disease: Mitral stenosis, pulmonary embolism (PE), pulmonary edema
        d) Autoimmune disorders: Wegener's granulomatosis, Goodpasture's syndrome
    (6) Suspect neoplasm if hemoptysis occurs in a patient without prior respiratory symptoms.
(e) Chest pain: As a reflection of the respiratory system, does not originate in the lung, because the lung is free of sensory nerve fibers
    (1) Chest wall pain: Arises from the parietal pleura, intercostal muscles, ribs, or overlying skin
        a) Well localized
        b) Often exacerbated by deep inspiration
    (2) Diaphragm pain: Often caused by an inflammatory process; pain often referred to the ipsilateral shoulder
    (3) Mediastinal pain: Caused by a mass or air under the mediastinum (pneumomediastinum); pain is substernal and dull

ii. Miscellaneous symptoms of respiratory disease: Postnasal drip, sinus pain, epistaxis, hoarseness, general fatigue, weight loss, fever, sleep disturbances, night sweats, anxiety, nervousness, anorexia

iii. Past medical history
(a) Question the patient regarding the presence of any allergy to either medications (herbal, over the counter) or food. Obtain a description of the type and severity of the reaction.
(b) Determine past instances of the present illness, with treatment and outcome. Assess for previous episodes of TB, exposure to TB, or positive TB skin test result. Assess for childhood lung diseases or infections such as asthma, pneumonia, and whooping cough. Record the treatment given (if any) and the length of time the patient followed the medication regimen.

    (c) Identify past surgeries or hospitalizations: dates, diagnosis, and complications; previous use of O_2 or mechanical ventilation.

    (d) Question about previous chest radiographs: dates, reasons, findings.

    (e) Determine whether any pulmonary function tests were performed previously and the results if known.

b. Family history (extremely important)

    i. Assess for similar illness or signs and symptoms in the patient's parents, siblings, and grandparents.

    ii. Determine the current state of health or cause of death for parents, siblings, and grandparents.

    iii. Find out if there is a family history of diseases such as asthma, cystic fibrosis, bronchiectasis, and α_1-antitrypsin deficiency (emphysema).

    iv. Determine whether a family member ever had TB with consequent exposure of the patient.

c. Social history and habits

    i. Personal status: Assess education, socioeconomic class, marital status, general life satisfaction, interests

    ii. Health habits

        (a) Smoking

            (1) Determine whether the patient is a current or past smoker of cigarettes, cigars, or pipe.

                a) Calculate pack-year history:

$$\text{No. of packs/day} \times \text{No. of years smoked} = \text{Pack-years}$$

                b) Determine whether the patient has tried to quit and, if so, what methods were used and whether the effort was successful. If the patient is a former smoker, determine the time since the last cigarette; otherwise, determine the desire for information on smoking cessation resources and readiness to quit.

            (2) Ascertain whether the patient has smoked marijuana or another inhaled recreational drug (e.g., crack cocaine). If so, attempt to quantify the amount and frequency of drug use.

            (3) Determine whether the patient chews tobacco. If so, quantify the type chewed and the amount per day.

        (b) Drinking habits: Determine the frequency and amount consumed, and the type of alcoholic and caffeine-containing beverages

        (c) Eating habits: Assess the quality of meals (adequacy or excess) and determine whether any respiratory symptoms occur with eating (i.e., meal-induced dyspnea or cough)

        (d) Sexual history: Question about sexual activity and orientation

    iii. Home conditions: Assess economic conditions, housing quality, presence of any pets and their health, presence of allergens

    iv. Occupational history: Assess past and present work conditions

        (a) Determine whether the patient was exposed to heat and cold, industrial toxins, or pollutants during work or military duty.

        (b) Assess the duration of exposure and the use of protective devices.

d. Medication history (prescription and over-the-counter medications or home remedies)

    i. Determine current and recent medications, dosage, and the reason for prescribing.

    ii. Assess whether the patient is using any inhaled medications.

        (a) Identify the device used: metered-dose inhaler (MDI), nebulizer, or other delivery device (e.g., Spinhaler, HandiHaler).

        (b) Assess the frequency of use: on an as-needed basis or on a regular schedule.

        (c) If possible, have the patient demonstrate the technique for inhaling medication. Many patients use an incorrect technique when inhaling their medications, which results in reduced deposition of the drug in the lung and reduced efficacy. Patients should exhale completely, inhale the drug slowly and deeply, and then hold the breath for 10 seconds if possible.

        (d) Preferred delivery methods are powder delivery devices (nonaerosol), MDI with spacer, nebulizer, MDI with open mouth, MDI with closed mouth (least amount of medication delivered).

2. Nursing examination of patient

    a. Physical examination data

      i. Inspection

        (a) Nurse must have a thorough knowledge of anatomic landmarks and lines (Figure 2-9).

          (1) Manubrium, body, and xiphoid process of the sternum, right and left sternal borders

          (2) Angle of Louis, point of maximal impulse, suprasternal notch

          (3) Interspaces, ribs, costal margins, costal angle, and spinous processes

          (4) Pulmonary lobes and areas of contact with the chest wall (Figure 2-10)

          (5) Lines: Midclavicular, midsternal, anterior-axillary, midaxillary, posterior-axillary, vertebral, and midscapular

        (b) Observe general condition and musculoskeletal development.

          (1) State of nutrition, debilitation, evidence of chronic disease

          (2) Pectus carinatum: Sternum protrudes instead of being lower than the adjacent hemithoraces

          (3) Pectus excavatum: Sternum is abnormally depressed between the anterior hemithoraces

          (4) Kyphosis: Exaggerated A-P curvature of the spine

          (5) Scoliosis: Lateral curvature of the spine, causing widened intercostal spaces on the convex side and crowding of the ribs on the concave side; when accompanied by kyphosis, it is called kyphoscoliosis. If severe, it can result in restrictive lung disease.

        (c) Observe the A-P diameter of the thorax; normal A-P diameter is approximately one third the transverse diameter. In patients with obstructive lung disease, the A-P diameter may be as great as or greater than the transverse diameter ("barrel chest").

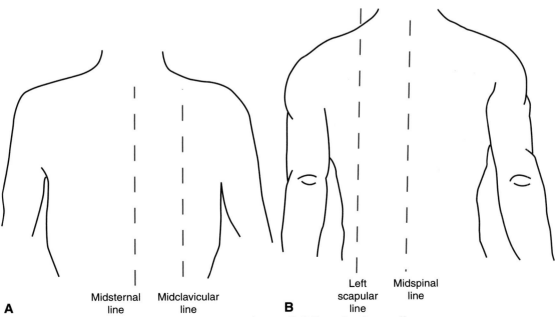

A   Midsternal   Midclavicular   **B**   Left   Midspinal
             line   line   scapular line
                                           line

FIGURE 2-9 ■ Landmarks of the chest. **A,** Anterior chest wall. **B,** Posterior chest wall.

(Continued)

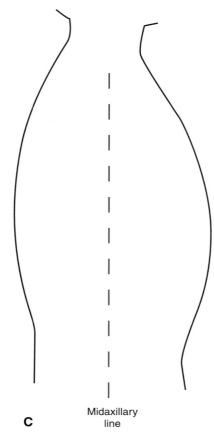

C

Midaxillary
line

FIGURE 2-9—Cont'd ▪ **C,** Lateral chest wall. (Courtesy American Association of Critical-Care Nurses, Aliso Viejo, Calif.)

(d) Observe the general slope of the ribs.
   (1) Ribs are normally at a 45-degree angle in relation to the spine.
   (2) In patients with emphysema, the ribs may be nearly horizontal.
(e) Observe for asymmetry.
   (1) One side may be larger because of tension pneumothorax or pleural effusion.
   (2) One side may be smaller because of atelectasis or unilateral fibrosis.
   (3) If asymmetry is present, the abnormal side will move less than the normal side.
(f) Look for retraction or bulging of the interspaces.
   (1) Retraction of the interspaces, which can be observed during inspiration, indicates more negative intrapleural pressure due to obstruction of the inflow of air or increased work of breathing.
   (2) Bulging of the interspaces may result from a large pleural effusion or pneumothorax, often seen during a forced expiration in patients with asthma or emphysema.
(g) Observe the ventilatory pattern.
   (1) Assess the level of dyspnea and the work of breathing.
      a) Position in which the patient can breathe most comfortably. Patients with chronic obstructive pulmonary disease (COPD) often assume a forward-leaning position, resting the arms on the knees or a bedside table.
      b) Use of accessory muscles of breathing
      c) Use of pursed-lip breathing
      d) Flaring of the ala nasi during inspiration, a common sign of air hunger, especially in ventilated patients
      e) Paradoxical movement of the diaphragm

    (2) Assess for inspiratory stridor—low-pitched or crowing inspiratory sounds that occur when the trachea or major bronchi are obstructed for one of the following reasons:

       a) Tumor (intrinsic or extrinsic), foreign body

       b) Severe laryngotracheitis or crushing injury

       c) Goiter, scar, or granulation tissue

    (3) Observe for expiratory stridor—low-pitched crowing sound heard on expiration. Causes include foreign body or intrathoracic, tracheal, or main-stem tumor.

    (4) Observe for unusual movements with breathing; on inspiration, the chest and abdomen should expand or rise together. Paradoxical breathing occurs with respiratory muscle fatigue: On inspiration, the chest rises and the abdomen is drawn in because the fatigued diaphragm does not descend on inspiration as it should. Instead, the diaphragm is drawn upward by the negative intrathoracic pressure during inspiration.

    (5) Observe and assess the ventilatory pattern.

       a) Eupnea: Normal, quiet respirations

       b) Bradypnea: Abnormally slow rate of ventilation

       c) Tachypnea: Rapid rate of ventilation

       d) Hyperpnea: Increase in the depth and, perhaps, in the rate of ventilation. Overall result is increased tidal volume and minute ventilation.

       e) Apnea: Complete or intermittent cessation of ventilation

       f) Biot's breathing: Two to three short breaths alternating with long, irregular periods of apnea

       g) Cheyne-Stokes respiration: Periods of increasing ventilation, followed by progressively more shallow ventilations until apnea occurs; pattern typically repeats itself. Sometimes occurs in normal persons when asleep and usually indicates CNS disease, heart failure, or sleep apnea.

    (6) Splinting of respirations—act of resisting full inspiration in one or both lungs as a result of pain

    (7) Flail chest—inward movement of a portion of the chest on inspiration, usually associated with trauma to the chest; from fracture of the rib cage in two or more sections

(h) Other observations

    (1) General state of restlessness, pain, altered mental status, fright, or acute distress. Earliest signs of hypoxemia often include a change in mental status and restlessness.

    (2) If O_2 is being administered, record the amount (flow in liters per minute), type of device (liquid, compressed gas), method of delivery (nasal cannula, Oxymizer, mask).

    (3) Inspect the extremities.

       a) Clubbing of the fingers is a late sign of a chronic pulmonary or cardiac disease.

       b) Cigarette stains on the fingers suggest a current smoking habit.

       c) Lower-extremity edema indicates possible right-sided heart failure from chronic pulmonary disease and hypoxemia-induced pulmonary hypertension.

    (4) Observe for cyanosis.

       a) Fundamental mechanism of cyanosis is an increase in the amount of reduced (deoxygenated) Hb in the vessels of the skin caused by one of the following:

          1) Decrease in the O_2 saturation of the capillary blood

          2) Increase in the amount of venous blood in the skin as a result of the dilation of venules and capillaries

       b) Visible cyanosis requires the presence of at least 5 g of reduced Hb per deciliter of blood.

          1) This is an absolute, not a relative, value. It is not the percentage of deoxygenated Hb that causes cyanosis but the amount of deoxygenated Hb without regard to the amount of oxyhemoglobin. Presence or absence of cyanosis may be an unreliable clinical sign.

2) In anemia, cyanosis may be difficult to detect because the absolute amount of Hb is too low. Conversely, patients with polycythemia may be cyanotic at higher levels of arterial O_2 saturation than those with normal Hb levels.

c) Discoloration suggestive of cyanosis may occur in patients with abnormal blood or skin pigments (methemoglobinemia, sulfhemoglobin, argyria).

d) Factors influencing cyanosis include the rate of blood flow, perfusion, skin thickness and color, the amount of Hb, cardiac output, and the perception of the examiner.

e) Central versus peripheral cyanosis compare as follows:

1) Central cyanosis implies arterial O_2 desaturation or an abnormal Hb derivative. Both mucous membranes and skin are affected.

2) Peripheral cyanosis without central cyanosis may result from the slowing of perfusion to the tissues (cold exposure, shock, decreased cardiac output). O_2 saturation may be normal.

f) In carbon monoxide poisoning, O_2 saturation may be dangerously low without obvious cyanosis because carboxyhemoglobin causes the skin to turn a cherry red.

(i) Assess for neck vein distention, neck masses, and enlarged nodes.

(j) Look for superior vena caval syndrome: distention of the neck veins and edema of the neck, eyelids, and hands; often seen with lung cancer.

(k) In elderly patients, examination shows flattening of the ribs and diaphragm, decreased chest expansion, use of accessory muscles, marked bony prominences, loss of subcutaneous tissue, pronounced dorsal curve of the thoracic spine, increased A-P diameter relative to lateral diameter, dyspnea on exertion, dry mucous membranes, decreased ability to clear mucus, and hyperresonance from increased distensibility of the lung.

ii. Palpation

(a) Palpation of the thoracic muscles and skeleton, feeling for any of the following: pulsations, palpable fremitus, tenderness, bulges, or depressions in the chest wall

(b) Expansion of the chest wall

(1) Examiner's hands should be placed over the lower lateral aspect of the chest, with the thumbs along the costal margin anteriorly or meeting posteriorly in the midline.

(2) Movement of the hands is noted on inspiration and expiration. Asymmetry of movement is always abnormal. Reduced chest wall movement is often seen in patients with barrel chest and emphysema.

(c) Position and mobility of the trachea

(1) Deviations of the trachea toward the defect are seen in atelectasis, unilateral pulmonary fibrosis, pneumonectomy, hemidiaphragm paralysis, and the inspiratory phase of flail chest.

(2) Deviation of the trachea to the side opposite the lesion is seen with neck tumors, thyroid enlargement, tension pneumothorax, pleural effusion, mediastinal mass, and the expiratory phase of flail chest.

(d) Point of maximal impulse: Deviates with mediastinal shift

(e) Palpation of ribs and chest for tenderness, pain, or air in subcutaneous tissue (crepitus)

(f) Vocal fremitus, palpable vibration of the chest wall, produced by phonation

(1) Patient should be instructed to say the word *ninety-nine* loud enough so that the fremitus can be felt with uniform intensity. Some soft-spoken women may need to falsely lower their voice so that the fremitus can be felt. Examiner should place the hands on the patient's chest wall.

(2) Diminished fremitus is seen in any condition that interferes with the transference of vibrations through the chest.

a) Pleural effusion or thickening, pleural tumors

b) Pneumothorax with lung collapse or emphysema

c) Obstruction of the bronchus (sputum plugs or tumors)

        (3) Increased fremitus results from any condition that increases the transmission of vibrations through the chest, such as the following:
            a) Pneumonia, consolidation
            b) Atelectasis (with open bronchus)
            c) Pulmonary infarction or pulmonary fibrosis
            d) Secretions with a patent airway

(g) Pleural friction fremitus
    (1) Occurs when inflamed pleural surfaces rub together during ventilation, producing a "grating" sensation that coincides with the respiratory excursion
    (2) May be palpable during both phases of ventilation but sometimes is felt only during inspiration

(h) Rhonchal fremitus
    (1) Produced by the passage of air through thick exudate, secretions, or an area of stenosis in the trachea or major bronchi
    (2) Unlike friction fremitus, can be relieved by coughing, suctioning, or clearing the secretions from the tracheobronchial tree

(i) Subcutaneous emphysema: Indicates a leak of air under the skin due to a communication with the airway, mediastinum, or pneumothorax
    (1) May be palpated over the area
    (2) On auscultation, may be mistaken for crackles (rales)

iii. Percussion: Tapping or thumping of parts of the body to produce sound. Nature of the sound produced depends on the density of the structures immediately under the area percussed.

(a) Sound vibrations produced by percussion probably do not penetrate more than about 4 to 5 cm below the surface; therefore, solid masses deep in the chest cannot be outlined with percussion. In addition, because a lesion must be several centimeters in diameter to be detectable by percussion, only large abnormalities can be located.

(b) Procedure is accomplished by striking the dorsal distal third finger of one hand, which is held against the thorax, with the distal tip of the flexed middle finger of the other hand
    (1) Striking finger must strike only the stationary finger instantaneously and then be immediately withdrawn.
    (2) All movement is executed at the wrist.
    (3) Examiner must be sensitive to the sounds that are received from the chest wall.
    (4) One side of the chest is compared with the other side.
    (5) Percussion of the posterior chest is done as patient inclines the head forward and rests the forearms on the thighs to move the scapulae laterally.
    (6) Percussion begins at the apices and continues downward to the bases, alternating side to side.

(c) Percussion sounds over the lung include the following:
    (1) Resonance: Sound heard normally over the lungs
    (2) Hyperresonance: Sound heard over the lungs in normal children, in the apices of the lungs relative to the base in an upright adult, and throughout the lung fields in adults with emphysema or pneumothorax
        a) Lower in pitch than normal resonance
        b) Relatively intense and easy to hear
        c) Indicates increased air (less dense)
    (3) Tympany: Produced by air in an enclosed chamber; does not occur in the normal chest except below the dome of the left hemidiaphragm, where it is produced by air in the underlying stomach or bowel
        a) Relatively musical sound
        b) Usually higher pitched than normal resonance; the higher the tension within the viscus, the higher the pitch
    (4) Dullness: Sound that is heard with lung consolidation, atelectasis, masses, pleural effusion, or hemothorax
        a) Short, not sustained

b) Soft, not loud; similar to a dull thud

c) Indicates that more dense material (fluid or solid) is in the underlying thorax

d) Normally heard over the liver and heart

(d) Percussion for diaphragmatic excursion: Range of motion of the diaphragm may be estimated with percussion

(1) Instruct the patient to take a deep breath and hold it.

(2) Determine the lower level of resonance-to-dullness change (the level of the diaphragm) by percussing downward until a definite change is heard in the percussion note. Mark the spot with a felt-tipped marker.

(3) After instructing the patient to exhale and hold the breath, repeat the procedure.

(4) Distance between the levels at which the tone change occurs is the diaphragmatic excursion.

a) Normal diaphragmatic excursion is about 3 to 4 cm; partial descent or hemidescent of the diaphragm may be due to paralysis of the diaphragm or hemidiaphragm. Suspect nerve injury in postoperative patients with these signs after thoracic surgery.

b) Diaphragm is normally higher on the right than the left.

c) Diaphragm is elevated in conditions that increase intra-abdominal pressure (pregnancy, ascites) and conditions that decrease thoracic volume (atelectasis).

d) Diaphragm is fixed and lower than normal in emphysema.

e) It is difficult to differentiate between an elevated diaphragm and a thoracic disease that causes dullness to percussion (e.g., pleural effusion). Paralysis of one or both hemidiaphragms may be present.

iv. Auscultation: Listening to sounds produced within the body

(a) Basic points

(1) Examiner should always compare one lung with the other by moving the stethoscope back and forth across the chest starting at the top of the thorax and moving downward.

(2) Listening to the anterior chest will cover the upper and middle lobes; listening to the back covers the bases (see Figure 2-10).

(3) Patient should be asked to breathe through the mouth a little more deeply than usual. This minimizes turbulent flow sounds produced in the nose and throat.

(4) Diaphragm of the stethoscope is more sensitive to higher-pitched tones and is thus best for hearing most lung sounds.

(5) Stethoscope earpieces should fit snugly to exclude extraneous sounds but should not be so tight that they are uncomfortable.

(6) Stethoscope tubing should be no longer than 20 inches. Optimal length is 12 to 14 inches.

(7) Place the stethoscope firmly on the chest to exclude extraneous sounds and eliminate sounds that result from light contact with the skin or air. Confusing sounds may be produced by moving the stethoscope on the skin or hair, breathing on the tubing, sliding the fingers on the tubing or chest piece, or listening through clothing.

(b) Normal breath sounds, which vary according to the site of auscultation

(1) Vesicular (always normal)

a) Soft sounds heard over the anterior, lateral, and posterior chest

b) Heard primarily during inspiration

(2) Bronchial (may be normal or abnormal, depending on the location of the sounds)

a) Heard normally over the trachea

b) High-pitched, harsh sound with long and loud expirations

c) When heard over the lung fields, has abnormal sound and suggests consolidation

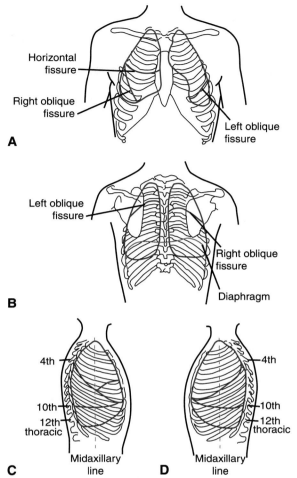

FIGURE 2-10 ■ Topographic position of lung fissures. **A,** Anterior chest. **B,** Posterior chest. **C** and **D,** Lateral chest. (From Ahrens TS. Pulmonary data acquisition. In: Kinney MR, Packa DR, Dunbar SB, eds. *AACN's Clinical Reference for Critical Care Nursing.* 3rd ed. St Louis, MO: Mosby; 1993:690.)

       (3) Bronchovesicular (normal or abnormal, depending on the location)
          a) Heard over large bronchi (near the sternum, between the scapulae, over the right upper lobe apex)
          b) Abnormal when heard over the lung fields; signifies consolidation
    (c) Abnormalities of breath sounds
       (1) Absent or diminished sounds caused by decreased airflow (airway obstruction, COPD, muscle weakness, splinting) or increased insulation blocking the transmission of sounds to the stethoscope (obesity, pleural disease or fluid, pneumothorax)
       (2) Bronchial sounds heard over the lung fields suggest consolidation or increased density of lung tissue (e.g., atelectasis, pulmonary infarction, pneumonia, large tumors with no airway obstruction)
    (d) Adventitious sounds: Abnormal sounds that are superimposed on underlying breath sounds
       (1) Evaluate whether position and coughing affect the sounds
       (2) Terminology
          a) Crackles (rales): Signify the opening of collapsed alveoli and small airways
            1) Crackles are described as fine or coarse.

2) Sound is heard as small pops or crackles; the sound of fine crackles can be mimicked by rubbing together a few pieces of hair near one's ear. Sound of coarse crackles can be mimicked by pulling open hook-and-loop (Velcro fastener) material.

3) Fine crackles occurring late in inspiration imply conditions that cause restrictive ventilatory defect.

4) Fine crackles heard early in inspiration are often atelectatic, because of small airway closure.

5) Coarse early inspiratory crackles are associated with bronchitis or pneumonia.

b) Wheeze: Indicates an obstruction to airflow or air passing through narrowed airways

1) Continuous high-pitched sound with musical quality; also called "sibilant" wheeze

2) Commonly heard during expiration but may be heard during inspiration

3) Causes: Asthma, bronchitis, foreign body, tumor, pulmonary edema, pulmonary emboli, poorly mobilized secretions

c) Gurgles (rhonchi): Result from the passage of air through secretions in the large airways

1) Low-pitched, continuous sounds

2) May have a snoring quality when very large airways are involved ("sonorous" wheezes)

3) Tend to improve or disappear after coughing

d) Pleural friction rub: Indicates inflammation and loss of pleural fluid

1) Grating, harsh sound in inspiration and expiration; disappears with breath holding. Sound can be mimicked by cupping a hand over one's ear and rubbing the fingers of the other hand over the cupped hand.

2) Heard with pleural infections, infarction, pulmonary emboli, fractured ribs. Located in the area of most intense chest wall pain.

e) Mediastinal crunch: Indicates air in the pericardium, mediastinum, or both. Heard synchronously with systole; often associated with pericardial friction rubs.

f) Pericardial friction rub

1) Occurs at atrial and ventricular systole with or without a diastolic component

2) Sounds persist with breath holding; heard most clearly at the left lower sternal border

(e) Voice sounds: Spoken words are modified by disease in a manner similar to breath sounds, which results in the increased or decreased conduction of sound

(1) Increased conduction occurs when normal lung tissue is replaced with denser, more solid tissue; it is associated with bronchial breathing.

a) Bronchophony: Spoken word (e.g., *ninety-nine*) is heard distinctly, but normal sound is muffled

b) Egophony: E sound changes to A; sound has the quality of sheep bleating

c) Whispered pectoriloquy: Whispered sounds are heard with clarity, as if the patient were speaking into the diaphragm of the stethoscope, but normal sound is muffled

(2) Decreased conduction of sound occurs in the presence of obstructed bronchi, pneumothorax, or large collections of fluid or tissue between the lung and the chest wall.

a) Decreased ability to hear voice sounds

b) Accompanied by decreased fremitus

b. Monitoring data

i. Pulse oximetry

(a) Noninvasive estimate of arterial O_2 saturation (SpO_2) using an infrared light source placed at the finger or other acceptable extremity, forehead, or earlobe

(b) Uses two principles for measurement

(1) Spectrophotometry measures the infrared light absorption of Hb (to distinguish saturated from reduced Hb).

(2) Photoplethysmography uses light to measure the arterial pressure waveforms generated by the pulse (pulse rate and strength) in the capillaries of the tissue at the measurement site.

(c) Pulse oximeters generally accurate in the SpO_2 range of 70% to 100% but inaccurate in states of low blood flow (decreased perfusion due to hypovolemia, hypotension, or vasoconstriction)

(d) SpO_2 reading adversely affected by the following:

(1) Motion of the extremity (false pulse rate and waveform artifact)

(2) Light dilution (interferes with the probe's ability to detect the correct light wavelength)

(3) Abnormal Hb (device cannot distinguish between oxyhemoglobin and carboxyhemoglobin and thus overestimates saturation); methemoglobin may interfere with light absorption

(4) IV dyes, some fingernail polish colors (e.g., metallic, dark colors such as black), or abnormal skin pigmentation (interfere with light absorption)

(5) Anemia (Hb level below $5 \, g/dl$ may result in insufficient signal to process readings)

(e) Useful for identifying the trend of changes in PaO_2 or acute desaturation episodes, especially when weaning from a ventilator

(f) Necessitates exercise of extreme caution not to overrely on a normal SpO_2 level to indicate normal oxygenation in all cases. If in doubt, get an ABG.

 ii. Blood gas analysis

(a) Acid-base balance (pH, $PaCO_2$, HCO_3^-): See Tables 2-3 and 2-4

(b) Oxygenation status (PaO_2, SaO_2, CaO_2)

3. **Appraisal of patient characteristics: Patients with acute pulmonary problems may present in progressive care units with an array of clinical findings that represent the highest priority of patient needs. Their clinical course may resolve quickly, slowly, or not at all. Important clinical features that the nurse needs to assess when providing care for these patients include the following:**

a. Resiliency

i. Level 1—*Minimally resilient:* A 75-year-old woman, with a history of diabetes, hypertension, and emphysema, admitted with an ischemic stroke and possible aspiration

ii. Level 3—*Moderately resilient:* A 65-year-old man on day 1 after abdominal surgery with rapid, shallow respirations who continues to refuse to cough, deep breathe, or ambulate postoperatively

iii. Level 5—*Highly resilient:* A 21-year-old woman admitted with a traumatic pneumothorax following a rib fracture from a fall

b. Vulnerability

i. Level 1—*Highly vulnerable:* A 32-year-old woman, who is 5 feet 2 inches tall and weighs 394 lb, being admitted for possible aspiration during extubation after appendectomy

ii. Level 3—*Moderately vulnerable:* A 25-year-old woman, with a history of cystic fibrosis, admitted with pneumonia requiring IV antibiotics and low-flow O_2 therapy

iii. Level 5—*Minimally vulnerable:* A 62-year-old man, with a history of COPD, admitted with a secondary pneumothorax requiring a chest tube

c. Stability

i. Level 1—*Minimally stable:* An 85-year-old man admitted with pneumonia who is requiring 100% O_2 via nonbreather mask to maintain SpO_2 >90%

ii. Level 3—*Moderately stable:* A 67-year-old man with a history of diabetes and hypertension recovering from acute respiratory failure and showing slowly improving ABGs after liberation from mechanical ventilation

iii. Level 5—*Highly stable:* A 55-year-old man with a history of sleep apnea admitted after a laparoscopic cholecystectomy for monitoring overnight

d. Complexity

      i. *Level 1—Highly complex:* A 72-year-old man recovering from acute respiratory failure requiring prolonged mechanical ventilation via tracheostomy tube and tube feedings via a gastrostomy tube who is undergoing weaning trials

      ii. *Level 3—Moderately complex:* A 60-year-old woman with a history of diabetes and severe rheumatoid arthritis complaining of moderate chest pain and dyspnea shortly after arriving on a flight from Hong Kong

      iii. *Level 5—Minimally complex:* A 23-year-old woman admitted after an asthma attack that occurred as a result of a visit to a recently painted and carpeted apartment and failure to get her inhaler to work

  e. Resource availability

      i. *Level 1—Few resources:* A 58-year-old Vietnam veteran with chronic bronchiectasis admitted after two episodes of hemoptysis. He does not qualify for Veterans Affairs benefits, is estranged from his only sibling, and subsists on meals at the local shelter.

      ii. *Level 3—Moderate resources:* A 49-year-old male cab driver recovering from ARDS after a motor vehicle crash and who will need continued pulmonary therapy after discharge. His son, a respiratory therapist, will visit his father twice daily to provide that care.

      iii. *Level 5—Many resources:* A 67-year-old man in whom pneumonia developed when influenza was superimposed on his COPD. His spouse has contacted the discharge planner to make any necessary care arrangements.

  f. Participation in care

      i. *Level 1—No participation:* A 43-year-old woman in a persistent vegetative state requiring prolonged ventilatory support via tracheostomy tube

      ii. *Level 3—Moderate level of participation:* A 92-year-old man recovering from community-acquired pneumonia who is eager to ambulate and use the incentive spirometer but requires assistance with the former and repeated instruction in the latter

      iii. *Level 5—Full participation:* A 28-year-old man admitted with a PE after a deep vein thrombosis (DVT) that developed after he was on an airplane for 17 hours who is requesting information related to the prevention of DVT

  g. Participation in decision making

      i. *Level 1—No participation:* A 29-year-old man who is comatose after a head injury and is being weaned from a tracheostomy before placement in a skilled nursing facility

      ii. *Level 3—Moderate level of participation:* A 72-year-old woman admitted immediately after a lobectomy who remains very sleepy but arousable

      iii. *Level 5—Full participation:* A 27-year-old woman who had a severe asthma attack and is requesting information regarding advanced directives

  h. Predictability

      i. *Level 1—Not predictable:* A 86-year-old woman admitted with an ischemic stroke who has become increasingly confused and tachypneic after lunch

      ii. *Level 3—Moderately predictable:* A 52-year old man admitted with a compound fracture of the left clavicle, as well as rib fractures with pneumothorax

      iii. *Level 5—Highly predictable:* A 74-year-old former smoker in whom pneumonia develops whenever a new strain of influenza appears

4. Diagnostic studies

  a. Laboratory

      i. Sputum examination

        (a) Obtain a specimen through voluntary coughing and expectoration, induction of sputum by inhalation of an aerosol, nasotracheal or endotracheal suctioning, transtracheal aspiration, or bronchoscopy.

        (b) Assess characteristics and compare with the patient's normal state.

          (1) Color and consistency: Green—*Pseudomonas* infection; yellow—bacterial infection; rust colored—pneumococcal infection

          (2) Volume: More than 25 ml/day is excessive

          (3) Odor: Should be odorless

            a) Foul smell may indicate an anaerobic putrefactive process.

            b) Musty odor may indicate *Pseudomonas* infection.

          (4) Microscopic examination

            a) Cytologic study for malignant cells

b) Smear for examination for bacteria (e.g., Gram stain) or fungi

c) Sputum cultures to diagnose infection and assess drug resistance

d) Stains on cultures for mycobacteria (acid-fast bacilli), *Pneumocystis carinii*, *Legionella pneumophila*

ii. Pleural fluid examination

(a) Diagnostic thoracentesis or pleural biopsy is performed to obtain a specimen.

(b) Determination of whether the fluid is a transudate or an exudate is based on the protein and lactate dehydrogenase (LDH) levels in the pleural fluid and blood.

(c) Specimen is examined for cell counts, protein and LDH levels, glucose level, amylase level, and pH; Gram staining for bacteria is performed; cytologic analysis for malignant cells and microorganisms is conducted.

(d) Biopsy of parietal pleura may be performed.

iii. Skin tests

(a) Type I hypersensitivity (mediated by immunoglobulin E): To pollens, molds, grass

(b) Type II hypersensitivity (mediated by T lymphocytes): Purified protein derivative testing for TB

(c) Fungal diseases

(d) As controls to assess anergy: Mumps, *Candida* infection

iv. Serologic tests used to determine the causative pathogen in bacterial, viral, mycotic, and parasitic diseases

b. Radiologic

i. Chest radiographic examination precedes all other studies.

(a) Posteroanterior and lateral views most common

(b) Portable A-P views are obtained in the intensive care unit (ICU) when the patient cannot be moved. These radiographs are generally of lesser quality than an erect posteroanterior film for the following reasons:

(1) There is difficulty in positioning the patient.

(2) Film distance from the chest is short; variable distances in serial films.

(3) X-ray generator is less powerful; there is interference from attached tubes, lines, equipment.

(c) Lateral decubitus views are used if fluid levels need to be identified (as with pleural effusions and abscesses).

(d) Oblique views may be used to localize lesions and infiltrates.

(e) Lordotic views are used to evaluate the apical portion of the lung and the middle lobe or lingula and can help determine whether a lesion is anterior or posterior.

(f) Expiratory films are used for visualizing pneumothorax or air trapping.

ii. Fluoroscopy

(a) Shows the movement of pulmonary and cardiac structures and the diaphragm, localizes pulmonary lesions

(b) Used to monitor during special procedures—catheter or chest tube insertion, bronchoscopy, thoracentesis

(c) Greater exposure of the patient to radiation during fluoroscopy than during a standard radiographic examination

iii. Tomography: Provides views at different planes through the lungs

(a) Gives better definition of small or questionable lesions; particularly useful for determining whether a lesion has calcification. Plain tomography is rarely used.

(b) Computed tomography (CT) scan: All chest CTs are spiral CTs now

(1) To scan axial cross sections of the body

(2) Particularly useful in detecting subtle differences in tissue density

(3) High-resolution CT (HRCT) for three-dimensional images of the lung to detect a pattern of emphysema, progression of fibrosis

iv. Magnetic resonance imaging (MRI)

(a) Can distinguish tumors from other structures, such as blood vessels, spinal cord, and bronchial walls

(b) Can differentiate pleural thickening, pleural fluid, and chest wall tumors from each other

    v. Pulmonary angiography: Visualizes the pulmonary arterial tree through the injection of radiopaque dye

        (a) Useful to investigate thromboembolic disease of the lung, congenital circulatory abnormalities, masses

        (b) Some risks; dangerous to perform in pulmonary hypertension; O_2 desaturation has occurred in some patients with the injection of contrast medium. Hemodynamic parameters should be measured before the procedure.

    vi. Ventilation-perfusion lung scanning

        (a) Involves injection or inhalation of radioisotopes; performed to obtain information on pulmonary blood flow and ventilation

        (b) Can detect pulmonary emboli and assess regional lung function preoperatively

    vii. Ultrasonography

        (a) Useful in evaluating pleural disease

        (b) Can detect small amounts of pleural fluid and loculations within the pleural space

        (c) Can distinguish fluid from pleural thickening

        (d) Can localize the diaphragm and detect disease immediately below it, such as a subphrenic abscess

        (e) Not useful for defining structures or lesions within the pulmonary parenchyma (the ultrasonic beam penetrates air poorly)

  c. Pulmonary function studies: See Box 2-3 and Figure 2-11

  d. Lung biopsy

BOX 2-3
PULMONARY FUNCTION STUDIES

PURPOSE
- Classify pulmonary function as normal or exhibiting a restrictive or obstructive defect
- Describe disease early and in physiologic terms
- Follow the patient in quantitative terms for future comparisons
- Assist in evaluation of the risk of surgery

LUNG VOLUMES AND CAPACITIES
- Measured with the patient in the upright position; values obtained are compared with predicted values (see Figure 2-11)
- Volumes: There are four discrete and nonoverlapping lung volumes
  1. Tidal volume (V_T): Volume of gas inspired and expired during each respiratory cycle
  2. Inspiratory reserve volume (IRV): Maximal volume of gas that can be inspired after a tidal breath is taken
  3. Expiratory reserve volume (ERV): Maximal volume of gas that can be expired from the end-expiratory position
  4. Residual volume (RV): Volume of gas remaining in the lungs at end of a maximal expiration
- Capacities: There are four capacities, each of which includes two or more of the primary volumes
  1. Total lung capacity (TLC): Volume of gas contained in the lung at the end of a maximal inspiration

$$TLC = V_T + IRV + ERV + RV$$

  2. Vital capacity (VC): Maximal volume of gas that can be expelled from the lungs following a maximal inspiration

$$VC = V_T + IRV + ERV$$

  3. Inspiratory capacity (IC): Maximal volume of gas that can be inspired from the resting expiratory level

$$IC = V_T + IRV$$

  4. Functional residual capacity (FRC): Volume of gas remaining in the lungs at resting end-expiration

$$FRC = ERV + RV$$

VENTILATORY MECHANICS
- Provide information about dynamic lung function. Subjects perform forced breathing maneuvers.
- Forced expiratory spirograms

FVC: Forced vital capacity; reduced in restrictive disease or in obstructive disease if there is air trapping

FEV_t: Forced expiratory volume in t (seconds); usually measured at 0.5, 1, and 3 seconds. Reduced in obstructive disease. Most useful measurements are FEV_1 and FEV_6.

$FEV_1/VC\%$: Forced expiratory volume at 1 second as a percentage of vital capacity. Evaluates obstruction to flow. FEV_1/VC: Normally >75% in adults.

FEF: Forced expiratory flows ($FEF_{25\%-75\%}$, $FEF_{75\%-85\%}$). These tests assess flows over a range of lung volumes. Values for timed flow studies are decreased out of proportion to vital capacity in obstructive disease.

- Flow-volume loop studies: Volume and flow during inspiration and expiration are graphically plotted. Obstructive disease produces abnormal flow-volume loops; restrictive disease produces normal-appearing but smaller flow-volume loops.
- Maximum voluntary ventilation (MVV)
  1. Volume of air ventilated with maximal effort over a short period of time
  2. May be used to predict the patient's ability to undergo procedures that require ventilatory reserve (i.e., surgery, extubation)

LUNG COMPLIANCE STUDIES

- Assess the distensibility of the lungs; lung compliance (C_L) is the reciprocal of elastance
- Expressed as the increase in volume (V) per increase in transpulmonary pressure (P)

$$C_L = \frac{\Delta V}{\Delta P}$$

- Static compliance (C_{st}) is measured in the absence of airflow.
  1. In the patient on a ventilator, it is measured by dividing V_T by the plateau pressure (minus positive end-expiratory pressure [PEEP]) and is called the *effective static compliance*.
  2. Normal values are around 100 ml/cm H_2O.
- Dynamic compliance (C_{dyn}) is measured under conditions of flow.
  1. In patients on a ventilator, it is measured by dividing V_T by the peak inspiratory pressure (minus PEEP) and is called the *effective dynamic compliance*.
  2. Normal range is between 40 and 50 ml/cm H_2O.
- Compliance is decreased in conditions that make the lungs or thorax stiffer or reduce expansibility. Such conditions include atelectasis, pneumonia, pulmonary edema, fibrotic changes, pleural effusion, pneumothorax, kyphoscoliosis, obesity, abdominal distention, flail chest, and splinting due to pain.
- Increases in compliance occur with age or emphysema.
- Compliance curves (serial changes in volume plotted against changes in pressure) are useful in monitoring patients on volume ventilators. Determinations of the best pressure-volume combinations for the patient may be made. Comparisons of static and dynamic pressure-volume curves help to determine which component (airway, lung, or chest wall) is contributing to changes in compliance.

GAS TRANSFER AND EXCHANGE STUDIES

- Blood gas and acid-base analysis
  1. Fundamental to the diagnosis and management of pulmonary problems
  2. See Physiologic Anatomy
- Diffusing capacity (D_L)
  1. Measures the amount of functioning alveolar-capillary surface area available for gas exchange
  2. Values decrease with ventilation-perfusion mismatching and membrane problems and with decreases in pulmonary capillary blood volume.

GUIDELINES FOR INTERPRETATION OF PULMONARY FUNCTION TEST RESULTS

- Values are compared with predicted values for age, height, and gender.
- Restrictive pulmonary impairment generally results in decreased volumes and capacities.
- Decreased static lung compliance suggests parenchymal disease.
- Obstructive defect generally results in decreased values on tests of dynamic ventilatory function. This change may be reversible with the use of bronchodilators.
- Chronic obstructive pulmonary disease with long-term air trapping and destruction of parenchyma results in increased FRC, residual volume, and TLC.
- Patient preparation and cooperation are necessary to obtain reliable and valid data for most pulmonary function tests.

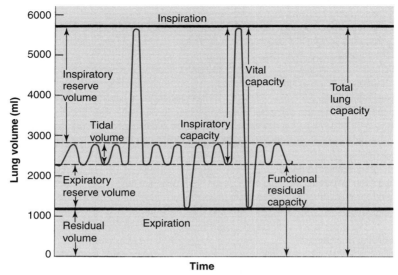

FIGURE 2-11 ■ Diagram showing respiratory excursions during normal breathing and during maximal inspiration and maximal expiration. (From Guyton AC, Hall JC. *Textbook of Medical Physiology*. 9th ed. Philadelphia, PA: Saunders; 1996:483.)

      i. Needle biopsy is used for the diagnosis of malignancy or infection; pneumothorax may be a complication.

      ii. Open lung biopsy requires a thoracotomy or thoracoscopic examination but has better diagnostic yields.

  e. Bronchoscopy: Insertion of a fiberoptic scope into the airways for direct visualization and possible obtaining of specimens

      i. Procedure is indicated for diagnosis of lung malignancy, evaluation of hemoptysis, removal of foreign body or secretions, and sampling of lung tissue via washings, brushings, or biopsy.

      ii. After the procedure, the patient must be observed for respiratory depression (due to sedatives), decreased ventilation, and hypoxemia.

      iii. Supplemental O_2 is administered during the procedure.

      iv. If transbronchial biopsy is performed, hemoptysis or pneumothorax is a possible complication.

  f. Mediastinoscopy: Performed for the diagnostic exploration of the mediastinum and to obtain biopsy specimens

Patient Care

1. Inability to establish or maintain a patent airway

  a. Description of problem: Blocked airway due to physiologic or mechanical obstruction and the inability of the patient to clear or maintain the airway. Clinical findings vary with the degree of obstruction and include abnormal breath sounds, altered respiratory rate or depth, cough, cyanosis (late), dyspnea.

  b. Goals of care

      i. Airway patency is maintained.

      ii. Breath sounds are clear with no adventitious sounds.

      iii. Secretions are easily expectorated or suctioned.

  c. Collaborating professionals on health care team: Nurse, physician, anesthesiologist, respiratory therapist

  d. Interventions

      i. Assist the patient to deep breathe.

         (a) Position to maximize inspiratory muscle length and to maximize ventilation (semi-Fowler's to high Fowler's position, depending on patient comfort).

(b) Ask the patient to take slow, deep breaths; assess volume (i.e., functional residual capacity [FRC] to total lung capacity [TLC]); ask the patient to hold the breath several seconds.

(c) Provide the patient with cues or devices to motivate independent deep-breathing exercises (e.g., incentive spirometer).

ii. Position the patient to facilitate coughing.

    (a) Help the patient assume a comfortable cough position (high Fowler's), with knees bent and a lightweight pillow over the abdomen to augment the expiratory pressures and minimize discomfort.

    (b) Teach the patient alternate cough techniques (controlled cough, the forced expiratory technique known as "huff coughing" or quad-assist cough). For controlled cough, the patient takes a slow maximal inspiration, holds the breath for several seconds, and follows with two or three coughs. Huff cough consists of one or two forced exhalations (huffs) from middle to low lung volumes with the glottis open.

    (c) Guaifenesin (an expectorant) may help to liquefy secretions.

iii. Provide an artificial airway and ventilation if indicated.

    (a) Oropharyngeal airway

      (1) Maintains the airway by holding the tongue anteriorly

      (2) Technique: Correct size measures from the corner of the patient's mouth to the angle of the jaw following the natural curve of the airway. Apply a jaw lift to help displace the tongue. Rotate the airway 180 degrees before insertion. As the tip of the airway reaches the hard palate, rotate the airway again by 180 degrees, aligning it as before in the pharynx.

      (3) Complications: Vomiting and aspiration with an intact gag reflex; malpositioning due to improper length; worsening of obstruction by pushing the tongue back further into the pharynx due to incorrect placement

    (b) Nasopharyngeal airway

      (1) Purpose: Useful in facial and jaw fractures when an oral airway cannot be used; more readily tolerated than the oropharyngeal airway

      (2) Complications: Nosebleed, nasal mucosa irritation

      (3) Adequate humidification: Essential to ensure the patency of a narrow lumen

      (4) Care: Airway should be taped in place to prevent inadvertent displacement. Tube should be removed periodically to prevent skin breakdown.

    (c) Endotracheal intubation: see Figure 2-12

      (1) **ETTs are generally managed in the ICU, but the progressive care unit registered nurse should be familiar with the procedure for intubation in the event of an emergency.**

      (2) Gather all the necessary equipment and inspect to ensure it is in working order.

        a) Suction system with catheters and tonsil (Yankauer) suction

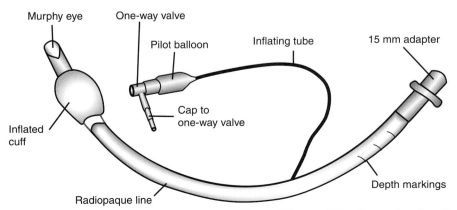

FIGURE 2-12 ■ Components of the endotracheal tube. (From Kirsten LD. *Comprehensive Respiratory Nursing: A Decision Making Approach.* Philadelphia, PA: Saunders; 1989:637.)

b) A manual resuscitation bag with a mask connected to 100% O_2
c) A laryngoscope handle with assorted blades
d) A variety of sizes of ETTs and a stylet

(3) Ensure the patient has patent IV access and electrocardiogram (ECG) and pulse oximetry monitoring in place.

(4) Administer sedation as ordered. Paralytics may also be used.

(5) Position the patient with the neck flexed and head slightly extended in the "sniff" position.

(6) Suction secretions from the oral cavity and pharynx and remove any dental devices.

(7) Preoxygenate and ventilate the patient using the manual resuscitation bag and mask with 100% O_2.

(8) Limit each intubation attempt to 30 seconds.

(9) Once the ETT is inserted, assess the patient for bilateral breath sounds and chest movement.
a) Feel air movement through the tube opening.
b) Assess for bilateral chest excursion during inspiration and expiration.
c) Auscultate both sides of the chest peripherally, as well as the abdomen.
d) Absence of breath sounds is indicative of an esophageal intubation.
e) Breath sounds heard over only one side are indicative of a mainstem intubation.

(10) Verify correct airway placement with a disposable end-tidal CO_2 detector or esophageal balloon.

(11) Inflate the cuff and secure the tube.

(12) Obtain a chest x-ray film to confirm placement.
a) The tip of the ETT should be approximately 3 to 5 cm above the carina.
b) Note the level of insertion (marked in centimeters on the side of the tube) at the teeth.

(13) Complications include nasal and oral trauma, pharyngeal and hypopharyngeal trauma, vomiting with aspiration, and cardiac arrest. Hypoxemia and hypercapnia can also occur, resulting in bradycardia, tachycardia, dysrhythmias, hypertension, and hypotension.

(d) Tracheostomy

(1) Purpose and indications
a) To facilitate removal of secretions from the tracheobronchial tree
b) To decrease dead space ventilation
c) To bypass an upper airway obstruction or provide an alternative airway
d) To prevent or limit the aspiration of oral or gastric secretions (cuffed tubes)
e) To aid in patient comfort when assisted or controlled ventilation is needed for an extended period of time

(2) Principles of care
a) Stoma is kept clean and dry.
b) Frequency of inner cannula tube exchanges with disposable tubes and of routine cleaning of inner cannulas with reusable inner cannulas follows hospital or institutional guidelines.
1) Be prepared for complications during any cleaning procedure.
2) Keep the following equipment at the bedside:
a) Self-inflating manual resuscitation bag and mask
b) Suction equipment (include catheters, O_2 flowmeter, tubing)
c) Tracheal tube and stoma cleaning supplies
3) Have an extra tracheostomy tube of the same size and type at the bedside.
c) Uncuffed tubes are commonly used in children and adults with laryngectomies and are sometimes used during decannulation or weaning (progressive downsizing of tube).
d) Cuffed tubes are typically used when the patient is receiving artificial ventilation (Figure 2-13). Tube may have an air-filled or self-inflating foam cuff, depending on the brand.

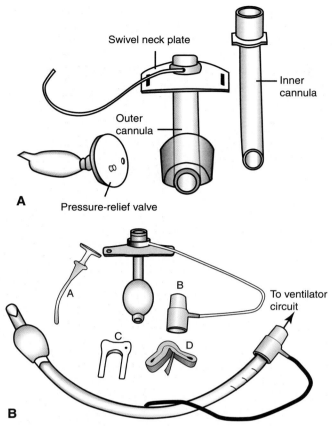

FIGURE 2-13 ■ Tracheostomy tubes. **A,** Shiley tracheostomy tube with disposable inner cannula. **B,** Bivona foam-cuffed tubes. *A,* Obturator; *B,* sideport airway connector; *C,* wedge; *D,* fabric tape. (From Kirsten LD. *Comprehensive Respiratory Nursing: A Decision Making Approach.* Philadelphia, PA: Saunders; 1989:656, 659.)

     e) Suctioning is always a sterile procedure except at home, where a clean technique may be used.

  (3) Weaning from the tracheostomy tube

     a) Decannulation will depend on whether the underlying patient condition that led to the need for the artificial airway has improved or reversed to the extent that the tracheostomy tube is no longer necessary.

     b) Patient must demonstrate physiologic and psychologic independence from an artificial airway. Techniques include the use of the following:

       1) Cuff deflation periods, with the tube opening capped to allow breathing through the upper airway

       2) Tracheostomy button

       3) Fenestrated tube with the cuff inflated or deflated, with the external tube opening capped or occluded to permit airflow to be directed to the upper airway

       4) Progressive downsizing of the tube from the original size to a smaller one

     c) Patient is monitored carefully to see how weaning is tolerated; blood gas studies and clinical observations are used.

     d) Complete sealing of the tracheotomy incision may occur within 72 hours of decannulation. Patients cannot produce adequate coughing pressure until this is accomplished.

iv. Prevent complications of airway intubation: See Box 2-4

▒ BOX 2-4
▒ **PREVENTION OF COMPLICATIONS OF AIRWAY INTUBATION**

PHYSIOLOGIC ALTERATIONS CAUSED BY AIRWAY DIVERSION
- Inspired air is inadequately conditioned and is irritating to delicate pulmonary membranes.
- Plastic or metal tubes are foreign bodies; they cause greater mucus production and impair ciliary movement.
- Accumulated oral bacteria and secretions provide a good medium for bacterial growth and may precipitate ventilator-associated pneumonia.
- Bypassing the larynx produces aphonia.
- Eliminating the glottis from the air route prevents the development of increased intrathoracic pressures, which makes effective coughing difficult.

COMPLICATIONS OCCURRING WHILE THE TUBE IS IN PLACE
OBSTRUCTION DUE TO
- Plugging with secretions that have become dried and inspissated; this is entirely preventable by systemic hydration and proper use of humidification and suctioning
- Herniation of the cuff over the end of the tube
- Kinking of the tube
- Cuff overinflation

TRACHEAL TUBE CUFFS
- Cuff design characteristics
  1. Low sealing pressure; intracuff pressure should not exceed the capillary filling pressure of the trachea (≤ 25 cm H_2O or ≤ 20 mm Hg) to avoid tracheal mucosal injury
  2. Cuff pressure is distributed over a large contact area.
  3. Large volumes of air are accepted with minor increases in balloon tension.
  4. Provides sufficient pressure to maintain an adequate seal during inspiration and expiration (necessary to allow positive pressure ventilation and the use of PEEP). Also may help prevent pulmonary aspiration of large food particles but does not protect against aspiration of liquids, such as water and enteral formula feedings.
  5. Does not distort tracheal wall
- Low-pressure, high-volume cuffs generally meet the desired characteristics and have replaced low–residual-volume, high-pressure cuffs.
- Special cuffs (e.g., Fome-Cuf, Bivona) are available for both endotracheal and tracheal tubes (see Figure 2-13). These devices inflate passively to fill a spongelike cuff that produces little or no pressure against the trachea. May be difficult to maintain a seal with positive pressure ventilation and increased PEEP or peak pressures.
- Principles of cuff inflation and deflation
- Inflation of low-pressure cuffs:
  Inflate with sufficient air to ensure no leak (minimal occlusive volume technique) or only minimal leak during peak inspiration (minimal leak technique).
  Need for increasing amounts of air to obtain a seal may be due to tracheal dilation or to a leak in the cuff or pilot balloon valve; the condition should be corrected.
- Routine deflation is not necessary. Periodic deflation may be useful so that the patient can breathe around the tube to facilitate speech (often difficult to accomplish when the patient is receiving mechanical ventilation).
  Regardless of cuff design or pressure characteristics, all cuff pressures should be routinely measured at least every 8 to 12 hours and whenever the cuff is reinflated or the tube position is changed.

DISPLACEMENT OR DISLODGMENT
Displacement or dislodgment out of the trachea (endotracheal or tracheostomy tube) and inadvertent movement into a false passage or pretracheal space (tracheostomy tube)
- Especially hazardous during the first 3 to 7 days of tracheostomy. Avoid by using a tube of the proper length and fixing it securely to the patient. Although securing the tube is important, care of the stoma and surrounding skin to prevent skin breakdown or pressure sores from the tube neck plate is also important.
- Dislodgment out of the trachea into tissue causes mediastinal emphysema, subcutaneous emphysema, and pneumothorax. Diagnosis is determined by observation of reduced or absent airflow movement from the tube opening, deterioration in blood gas values and/or vital signs, observations of neck and local tissue swelling with crepitations by palpation, poor chest excursion and respiratory distress, and inability to pass a suction catheter properly through the tube.

- Low tube placement into one bronchus or at the level of the carina results in obstruction or atelectasis of the nonventilated lung. Check the placement of the endotracheal tube by auscultation, followed by radiographic examination or use of a fiberoptic scope.
    1. Displacement into one bronchus: Signs and symptoms are as follows:
    Decreased or delayed motion on one side of the chest
    Unilateral diminished breath sounds
    Excessive coughing
    Localized expiratory wheeze
    2. Placement at the level of the carina: Signs and symptoms are as follows:
    Excessive coughing
    Localized expiratory wheeze
    Difficulty in introducing the suction catheter
    Bilateral diminished breath sounds

OTHER COMPLICATIONS

- Poor oral hygiene; mouth care is absolutely essential
- Local infection of tracheostomy wound, tracheal tissue, or lungs; tracheostomy should be treated as a surgical wound and specimens for culture should be obtained if active infection is suspected
- Massive hemorrhage resulting from erosion of the tracheostomy tube into the innominate vessels; may be fatal. Occurs most often with low placement of the tube, excessive "riding" of the tube within the trachea, or pulling torsion on the tube; watch for pulsations moving the tube with the heartbeat.
- Disconnection between the tracheal tube and ventilator
    1. Most likely to occur when the patient is being turned
    2. All ventilators must have adequate alarms.
    3. Frequent checking of all connections should be routine.
- Leaks caused by broken or malfunctioning cuff balloon or pilot valve
    1. Diagnosis is confirmed by the ability of a previously aphonic patient to talk, detection of air movement at the nose and mouth, pressure changes on the ventilator, and decreased exhaled volumes as measured with a handheld portable respirometer or ventilator spirometer.
    2. Tube must be removed and replaced. Always check the cuff for leaks before inserting; note the cuff pressure and amount of air required to fill the cuff and compare with later values.
- Tracheal ischemia, necrosis, dilation
    1. Because of the oval shape of the trachea and the round shape of the tube, there is a tendency for erosion in the anterior and posterior trachea.
    2. Diagnosis is indicated by the necessity to use larger and larger amounts of air to inflate the balloon to maintain the seal.
    3. May progress to tracheoesophageal fistula; this is indicated if food is aspirated through the trachea or air is in the stomach or if the results of a methylene blue dye test are positive
    4. Prevention is through the use of low-pressure cuffs and routine monitoring of cuff pressures.

EARLY POSTEXTUBATION COMPLICATIONS
ACUTE LARYNGEAL EDEMA

- Most frequently seen in children
- In adults, is commonly associated with the use of an oversized tube or with preexisting inflammation of the upper airway
- Prevention
    1. Close observation for several hours after extubation
    2. Patient may require supplemental O_2 after prolonged intubation; use of a bland aerosol, such as highly humidified air via a face mask or face tent, is controversial and of no proven benefit.
- Treatment
    1. Oxygen, steroids
    2. Introduction of a smaller endotracheal tube, tracheotomy
    3. Racemic epinephrine administered via small-volume nebulizer; intent is to reduce subglottic edema by inhalation of a potent vasoconstrictor

HOARSENESS

- Common following either short-term or long-term endotracheal intubation
- Usually disappears during the first week

Continued

■ **BOX 2-4**
■ **PREVENTION OF COMPLICATIONS OF AIRWAY INTUBATION—Cont'd**

ASPIRATION
- Aspiration of food, saliva, or gastric contents if the swallowing mechanism is impaired
- Presence of the tube over extended periods results in a loss of the usual protective reflexes of the larynx.
- Monitor the patient carefully during feedings; watch for excessive coughing; start with clear liquids after tube removal.

DIFFICULTY IN REMOVING THE TRACHEOSTOMY TUBE
- More frequently seen in infants but occurs in adults as well
- Related to the narrow lumen of the trachea, which is further reduced by swelling

LATE POSTEXTUBATION COMPLICATIONS
FIBROTIC STENOSIS OF THE TRACHEA
- Caused by prolonged use of any tube with a rigid inflatable cuff
- Follows earlier ulceration and necrosis of the site
- Lesions may become advanced before the appearance of clinical evidence (dyspnea, stridor); a tracheoesophageal fistula may form.
- Prevented by the use of low-pressure cuffs and proper monitoring of cuff pressures

STENOSIS OF THE LARYNX
- Caused by the discrepancy between the anatomy of the larynx and the size and shape of the tube
- Treatment
  1. Dilation or surgical intervention
  2. Permanent tracheostomy

e. Evaluation of patient care
   i. Breath sounds are clear bilaterally with no adventitious sounds.
   ii. Patient is able to expectorate or suction secretions.
   iii. ABG levels are within acceptable limits.
   iv. Patient or caregiver is able to care for the artificial airway.
2. **Impaired respiratory mechanics**
   a. Description of problem: Patient is unable to maintain adequate oxygen supply because of structural impediments (e.g., airway constriction, closure, or obstruction by secretions; a flattened diaphragm; respiratory muscle fatigue; loss of structural integrity of the thoracic cage). Clinical findings may include dyspnea, tachypnea, fremitus, abnormal ABG values, cyanosis (late finding), cough, nasal flaring, use of accessory muscles of respiration, assumption of a three-point position or the use of pursed-lip breathing, prolonged expiratory phase, increased A-P chest diameter, and altered chest excursion.
   b. Goals of care
      i. Respiratory rate, tidal volume, and maximal inspiratory pressure are within normal limits for the patient.
      ii. Dyspnea at rest is minimal; exertional dyspnea is decreased.
      iii. Patient takes bronchodilator medications as prescribed.
      iv. Patient is able to pace the activities of daily living (ADLs) in line with ventilatory function.
   c. Collaborating professionals on health care team: Physician, pulmonologist, nurse, respiratory therapist, possibly physical or occupational therapist
   d. Interventions
      i. Teach pursed-lip breathing, abdominal stabilization, and directed or controlled coughing techniques to minimize the energy expenditure of respiratory muscles. Pursed-lip breathing forces the patient to breathe slowly and establishes a back pressure in the airway, which helps to stabilize the airway and diminish dyspnea, especially after exertion.

    ii. Evaluate the status of the inspiratory muscles and, if appropriate, initiate inspiratory muscle training.
- (a) Inspiratory muscle training may improve the conscious control of the respiratory muscles and decrease the anxiety associated with increased respiratory effort.
- (b) Improved respiratory muscle strength may improve exercise tolerance and decrease dyspnea.
- (c) Monitor O_2 saturation via pulse oximetry as a measure of tolerance during training.

    iii. Teach the patient medication names, doses, method of administration, schedule, and appropriate behavior should an adverse effect occur. Instruct in the consequences of improper use of medications.
- (a) β-Agonists and anticholinergics are bronchodilators commonly prescribed to decrease airflow resistance and the work of breathing.
- (b) Patient should be able to demonstrate the proper technique for MDI self-administration. Spacer may be attached to the MDI to optimize medication delivery. If technique is poor or the patient is unable to use an MDI, assess the need for an alternative delivery device, such as a small-volume nebulizer.

    iv. Teach the patient to modify ADLs within ventilatory limits.
- (a) Encourage periodic hyperinflation of the lungs with a series of slow, deep breaths.
- (b) Hyperinflation therapy helps to prevent atelectasis and reduced lung compliance by expanding the alveoli, which are partially closed, and by mobilizing airway secretions.

    v. Monitor the rate and pattern of respiration, breath sounds, use of accessory muscles of respiration, and sensation of dyspnea. Clinical manifestations of respiratory muscle fatigue include the following:
- (a) Shallow, rapid breathing in early stages
- (b) Use of accessory muscles and a paradoxical breathing pattern
- (c) Active use of expiratory muscles, magnified sense of dyspnea
- (d) Respiratory alternans

  e. Evaluation of patient care
- **i.** Rate, depth, and pattern of ventilation are in the normal range for the patient.
- **ii.** Patient reports decreased dyspnea at rest and with exertion.
- **iii.** When inspiratory muscle training is appropriate, the patient's use of this training improves maximal inspiratory pressures.
- **iv.** Patient demonstrates safe and correct inhalation of respiratory medications and identifies side effects to be reported.

3. Impaired alveolar ventilation

  a. Description of problem: Inability to maintain spontaneous ventilation. Clinical findings include an ineffective breathing pattern, dyspnea, tachypnea or apnea, accessory muscle use, abnormal ABG levels, excess work of breathing.

  b. Goals of care
- **i.** Respiratory rate and breathing pattern are normal for the patient.
- **ii.** ABG levels are within acceptable limits for the patient.
- **iii.** Dyspnea is decreased with no air trapping at the end of expiration.
- **iv.** No evidence of ventilator-related complications is apparent.

  c. Collaborating professionals on health care team: Nurse, physician, anesthesiologist, respiratory therapist, infection control specialist, home care service aide

  d. Interventions
- **i.** Promote normal rest and sleep patterns. Plan activities to allow rest periods. Rest allows energy reserves to be replenished. Sleep deprivation blunts the patient's respiratory drive.
- **ii.** Provide an appropriate level of mechanical ventilatory support as warranted (Box 2-5).
- **iii.** Prevent the development of complications associated with the use of positive pressure ventilation (Box 2-6).
- **iv.** Provide optimal methods for weaning (also called liberating) patients from continuous mechanical ventilation.

■ **BOX 2-5**
■ **LEVELS OF VENTILATORY SUPPORT**

OBJECTIVES OF MECHANICAL VENTILATION
PHYSIOLOGIC OBJECTIVES
- To support or otherwise manipulate pulmonary gas exchange
  1. Alveolar ventilation (e.g., arterial partial pressure of carbon dioxide [Pa_{CO_2}] and pH)
  2. Arterial oxygenation (e.g., partial pressure of oxygen [Pa_{O_2}], arterial oxygen saturation [Sa_{O_2}], and oxygen content [Ca_{O_2}])
- To increase lung volume
  1. End-inspiratory lung inflation
  2. Functional residual capacity
- To reduce or otherwise manipulate the work of breathing

CLINICAL OBJECTIVES
- To reverse hypoxemia
- To reverse acute respiratory acidosis
- To relieve respiratory distress
- To prevent or reverse atelectasis
- To reverse ventilatory muscle fatigue
- To permit sedation and/or neuromuscular blockade
- To decrease systemic or myocardial oxygen consumption
- To reduce intracranial pressure
- To stabilize the chest wall

POSITIVE PRESSURE VENTILATORS
- Most common type of ventilatory support used in critical care. Apply positive pressure to the airways during the clinician-selected pattern of ventilation.
- Response of the breath delivery system to patient efforts
  1. Triggering: Initiation of gas delivery. Significant ventilatory loads can be imposed by insensitive or unresponsive ventilator triggering systems. Oversensitive valves can result in spontaneous ventilator cycling independent of patient effort.
  2. Gas delivery: Flow from the ventilator is governed (or limited) by a set flow (flow limited) or set pressure (pressure limited) on most machines
  3. Cycling: Gas delivery can be terminated at a preset volume, time, or flow
- Response of patient efforts to ventilator settings
  1. Alteration of the activity of mechanoreceptors in the airways, lungs, and chest wall
  2. Alteration of arterial blood gas (ABG) values
  3. Elicitation of respiratory sensations in conscious or semiconscious patients
  4. Result is a change in rate (ventilatory demand), depth, and timing of respiratory efforts (synchrony between patient and ventilator) through neural reflexes and chemical (chemoreceptors), and behavioral responses.

STANDARD MODES OF MECHANICAL VENTILATION
Modes of mechanical ventilation are classified according to initiation of the inspiratory cycle.
- *Assist control (A/C):* Every breath is supported by the ventilator. Backup control ventilatory rate is set, but the patient may choose any rate above the set rate. Most ventilators deliver A/C ventilation using volume-cycled or volume-targeted breaths. Pressure-limited or pressure-targeted A/C is available on certain ventilators.
- *Synchronized intermittent mandatory ventilation (SIMV):* Mode of ventilation and weaning that combines a preset number of ventilator-delivered mandatory breaths of predetermined tidal volume with the capability for intermittent patient-generated spontaneous breaths. The mandatory breath is delivered in synchrony with the patient's effort.
- *Pressure support ventilation (PSV):* Pressure-targeted, flow-cycled mode of ventilation in which each breath must be triggered by the patient. Application of positive pressure to the airway is set by the clinician. This augmentation to inspiratory effort starts at the initiation of inhalation and typically ends when a minimum inspiratory flow rate is reached. There are two applications for this mode:
  1. Used in conjunction with SIMV to improve patient tolerance and decrease the work of spontaneous breaths, especially from demand-flow systems and endotracheal tubes with a narrow inner diameter
  2. Used as a stand-alone ventilatory mode for patients under consideration for weaning or during the stabilization period

- *Continuous positive airway pressure (CPAP):* Designed to elevate end-expiratory pressure to above atmospheric pressure to increase lung volume and oxygenation. All breaths are spontaneous, and therefore an intact respiratory drive is required. Can be used in intubated, as well as nonintubated, patients via a face or nasal mask. Depending on machine type, CPAP is delivered via a continuous flow or demand valve system.
- *Bilevel positive airway pressure* (BiPAP, Respironics, Inc.): This noninvasive ventilatory assist device employs a spontaneous breathing mode with the baseline pressure elevated above zero. Unlike CPAP, BiPAP allows separate regulation of inspiratory and expiratory pressures. Application of BiPAP is essentially a combination of PSV with CPAP. The differences between inspiratory and expiratory positive airway pressures (IPAP and EPAP, respectively) contribute to the total ventilation. Enhances the capabilities of home CPAP for obstructive sleep apnea to provide nocturnal support in a variety of restrictive and obstructive disorders. Affords a noninvasive means of augmenting alveolar ventilation in hypercapnic respiratory failure.

GUIDELINES FOR VENTILATOR ADJUSTMENT DURING VOLUME-TARGETED (VOLUME-CYCLED) VENTILATION

All ventilator controls and settings are adjusted according to the patient's underlying disease process and the results of ABG analysis.

- *Minute ventilation:* Usually 6 to 10 L/min but may be much higher, depending on patient needs
- *Tidal volume:* Governed by estimated tidal volume; normally varies from 8 to 10 ml/kg ideal body weight to prevent lung overinflation and potential stretch injury to the lung tissue. Preset tidal volume may be reduced to 6 to 8 ml/kg. Intentional use of lower tidal volumes may cause an increase in arterial CO_2 levels and is therefore referred to as permissive hypercapnia. Low tidal volume has been shown to lower mortality in some settings. Use of intermittent sighs during mechanical ventilation is no longer routinely recommended.
- *Respiratory rate:* Varies from 8 to 12 breaths/min for most clinically stable patients; rates above 20 breaths/min are sometimes necessary
- *Flow rate:* Adjusted so that inspiratory volume delivery can be completed in a time frame that allows adequate time for exhalation. Inspiratory flow rate range of about 40 to 100 L/min is most commonly employed. Slow flow rates are preferred for optimal air distribution in normal lungs; faster flow rates are beneficial in patients with obstructive lung disease. Altering the flow rate may reduce the work of breathing, improve patient-ventilator synchrony, and increase the comfort of patients who are restless while undergoing mechanical ventilation.
- *I/E ratio:* Normal ratio is 1:2 to 1:3
- Inspiratory flow of gas from the ventilator: Depending on the model, can be delivered using one of several flow patterns, such as decelerating, square wave, or sine wave
- *Oxygen concentration:* Initially, the fraction of inspired oxygen (F_{IO_2}) is deliberately set at a high value (often 1.0) to ensure adequate oxygenation. An ABG sample is obtained, and the F_{IO_2} is adjusted according to the patient's arterial partial pressure of oxygen (Pa_{O_2}) and Sa_{O_2}. Inspired partial pressure of O_2 is adjusted so that Pa_{O_2} is acceptable for the patient's condition. This is usually a Pa_{O_2} higher than 55 mm Hg or an Sa_{O_2} of 88% or higher. Excessively high levels for prolonged periods can cause oxygen toxicity. The lowest F_{IO_2} that achieves an acceptable Pa_{O_2} and Sa_{O_2} should be used.
- *Positive end-expiratory pressure (PEEP):* Used as appropriate to reduce the F_{IO_2} to safe levels
- *Humidification:* Continuous humidification is mandatory, with inspired air warmed to near body temperature. Standard humidifiers using a water feed system must be monitored closely for water condensation in the tubing and emptied routinely. Heat and moisture exchanges (HME) are sometimes used.
- *Sensitivity:* Established parameters are followed for sensitivity settings (when the patient can trigger the machine for "assistance"); sensitivity is adjusted so that minimal patient effort is required, usually −0.50 to −1.5 cm H_2O; certain ventilators allow for a flow-triggering mechanism and should be set to their maximum sensitivity (1 to 3 L/min)
- *Pressure limit alarms:* Should be set at approximately 10 to 15 cm H_2O above the patient's normal peak inflation pressure (PIP) or airway pressure. Goal is to keep PIP below 35 to 40 cm H_2O if possible. Peak inspiratory plateau is equal to or less than 35 cm H_2O. Certain ventilators provide a low–airway-pressure alarm feature. Check that all other alarms are operational and on at all times.

ASSESSMENT OF THE EFFECTIVENESS OF MECHANICAL VENTILATION

- Some general measures include the following:
  1. All patients on life support equipment should be monitored and clinically observed routinely according to institutional policy.
  2. Physical assessment should be performed each shift.
  3. Ventilator system and its current settings should be assessed.

Continued

■ **BOX 2-5**
■ **LEVELS OF VENTILATORY SUPPORT—Cont'd**

4. Manual self-inflating resuscitation bag should be open and ready for use.
5. Suction equipment should be in working order and ready for use.
6. When medications are to be given, orders must be written clearly and precisely (e.g., a bronchodilator can be administered continuously by aerosol or via the ventilator circuit by metered dose inhaler).
7. Many patients have an arterial line, cardiac monitor, intravenous line, and urinary catheter if they are on continuous ventilatory support.

■ General monitoring for patients on continuous ventilatory support
1. Hemodynamic monitoring (arterial or pulmonary artery catheter) if indicated
2. Cardiac monitoring, heart sounds, pulses, pulse pressures, electrocardiogram as needed or as part of standard intensive care unit routine
3. Pulmonary function studies: Vital capacity, negative inspiratory pressure, minute ventilation, maximum voluntary ventilation, as required
4. Biochemical, hematologic, and electrolyte studies
5. Cardiac output assessment, blood volume status
6. Measurement of intake and output, body weight
7. Respiratory pattern assessment, breath sounds, symmetry in chest movement, vital signs
8. Inspection of dressings and drainages, tubes, and suction apparatus
9. Assessment of neurologic state, level of consciousness, pain, level of anxiety
10. Evaluation of response to treatments and medications

VENTILATORY MONITORING OF ANY PATIENT ON CONTINUOUS VENTILATION
■ Ventilation checks performed routinely
1. When blood gas samples are drawn
2. When changes are made in ventilator settings
3. Hourly or more frequently for any patient in unstable condition
4. Routinely throughout each shift
■ Components of the ventilator sheet to be recorded on the nursing flow sheet
1. Blood gas values
Record source (arterial, mixed venous) with ventilator settings and measurements so that decisions about changes may be made.
It often is valuable to document the patient's position at the time of the blood gas drawing, because position changes (side lying, upright, supine) influence ventilation-perfusion relationships and, hence, blood gas analysis results.
2. Ventilator settings to be read from the machine
Ventilator mode (e.g., SIMV or A/C)
Tidal volume, machine preset rate, pressure support level (if used), preset minute volume, inspiratory flow rate or time, and preset I/E ratio (depending on mode and ventilator)
Temperature of the humidification device, temperature of the inspired gas
Oxygen concentration
Peak inflation airway pressure limit
PEEP level set
Alarms on
3. Ventilator measurements to be taken
PIP, plateau, and/or mean airway pressures if requested, and PEEP level (measurement of auto-PEEP may be required for some patients)
Fio_2, alveolar to arterial gradient or Pao_2/Fio_2 ratio, shunt fractions (if ordered)
Minute ventilation (exhaled), respiratory rate (both patient and machine), tidal volume (exhaled)
Effective compliance, static and dynamic; compliance curves (depending on institutional policy)
I/E ratio (displayed), dead space/tidal volume ratio (if requested)
4. Respiratory monitoring techniques during mechanical ventilation
Pulse oximetry: Noninvasive estimate of arterial oxygen saturation (Spo_2). See discussion in Monitoring Data under Patient Assessment.
End-tidal CO_2 ($Petco_2$) monitoring: Noninvasive sampling and measurement of exhaled CO_2 tension at the patient-ventilator interface. See discussion in Monitoring Data under Patient Assessment.

■ **BOX 2-6**
■ **COMPLICATIONS ASSOCIATED WITH POSITIVE PRESSURE VENTILATION**

CARDIAC EFFECTS
DECREASED CARDIAC OUTPUT
- Caused by decreased venous return to the heart and reduced transmural pressures (intracardiac minus intrapleural pressures). In addition, there are increases in pulmonary vascular resistance and juxtacardiac pressure from the surrounding distended lungs.
- Pulse changes, decreased urine output and blood pressure
- Treatment
  1. Positioning with the head flat and legs elevated (modified Trendelenburg's position)
  2. Administration of fluids to increase preload
  3. Adjustment of volumes delivered by ventilator
  4. Careful positive end-expiratory pressure (PEEP) titration; avoidance of auto-PEEP

POSSIBLE DYSRHYTHMIAS
- Causes: Hypoxemia and pH abnormalities
- Patients in unstable condition on ventilators should have cardiac monitoring.

PULMONARY EFFECTS
BAROTRAUMA (PNEUMOTHORAX, PNEUMOMEDIASTINUM, SUBCUTANEOUS EMPHYSEMA)
- Occurs when a high pressure gradient between the alveolus and adjacent vascular sheet causes the overdistended alveolus to rupture. Gas is forced into the interstitial tissue of the underlying perivascular sheet. The gas may dissect centrally along the pulmonary vessels to the mediastinum and into the fascial planes of the neck and upper torso; high inflation volumes, or volutrauma, have also been described as an important risk factor.
- Positive pressure ventilation, especially with PEEP, subjects patients to the risk of pneumothorax, particularly if high pressures and volumes are used.
- Barotrauma can occur with main-stem intubation, in patients with acute lung injury (ALI) or chronic obstructive pulmonary disease (COPD), and in other patients with acute lung injury.
- Diagnosis
  1. Increases in airway peak pressure
  2. Decreased breath sounds and chest movement on the affected side
  3. Changes in vital signs, restlessness, possible cyanosis
  4. Chest radiographic changes

ATELECTASIS
- Collapse of lung parenchyma from the occlusion of air passage, with reabsorption of gas distal to the occlusion
- Causes
  1. Obstruction
  2. Possible lack of periodic deep inflations in patients ventilated with small tidal volumes
- Diagnosis
  1. Diminished breath sounds or bronchial breath sounds, rales, or crackles
  2. Chest radiographic evidence
  3. Alveolar to arterial (A-a) gradient increases, ratio of arterial partial pressure of oxygen (Pa_{O_2}) to fraction of inspired oxygen ($F_{I_{O_2}}$) decreases, and compliance decreases
- Prevention
  1. Use of lower tidal volumes
  2. Humidification, vigorous tracheal suctioning based on need
  3. Chest physical therapy, repositioning

INABILITY TO LIBERATE (WEAN) FROM VENTILATOR
- Can occur in any patient, particularly those with COPD, cystic fibrosis, debilitation, malnutrition, and musculoskeletal disorders
- Mechanical ventilation eases the work of breathing for these patients, which makes the transition to breathing off the ventilator (i.e., weaning) difficult.

Continued

■ **BOX 2-6**
■ **COMPLICATIONS ASSOCIATED WITH POSITIVE PRESSURE VENTILATION—Cont'd**

HYPERCAPNIA—RESPIRATORY ACIDOSIS
- Inadequate ventilation leads to acute retention of carbon dioxide and decreased pH.
- Patients can tolerate increased arterial partial pressure of carbon dioxide ($Paco_2$) and decreased pH under certain circumstances.
- Corrected by improving alveolar ventilation and treating the underlying cause

HYPOCAPNIA—RESPIRATORY ALKALOSIS
- Due to hyperventilation, which causes increased elimination of carbon dioxide and increased pH
- If carbon dioxide is decreased too rapidly, shock or seizures may result, particularly in children.
- Maintain ventilation to produce a normal pH, not necessarily a normal partial pressure of carbon dioxide ($Paco_2$).
- Treatment
  1. Decrease the respiratory rate.
  2. Decrease the tidal volume if inappropriately high.
  3. Add mechanical dead space.

FLUID IMBALANCE
- Fluid retention: Due to overhydration by airway humidification and decreased urinary output because of possible antidiuretic hormone effects. Symptoms include the following:
  1. Increased A-a gradient, decreased Pao_2/Flo_2 ratio
  2. Decreased vital capacity and compliance
  3. Weight gain, intake greater than output
  4. Increased dead space/tidal volume ratio
  5. Hemodilution (decreased hematocrit and decreased sodium values)
  6. Increased bronchial secretions
- Dehydration related to decreased enteral or parenteral intake in relation to urinary and/or gastrointestinal output, and overdiuresis. In addition, insensible losses average 300 to 500 ml/day and increase with fever. See Chapters 5 and 6 for clinical findings.
- Signs and parameters to be monitored
  1. Daily weight changes (often more accurate than intake and output measurement)
  2. Skin turgor, moistness of the oral mucosa
  3. Hemoglobin and hematocrit values
  4. Character of pulmonary secretions
  5. Airway humidification

INFECTION AND VENTILATOR-ASSOCIATED PNEUMONIA
- Patients at risk: Debilitated, aged, immobile, early postoperative, or immunocompromised individuals
- Intubation bypasses normal upper airway defenses and makes oral care more difficult.
- Ventilatory equipment and therapy, particularly aerosols, may be the carrier.
- Suctioning technique may not be sterile.
- There may be cross-contamination between patients and staff or autocontamination.
- Pulmonary patients may have indwelling catheters of various types.
- Nonsterile solutions may be left out in open containers.
- Patients may be improperly positioned so that aspiration is possible, or the endotracheal tube cuff may not be inflated to minimal occlusive volume.
- Preventive measures
  1. Aseptic airway and tracheostomy technique
  2. Sterile suction technique using an open-suction or closed-suction catheter system
  3. Elevation of the head of the bed to 30 to 45 degrees continuously or as patient condition warrants
  4. Rigorous hand washing, which is mandatory and critical, as well as the use of personal protective equipment as necessary
  5. Meticulous oral care to assist in prevention, including teeth brushing to remove dental bacteria, which should be performed regularly and frequently
  6. Bronchial hygiene, chest physical therapy as indicated
  7. Isolation techniques as needed

8. Routine cultures of specimens from patients and machines
9. Avoidance of routine tracheal instillation of normal saline for lavage
10. Antibiotics as indicated
11. Restriction of the number of patient contacts (staff and visitors)
12. Early recognition and response to clinical and laboratory signs of infection
13. Change of ventilator tubing, including humidifier reservoirs, according to institutional policy; verify the length of time that the ventilator circuit is left in place before changing
14. Emptying and changing of reservoir water per institutional policy; empty water in tubing into a waste receptacle every 1 to 2 hours and as needed

GASTROINTESTINAL EFFECTS
COMPLICATIONS
- Stress ulcer and bleeding
- Adynamic ileus
- Gastric dilatation from loss of adequate nerve supply; fluid shifts may lead to shock

PREVENTION AND TREATMENT
- Routine auscultation of bowel sounds
- Antacids, histamine antagonists
- Hemoccult or Gastroccult and pH stomach aspirate testing; stool check for blood

PATIENT "FIGHTING" OF THE VENTILATOR, AGITATION, AND DISTRESS
CAUSES
- Incorrect ventilator setup for the patient's needs (e.g., inspiratory flow rate less than needed)
- Acute change in patient status
- Obstructed airway, pneumothorax
- Ventilator malfunction
- Acute anxiety
- Acute pain

MANAGEMENT
- Perform a rapid bedside check of the patient and ventilator.
- Disconnect the patient from the ventilator and provide manual ventilation with 100% oxygen via a self-inflating bag.
- Check vital signs, chest expansion, and bedside monitoring equipment.
- Suction the airway and check the patency of the endotracheal or tracheostomy tube.
- Obtain arterial blood gas values.
- Sedate the patient if indicated and order for acute anxiety, and give analgesics if pain is present; observe for hypoventilation and be prepared to adjust the ventilator setting to meet the patient's needs.

PRINCIPLES FOR MATCHING VENTILATION TO PATIENT NEEDS
- Do not assume that the patient will adjust to the ventilator; the reverse is desirable.
- Vary the cycle frequency, tidal volume, triggering sensitivity, and inspiratory flow rate until the correct combination is achieved.
- Provide calm reassurance and moderate sedation as indicated.

(a) Indications for weaning or liberation (term usually reserved for the gradual withdrawal of ventilatory support, although it includes the overall process of discontinuing ventilator support)
   (1) Underlying disease process is resolved; original signs of the need for ventilatory support are no longer present.
   (2) Patient's strength, vigor, and nutritional status are adequate.
   (3) Patient does not require more than 5 cm H_2O of positive end-expiratory pressure (PEEP) or an FIO_2 greater than 0.5 to maintain an acceptable PaO_2 (usually at least 55 to 60 mm Hg).

    (4) Patient has stable, acceptable hemodynamic parameters and Hb level.

    (5) Patient has stable and acceptable values for ABGs, V_T, vital capacity, respiratory rate, minute ventilation, maximum inspiratory and expiratory pressures, A-a gradient or Pao_2/Fio_2 ratio, and compliance; V_D/V_T ratio is within minimal acceptable range (<0.6).

    (6) Level of consciousness is acceptable.

    (7) Patient is psychologically prepared, emotionally ready, and cooperative.

    (8) Predictors of successful weaning and criteria for liberation trial include the following:

        a) Resting minute volume ($\dot{V}_E$) of less than 10 L and ability to double this value during a maximum voluntary ventilation effort

        b) Maximum inspiratory pressure more negative than -20 cm H_2O

        c) Spontaneous V_T greater than 5 ml/kg

        d) Spontaneous respiratory frequency (f) equal to or less than 30 breaths/min

        e) Vital capacity above 10 ml/kg body weight

        f) Pao_2/Fio_2 ratio higher than 200

        g) f/V_T ratio less than 105 (rapid shallow breathing index)

        h) Acceptable scores on integrative indices such as the Burns Wean Assessment Program (BWAP), CROP index (compliance, rate, oxygenation, pressure)

(b) Principles of liberation

    (1) Explain the procedure. Place the patient in an upright position for better lung expansion. Obtain baseline measurements of vital signs.

    (2) Obtain ventilatory measurements or weaning parameters while the patient is off the ventilator. Measure minute ventilation, rate, V_T, maximum inspiratory pressure, vital capacity (V_C), and maximum voluntary ventilation.

    (3) Be prepared to give periodic manual ventilations.

    (4) Consider returning the patient to the ventilator with baseline settings if signs of patient intolerance or tiring occur, including the following:

        a) Decreased V_T, increased respiratory rate

        b) Increasing $Paco_2$ and/or decreasing pH

        c) O_2 desaturation by blood gas analysis or pulse oximetry

        d) Patient apprehension, diaphoresis, fatigue, decreasing level of consciousness

        e) Cardiac dysrhythmias, changes in blood pressure or heart rate, or hemodynamic changes

    (5) Mechanisms contributing to failure to wean include insufficient ventilatory drive, hypoxemia, high ventilatory requirement, respiratory muscle weakness, low compliance, and excessive work of breathing. The longer it takes to resolve the problem that precipitated the need for ventilatory support, the more difficult it may be to wean.

(c) Techniques of discontinuing ventilator support (T tube, intermittent mandatory ventilation, pressure-supported ventilation, continuous positive airway pressure [CPAP]): See Box 2-7

(d) Treatment of the difficult-to-wean patient

    (1) Some patients pose significant problems in terms of costs, health care resources, and ethical dilemmas when ventilator removal is attempted.

    (2) Evaluate for and, if appropriate, initiate inspiratory muscle training (the benefit of this step is controversial).

    (3) Monitor O_2 saturation via oximeter during the training session to verify that the patient's blood does not desaturate.

    (4) Monitor the color, consistency, and volume of sputum. Change in sputum characteristics may indicate infection, which may increase the work of breathing.

    (5) Physical therapy and rehabilitation efforts are very important (with both physical and psychologic advantages).

    (6) Monitor the rate and depth of respiration, breath sounds, use of accessory muscles of respiration, and dyspnea.

▓ BOX 2-7
▓ TECHNIQUES FOR DISCONTINUING VENTILATOR SUPPORT

T-TUBE TRIAL

T-tube trial is also known as a Briggs, T-piece, or T-bar adapter trial. Patient is disconnected from the ventilator and attached to a high-humidity oxygen or air source by a T-shaped airway adapter.

- Total unassisted spontaneous breathing occurs, usually for 5 to 120 minutes depending on tolerance, followed by periods of rest.
- Optimal duration of the T-tube trial has not been standardized; patients are usually extubated once they can tolerate several hours of unassisted breathing.
- Arterial blood gas (ABG) levels are periodically measured to assess alveolar ventilation status.
- Careful visual observation is required because the ventilator is on standby status and without integral alarms in case of T-tube system disconnection.

INTERMITTENT MANDATORY VENTILATION

In intermittent mandatory ventilation (IMV), the amount of support provided by the ventilator is gradually reduced, and the amount of respiratory work done by the patient is progressively increased.

- Transition period may be several hours to several days, depending on the length of time ventilatory support was required, as well as institutional policy.
- Pace of decreasing the IMV rate is determined by clinical assessment and ABG analysis.
- Pressure support ventilation (PSV) is often used with IMV in lower amounts (5 to 10 cm H_2O); the IMV rate is reduced while the PSV level is held constant.

PRESSURE SUPPORT VENTILATION

Stand-alone mode of PSV is also used as a means of gradually reducing the level of ventilator support.

- PSV level is initially titrated to a spontaneous tidal volume of 10 to 12 ml/kg and then reduced in increments of 3 to 6 cm H_2O on the basis of clinical assessment and ABG analysis.
- PSV is titrated down until a low level of support is reached (5 to 10 cm H_2O).

CONTINUOUS POSITIVE AIRWAY PRESSURE

With continuous positive airway pressure (CPAP) ventilatory support, the patient breathes spontaneously (with no mechanical assistance) against a threshold resistance, with pressure above atmospheric levels maintained at the airway throughout breathing.

- CPAP level is initially set at 3 to 5 cm H_2O.
- May be helpful for patients with dynamic hyperinflation and auto–positive end-expiratory pressure
- When weaning trials are completed, the patient is usually extubated from CPAP at 3 to 5 cm H_2O.

In theory, CPAP prevents or limits the deterioration in oxygenation that often occurs when patients switch from mechanical ventilation to spontaneous breathing. Some data refute this notion.

(7) Monitor the patient for clinical signs of respiratory muscle fatigue, including shallow, rapid breathing (early); increased $Paco_2$, decreased respiratory rate (late).

(8) Observe for abnormal chest wall motion as an indication of respiratory muscle dysfunction.

    a) Paradoxical motion of the chest wall is characterized by expansion of the rib cage and inward motion of the abdomen during inspiration.

    b) Asynchronous chest wall motion is characterized by disorganized and uncoordinated respiratory motion.

(9) Administer appropriate drug therapy for maintenance of ventilation (Box 2-8).

  v. Assist the patient in maintaining adequate nutrition.

    (a) Assess nutritional status (see Chapter 8).

    (b) Provide nutritional support.

      (1) Oral feedings with calorie supplements; small, frequent feedings are often better tolerated by dyspneic patients

      (2) Enteral feedings via nasogastric, small-bore nasoenteral, or gastric feeding tubes for patients who cannot eat but have a functional gastrointestinal tract or have ETTs and cannot take oral feedings

■ BOX 2-8
■ DRUG THERAPY FOR MAINTENANCE OF VENTILATION

NARCOTICS
- Morphine sulfate, meperidine, and fentanyl, dosed to effect
- Act as a respiratory depressant; good euphoric agents and excellent analgesics
- Provide sedation and good control of ventilation without adverse side effects in a well-ventilated, well-oxygenated, acid-base–balanced patient; often used in combination with a benzodiazepine for sedative effects
- Sensation of dyspnea is reduced.
- Large dosages may cause increased venous capacitance.
- Drug tolerance may develop with prolonged use.

BENZODIAZEPINES
- Lorazepam and midazolam are the most commonly used agents in the critical care setting.
- These drugs cause a central nervous system (CNS)–depressant effect, which can lead to alveolar hypoventilation and respiratory acidosis, particularly in geriatric patients and in those with liver disease.
- Severe respiratory depression and apnea can result if they are used with other CNS-depressant drugs.
- As with any sedative agent, the routine use of a validated sedation scale for monitoring and assessing the degree of sedation is important.

BRONCHODILATORS
β-AGONISTS
- Stimulate β-receptors in the bronchial smooth muscle, which results in bronchial smooth muscle relaxation; the most potent bronchodilators currently available
- Epinephrine: Stimulates β_1- and β_2-receptors; given by inhalation or parenterally, with rapid action either way; duration of action is 0.5 to 2 hours
- Metaproterenol: Has equal β_1 and β_2 effects; given in inhaled or oral form; duration of action is 3 to 4 hours
- Isoetharine: Mainly β_2 effects; given by inhalation; duration of action is 3 to 4 hours
- Terbutaline: Mainly β_2 actions; given subcutaneously, orally, or inhaled; duration of action is 2 to 4 hours for subcutaneous route, 3 to 7 hours inhaled, 5 to 8 hours orally; however, side effects are worse with oral doses
- Albuterol: Mostly β_2 selective; given in inhaled and oral forms; duration of action is 4 to 6 hours inhaled and 5 to 8 hours in oral form
- Bitolterol: Mostly β_2 selective; given in inhaled and oral forms; duration of action is 4 to 8 hours
- Pirbuterol: Mostly β_2 selective; given by inhalation; duration of action is 4 to 6 hours
- Salmeterol and formoterol: Mostly β_2 selective; given by inhalation; duration of action is 12 hours; because of the delay in the onset of action, this drug is never to be used in an acute bronchospasm attack

ANTICHOLINERGIC BRONCHODILATORS
- Block cholinergic constricting influences on bronchial muscle
- Work predominantly on the large airways
- Atropine and ipratropium: Given in inhaled form
- Tiotropium (Spiriva): 24-hour duration of action, given by powder inhalation

ANTIALLERGY MEDICATIONS
- Block immunoglobulin E–dependent mast cell release of mediators of bronchoconstriction, such as histamine and leukotrienes
- Cromolyn sodium: Does not actively bronchodilate but prevents bronchoconstriction; inhaled liquid given by metered dose inhaler, inhaled powder given by Spinhaler, or liquid nasal spray
- Nedocromil sodium: Given by inhalation aerosol (similar to cromolyn sodium)
- Montelukast: Given orally in the evening to counteract hormonal variation in bronchoconstriction

STEROIDS
- Augment the effects of β-agonist bronchodilators and are anti-inflammatory; often started at high dosage, then tapered off
- Dosage should be kept low to minimize adrenocortical and pituitary suppression and side effects.
- Prednisone: Oral dose often given once daily, in the early morning to minimize systemic side effects

- Hydrocortisone: Methylprednisolone given intravenously
- Inhaled steroids (beclomethasone, flunisolide, fluticasone triamcinolone): Given after inhaled β-agonists
- Provide beneficial pulmonary steroid effects with minimal systemic absorption
- When steroids are taken by inhalation, the patient must use a spacer device and rinse the mouth with water after each use to prevent fungal infection (candidiasis) of the oropharynx or larynx.

        (3) Total parenteral nutrition (TPN): Indicated for patients with a nonfunctional gastrointestinal tract

    (c) Provide general patient care and personal hygienic measures (especially meticulous oral care), which may improve the patient's appetite.

  e. Evaluation of patient care

    i. Acid-base and oxygenation parameters remain within normal limits.

    ii. Patient is comfortable and well rested on the ventilator with no air trapping or auto-PEEP.

    iii. No clinical evidence of ventilator-associated infections or complications is present.

4. Impaired respiratory gas exchange

  a. Description of problem: Inability to maintain adequate respiratory gas exchange. Clinical findings include confusion, anxiety, somnolence, restlessness, irritability, inability to mobilize secretions, hypercapnia, hypoxemia, hypoxia, dyspnea, cyanosis, tachycardia, and dysrhythmias.

  b. Goals of care

    i. Hypoxemia resolves or improves.

    ii. Eucapnia is present or the patient's usual compensated $Paco_2$ and pH levels are observed.

    iii. Patient performs ADLs and modifies self-care activity with or without supplemental O_2.

    iv. Patient indicates that he or she is able to breathe comfortably.

  c. Collaborating professionals on health care team: Nurse, physician, respiratory therapist, dietitian, physical therapist, social worker, discharge coordinator

  d. Interventions

    i. Assess oxygenation status.

      (a) Hypoxia-hypoxemia relationships

        (1) Hypoxia: Decrease in oxygenation at the tissue level (a clinical diagnosis); must be corrected; in some cases O_2 therapy alone may not correct tissue hypoxia

        (2) Hypoxemia: Decrease in arterial blood O_2 tension (a laboratory diagnosis). A normal Pao_2 alone does not guarantee adequate tissue oxygenation.

        (3) Organs most susceptible to lack of O_2: Brain, adrenal glands, heart, kidneys, liver, and retina of the eye

        (4) Factors governing effective oxygenation

          a) Sufficient O_2 supply in inspired air

          b) Sufficient ventilation to enable gas exchange between the atmosphere and the alveoli of the lungs

          c) Ready diffusion of gases across the alveolar-capillary membrane

          d) Adequate circulation of blood from the lungs to tissues; adequate volume of blood and Hb level. Falling cardiac output leads to a compensatory rise in O_2 extraction at the tissue level.

          e) O_2 brought to tissues must be readily released from the Hb molecule and be readily diffused into and taken up by various tissues.

      (b) Assessment of hypoxemia-hypoxia

        (1) Clinical signs and symptoms: See Description of Problem discussed previously; may also include apprehension, headache, angina, impaired judgment, hypotension, abnormal respirations, hypoventilation, yawning

        (2) ABG analysis, including oxyhemoglobin saturation, and content; Hb level; arteriovenous O_2 content differences (if pulmonary artery catheter is in place)

        (3) Noninvasive O_2 monitoring

          a) Pulse oximetry (Spo_2): See Patient Assessment

ii. Provide O_2 therapy.
   (a) Principles of O_2 therapy
      (1) Remember the airway; no O_2 treatment is of any use without a patent and adequate airway.
      (2) O_2 is a drug and should be administered in a prescribed dose (the FIO_2 is the dose).
      (3) Response to O_2 administration should be interpreted in terms of its effect on tissue oxygenation rather than only its effect on ABG values.
      (4) Disease pathology is the major determinant of the effectiveness of O_2 therapy.
      (5) Delivered concentration of gas from any appliance is subject to the condition of the equipment, the application technique, and the cooperation and ventilatory pattern of the patient.
      (6) Low-flow O_2 systems do not provide the total inspired gas (the patient breathes some room air) and therefore are adequate only if tidal volume is adequate, respiratory rate is not excessive, and ventilator pattern is stable. Variable O_2 concentrations (21% to 90%) are provided, but FIO_2 varies greatly with changes in tidal volume and ventilatory pattern.
      (7) High-flow O_2 systems provide the total inspired gas (the patient breathes only gas supplied by the apparatus) and are adequate only if flow rates exceed the inspiratory flow rate and minute ventilation. Both high and low O_2 concentrations (24% to 100%) may be delivered.
   (b) Rationale for the use of low-flow O_2 systems in patients with COPD and chronic CO_2 retention
      (1) Central chemoreceptors become desensitized to chronically high blood CO_2 levels, so CO_2 no longer serves as a respiratory stimulus; the only remaining stimulus to increase ventilation is hypoxemia. As a result, high concentrations of O_2 depress the ventilatory drive, which leads to $\dot{V}/\dot{Q}$ mismatching, the Haldane effect, depressed minute ventilation, and increased $Paco_2$.
      (2) Nursing implications
         a) Administer only enough O_2 to keep Pao_2 at adequate levels for the patient (50 to 60 mm Hg).
         b) Safety lies in the use of controlled low flow rates, monitoring of ABG levels, and careful observation.
   (c) Hazards of O_2 therapy
      (1) O_2-induced hypoventilation
         a) Prevent by the use of low flow rates and O_2 concentrations (FIO_2 of 0.24 to 0.30).
         b) Patient is at greatest risk when the $Paco_2$ is chronically elevated above normal.
         c) Use O_2 therapy with caution in patients with chronic CO_2 retention (see earlier); priority is to correct hypoxemia; if $Paco_2$ increases and pH decreases, may need to intubate or use bilevel positive airway pressure (BiPAP).
      (2) Absorption atelectasis: Due to the elimination of nitrogen (nitrogen washout) and the effect of O_2 on pulmonary surfactant
      (3) O_2 toxicity: Rarely seen in adults
         a) Due to lung exposure to a high concentration (exact level is controversial; usually considered to be FIO_2 >0.50 to 0.70) over an extended time (longer than 48 to 72 hours)
         b) May be mild or fatal
         c) Early signs and symptoms
            1) Retrosternal distress, dyspnea, coughing
            2) Restlessness, paresthesias in the extremities
            3) Nausea, vomiting, anorexia
            4) Fatigue, lethargy, malaise
         d) Late signs and symptoms: Progressive respiratory difficulty to asphyxia, cyanosis

e) Pathologic process

1) Local toxicity to the capillary endothelium leads to interstitial edema, which thickens the alveolar-capillary membrane. Type I alveolar cells are destroyed by an exudative response. In the end stages, hyaline membranes form in the alveolar region, followed by fibrosis and pulmonary hypertension.

2) Biochemical changes are most likely due to the overproduction of oxygen free radicals, which produce oxidation reactions that inhibit enzyme functions and/or kill cells. High Po_2 values can also release additional free radicals from neutrophils and platelets, which instigate the capillary endothelial damage described.

f) Both the concentration and duration of O_2 administration are critical (50% O_2 or higher over several days is potentially dangerous). Even low-flow O_2 (1 to 2 L/min) has been shown to produce cellular changes over time.

g) Clinical changes in O_2 toxicity: Decreased compliance and vital capacity, increased A-a gradient, reduced Pao_2/Fio_2 ratio

(4) Prevention of complications caused by O_2 therapy

a) O_2 is a potent drug that should be used only when indicated and according to preestablished goals of therapy.

b) If high concentrations are necessary, the duration of administration should be kept to a minimum and the concentration reduced as soon as possible.

c) Objective is to maintain Pao_2 of at least 55 to 60 mm Hg to produce an acceptable Sao_2 of 88% to 90% without causing lung injury or inducing CO_2 retention.

d) Reassessment of ABG levels is mandatory during the initial titration of O_2 therapy and when pulse oximetry values are questionable.

e) Depending on the O_2 delivery device used, the exact concentration of Fio_2 should be measured when appropriate with an O_2 analyzer.

f) Patients should never be exposed to dangerous levels of hypoxemia for fear of development of O_2 toxicity. Hypoxia is far more common than O_2 toxicity and must be corrected. Pure O_2 (100%) should never be withheld in an emergency.

(d) Methods of O_2 delivery (low-flow and high-flow systems): See Box 2-9

iii. Administer PEEP: Major oxygenation adjunct treatment modality

(a) Pressure above the atmospheric level is maintained at the airway opening at the end of expiration to prevent alveolar collapse.

(b) At the end of quiet expiration, lung volume is increased; therefore, FRC is increased. Increase in FRC depends on both the amount of PEEP used and the functional state of the lungs. Alveolar volume is increased; recruitment of alveoli occurs.

(c) Major goal of PEEP is enhanced O_2 transport by improvement in Pao_2 and Sao_2. PEEP reduces the shunt effect of collapsed alveoli and may increase Pao_2 dramatically. Another important goal of PEEP is to avoid increasing Fio_2, which could lead to O_2 toxicity.

(d) Clinical use of PEEP includes the following:

(1) ALI and the presence of diffuse pulmonary infiltrates, characterized by closure of the airways or the collapse of alveoli at end expiration, which results in refractory hypoxemia and increased Fio_2 requirements

(2) ARF that has caused a persistent hypoxemia with an Fio_2 of 0.5 or greater

(3) Cardiogenic pulmonary edema

(4) Avoidance of pulmonary O_2 toxicity from high Fio_2 values

(e) For dosing, the amount of PEEP is tailored to the patient's need; there is no arbitrary upper limit. Determination of the optimal level requires accurate assessment of cardiopulmonary function, including measurement of peak and plateau airway pressures, blood pressure, and cardiac output when available. PEEP levels above 10 to 12 cm H_2O are generally considered high.

(f) Side effects of PEEP include the following:

■ **BOX 2-9**
■ **METHODS OF OXYGEN DELIVERY**

MASKS
GENERAL POINTS
- Useful if O_2 is needed quickly and for short periods
- Concentrations of 24% to 100% O_2 are delivered, depending on the device

DISADVANTAGES
- Uncomfortable and hot
- Irritation of the skin caused by tight fit
- Difficult to control the fraction of inspired O_2 (FIO_2) precisely, except when the Venturi mask is used
- Must be removed when the patient eats, so that O_2 delivery is lost

POSSIBLE COMPLICATIONS
- Patients who are prone to vomit may experience aspiration.
- Obstruction by a flaccid tongue may occur in comatose patients; use an oral airway and secure it.
- May cause CO_2 retention and hypoventilation if the flow is too low and exhalation ports are obstructed

TYPES OF MASK
- Simple
  1. 35% to 60% O_2 at flows of 6 to 10 L/min
  2. FIO_2 varies considerably with changes in tidal volume, ventilatory pattern, and inspiratory flow rate and with a tight or loose fit of the mask.
- Partial rebreathing
  1. Delivers 35% to 60% O_2 or higher at flows of 6 to 10 L/min
  2. Portion of exhaled breath enters the reservoir bag to be rebreathed with incoming 100% O_2 in the next breath.
  3. Flows must be adjusted so that the reservoir bag does not completely collapse during inspiration; otherwise, CO_2 retention may occur.
- Nonrebreathing
  1. Delivers 90% or more O_2 concentration, provided there are no leaks in the system; a one-way valve between the reservoir bag and mask prevents rebreathing from the 100% O_2 gas source
  2. Ideal method of delivering a high O_2 gas concentration for the short term
  3. Reservoir bag must not collapse during inspiration.
- Air entrainment (Venturi mask)
  1. Adjustments allow for the delivery of precise O_2 concentrations of 24% to 50%.
  2. Total airflow must be adequate for the ventilatory needs of the patient.
  3. Best suited to patients who must have a consistent FIO_2

NASAL CANNULA
- Low O_2 concentrations are delivered (<40%), but level depends on the patient's tidal volume.
- FIO_2 can be estimated as a 4% increase in FIO_2 for each liter of O_2 flow; generally not run at flow rates beyond 5 or 6 L/min.
- Humidifier is not necessary unless flow rates exceed 4 L/min.

ADVANTAGES
- Easy to apply
- Light
- Economical
- Disposable
- Patient mobility allowed

DISADVANTAGES
- Easily dislodged
- High flow rates uncomfortable (dryness and bleeding)
- Possible skin breakdown around the ears caused by tubing, nasal dryness, and breakdown of mucous membranes from the prongs

NASAL CATHETER

- Low O_2 concentrations delivered (<40%)
- Catheter should not be forced through the nose; periodic rotation of a new catheter to the opposite nares should be done at least every 8 hours; rarely used in adults.
- Eventual delivery of O_2 to blood is not significantly different regardless of whether a cannula or a catheter is used or whether the patient's mouth is open or closed. Variability in F_{IO_2} is caused by the O_2 flow rate setting and the patient's rate and depth of respiration.

DISADVANTAGES

- Technique of insertion
- Potential for gastric distention
- Potential for nasopharyngeal injury

RESERVOIR CANNULA

Combines the concepts of low flow and reservoir delivery systems. Reservoir cannula stores about 20 ml of O_2 during exhalation. Pendant reservoir delivery system is situated over the anterior chest wall.

ADVANTAGES

- Decreased flow needed for a given F_{IO_2}
- Reduced O_2 costs
- Allows longer periods away from a stationary O_2 source

DISADVANTAGES

- Patients may object to the appearance of a reservoir "mustache" cannula.
- F_{IO_2} variability still exists.
- Amount of O_2 savings varies greatly, depending on individual patient needs.

AIR ENTRAINMENT NEBULIZER

Air entrainment nebulizer, a pneumatically powered device containing sterile water, is capable of providing high-level humidification in the form of an aerosol and a heat control, as well as delivering O_2 at a preset F_{IO_2}. Dilution of the 100% O_2 source from the flow meter occurs via a fixed or adjustable air entrainment port located on the nebulizer canister. F_{IO_2} can be set from 0.21 to 1.0.

ADVANTAGES

- Ideal for providing humidification for a patient with an artificial airway
- Humidified air or O_2 is delivered by using a variety of attachments, including the following:
  1. Aerosol mask
  2. Face tent
  3. Tracheostomy collar
  4. T-tube or Briggs adapter

DISADVANTAGES

- Air entrainment nebulizers generate consistent F_{IO_2} delivery to the patient only when their output flow meets or exceeds the patient's inspiratory flow demands.
- Because water condensation in large-bore tubing obstructs total flow and decreases air entrainment, F_{IO_2} increases.
- Delivered F_{IO_2} is more variable at O_2 concentrations above 40%.

(1) Exacerbation of the same hemodynamic consequences that occur with positive pressure breathing (see Box 2-6). Patients with poor cardiovascular dynamics are at most risk. Adequate intravascular volume is essential.

(2) Barotrauma or volutrauma: Rupture of lung tissue at high PEEP levels, especially in patients with acute lung injury (ALI). Associated with high peak and plateau inflation pressures and high mean airway pressures.

   (g) Monitoring guidelines are as follows:
      (1) It is essential to monitor the parameters that indicate the status of cardiac output and tissue perfusion (see Chapter 3).
      (2) Urinary output should be closely monitored.
      (3) If a significant drop in cardiac output occurs, PEEP may need to be reduced, or vasoactive drug support for blood pressure may be indicated. Hypovolemia, if present, must be corrected when this is a contributing factor to decreased cardiac output. Short-term inotropic therapy may sometimes be employed to correct decreased cardiac output in a normovolemic patient with known or suspected ventricular dysfunction.
      (4) PEEP is lost if the patient is disconnected from the ventilator for suctioning. For this reason, closed-suction catheter systems are often used for mechanically ventilated patients to maintain PEEP levels during suctioning. If a precipitous drop in SpO_2 occurs during suctioning, preoxygenation before the procedure becomes critical.
   iv. Administer CPAP (see Boxes 2-5 and 2-7).
      (a) Similar to PEEP but used in spontaneously breathing patients via a nasal mask. May also be used in ventilator-dependent patients to improve Pao_2 and saturation levels.
      (b) Used during weaning from mechanical ventilation, for obstructive sleep apnea, and in select pediatric patients
   v. Encourage the patient to take deep breaths (see Inability to Establish or Maintain a Patent Airway).
   vi. Position the patient to facilitate $\dot{V}/\dot{Q}$ matching ("good side down").
   vii. Provide rest periods between activities to minimize O_2 demands.
   viii. Alleviate or minimize anxiety, which may increase O_2 demands.
   ix. Monitor the patient's response to any activity. If deterioration occurs, assist the patient with care, including helping with turning and transfer, and passive range-of-motion exercises.
   x. Teach the patient and significant others techniques of self-care that will minimize O_2 consumption.
   xi. Maintain body temperature at a normal level; avoid patient shivering.
   e. Evaluation of patient care
   i. ABG and vital sign values are within normal limits for the patient with or without supplemental O_2 or mechanical ventilation.
   ii. Cyanosis and dyspnea are absent.
   iii. Patient performs techniques that maximize ventilation-perfusion matching.

SPECIFIC PATIENT HEALTH PROBLEMS

Acute Respiratory Failure

1. **Pathophysiology**
   a. Respiratory system cannot carry out its two major functions: (1) delivery of an adequate amount of O_2 into the arterial blood and (2) removal of a corresponding amount of CO_2 from mixed venous blood. As an "acute" disorder, the onset must be relatively sudden; however, the onset can occur over days, as may be seen in patients with preexisting lung disease, or within minutes to hours, as may be seen in patients with no preexisting lung disease.
   b. ARF can be categorized according to the extent to which ABG values are abnormal. Abnormalities can exist in Po_2, Pco_2, or both; the more severe the hypoxemia or hypercapnia, the greater the consensus about categorization. However, the interpretation of ABGs must take into consideration two important aspects of the clinical situation: Blood gas values before the onset of ARF (which depend on whether preexisting lung disease was present) and the rapidity with which the ABG abnormalities developed.

c. As mentioned, the abnormalities in ABG levels may be in P_{O_2} (hypoxemic respiratory failure), in P_{CO_2} (hypercapnic respiratory failure), or in both. Critical value for the diagnosis based on arterial hypoxemia is Pa_{O_2} lower than 55 mm Hg or Sa_{O_2} lower than 88%; lower values can cause a marked decrease in oxyhemoglobin saturation and, therefore, a considerable drop in O_2 content. Corresponding critical value for the diagnosis of acute hypercapnic respiratory failure is Pa_{CO_2} above 50 to 55 mm Hg (with an accompanying acidemia, or pH of <7.30).

d. Three major pathophysiologic mechanisms cause ARF—hypoventilation, ventilation-perfusion mismatching, and intrapulmonary shunting. These physiologic abnormalities result from structural processes that comprise the pathologic background for the abnormalities of gas exchange. Two major processes involved are the following:

  i. Increase in extravascular lung water
    (a) Characterized by severe hypoxemia with normal to low Pa_{CO_2}
    (b) Occurs in patients with cardiogenic or noncardiogenic pulmonary edema and other parenchymal infiltrates

  ii. Impaired ventilation
    (a) Characterized by elevated Pa_{CO_2} and decreased Pa_{O_2}
    (b) Occurs with intrapulmonary disorders (airway disease) or extrapulmonary problems (neuromuscular or chest wall diseases, alterations in respiratory drive). Other causes include low partial pressure of inspired oxygen (P_{IO_2}) due to high altitude or inhalation of toxic gases and low mixed-venous oxygenation secondary to anemia, hypoxemia, inadequate cardiac output, or increased O_2 consumption.

2. **Etiology and risk factors**
  a. Increase in extravascular lung water (ALI, pulmonary edema, aspiration, pneumonia, atelectasis)
  b. Impaired ventilation
    i. Intrapulmonary problems (see causes listed under Impaired Respiratory Mechanics and Impaired Alveolar Ventilation)
    ii. Extrapulmonary problems: Pleural effusion, kyphoscoliosis, multiple rib fractures, thoracic surgery, peritonitis; neuromuscular defects such as polio, Guillain-Barré syndrome, multiple sclerosis, myasthenia gravis, brain or spinal injuries; drug effects (narcotics, barbiturates, tranquilizers, anesthetic agents); cerebral infarction
  c. Patient history
    i. Past medical history—Chronic airway obstruction, restrictive defects, neuromuscular defects, or respiratory center damage; history of conditions that impair gas exchange and diffusion
    ii. Family history—Any significant pulmonary disease in parents, grandparents, or siblings. One form of emphysema caused by a deficiency of the enzyme α_1-antitrypsin is an inherited disorder.
    iii. Social history—Current or past smoking; calculate the pack-year history for smokers (number of cigarettes smoked per day times the number of years smoked)
    iv. Medication history—Prescribed and over-the-counter medications, their dosages, and last time taken. Assess for evidence of noncompliance in taking prescribed medications (i.e., missed doses or overdoses).

3. **Signs and symptoms**
  a. Patient's chief complaint
    i. Most often dyspnea or increased work of breathing
    ii. Other symptoms
      (a) Increased pulmonary secretions
      (b) Manifestations of hypoxemia
      (c) Manifestations of hypercapnia with acidemia: Headache, confusion, inability to concentrate, irritability, somnolence, dizziness
  b. Nursing examination of patient
    i. Inspection
      (a) General observations

(1) Posture, skin color, cyanosis, tissue perfusion, lung expansion

(2) Signs of right-sided heart failure, such as pitting edema of the lower extremities, jugular venous distention

(3) Signs of hypercapnia with acidemia: Muscle twitching, asterixis, miosis, papilledema, engorged fundal veins, diaphoresis

(b) Thoracic abnormalities such as increased A-P diameter (barrel chest), intercostal retractions, bulging interspaces on expiration (obstruction to air outflow), pectus carinatum or excavatum, spinal deformities

(c) Pattern of ventilation

(1) Use of accessory muscles of respiration

(2) Abnormal rate, depth, or rhythm of breathing

(3) Inspiration-to-expiration ratio (normal ratio is 1:2 or 1:3)

(4) Inspiratory and/or expiratory stridor, indicative of upper airway airflow obstruction

ii. Palpation

(a) Skin temperature and texture

(b) Vocal fremitus

iii. Percussion

(a) Dullness over dense lung tissue (consolidation or pulmonary edema)

(b) Hyperresonance with air trapping (COPD) or pneumothorax

iv. Auscultation

(a) Decreased breath sounds with less air movement or less dense lung tissue (COPD)

(b) Bronchial and bronchovesicular breath sounds over areas of consolidation, atelectasis, pulmonary edema

(c) Adventitious sounds: Crackles or rales, rhonchi or gurgles, wheezes, pleural friction rub with pleuritis

4. **Diagnostic study findings**

a. Laboratory: ABG analysis

i. Respiratory failure is defined by ABG measurements as hypoxemic (decreased Pao_2) and/or hypercapnic (increased $Paco_2$ and decreased Pao_2)

ii. Criteria: Pao_2 below 55 mm Hg, $Paco_2$ above 50 mm Hg, or both

(a) Acute: Acidosis, normal or mildly increasing blood buffer (HCO_3^-) levels

(b) Chronic: Relatively normal pH, elevated blood buffer levels

iii. Shunt studies: Demonstrate intrapulmonary shunt greater than 15%

b. Radiologic: Findings depend on the primary disease

5. **Goals of care**

a. Impaired respiratory gas transport: Fio_2 is sufficient for the patient's O_2 supply needs; respiratory rate, tidal volume, ABG levels are within normal limits for the patient

b. Impaired alveolar ventilation

i. Respiratory rate and breathing pattern are normal for the patient.

ii. Patient has a minimal sensation of dyspnea with no auto-PEEP.

iii. No ventilator-associated infections or other complications are present.

c. Impaired respiratory gas exchange

i. Hypoxemia resolves or improves.

ii. Eucapnia or the usual compensated $Paco_2$ and pH levels are observed.

iii. Mental status is normal, and the patient is breathing comfortably.

iv. Patient performs techniques that maximize $\dot{V}/\dot{Q}$ matching.

6. **Collaborating professionals on health care team: Nurse, physician, respiratory therapist, infection control specialist, dietitian, clinical pharmacologist**

7. **Management of patient care**

a. Anticipated patient trajectory

i. Delivery of care: Depending on the severity of the patient's signs and symptoms or the frequency or type of interventions required, the patient may need to be transferred to the ICU for treatment

ii. Positioning: Keep the head of the bed elevated at least 30 degrees to maximize ventilation and prevent aspiration; turn as warranted to maximize $\dot{V}/\dot{Q}$ matching

     iii. Skin care: Turn the patient frequently to mobilize secretions and maintain skin integrity

     iv. Pain management: Administer pain medication or sedative to relieve the discomfort of tubes and treatment and prevent treatment interference

     v. Nutrition: Obtain dietary consult and collaboration; provide adequate nutrition to maintain cellular function and healing with the increased work of breathing

     vi. Infection control: Follow all measures to avoid ventilator-associated pneumonia, including thorough oral care with brushing at regular intervals; hand washing hygiene; and meticulous care with vascular lines, airways, humidification systems, and the like to prevent hospital-associated infection. Maintain the integrity of invasive line systems and urinary drainage system; use aseptic technique as warranted.

     vii. Transport: Ensure that optimal levels of patient care, patient monitoring, O_2 supply, humidification, and positioning are maintained throughout transport.

     viii. Discharge planning: Initiate early with the patient and family, especially if the patient will require continued care at home; evaluate the need for support and rehabilitation on discharge; anticipate home care equipment needs; provide a social services consult to arrange for the transition to home care, if warranted

     ix. Pharmacology: Antibiotics, sedatives, and analgesics as warranted. Instruct the patient and family in medications, inhalers, spirometry, and so on, to be used at home.

     x. Psychosocial issues: Degree, nature, and extent of support must be tailored to patient and family needs and incorporate as wide an array of health care services as warranted.

     xi. Treatments
        (a) Noninvasive
           (1) BiPAP, CPAP
           (2) O_2 delivery systems
        (b) Invasive
           (1) Intubation and mechanical ventilation
           (2) IV medications, vascular monitoring lines, drainage systems
           (3) Nutrition via nasogastric feeding tube, percutaneous endoscopic gastrostomy (PEG) tube, or small-bore feeding tube

     xii. Ethical issues: Issues related to the use and withdrawal of artificial means of ventilation represent a common source of ethical decision-making requirements involving the patient (with or without an advance directive in place), family members, members of the health care team, and possibly others such as a hospital ethics committee (see Chapter 1 coverage of these issues)

  b. Potential complications

     i. Hospital-associated infections: Aspiration, urinary tract infection, pneumonia
        (a) Mechanism: Patient vulnerable because of position changes and possible need for enteral feedings, probable use of a urinary catheter, foreign airway object, recumbency, and the need for cleansing and removal of oropharyngeal secretions
        (b) Management: See Positioning, Skin Care, and Infection Control (covered earlier)

     ii. Complications related to the therapies used for ventilatory support (i.e., O_2 toxicity, barotrauma, volutrauma, tracheal damage, gastric ulcers, inability to wean from the ventilator)
        (a) Mechanism: See Box 2-6
        (b) Management: See Box 2-6

     iii. Ethical issues: See coverage in Chapter 1

8. Evaluation of patient care

  a. Arterial and mixed-venous blood gas values are within the desired range for the patient.

  b. Ventilatory parameters are within acceptable limits for the patient.

  c. Rate, depth, and pattern of ventilation remain within normal limits for the patient with minimal or no use of accessory muscles of respiration.

  d. Patient reports decreased dyspnea at rest and with exertion.

  e. When inspiratory muscle training is appropriate, the patient's use of the training results in improved maximal inspiratory pressures.

    f. Patient demonstrates correct and effective administration of inhaled respiratory medications and identifies side effects that need to be reported to a health care provider.

    g. No signs of ventilator-associated infections or other complications are noted.

    h. Patient performs ADLs with or without supplemental O_2.

Acute Lung Injury

1. Pathophysiology

    a. ALI refers to a group of manifestations of an evolving severe diffuse lung injury. Acute form of ALI nearly always occurs suddenly. Some patients survive and recover completely, although may have some residual impairment, however slight. Others—notably those with sepsis (particularly of abdominal origin)—have a high mortality because their ALI evolves into a chronic form.

        i. The severest form of ALI is called acute (formerly called "adult") respiratory distress syndrome (ARDS). ARDS is identified by the same diagnostic criteria as ALI except that the ratio of Pao_2 to Fio_2 is less than or equal to 200 mm Hg.

    b. Acute phase of ALI is characterized by damaged integrity of the blood-gas barrier. There is extensive damage to type I alveolar epithelial cells with increased endothelial permeability. Interstitial edema is found along with the leakage of protein-containing fluid into the alveoli. This alveolar fluid contains erythrocytes and leukocytes in addition to amorphous material comprising strands of fibrin. There is also impaired production and function of surfactant. Resultant physiologic abnormalities are as follows:

        i. Shunting of blood through atelectatic or fluid-filled lung units causes a widening of the A-a difference in Po_2; the resultant hypoxemia is resistant to high Fio_2 but is often responsive to PEEP.

        ii. Physiologic dead space is increased, frequently exceeding 60% of each breath; consequently, very large minute ventilation may be required to maintain acceptable levels of arterial Pco_2.

        iii. Compliance of certain portions of lung parenchyma is reduced. Increased stiffness of the lungs is associated with decreased FRC and a requirement for high peak inspiratory pressures during mechanical ventilation. Other lung areas have relatively normal specific compliance and thus are not so much stiff as they are small.

        iv. Resistance to blood flow through the lungs is increased by narrowing or obstruction of pulmonary vessels. As a result, peak airway pressure (PAP) is often increased while pulmonary capillary occlusive pressure (PCOP) remains normal or low. Chest radiographs reveal diffuse bilateral infiltrates suggesting noncardiogenic pulmonary edema (i.e., filling pressures in the left side of the heart are low or normal).

    c. Chronic phase of ALI is characterized by thickening of the endothelium, epithelium, and interstitial space. Type I cells are destroyed and replaced by type II cells (neutrophils), which proliferate but do not differentiate into type I cells as normal. Interstitial space is greatly expanded by edema fluid, fibers, and a variety of proliferating cells. Fibrosis commences after the first week. Within the alveoli, the protein-rich exudate may organize to produce the characteristic "hyaline membrane," which effectively destroys the structure of the alveoli.

    d. Resultant physiologic abnormalities are the following:

        i. Increased vascular resistance

        ii. Hypoxemia due to $\dot{V}/\dot{Q}$ mismatch or possible diffusion defect

        iii. Decreased tissue compliance

2. Etiology and risk factors

    a. Direct injury: Pulmonary contusion, gastric aspiration, near drowning, inhalation of toxic gases and vapors, some infections, fat embolus, amniotic fluid embolus, radiation, bleomycin

    b. Indirect injury: Septicemia, shock or prolonged hypotension, nonthoracic trauma, cardiopulmonary bypass, drug overdose, head injury, pancreatitis, diabetic coma, multiple blood transfusions

3. Signs and symptoms

    a. Patient's chief complaint: Severe dyspnea

    b. Increased work of breathing manifested by tachypnea, hyperpnea, nasal flaring, intercostal retractions, use of accessory muscles

    c. Production of frothy, pink sputum, dullness to percussion, bronchovesicular breath sounds over most lung fields, and diffuse crackles and gurgles over all lung fields if substantial pulmonary edema is present

    d. Diminished lung expansion

    e. Diminished level of consciousness if hypoxemia is severe

4. Diagnostic study findings: To exclude other causes of pulmonary edema

    a. Laboratory: ABG analysis

        i. Hypoxemia is the hallmark of ALI and is due to intrapulmonary shunting. Hypoxemia is refractory to O_2 therapy (i.e., Pao_2 is below 60 mm Hg or Sao_2 is below 90% with Fio_2 above 0.5).

        ii. Respiratory alkalosis occurs in the early phases of ALI because of hyperventilation.

        iii. Hypercapnia is not usually seen initially; it is an ominous sign if present.

        iv. Shunt studies demonstrate large right-to-left shunt (usually >20% of cardiac output) measured during 100% O_2 breathing.

        v. A-a gradient is increased, and Pao_2/Fio_2 ratio is reduced.

    b. Radiologic: Chest radiograph demonstrates diffuse bilateral interstitial and alveolar infiltrates without cardiomegaly or pulmonary vascular redistribution in the acute phase; a fine or coarse reticular pattern evolves in the chronic phase

    c. Pulmonary function

        i. Reduced pulmonary compliance and FRC

        ii. Reduced FRC secondary to microatelectasis and edema

        iii. Increased dead space ventilation (V_D/V_T)

    d. Hemodynamic monitoring: Pulmonary artery occlusive pressure may be normal or low, but PAP is often elevated

5. Goals of care

    a. Hypoxemia resolves or improves with or without O_2 supplementation or mechanical ventilation.

    b. Respiratory rate, depth, and breathing pattern are normal for the patient.

    c. Arterial pH, Pco_2, and Po_2 normalize to acceptable values.

    d. Patient has minimal or no sensation of dyspnea.

    e. There is no clinical evidence of any complications related to equipment or therapies.

6. Collaborating professionals on health care team: Nurse, advanced practice nurse, home care nurse, physician, intensivist, pulmonologist as warranted, respiratory therapist, dietitian, clinical pharmacologist, infection control specialist, discharge coordinator, home care aide, social service personnel, occupational and/or physical therapist, as indicated

7. Management of patient care

    a. Anticipated patient trajectory: See also Acute Respiratory Failure and Patient Care

        i. Delivery of care: Depending on the severity of the patient's signs and symptoms or the frequency or type of interventions required, the patient may need to be transferred to the ICU for treatment

        ii. Treatments (additional)

            (a) ABG monitoring: Notify the physician immediately if Pao_2 drops below 60 mm Hg or if $Paco_2$ shows an upward trend

            (b) BiPAP, CPAP

            (c) Decreased V_T to protect lung; permissive hypercapnia may be used

    b. Potential complications (see also Acute Respiratory Failure)

        i. Fluid overload

            (a) Mechanism: Same mechanisms responsible for producing pulmonary infiltrates

            (b) Management: Monitor input and output closely; observe for signs of fluid overload; use the lowest intravascular volume compatible with adequate tissue perfusion

8. Evaluation of patient care: Underlying condition(s) that precipitated the development of ALI is (are) reversed or effectively managed; see also Acute Respiratory Failure

Chronic Obstructive Pulmonary Disease

1. **Pathophysiology**
   a. COPD is an inclusive and nonspecific term referring to a condition in which patients have chronic cough and expectoration and various degrees of dyspnea either at rest or with exertion, with a significant and progressive reduction in expiratory airflow as measured by the forced expiratory volume in 1 second (FEV_1). This airflow abnormality does not show major reversibility in response to pharmacologic agents. Terms such as chronic obstructive airway disease, chronic obstructive lung disease, chronic airflow obstruction or chronic airway obstruction, and chronic airflow limitation all mean the same thing.
   b. COPD is usually divided into two subtypes: chronic bronchitis and emphysema. However, other diseases such as cystic fibrosis, bronchiectasis, or bronchiolitis obliterans are associated with chronic airflow limitation. The separate pathophysiology of these subtypes (chronic bronchitis and emphysema) is described here, but most patients exhibit signs and symptoms of both clinical conditions. Asthma has an obstructive component but is no longer classified with COPD.
      i. Chronic bronchitis: Clinical diagnosis defined as the presence of chronic cough with sputum production on a daily basis for a minimum of 3 months a year for not less than 2 successive years. Many patients exhibit chronic hypoxemia with resultant episodes of cor pulmonale. They may also have reduced responsiveness of the respiratory center to hypoxemic stimuli, a trait that is probably inherited. Some of the pathophysiologic findings of chronic bronchitis are the following:
         (a) Increase in the size of the tracheobronchial mucus glands (increased Reid index) and goblet cell hyperplasia, which results in increased sputum production
         (b) Epithelial mucus cell metaplasia, which results in a decreased number of cilia. Hypersecretion of mucus and impaired cilia lead to a chronic productive cough.
         (c) Increase in bronchial wall thickness with progressive obstruction to airflow (chronic obstructive bronchitis)
         (d) Exacerbations usually due to infection, with the following clinical picture:
            (1) Increased amount of sputum and retained secretions
            (2) Increased $\dot{V}/\dot{Q}$ abnormalities, which increase hypoxemia, CO_2 retention, and acidemia
            (3) Pulmonary vessel constriction increased by hypoxemia and acidemia, raising PAP and ultimately leading to right-sided heart failure (cor pulmonale)
      ii. Emphysema: Anatomic alteration of the lung characterized by an abnormal enlargement of the air spaces distal to the terminal, nonrespiratory bronchioles, accompanied by destructive changes in the alveolar walls. Patients with emphysema often exhibit increased dyspnea and breathing effort owing to an inherent increased responsiveness to hypoxemia. Resultant clinical picture is typically that of a well-oxygenated and dyspneic patient. Pulmonary abnormalities seen in emphysema are the following:
         (a) Gas exchange surface of the respiratory bronchioles, alveolar ducts, and alveoli is reduced.
         (b) Air trapping is increased because of the loss of elastic recoil in airway support structures (causes increased A-P diameter).
         (c) Air sacs are replaced by bullae, and capillary area is proportionately diminished.
         (d) $\dot{V}/\dot{Q}$ inequality occurs and FRC is increased.
         (e) Increased work of breathing results in greater resting O_2 consumption
2. **Etiology and risk factors (chronic bronchitis and emphysema)**
   a. Cigarette smoking—The most important factor and the major toxic stimulus
   b. Environmental pollution, occupational exposure
   c. Predisposition due to genetic makeup, especially if there is known α_1-antitrypsin deficiency. Should be considered in nonsmokers or young patients (<50 years of age) with emphysema. Current guidelines recommend testing every patient with COPD for this genetic finding.
3. **Signs and symptoms: These diseases may present as pure entities, but it is common for patients to have a combination of the symptoms of the two**

  a. Chronic bronchitis

    i. Chief complaint is usually chronic cough and sputum production.

    ii. Wheezing, peripheral edema are present.

    iii. Observe for signs of right-sided heart failure: peripheral edema, distended neck veins, skin color that is dusky or cyanotic. Patients with chronic bronchitis show little sign of respiratory distress or dyspnea at rest.

    iv. Chest expansion may be normal; vocal fremitus may be normal or increased because of copious bronchial secretions.

    v. Resonance may be heard on percussion if there are no areas of secretion retention or consolidation.

    vi. Dullness to percussion is heard in areas of increased lung density (consolidation).

    vii. Coarse crackles and gurgles, expiratory wheezes are commonly heard.

  b. Emphysema

    i. Chief complaint: Dyspnea on exertion (early symptom) and eventually dyspnea at rest

    ii. Skin color often pinkish because the patient is well oxygenated

    iii. Weight loss, inability to perform ADLs

    iv. Barrel chest; note posture and work of breathing both at rest and during exercise; use of accessory muscles of respiration is common

    v. Pursed-lip breathing

    vi. Reduced chest excursion due to hyperinflated lungs and flattened diaphragm from chronic air trapping

    vii. Reduced vocal fremitus due to less dense, more hyperinflated lungs

    viii. Hyperresonance throughout all lung fields

    ix. Distant, quiet breath sounds due to reduced air movement and air trapping; wheezes heard on occasion

4. Diagnostic study findings

  a. Chronic bronchitis

    i. Laboratory

      (a) ABG analysis: Hypoxemia and often hypercapnia with compensated respiratory acidosis

      (b) Other laboratory findings: Polycythemia on complete blood cell count (CBC) in some patients

    ii. Pulmonary function: Reduction in FEV_1 and all other measures of expiratory airflow; some reversibility after bronchodilator therapy in selected patients

  b. Emphysema

    i. Laboratory: ABG analysis—may be normal or abnormal, depending on the type and severity of $\dot{V}/\dot{Q}$ abnormalities. Hypoxemia, if present, may be mild with normal $Paco_2$; greatest during sleep.

    ii. Radiologic: Chest radiographs often show low, flattened diaphragms. In severe emphysema, lung fields may be hyperlucent and show hyperinflation, with diminished vascular markings and bullae. Disease is most prominent in the upper lung zones except in α_1-antitripsin deficiency, in which a basilar predominance may be seen. Chest radiographs are of value during acute exacerbation to exclude complications such as pneumonia and pneumothorax.

    iii. Pulmonary function: Increased FRC, residual volume, and TLC. Reduced FEV_1 with the ratio of FEV_1 to forced vital capacity (FVC) of less than 75% (greater than 80% is normal) and reduction in other expiratory airflow measures, which is typically nonreversible after administration of bronchodilators. Increased lung compliance and decrease in static recoil. Decreased diffusion capacity indicating a reduction in alveolar capillary gas exchange area (not a specific indicator of emphysema, however).

5. Goals of care

  a. Both disorders

    i. Major through terminal airways remain patent and free of secretions.

    ii. Oxygenation improves.

    iii. Alveolar ventilation improves.

    iv. Work of breathing is minimized; ABG levels, vital signs, and tidal volume are within normal limits for the patient.

b. Chronic bronchitis

    i. Constricted airways are dilated.

    ii. Patient is able to effectively clear secretions.

    iii. There are minimal to no signs and symptoms of right-sided heart failure.

    iv. Patient reports taking bronchodilator medications as prescribed.

c. Emphysema

    i. Breathing pattern is normal for the patient.

    ii. Sensation of dyspnea is decreased.

    iii. There is no air trapping at the end of expiration (auto-PEEP).

6. Collaborating professionals on health care team: See Acute Respiratory Failure

7. Management of patient care

    a. Anticipated patient trajectory

        i. Delivery of care: Depending on the severity of the patient's signs and symptoms or the frequency or type of interventions required, the patient may need to be transferred to the ICU for treatment

        ii. Positioning: Keep the head of the bed elevated 30 to 45 degrees unless medically contraindicated to improve ventilation and prevent aspiration. Allow the patient to assume a position of comfort for breathing to diminish dyspnea. Patients with emphysema may need an overbed table for best positioning.

        iii. Skin care: Many of these patients have little adipose tissue owing to the increased work of breathing associated with these disorders. Others may exhibit peripheral edema related to right-sided heart failure. In either case, skin integrity warrants frequent monitoring and active care so that pressure ulcers or other breaks do not lead to infection.

        iv. Nutrition: Labored ventilation and the increased work of breathing associated with these disorders often precipitate the need for dietary consultation to ensure that sufficient protein and calorie intake are paired with judicious fluid intake.

        v. Infection control: These patients are especially vulnerable to hospital-associated infections; see coverage in Acute Respiratory Failure. Consultation with an infection control specialist on an ongoing basis may be warranted.

        vi. Transport: Ensure that optimal levels of patient care, patient monitoring, O_2 supply, humidification, and positioning are maintained throughout transport.

        vii. Discharge planning: See Acute Respiratory Failure. In addition, discuss the need for smoking cessation; instruct in the proper use of an inhaler, effective coughing techniques, follow-up care at home. Secure consultation with social services to address the medical and social services support needed.

        viii. Pharmacology: Bronchodilators, steroids, and antibiotics as needed; sedatives and pain medication sufficient to enable therapies to be performed and to keep the patient comfortable. For patients with documented α_1-antitrypsin deficiency receiving α_1-proteinase inhibitor (Prolastin), provide medication monitoring instruction.

        ix. Psychosocial issues: Degree, nature, and extent of support must be tailored to patient and family needs and incorporate as wide an array of health care services as warranted. As COPD can have a major impact on family roles, dynamics, and income, it is important to identify issues and communicate these to the social worker.

        x. Treatments (see also Acute Respiratory Failure)

            (a) Carefully administer O_2 using the lowest F_{IO_2} that produces adequate oxygenation; observe for CO_2 retention.

            (b) Observe for signs of fluid overload; monitor intake and output closely.

            (c) Monitor ABG levels; notify the physician immediately if Pa_{O_2} drops below the patient's known baseline or target level (usually Pa_{O_2} of 55 to 60 mm Hg or higher) or if Pa_{CO_2} rises significantly beyond the established baseline value. In a patient with chronic CO_2 retention, monitoring Pa_{CO_2} is less important than observing pH changes. Be prepared for the possibility of endotracheal intubation and the need for mechanical ventilatory support.

(d) Consider administration of influenza and pneumococcal vaccine.
- **xi.** Ethical issues: See Acute Respiratory Failure; determine whether an advance directive is in place because intubation may be a terminal event
- **b.** Potential complications
  - **i.** Hospital-associated infections: See Acute Respiratory Failure
  - **ii.** Inability to wean or liberate from the ventilator: See prior coverage
  - **iii.** Deconditioning secondary to steroid use or lack of muscle work
    - (a) Mechanism: Chronic increased work of breathing may not be compensated sufficiently by diet and—together with right-sided heart failure—may make ambulation virtually impossible; therefore patients with COPD have a tenuous ability to maintain muscle strength
    - (b) Management: Dietary consult to develop a comprehensive plan to replace the nutritional deficit and enable the patient to regain muscle strength; physical and/or occupational therapy to provide strength training
  - **iv.** Cor pulmonale
    - (a) Mechanism: Right-sided heart failure develops secondary to increased resistance to blood flow and increased pressures in the right side of the heart, the pulmonary artery, and the venous circuit owing to COPD
    - (b) Management: Symptomatic management of problems such as fluid balance, peripheral edema, cough
8. **Evaluation of patient care**
   - **a.** Airways are clear with minimal constriction and secretions.
   - **b.** Patient experiences minimal dyspnea at rest, lessened dyspnea on exertion.
   - **c.** ABG levels and pulmonary parameters are within acceptable ranges for the patient.
   - **d.** Tidal volume and respiratory excursion are optimal for the patient.
   - **e.** Overt signs and symptoms of right-sided heart failure are minimal or absent.
   - **f.** No ventilator-associated infections or other complications are present.

Asthma and Status Asthmaticus (Severe Asthmatic Attack)

1. **Pathophysiology**
   - **a.** Asthma: Chronic disease of variable severity characterized by airway hyperreactivity that produces airway narrowing of a reversible nature
     - **i.** Increased responsiveness of the airways to various stimuli
     - **ii.** Widespread narrowing of the airway with changes in severity; airway closure may occur
     - **iii.** Cellular infiltration and mucosal edema
     - **iv.** Airway hyperreactivity, with smooth muscle contraction and excessive mucus production and diminished secretion clearance
     - **v.** $\dot{V}/\dot{Q}$ abnormalities
     - **vi.** Increased work of breathing and airway resistance
     - **vii.** Hyperinflation of the lung, with an increase in residual volume
     - **viii.** Host defect of altered immunologic state
     - **ix.** Development of airway remodeling in some patients, then response as in COPD
   - **b.** Status asthmaticus: Severe asthma attack that is refractory to bronchodilator therapy, including β-adrenergic agents and IV aminophylline
     - **i.** Severely reduced spirometric values for peak expiratory flow rate (PEFR), FVC, and FEV_1
     - **ii.** Presence of hypoxemia with a reduced Pa_{O_2}/F_{IO_2} ratio
     - **iii.** Airway narrowing due to the following:
       - (a) Bronchial smooth muscle spasm (minor component)
       - (b) Inflammation of bronchial walls, which leads to increased mucosal permeability and basement membrane thickening
       - (c) Mucus plugging from airways due to increased production and reduced clearance of secretions. Mucus plugging, mucosal edema, and inspissated secretions account for the apparent resistance to bronchodilator therapy in patients in status asthmaticus.

2. **Etiology and risk factors (for development of an asthma attack)**
   a. Respiratory infection
   b. Allergic reaction to inhaled antigen (pollen, grass, perfume, smoke)
   c. Inappropriate bronchodilator management
   d. Idiosyncratic reaction to aspirin or other nonsteroidal anti-inflammatory drugs
   e. Emotional stress, exercise
   f. Occupational or environmental exposure (air pollution, ingestion of metabisulfite [food preservative])
   g. Use of nonselective β-blocking agents (propranolol, timolol maleate)
   h. Mechanical stimulation (coughing, laughing, and cold air inhalation)
   i. Sinusitis, reflux esophagitis
   j. Genetic predisposition
3. **Signs and symptoms**
   a. Chief complaints usually dyspnea, wheezing, cough, and chest tightness; severity ranges from intermittent, mild symptoms to severe respiratory symptoms despite intensive therapy
   b. Physical exhaustion, inability to sleep or rest, anxiety
   c. Difficulty speaking in sentences, minimal chest excursion with inspiration
   d. Production of thick, tenacious sputum
   e. Increased work of breathing evidenced by the following:
      i. Posture—Habitus often leaning forward, with head lowered
      ii. Respiratory distress, tachypnea, hyperpnea at rest, expiratory stridor
      iii. Use of pursed-lip breathing with prolonged expiration
      iv. Nasal flaring, bulging of interspaces on expiration, diaphoresis
   f. Possible presence of pulsus paradoxus; pulse rate higher than 110 beats/min with pulsus paradoxus greater than 12 mm Hg in the presence of tachypnea (respiratory rate of >30/min) indicates a severe episode
   g. Signs of dehydration
   h. Possible decrease of vocal fremitus (decreased density with lung hyperinflation); rhonchal fremitus with copious secretions
   i. Hyperresonance throughout the lung fields, low diaphragm, and limited diaphragmatic excursion on percussion
   j. Expiratory wheezes or rhonchi (as air and secretions move through narrowed airways). Severe wheezing may be audible without a stethoscope.
   k. Decreased breath sounds throughout constitute an ominous sign. Asthmatic patient is then not moving enough air and will likely need to be intubated.
4. **Diagnostic study findings**
   a. Laboratory
      i. Evidence of infection (i.e., positive sputum culture results), elevated white blood cell count
      ii. ABG analysis
         (a) ABG analysis may initially show low normal or decreased $Paco_2$, increased pH, and decreased Pao_2 (<60 mm Hg).
         (b) In severe asthmatic attacks, progression to a "normal" or increased $Paco_2$ level may be a sign of impending respiratory failure.
   b. Radiologic: Chest radiograph may be normal or hyperlucent. Used to confirm or rule out a diagnosis of pneumonia, atelectasis, pneumothorax, or other condition that mimics asthma.
   c. Pulmonary function: Reduced FEV_1 and PEFRs. Serial measurements of these parameters indicating the response to bronchodilators are essential to establish the severity of the obstruction and assess the adequacy of the response to therapy. In patients requiring hospitalization, PEFR may be less than 60 L/min initially or may not improve to more than 50% of the predicted value after 1 hour of treatment. FEV_1 may be less than 30% of the predicted value or may not improve to at least 40% of the predicted value after 1 hour of aggressive therapy.

5. **Goals of care**
   a. Diameter and patency of the airways are improved.
   b. Airway secretions and coughing are reduced.
   c. Dyspnea and the work of breathing are reduced.
   d. Oxygenation and ABG values are optimized.
6. **Collaborating professionals on health care team: See Acute Respiratory Failure**
7. **Management of patient care**
   a. Anticipated patient trajectory
      i. Delivery of care: Depending on the severity of the patient's signs and symptoms or the frequency or type of interventions required, the patient may need to be transferred to the ICU for treatment
      ii. Positioning: Keep the head of the bed elevated 30 to 45 degrees to maximize ventilation, enhance coughing effectiveness, and prevent aspiration. Assist the patient to his or her own position of comfort.
      iii. Nutrition: See coverage under Chronic Obstructive Pulmonary Disease. Dietary consult may be needed to arrange dietary supplements, treat any malnourishment, and restore positive nitrogen balance and adequate hydration.
      iv. Infection control: See Acute Respiratory Failure and Chronic Obstructive Pulmonary Disease. Patients are particularly susceptible to pulmonary infection because of the copious volume of thick secretions, inspissated secretions that plug the airways, and airway constriction.
      v. Transport: Ensure that optimal levels of patient care, patient monitoring, O_2 supply, humidification, and positioning are maintained throughout transport
      vi. Discharge planning: See Chronic Obstructive Pulmonary Disease. In addition, teach correct inhaler technique, teach peak flow and symptom monitoring, and instruct the patient and family on avoidance of allergens and situations that trigger episodes and on the importance of taking medications properly.
      vii. Pharmacology: Administer bronchodilators and monitor effects (use of salmeterol is contraindicated during an acute asthma attack because of its delayed onset of action; albuterol or some other bronchodilator with a rapid onset of action should be used); administer steroids and antibiotics as needed
      viii. Psychosocial issues: Degree, nature, and extent of support must be tailored to patient and family needs and incorporate as wide an array of health care services as warranted. Asthmatic attacks are stressful and frightening to the patient and family; the ICU environment may only add further anxiety. Need to work with the family as a unit because the ramifications of asthma may extend to the physical home environment and interpersonal dynamics, and ability to work and function in customary roles.
      ix. Treatments: See Chronic Obstructive Pulmonary Disease
         (a) Administer O_2 therapy, BiPAP or CPAP.
         (b) For cases in which intubation and mechanical ventilation become necessary: See Acute Respiratory Failure.
         (c) Administer fluids and humidification to keep airway secretions thin and easily expectorated.
         (d) Follow designed dietary plan for nutrition.
         (e) Perform close objective monitoring of ABG values, acid-base status, and ventilatory parameters (especially FEV_1 or peak flow rates if spirometry is not available).
   b. Potential complications: See Chronic Obstructive Pulmonary Disease. Note that because asthma is a reversible condition, avoidance of allergens and other triggers, sufficient fluid intake, effective coughing, air humidification, and proper use of an MDI should enable the patient to reverse most problems and resume normal activities.
8. **Evaluation of patient care**
   a. Airways remain patent and significantly less constricted.
   b. Airway secretions are diminished in volume and readily expectorated.
   c. Patient experiences minimal dyspnea at rest with significantly reduced work of breathing.
   d. ABG values and pulmonary parameters are acceptable for the patient.

Pulmonary Embolism

1. **Pathophysiology**
   a. PE, an obstruction of the pulmonary artery by an embolus, affects lung tissue, the pulmonary circulation, and the function of the right and left sides of the heart. Degree of compromise correlates with the extent of embolic vascular occlusion and the degree of preexisting cardiopulmonary disease.
   b. Most emboli (>90%) arise from DVTs in the iliofemoral system. Other sites include the right side of the heart and the pelvic area. Nonthrombotic emboli, such as fat, air, and amniotic fluid, also occur but are relatively uncommon.
   c. Factors favoring venous thrombosis (Virchow's triad) include the following:
      i. Blood stasis
      ii. Blood coagulation alterations
      iii. Vessel wall abnormalities
   d. Distribution of emboli is related to the size of emboli and blood flow. Very large emboli have an impact in a large artery; however, the thrombus may break up and block several smaller vessels. Lower lobes are frequently involved because they have greater blood flow.
   e. Pulmonary infarction (death of the embolized tissue) occurs infrequently. More often, there is distal hemorrhage and atelectasis, but alveolar structures remain viable. Infarction is more likely if the embolus completely blocks a large artery or if there is preexisting lung disease. Infarction results in alveolar filling with extravasated red blood cells and inflammatory cells and causes opacity on a radiograph. Occasionally, the infarct becomes infected, which leads to an abscess.
   f. Effects of acute pulmonary artery obstruction include the following:
      i. There is altered gas exchange due to right-to-left shunting and $\dot{V}/\dot{Q}$ inequalities. Possible etiologic mechanisms for these alterations include the following:
         (a) Overperfusion of the uninvolved lung, which lowers $\dot{V}/\dot{Q}$ ratios
         (b) Eventual reperfusion of atelectatic areas distal to the embolic obstruction
         (c) Development of postembolic pulmonary edema
      ii. Degree of hemodynamic compromise correlates with the degree of vascular occlusion in patients with no underlying heart or lung disease.
         (a) Initial hemodynamic consequence is acute reduction in the pulmonary vascular cross-sectional area with a subsequent increase in the resistance to blood flow through the lungs.
         (b) If cardiac output remains constant or increases, pulmonary arterial pressure must rise.
      iii. If cardiac or pulmonary disease exists and has already impaired the pulmonary vascular reserve capacity, a small degree of vascular occlusion will result in greater pulmonary artery hypertension and more serious right ventricular dysfunction.

2. **Etiology and risk factors (for DVT then PE)**
   a. Previous pulmonary embolus or venous disease of a lower extremity
   b. Surgery or anesthesia, prolonged immobilization
   c. Diabetes mellitus, polycythemia vera, dysproteinemia
   d. Central line disconnection (air embolus)
   e. Trauma (especially fractures of the spine, pelvis, or legs with fat emboli) or recent pelvic or lower abdominal surgery
   f. Heart failure, acute myocardial infarction
   g. Shock (bacteremic or nonbacteremic), burns
   h. Obesity, malignancy
   i. Estrogen administration, pregnancy, recent childbirth (amnionic fluid embolus)

3. **Signs and symptoms**
   a. Patient's chief complaint varies considerably, depending on the severity and type of embolism. Sudden onset of chest pain (usually pleuritic), cough, and hemoptysis (which suggests pulmonary infarction) are commonly reported.
   b. Massive PE (>50% vascular occlusion) is indicated by mental clouding, anxiety, feeling of impending doom and apprehension.
   c. Other symptoms may be vague and nonspecific.

     i. Dyspnea, tachypnea, increased work of breathing

     ii. Tachycardia, diffuse chest discomfort, reduced blood pressure

     iii. Anxiety, restlessness, apprehension, agitation, syncope

     iv. Asymmetric chest expansion due to pleuritic pain

     v. Petechiae over the thorax and upper extremities (fat emboli)

     vi. Diaphoresis, cold and clammy skin, and cyanosis

     vii. Increased fremitus with a large hemorrhagic pulmonary infarct; pleural friction fremitus may be palpated in patients with pleural inflammation distal to an infarct

     viii. Resonance heard throughout the lung fields except dullness to percussion over the area of infarction

     ix. Pleural friction rub; inspiratory crackles (rales) may be heard; increased intensity of the pulmonic second sound (P_2); fixed splitting of the second heart sound (S_2) is an ominous finding caused by marked right ventricular overload. Murmur is heard over the affected lung field, augmented by inspiration, and is generated by flow through a partially obstructed pulmonary artery. Murmur may be absent initially and then develop as an embolus resolves.

4. Diagnostic study findings

    a. Laboratory: ABG levels may indicate respiratory alkalosis (caused by hyperventilation) and hypoxemia; A-a gradient is increased; in a small percentage (6%) of patients, the A-a gradient may be normal

    b. Radiologic

     i. Chest radiograph: Nonspecific, frequently normal. Pleural effusion occurs in 30% to 50% of cases but is small; atelectasis and elevated hemidiaphragm on the affected side may be seen.

     ii. Lower-extremity Doppler ultrasonography: To evaluate for DVT as a possible cause. Negative findings on serial ultrasonographic scans reduce the likelihood of PE to less than 2%.

     iii. Pulmonary angiography: Most definitive test (gold standard) for PE; should be considered when results of noninvasive tests are equivocal or contradictory or as an initial diagnostic test if the patient is hemodynamically unstable

     iv. CT-angiography may also be done.

    c. ECG: Usually normal, but in massive PE may reveal "P pulmonale," right-axis deviation, or incomplete or new right bundle branch block. ECG often demonstrates sinus tachycardia or, less frequently, atrial fibrillation or flutter.

    d. Radionuclide testing: Lung $\dot{V}/\dot{Q}$ scan not definitive but suggestive of PE; less risky than angiography; performed for all clinically stable patients with suspected PE; about 60% of $\dot{V}/\dot{Q}$ scans will show indeterminate findings

5. Goals of care

    a. Pulmonary artery blood flow is restored.

    b. Hemodynamic parameters return to normal.

    c. Recurrence or worsening of embolization and thrombosis is prevented.

    d. Chest pain is relieved.

6. Collaborating professionals on health care team: Nurse, physician, pulmonologist, respiratory therapist, clinical pharmacologist

7. Management of patient care

    a. Anticipated patient trajectory

     i. Delivery of care: Depending on the severity of the patient's signs and symptoms or the frequency or type of interventions required, the patient may need to be transferred to the ICU for treatment

     ii. Positioning: Keep the head of the bed elevated at 30 to 45 degrees to enhance ventilation and prevent aspiration. Avoid using knee elevation on a Gatch bed; instruct the patient to avoid crossing the legs or sitting with the feet dependent for long periods. Vary position and do range-of-motion manipulations to enhance peripheral blood flow.

     iii. Skin care: Inspect skin integrity regularly, especially on the lower legs. Promptly report the patient's development of pain, swelling, tenderness, rubor, and localized warmth in a lower extremity (suggestive of phlebitis, possible thrombosis). Have the patient perform active or passive range-of-motion exercises, ambulate when able, wear antiembolism stockings as ordered.

    iv. Pain management: Administer analgesics for relief of chest pain (can be severe)

    v. Nutrition: Ensure adequate fluid intake to avoid dehydration and increased blood viscosity

    vi. Discharge planning: Provide patient education and follow-up related to the prevention of phlebitis and DVT, facilitation of venous return, and safe use of anticoagulants

    vii. Pharmacology: Administer anticoagulants as ordered; monitor for signs of bleeding; administer thrombolytic therapy, sedatives, and pain medication as ordered

    viii. Treatments

        (a) O_2 administration, as needed

        (b) Early ambulation, turning, promotion of coughing and deep breathing

        (c) Use of elastic stockings, pneumatic compression stockings (if not contraindicated with systemic anticoagulation), leg elevation

        (d) Adequate fluid intake

        (e) Thrombolytic and anticoagulant therapy, heparin or low-molecular-weight heparin

        (f) IV medications

        (g) Placement of filter device in inferior vena cava

        (h) Surgical embolectomy

  b. Potential complications

    i. Hospital-acquired infection: Aspiration; see Acute Respiratory Failure

    ii. Bleeding

        (a) Mechanism: Risk of anticoagulation therapy

        (b) Management: Judicious, closely monitored use of anticoagulants

8. Evaluation of patient care

  a. Respiratory rate, breathing pattern, and hemodynamic parameters are normal for the patient.

  b. Arterial pH, P_{CO_2}, and P_{O_2} indicate desired levels of oxygenation, ventilation, and acid-base balance for the patient.

  c. Coagulation profile is within the desired range for the patient.

  d. Patient reports a decrease in the sensation of dyspnea.

  e. Patient denies chest pain and dyspnea.

Pneumothorax

1. Pathophysiology

  a. A pneumothorax occurs as the result of the accumulation of air or other gas in the pleural space. Can be classified as spontaneous (without obvious cause or trauma), traumatic (direct or indirect chest trauma), iatrogenic, or tension.

    i. Spontaneous

        (a) Primary—Disruption of the visceral pleura that allows air from the lung to enter the pleural space; occurs spontaneously in patients *without* underlying lung disease

        (b) Secondary—Disruption of the visceral pleura that allows air from the lung to enter the pleural space; occurs spontaneously in patients *with* underlying lung disease

    ii. Traumatic

        (a) Open—Laceration in the parietal pleura that allows atmospheric air to enter the pleural space; occurs as a result of penetrating chest trauma

        (b) Closed—Laceration in the visceral pleura that allows air from the lung to enter the pleural space; occurs as a result of blunt chest trauma

    iii. Iatrogenic—Laceration in the visceral pleura that allows air from the lung to enter the pleural space; occurs as a result of therapeutic or diagnostic procedures, such as central line insertion, thoracentesis, and needle aspirations

      iv. Tension—Occurs when air is allowed to enter the pleural space but not exit it; as pressure increases inside the pleural space, the lung collapses and the mediastinum shifts to the unaffected side; may be a result of a spontaneous or traumatic pneumothorax

  b. Regardless of the etiology, once air enters the pleural space, the affected lung becomes compressed.

      i. As the lung collapses, the alveoli become underventilated, causing $\dot{V}/\dot{Q}$ mismatching and intrapulmonary shunting.

      ii. If the pneumothorax is large, hypoxemia ensues and ARF quickly develops.

      iii. In addition, increased pressure within the chest can lead to shifting of the mediastinum, compression of the great vessels, and decreased cardiac output.

2. Etiology and risk factors

  a. Disruption of the parietal pleura occurs as the result of penetrating trauma to the chest wall, which allows atmospheric air to enter the pleural space (traumatic open pneumothorax).

  b. Disruption of the visceral pleura occurs as the result of air entering the pleural space from the lung.

      i. Blunt chest wall trauma (traumatic closed pneumothorax)

      ii. Diagnostic or therapeutic procedures (traumatic iatrogenic pneumothorax)

      iii. Diseases of the pulmonary system (secondary spontaneous pneumothorax)

      iv. Ruptured subpleural blebs (primary spontaneous pneumothorax)

3. Signs and symptoms

  a. Chief complaint: Chest pain on the affected side and dyspnea are the two most prominent symptoms

  b. Inspection

      i. Decreased chest movement over the affected side

      ii. Shallow respirations and tachypnea

      iii. Use of accessory muscles, intercostal retractions

      iv. Open chest wound may be present because of penetrating chest trauma

      v. Position of the trachea may be displaced—toward the injured side in pneumothorax, toward the contralateral side in tension pneumothorax

  c. Palpation

      i. Subcutaneous emphysema

      ii. Decreased fremitus

  d. Percussion: Hyperresonance

  e. Auscultation: Decreased or absent breath sounds over affected area

4. Diagnostic study findings

  a. Laboratory: ABGs may demonstrate hypoxemia and hypercapnia depending on size of pneumothorax

  b. Radiologic

      i. Chest radiography

         (a) Pneumothorax: Increased translucency evident on the affected side

         (b) Tension pneumothorax: Shows a shift in the mediastinum to the unaffected side in addition to pneumothorax

5. Goals of care

  a. Patent airway is maintained.

  b. ABG levels and pulmonary parameters are restored to and maintained within acceptable limits for the patient.

  c. Chest wall integrity and stability are restored.

  d. Integrity of the pleural space is reestablished.

  e. Chest pain and dyspnea are minimized.

6. Collaborating professionals on health care team: See Acute Respiratory Failure

7. Management of patient care

  a. Anticipated patient trajectory

      i. Delivery of care: Depending on the severity of the patient's signs and symptoms or the frequency or type of interventions required, the patient may need to be transferred to the ICU for treatment

   ii. Positioning: Keep the head of the bed elevated 30 to 45 degrees to optimize ventilation and prevent aspiration; provide symptomatic treatment to ensure the ability to cough and deep breathe

   iii. Skin care: Reinforce dressings as necessary; provide wound care around chest tubes and at other invasive sites

   iv. Pain management: Pain medication and sedatives to relieve the discomfort of tubes and treatment and prevent treatment interference. Administer analgesia judiciously to avoid compromise of ventilation.

   v. Nutrition: Provide adequate nutrition to promote healing; secure pharmacologic and dietary consults for composition and administration of parenteral and/or enteral feeding. Maintain accurate input and output records and monitor fluid balance.

   vi. Infection control: Hand hygiene

   vii. Transport: Ensure that optimal levels of patient care, patient monitoring, O_2 supply, humidification, and positioning are maintained throughout transport

   viii. Discharge planning: Evaluate the need for rehabilitation on discharge; anticipate home care equipment needs

   ix. Pharmacology: Pain medications, sedatives, and antibiotics as needed

   x. Psychosocial issues: Degree, nature, and extent of support must be tailored to patient and family needs and incorporate as wide an array of health care services as warranted

   xi. Treatments
   (a) Placement of a percutaneous catheter attached to a Heimlich valve or insertion of a thoracic vent, or insertion of a chest tube with underwater-seal suction drainage
      (1) Heimlich valve—Small one-way valve device that is easily secured to a catheter placed in the chest, allows air to exit from the pleural space but not enter it
      (2) Thoracic vent—Similar to a Heimlich valve in that it is a one-way valve, but it comes attached to the catheter
   (b) Placement of chest tubes attached to drainage system, usually inserted in the fourth or fifth intercostal space on the midaxillary line
      (1) Observe for the absence or presence of bubbling in the water seal chamber.
      (2) If suction is ordered, maintain the appropriate suction setting.
      (3) Monitor and record the volume and nature of drainage; notify the physician if the volume of bloody drainage exceeds the limit set by protocol, unit routine, or written order.
      (4) Avoid kinks or dependent loops in chest drainage tubing to facilitate drainage.
      (5) Properly secure the chest tube insertion site.
      (6) Observe for signs of leaking pleural fluid or bleeding at the insertion site.
      (7) Routinely check the system for loose connections.
      (8) Preparation for an inadvertent break in a closed chest drainage system set for negative pressure; follow unit procedure in the event of a break in system integrity
   (d) Assistance with emergency decompression of tension pneumothorax through insertion of a large-bore needle or catheter into the second intercostal space at the midclavicular line of the affected side

   xii. Ethical issues: If relevant to the case, see discussion in Acute Respiratory Failure, Chronic Obstructive Pulmonary Disease; see also Chapter 1

b. Potential complications
   i. Hospital-associated infection via wound contamination
   ii. Air leak in the chest tube drainage system—unexpected bubbling in the water-seal chamber
   (a) Place a padded clamp on the drainage tubing as close to the dressing as possible.

(1) If the air bubbling stops, the air leak is located between the patient and the clamp either within the patient or at the insertion site. Remove the clamp, expose the chest tube site, and inspect the tube to ensure that all the eyelets are within the patient. Notify the physician if an eyelet is outside the chest. If all the eyelets are within the patient, the patient probably has an internal air leak.

(2) If the air bubbling does not stop when a clamp is placed on the chest tube, the leak is located between the clamp and the drainage collector. Release the clamp and move it down the tubing a few inches at a time to a point where the bubbling stops. Note the site as the point of the leak and place tape over the whole to reestablish a seal or replace the system.

    iii. If the chest tube system is inadvertently interrupted, place the chest tube into a bottle of sterile water or normal saline solution while the drainage system is reestablished.

8. **Evaluation of patient care**
   a. Respiratory rate, breathing pattern, and ABG values are normal for the patient.
   b. Chest wall motion and expansion are normal in both phases of ventilation.
   c. All blood, air, chyle, or other foreign matter is evacuated from the pleural space; negative pressure is restored; both lungs are fully expanded.
   d. Patient denies chest pain, shortness of breath, and dyspnea.

Acute Pneumonia

1. **Pathophysiology**
   a. Inflammatory process of the alveolar spaces caused by infection
   b. Possible pathogenic mechanisms for the development of pneumonia
       i. Aspiration
       ii. Inhalation
       iii. Inoculation
       iv. Direct spread from contiguous sites
       v. Hematogenous spread
       vi. Colonization in chronic lung disease (e.g., COPD, cystic fibrosis)
   c. Acquisition of infection depends on the nature of the infecting organism, the immediate environment, and the defense status of the host
   d. Important constituents of the pulmonary defense system
       i. Upper airway defenses: Adversely affected by nasotracheal intubation, endotracheal intubation, suction catheters, nasogastric tubes
          (a) Nasopharyngeal filtration
          (b) Mucosal adherence
          (c) Bacterial interference
          (d) Saliva
          (e) Secretory immunoglobulin A
       ii. Lower airway defenses: May be impaired or inactivated by old age; underlying diseases such as diabetes, chronic bronchitis, malnutrition; and drug or O_2 therapy
          (a) Cough reflex
          (b) Mucociliary clearance
          (c) Humoral factors
          (d) Cellular factors

2. **Etiology and risk factors**
   a. Normal host infected with usual organisms
       i. *Streptococcus pneumoniae* (pneumococcus): Most common cause, especially in older patients and those with a variety of chronic diseases
       ii. *Mycoplasma pneumoniae* ("walking pneumonia"): Spread by droplet nuclei; may occur in epidemics
       iii. *Haemophilus influenzae*: With encapsulated type B organisms, is more likely to cause bacteremia; nontypable *H. influenzae* is seen more in the elderly population

    iv. Viruses: Relatively uncommon cause of pneumonia in adults, accounting for 25% to 50% of nonbacterial pneumonias; influenza A virus is the most common cause; others include adenovirus and coxsackievirus; pneumonia caused by cytomegalovirus, respiratory syncytial virus, and herpes simplex virus are often seen in immunocompromised patients

    v. *Chlamydia pneumoniae*: Causes a spectrum of illnesses from mild upper respiratory symptoms to pneumonia

    vi. Fungi: Inhalation of *Histoplasma capsulatum* results in acute severe pulmonary histoplasmosis. Similar reactions occur in patients infected with *Blastomyces dermatitidis*, *Cryptococcus*, *Coccidioides immitis*, *Aspergillus fumigatus*, and *Candida albicans*. Geographic location is important in identifying certain organisms.

b. Normal host infected with unusual organisms

    i. *Legionella pneumophila* infections may be sporadic or occur in localized outbreaks in institutions.

    ii. *Bacillus anthracis* infects humans who have been in contact with anthrax-infected animals.

    iii. *Yersinia pestis* causes plague; transmitted from wild animals and their fleas, or via the respiratory route.

    iv. *Francisella tularensis* causes pleuropulmonary tularemia, endemic in certain parts of the United States; transmitted by ticks or, possibly, by inhalation from infected animals.

    v. Group A *Streptococcus* and *Meningococcus* bacteria reside in the upper respiratory tract; pneumonia occurs in individuals housed in groups, such as in military service. *Streptococcus pyogenes* causes pneumonia typically after outbreaks of viral infections.

    vi. *Mycobacterium tuberculosis* infection or atypical TB can produce life-threatening pulmonary complications in hosts whose only risk factor is age.

c. Abnormal host infected with usual organisms: Compromised states can result from the presence of chronic underlying disease, poor nutrition, trauma, or surgery, or subsequent to immunosuppression

    i. Pneumococcal pneumonia is more severe in this population.

    ii. Gram-negative bacilli, such as *Escherichia coli*, *Pseudomonas aeruginosa*, *Serratia*, *Proteus vulgaris*, *Acinetobacter* and *Klebsiella pneumoniae*, and *Moraxella catarrhalis*, can be the causative organisms.

    iii. Anaerobic bacteria, such as *Bacteroides*, cause severe pulmonary infections in the abnormal host.

    iv. *Staphylococcus aureus* pneumonia is seen in patients with diabetes, in patients with a recent history of influenza, and institutionalized or hospitalized patients.

    v. *K. pneumoniae* causes a virulent, necrotizing pneumonia often seen in alcoholic or debilitated patients; abscess formation is common.

d. Abnormal host infected with unusual organisms

    i. Enterococcal pneumonia is associated with the use of third-generation cephalosporins.

    ii. Group B *S. pneumoniae* pneumonia is often seen in older patients with underlying diseases.

    iii. Hospital-acquired *L. pneumophila* pneumonia occurs in patients with renal transplants and those who are debilitated and immunocompromised.

    iv. *Legionella micdadei*, the Pittsburgh pneumonia agent, may infect patients with renal transplants during corticosteroid therapy.

    v. Fungi, including *A. fumigatus* and *Aspergillus flavum*, produce pneumonia mostly in patients who have received high doses of steroids and broad-spectrum antibiotics.

    vi. *Nocardia asteroides* pneumonia is seen in patients with renal transplants and patients with hematologic malignancies.

    vii. *Pneumocystis carinii* infections, infections with typical and atypical mycobacteria, and cytomegalovirus infections are seen in patients with acquired immunodeficiency syndrome.

    e. Multidrug-resistant organisms, vancomycin-resistant enterococci, and penicillin-resistant *S. pneumoniae* are becoming more prevalent in the community; therefore, patients may enter facilities with the infection rather than acquire it in the hospital.

    f. Pneumonias can be categorized by their mode of origin as follows:

      i. Hospital-acquired pneumonia—Pneumonia that develops >48 hours after hospital admission and is not incubating at admission

      ii. Ventilator-associated pneumonia—Pneumonia in patients who have been receiving mechanical ventilation for ≥48 hours; a subset of hospital-acquired pneumonia

      iii. Health care–associated pneumonia—Pneumonia developing before hospital admission in patients in close contact with the health system

      iv. Community-acquired pneumonia—Pneumonia acquired outside of the hospitals or extended-care facility

3. Signs and symptoms

    a. Chief complaint varies, depending on the organism. Some common presentations include the following:

      i. Pneumococcal pneumonia: Abrupt shaking chills or rigor, fever, dyspnea, pleuritic pain, and cough productive of rusty sputum

      ii. Mycoplasma: Fever, myalgias, headache, minimally productive cough, and nonpleuritic chest pain

      iii. *H. influenzae:* Fever, chills, and cough with purulent sputum

      iv. *Klebsiella:* Sudden onset, blood-tinged sputum, and tachypnea

    b. Clinical features: See Acute Respiratory Failure; also hypoxemia, increased work of breathing, impaired alveolar ventilation, impaired respiratory gas exchange

      i. Asymmetric chest expansion with dullness or flatness to percussion over affected areas

      ii. Breath sounds may be decreased; fine inspiratory crackles or bronchial breath sounds over areas of consolidation (lobar pneumonia)

      iii. Bronchophony; whispered pectoriloquy and egophony may also be heard with consolidation

4. Diagnostic study findings

    a. Laboratory

      i. Sputum examination

        (a) Color and consistency vary with the pathogen

        (b) Initial Gram staining and microscopic examination

          (1) Good sputum specimen contains few (less than five) squamous epithelial cells picked up in transit through the upper respiratory tract. When sputum cannot be expectorated, a specimen may be obtained by other means such as suctioning, transtracheal aspiration, fiberoptic bronchoscopy, needle aspiration of the lung, or open lung biopsy.

          (2) Examination of expectorated sputum specimens has relatively poor sensitivity and specificity.

          (3) Staining demonstrates polymorphonuclear leukocytes (PMNs) and bacterial agents; large numbers of PMNs are seen in most bacterial pneumonias; fewer PMNs and more mononuclear inflammatory cells are seen in mycoplasmal and viral pneumonias.

          (4) Sputum cultures are done with initial Gram staining and microscopic examination; however, some bacteria are relatively difficult to grow, so the initial Gram stain result is just as important in making the etiologic diagnosis.

      ii. Blood cultures

        (a) Obtaining a blood sample is very important in patient evaluation because of the high specificity of a positive culture result, especially in hospitalized patients with pneumococcal pneumonia.

        (b) Blood and sputum cultures are obtained before antibiotic administration.

        (c) Patients with documented bacteremic pneumonia have a worse prognosis than those with nonbacteremic pneumonia.

        iii. Leukocyte counts
- (a) Often elevated in lobar pneumonia; may be normal with atypical pneumonia
- (b) Normal or reduced in the elderly, in immunocompromised patients, in patients with overwhelming infections, and in those with viral infection

        iv. ABG analysis: May indicate hypoxemia and hypocapnia in lobar pneumonia

  b. Radiologic: Chest radiographic findings vary with involvement
        i. Segmental or lobar consolidation, infiltrates
        ii. Particularly helpful in detecting parapneumonic effusions, abscesses, and cavities

  c. Thoracentesis: May be indicated when significant pleural effusion is present

5. Goals of care
- **a.** Pulmonary infection is halted and reversed.
- **b.** Oxygenation and ventilation are improved.
- **c.** Removal of airway secretions is facilitated.
- **d.** Vital signs, ABG values, and respiratory dynamics are restored to within normal limits for the patient.
- **e.** Dyspnea at rest and with exertion is minimized.
- **f.** Positive nitrogen balance is established and maintained to promote regaining of strength and healing.

6. Collaborating professionals on health care team: See Acute Respiratory Failure, Chronic Obstructive Pulmonary Disease

7. Management of patient care
- **a.** Anticipated patient trajectory
  - i. Delivery of care: Depending on the severity of the patient's signs and symptoms or the frequency or type of interventions required, the patient may need to be transferred to the ICU for treatment
  - ii. Positioning: See Acute Respiratory Failure, Chronic Obstructive Pulmonary Disease; change position to mobilize secretions; avoid the supine position
  - iii. Skin care: Turn frequently to drain lungs and maintain skin integrity
  - iv. Pain management: Pleuritic chest pain control may be achieved by anti-inflammatory agents, analgesics, or intercostal nerve blocks; pain medication and sedatives need to relieve the discomfort of tubes and treatment and prevent interference with turning, coughing, deep breathing, incentive spirometry, ambulation
  - v. Nutrition: Enlist assistance from a dietitian to ensure that nutritional intake is adequate to restore strength, facilitate ventilator weaning, and support healing and recovery; if possible, use the enteral route to reduce infection risk
  - vi. Infection control: Regular, thorough oral care with brushing (versus swabbing) and cleansing appears to reduce morbidity and mortality from pneumonia. Use strict infection control procedures; avoid unnecessary invasive procedures or limit their duration of use.
  - vii. Transport: Ensure that optimal levels of patient care, patient monitoring, O_2 supply, humidification, and positioning are maintained throughout transport
  - viii. Pharmacology: Administer antibiotics within 8 hours of admission, preferably within 4 hours, and monitor response; administer sedatives and pain medication as needed
  - ix. Treatments: See Acute Respiratory Failure
- **b.** Potential complications
  - i. Superimposed hospital-associated infection(s): See Acute Respiratory Failure
  - ii. Difficulty weaning or liberating from mechanical ventilation: See Impaired Alveolar Ventilation, Acute Respiratory Failure, Chronic Obstructive Pulmonary Disease

8. Evaluation of patient care
- **a.** No clinical, laboratory, or radiologic evidence of pulmonary infection is present.
- **b.** Secretions are minimal and the patient able to expectorate readily.
- **c.** Blood gas values and ventilatory parameters are within acceptable limits.
- **d.** Breath sounds are clear bilaterally, and no adventitious sounds are present.

Pulmonary Aspiration

1. **Pathophysiology (varies with the type of aspiration)**
   a. Pulmonary aspiration may result from vomiting or regurgitation. Vomiting is an active mechanism that interrupts breathing, causes the diaphragm to descend, contracts the anterior abdominal wall, elevates the diaphragm, closes the pylorus, and opens the esophageal sphincter, which results in ejection of contents from the stomach. Regurgitation is completely passive and may occur even in the presence of paralyzed muscles. Powerful laryngeal and cough reflexes normally prevent aspiration of gastric contents into the tracheobronchial tree. Any impairment or depression of these normal reflexes increases the risk of pulmonary aspiration.
   b. Large particles can obstruct major airways and cause immediate asphyxiation and death.
   c. If clear acidic liquid, pH of aspirated material largely determines the extent of pulmonary injury. If the pH decreases below 2.5 or if the volume of acidic fluid is large, the severity of lung injury increases.
      i. Chemical burns destroy type II alveolar cells that produce surfactant and increase alveolar capillary membrane permeability, with subsequent extravasation of fluid and blood into the interstitium and alveoli.
      ii. As fluid and blood accumulate in the alveolar space, the lung volume diminishes; thus, both FRC and compliance decrease. Reflex airway closure may also occur.
      iii. Alveolar ventilation decreases relative to perfusion, which results in intrapulmonary shunting. Hypoxia can occur minutes after acid aspiration.
      iv. Extensive irritation of the airways by acidic fluid may induce intense bronchospasm.
      v. Widespread peribronchial hemorrhage along with pulmonary edema and necrosis may occur.
   d. If clear nonacidic liquid, nature and extent of pulmonary damage depends on the volume of the aspirate and its composition.
      i. Aspiration of less-acidic or neutral pH liquids can induce hypoxia with acute respiratory decompensation. Reflex airway closure, pulmonary edema, and changes in the characteristics of surfactant may occur. There is little necrosis.
      ii. Sequelae are more frequently transient and more easily reversible than with aspiration of acidic liquid.
   e. Foodstuff or small particles may produce a severe subacute inflammatory pulmonary reaction with extensive hemorrhage.
      i. Within 6 hours of aspiration, there may be extensive hemorrhagic pneumonia.
      ii. Extravasation of fluid from the intravascular space into the lungs usually occurs but is generally not as intense or rapid as after acid aspiration.
      iii. Severe intrapulmonary shunting may result, and arterial P_{O_2} may be as low as or lower than that seen after the aspiration of acidic liquid.
      iv. Arterial P_{CO_2} is usually much higher after the aspiration of food. This may indicate a higher degree of hypoventilation.
      v. Aspiration of acidic foodstuff may produce even more tissue necrosis as a result of the combined effects of acid and foods.
   f. Aspiration of material grossly contaminated with bacteria (i.e., in bowel obstruction) can be fatal.
2. **Etiology and risk factors: Aspiration is usually associated with specific predisposing conditions**
   a. Altered consciousness: Drug or alcohol use, anesthesia, seizures, CNS disorders, shock, use of sedatives
   b. Altered anatomy: Tracheostomy, esophageal or tracheal abnormalities, nasogastric or nasointestinal tube, ETT, intestinal obstruction
   c. Protracted vomiting or coughing
   d. Improper positioning of the patient, especially if the patient is receiving enteral hyperalimentation

3. **Signs and symptoms**
   a. Patient's chief complaints: Cough, dyspnea, wheezing. With fluid or solid object aspiration, there can be an abrupt onset of acute respiratory distress.
   b. Hypoxemia: See Acute Respiratory Failure, Inability to Establish or Maintain a Patent Airway, Impaired Respiratory Mechanics
   c. Increased work of breathing (depends on the nature and extent of aspiration): See Chronic Obstructive Pulmonary Disease, Asthma
   d. Increased respiratory secretions, hypotension, tachycardia, tachypnea, fever
   e. Inspiratory stridor due to foreign body obstruction of a large bronchus; may be accompanied by cyanosis, tachypnea, use of accessory respiratory muscles
   f. Wheezing heard with aspiration of both liquids and solid objects. Crackles and possible wheezing heard in the affected lung with aspiration. Absent breath sounds if a major bronchus is occluded.

4. **Diagnostic study findings**
   a. Laboratory
      i. Sputum examination: Induced cough or tracheal suction to obtain specimens for stain and culture; cytologic examination is sometimes diagnostic. Fiberoptic bronchoscopy is sometimes used in infectious processes.
      ii. ABG analysis: May demonstrate hypoxemia
   b. Radiologic: Dependent lobe infiltrates and atelectasis. Gravity-dependent areas of the lungs most prone to aspiration include the superior segments of the lower lobes and the posterior segments of the upper and lower lobes. If a nasogastric or nasointestinal tube is in place, radiographs should verify their proper location and position, particularly if medications and/or enteral formula feedings are being administered.
   c. Pulmonary function: May show decreased compliance or decreased diffusing capacity
   d. Open lung biopsy: Reserved for patients who are unable to safely undergo transbronchial biopsy

5. **Goals of care**
   a. Patent airway is established and maintained.
   b. Oxygenation and alveolar ventilation return to normal values.
   c. Harmful effects of the aspirant on pulmonary function are minimized.
   d. Recurrence of aspiration is prevented.

6. **Collaborating professionals on health care team: See Acute Respiratory Failure, Chronic Obstructive Pulmonary Disease**

7. **Management of patient care**
   a. Anticipated patient trajectory: See also Acute Pneumonia, Acute Respiratory Failure
      i. Delivery of care: Depending on the severity of the patient's signs and symptoms or the frequency or type of interventions required, the patient may need to be transferred to the ICU for treatment
      ii. Positioning: Elevate head of the bed 30 to 45 degrees to prevent recurrence of aspiration; avoid the supine position or any posture that predisposes to regurgitation or aspiration, especially if enteral feedings are administered
      iii. Nutrition: See Acute Pneumonia. If the patient is being fed nasoenterally, carefully verify the location of the feeding tube and routinely assess for pulmonary aspiration by clinical findings, as well as routine testing of tracheal aspirates for the presence or absence of glucose. False-positive readings may be caused by blood or other unknown factors.
      iv. Infection control: Monitor carefully because many aspirants may cause chemical irritation and/or infection
      v. Transport: Ensure that optimal levels of patient care, patient monitoring, O_2 supply, humidification, and positioning are maintained throughout transport
      vi. Discharge planning: If the patient will return home with a feeding tube in place, provide patient and family education regarding safe administration of tube feedings; supervision by home care services may need to be arranged
      vii. Pharmacology: Antibiotics may be necessary if infection ensues; corticosteroids may be of benefit if given immediately after aspiration of acid

      viii. Treatments: See Pneumonia, Acute Respiratory Failure

    b. Potential complications: See Pneumonia, Acute Respiratory Failure

8. Evaluation of patient care

    a. Airway remains patent and free of secretions.

    b. ABG values and ventilatory parameters are within acceptable limits.

    c. No clinical evidence of complications from aspirated material is present.

Pulmonary Problems in Surgical Patients

1. Pathophysiology

    a. Surgery represents a stress to the respiratory system. Pulmonary problems are the major cause of morbidity after surgery.

    b. Changes in pulmonary function occur normally during the immediately postoperative period. These changes are most evident after abdominal or thoracic surgery.

        i. Reduction in FVC is consistent with a restrictive defect; it is significant but usually temporary.

        ii. Reduction in lung volumes, especially FRC, also occurs, in part because of pain and the supine position.

        iii. Reduced lung compliance is present, resulting in reduced tidal volume and increased respiratory frequency.

    c. Microatelectasis is the most common cause of hypoxemia; the increased respiratory frequency leads to respiratory alkalosis.

    d. Bacterial invasion of the lower airways and reduced clearance after surgery predispose to respiratory infection.

    e. Aspiration of gastric and oropharyngeal contents occurs after surgery in patients who have a disturbance in consciousness.

    f. Arterial hypoxemia due to $\dot{V}/\dot{Q}$ mismatching is common in the postoperative period in normal patients and is exaggerated in patients with COPD.

2. Etiology and risk factors

    a. History of COPD or cigarette smoking is the most important risk factor. Preoperative hypercapnia is a serious risk factor.

    b. Obesity results in decreased vital capacity.

    c. Very young and elderly persons are at increased risk for these complications.

    d. People with underlying chronic diseases are at greater risk.

    e. Prolonged anesthesia time increases risk.

    f. Thoracic and abdominal surgery are especially hazardous to patients at risk. Maximal inspirations are voluntarily limited because of pain, which thereby increases the risk of atelectasis.

3. Signs and symptoms

    a. Patient's chief complaint varies with the type of surgery but is often incisional pain.

    b. Cough with or without sputum production may occur and fear of or reluctance to cough, deep breathe, and move about after surgery.

    c. Tachypnea, shallow respirations due to splinting with incisional pain may progress to signs of respiratory distress, increased work of breathing, dyspnea.

    d. If atelectasis progresses to pneumonia, clinical signs include those related to fever and infection (e.g., crackles from small airway collapse due to shallow breathing, rhonchi or gurgles from secretions in the larger airways, wheezing indicating airflow obstruction, bronchial breath sounds with consolidation).

4. Diagnostic study findings

    a. Preoperative medical evaluation includes chest radiography, ECG, sputum examination, and pulmonary function tests.

        i. FEV_1, FVC, and PEFR values are used to predict the development of postoperative pulmonary complications.

        ii. Split pulmonary function studies estimate the amount of pulmonary function remaining after surgery.

        iii. Other diagnostic tests may be ordered before surgery, depending on preexisting pulmonary or cardiac disease. These include CT scan of the chest and $\dot{V}/\dot{Q}$ scan.

    b. For patients with abnormal pulmonary function study results, ABG analysis is performed before surgery. Presence of hypoxemia or CO_2 retention at baseline indicates that postoperative ABG levels should be followed closely.

    c. Cardiac stress test, possible cardiac catheterization are performed if the stress test results are positive.

5. Goal of care: Prevent or minimize postoperative pulmonary complications

6. Collaborating professionals on health care team: Nurse, physician, anesthesiologist, respiratory therapist

7. Management of patient care

    a. Anticipated patient trajectory: See Pulmonary Aspiration, Acute Pneumonia, Chronic Obstructive Pulmonary Disease

        i. Delivery of care: Depending on the severity of the patient's signs and symptoms or the frequency or type of interventions required, the patient may need to be transferred to the ICU for treatment

        ii. Positioning: After thoracic surgery

            (a) After a lobectomy the patient should be turned onto the nonoperative side. When the good lung is dependent (down), blood flow is greater to the area with better ventilation and $\dot{V}/\dot{Q}$ matching is better. When the affected (operative side) lung is dependent (down), blood flow is greater to an area with less ventilation and $\dot{V}/\dot{Q}$ mismatching results. The patient should be turned frequently to promote secretion removal but should have the affected lung dependent as little as possible.

            (b) After a pneumonectomy the patient should initially be positioned supine or turned onto the operative side. Turning onto the operative side promotes splinting of the incision and facilitates deep-breathing exercises. Tilting the patient slightly toward the unaffected side is possible, but the surgeon should indicate when free side-to-side positioning is safe.

        iii. Treatments

            (a) Provide preoperative training in effective techniques for turning, deep breathing, coughing, ambulation, activity exercises, and active and passive range-of-motion exercises; suggest oral hygiene care.

            (b) Encourage cessation of smoking at least 48 hours before surgery. If surgery can be postponed or is elective, cessation 4 to 6 weeks before surgery may be indicated.

            (c) Familiarize the patient with respiratory therapy equipment and techniques, such as incentive spirometry, chest physiotherapy, and the postoperative exercise program.

            (d) Provide early ambulation and leg exercises, chest physiotherapy, and postural drainage.

            (e) Guide the patient to perform intensive deep breathing exercises and incentive spirometry, and support chest and abdominal incisions during coughing.

    b. Potential complications (see previous coverage of each complication listed)

        i. Acute pneumonia

        ii. Acute respiratory failure

        iii. Difficulty weaning from ventilator

8. Evaluation of patient care

    a. Patient evidences no clinical signs of pulmonary complications after surgery.

    b. Patient's pulmonary function is equivalent to or better than preoperative function.

Obstructive Sleep Apnea

1. Pathophysiology

    a. *Apnea* is defined as cessation of airflow for more than 10 seconds. *Sleep apnea* is defined as repeated episodes of upper airway obstruction associated with obstructive apnea and hypopnea during sleep together with daytime sleepiness or altered cardiopulmonary function. Epidemiologic studies estimate that the condition affects 2% to 4% of middle-aged adults.

    b. Upper airway dysfunction and the specific sites of narrowing or closure are influenced by the underlying neuromuscular tone, upper airway muscle synchrony, and the stage of sleep.

i.   These events are most prominent during rapid eye movement sleep secondary to hypotonia of the upper airway muscles characteristic of this stage of sleep.

ii. Definitive event in obstructive sleep apnea is the posterior movement of the tongue and palate into apposition with the posterior pharyngeal wall, which results in occlusion of the nasopharynx and oropharynx.

iii. After the obstruction and resultant apnea, progressive asphyxia develops until there is a brief arousal from sleep, restoration of upper airway patency, and resumption of airflow. Patient quickly returns to sleep, only to experience the sequence of events over and over again.

iv. Patients with sleep apnea are at increased risk for diurnal hypertension, pulmonary hypertension, nocturnal dysrhythmias, right and left ventricular failure, myocardial infarction, and stroke.

v.   Hypoxemia, hypercapnia, polycythemia, and cor pulmonale may complicate the late stages of the disease.

2. **Etiology and risk factors**
   a. Obesity—Increased upper body obesity, as reflected by neck circumference (neck size 17 inches and larger in men, 16 inches and larger in women)
   b. Nasal obstruction such as severe septal deviation or nasopharyngeal infection or blockage
   c. Adenoidal or tonsillar hypertrophy (seen in children)
   d. Micrognathia, retrognathia, or macroglossia
   e. Vocal cord paralysis
   f. Genetically determined craniofacial features or abnormalities of ventilatory control (CNS)—May be the reason that sleep apnea is common in some families

3. **Signs and symptoms**
   a. Patient's chief complaint: Excessive daytime sleepiness
   b. Fatigue, as well as related personality changes and cognitive difficulties (patient may come to the hospital after an accident caused by daytime sleepiness)
   c. Chronic loud snoring
   d. Morning headaches
   e. Loss of libido

4. **Diagnostic study findings**
   a. Laboratory: ABG analysis is not diagnostic of sleep apnea but is performed as part of a diagnostic workup to determine baseline ventilation and oxygenation
   b. Polysomnography (sleep study) for sleep staging, airflow and ventilatory effort, arterial O_2 saturation, ECG, body position, and periodic limb movement evaluation
   c. Home evaluation and testing
      i. Pulse oximetry, portable (home) monitoring of cardiopulmonary channels, such as airflow, ventilatory effort, and heart rate may be evaluated.
      ii. Sensitivity and specificity of pulse oximetry findings alone for the diagnosis of sleep apnea are controversial.
   d. Pulmonary function studies: May be done to exclude or confirm concomitant intrinsic lung disease, such as obstructive or restrictive lung disease

5. **Goals of care: Apneic episodes during sleep are prevented**

6. **Collaborating professionals on health care team: Nurse; ear, nose, and throat physician; sleep study staff; respiratory therapist**

7. **Management of patient care**
   a. Anticipated patient trajectory
      i.   Positioning: Keep the head of the bed elevated 30 to 45 degrees; avoid the supine position; maintain a neutral position for head and neck alignment; avoid neck flexion
      ii. Nutrition: Obtain a dietary consult to initiate a weight reduction program if obesity is a contributing factor
      iii. Transport: Ensure that optimal levels of patient care, patient monitoring, O_2 supply, humidification, and positioning are maintained throughout transport
      iv. Discharge planning: Educate the patient regarding the proper use and care of oral or dental devices or CPAP equipment. Side effects of the use of oral or dental devices include excessive salivation and temporomandibular joint discomfort.

v.   Pharmacology: Instruct the patient to avoid alcoholic beverages and sedatives before sleep

vi.   Psychosocial issues: Degree, nature, and extent of support must be tailored to patient and family needs and incorporate as wide an array of health care services as warranted. Daytime demeanor and social interactions may improve considerably after the disorder is effectively treated.

vii.   Treatments

(a) O_2 delivery via a CPAP or BiPAP device as ordered

(1)   Instruct on the proper use and maintenance of equipment.

(2)   Teach care of the skin surrounding the nose area where the mask is applied.

(3)   Assess for intolerance to nasal CPAP machine noise and airway pressure.

(b)   Postoperative monitoring and instruction after surgical treatment or correction for sleep apnea if indicated

(1)   Perform preoperative and postoperative teaching for patients requiring tracheostomy; if the neck is thick, the decannulation process may be difficult.

(2)   Repeat the sleep study or nocturnal oximetry after tracheostomy tube placement, because the patient may still hypoventilate as a result of central sleep apnea or intrinsic lung disease.

(3)   Provide tracheostomy tube and stoma care instruction to the patient and family.

b.   Potential complications: Hospital-acquired infection. See Pulmonary Aspiration, Acute Pneumonia

8.   **Evaluation of patient care**

a.   Repeated sleep study verifies that no further episodes of obstructive sleep apnea have occurred.

b.   Patient reports feeling well rested with no headache on awakening.

c.   Patient's presenting symptoms and related signs of fatigue no longer persist.

REFERENCES AND BIBLIOGRAPHY

Physiologic Anatomy

Albertine KH, Williams MC, Hyde DM. Anatomy of the lungs. In: Mason RJ, Murray JF, Broaddus VC, Nadel JA, eds. *Murray & Nadel's Textbook of Respiratory Medicine.* 4th ed. Philadelphia, PA: Elsevier; 2005.

Boron WF, Boulpaep EL. *Medical Physiology: A Cellular and Molecular Approach.* Philadelphia, PA: Elsevier; 2005.

Brashers VL. Structure and function of the pulmonary system. In: McCance KL, Huether SE, eds. *Pathophysiology: The Biologic Basis for Disease in Adults and Children.* 5th ed. St Louis, MO: Mosby; 2006.

Guyton AC, Hall JE. *Textbook of Medical Physiology.* 11th ed. Philadelphia, PA: Saunders; 2005.

Hicks GH. The respiratory system. In: Wilkins RL, Stoller JK, Kacmarek RM, eds. *Egan's Fundamentals of Respiratory Care.* 9th ed. St Louis, MO: Mosby; 2008.

Ruppel GL. Ventilation. In: Wilkins RL, Stoller JK, Kacmarek RM, eds. *Egan's Fundamentals of Respiratory Care.* 9th ed. St Louis, MO: Mosby; 2008.

Wagner PD, West JB. Ventilation, blood flow, and gas exchange. In: Mason RJ, Murray JF, Broaddus VC, Nadel JA, eds. *Murray & Nadel's Textbook of Respiratory Medicine.* 4th ed. Philadelphia, PA: Elsevier; 2005.

Wilkins RL. Gas exchange and transport. In: Wilkins RL, Stoller JK, Kacmarek RM, eds. *Egan's Fundamentals of Respiratory Care.* 9th ed. St Louis, MO: Mosby; 2008.

Zakynthinos SG, Koulouris NG, Roussos C. Respiratory system mechanics and energetics. In: Mason RJ, Murray JF, Broaddus VC, Nadel JA, eds. *Murray & Nadel's Textbook of Respiratory Medicine.* 4th ed. Philadelphia, PA: Elsevier; 2005.

Patient Assessment

Beckos V, Marini J. Monitoring the mechanically ventilated patient. *Crit Care Clin.* 2007;23:575–611.

Bidwell JL, Pachner RW. Hemoptysis: diagnosis and management. *Am Fam Physician.* 2005;72(7):1253-1260.

Brightling CE. Clinical applications of induced sputum. *Chest.* 2006;129(5):1344-1348.

★ Fitzgerald MA. Perfecting the·art. The physical exam. *RN.* 1991;54(11):34-39.

Giulliano KK, Higgins TL. New-generation pulse oximetry in the care of critically ill patients. *Am J Crit Care.* 2005;14:26-39.

Grap MJ. Pulse oximetry monitoring. In: Burns SM, ed. *Noninvasive Monitoring*. 2nd ed. Sudbury, MA: Jones and Bartlett; 2007.

Irwin RS. Assessing cough severity and efficacy of therapy in clinical research: ACCP evidence-based clinical practice guidelines. *Chest*. 2006;129 (1 Suppl):232S-237S.

Johnson KL. Diagnostic measure to evaluate oxygenation in critically ill adults: implications and limitations. *AACN Clin Issues*. 2004;15:506.

O'Rourke ME. Clinical dilemma: dyspnea. *Semin Oncol Nurs*. 2007;23(3):225-231.

Ruholl L. Arterial blood gases: analysis and responses. *Medsurg Nurs*. 2006;15:343.

Scanlan CL, Wilkins RL. Gas exchange and transport. In: Wilkins RL, Stoller JK, Kacmarek RM, eds. *Egan's Fundamentals of Respiratory Care*. 9th ed. St Louis, MO: Mosby; 2008.

Seidel HM, Ball JW, Dains JE, Benedict GW. *Mosby's Guide to Physical Examination*. 6th ed. St Louis, MO: Mosby; 2006.

Shiber JR, Santana J. Dyspnea. *Med Clin North Am*. 2006;90(3):453-479.

Stiesmeyer JK. A four-step approach to pulmonary assessment. *Am J Nurs*. 1993;93(8):22.

Wilkins RL. Bedside assessment of the patient. In: Wilkins RL, Stoller JK, Kacmarek RM, eds. *Egan's Fundamentals of Respiratory Care*. 9th ed. St Louis, MO: Mosby; 2008.

Wilkins RL, Hodgkin JE, Lopez B. *Fundamentals of Lung and Heart Sounds*. 3rd ed. St Louis, MO: Mosby; 2004.

Woodruff D. Six steps to ABG analysis. *Nursing*. 2007;2:48.

Patient Care

Barreiro TJ, Gemmel DJ. Noninvasive ventilation. *Crit Care Clin*. 2007;23(2):201-222.

Burns SM. Weaning from mechanical ventilation. In: Burns SM, ed. *Care of Mechanically Ventilated Patients*. 2nd ed. Sudbury, MA: Jones and Bartlett; 2007.

Calfee CS, Matthay MA. Recent advances in mechanical ventilation. *Am J Med*. 2005;118(6):584-591.

Donahoe M. Basic ventilator management: lung protective strategies. *Surg Clin North Am*. 2006;86(6):1389-1408.

Frazier SK. Cardiovascular effects of mechanical ventilation and weaning. *Nurs Clin North Am*. 2008;43(1):1-15.

Gardner A, Hughes D, Cook R, Henson R, Osborne S, Gardner G. Best practice in stabilisation of oral endotracheal tubes: a systematic review. *Aust Crit Care*. 2005;18(4):158-165.

Haitsma JJ. Physiology of mechanical ventilation. *Crit Care Clin*. 2007;23(2):117-134.

MacIntyre N. Discontinuing mechanical ventilatory support. *Chest*. 2007;132(3):1049-1056.

MacIntyre NR, Branson RD. *Mechanical Ventilation*. 2nd ed. St Louis, MO: Saunders; 2009.

Munro N. Weaning smokers from mechanical ventilation. *Crit Care Nurs Clin North Am*. 2006;18(1):21-28.

Pilbeam SP, Cairo JM. *Mechanical Ventilation: Physiology and Clinical Applications*. 4th ed. St Louis, MO: Mosby; 2006.

Pierce LNB. Invasive and noninvasive modes and methods of mechanical ventilation. In: Burns SM, ed. *Care of Mechanically Ventilated Patients*. 2nd ed. Sudbury, MA: Jones and Bartlett; 2007.

Pierce LNB. *Management of the Mechanically Ventilated Patient*. 2nd ed. St Louis, MO: Saunders; 2007.

Prinianakis G, Kondili E, Georgopoulos D. Patient-ventilator interaction: an overview. *Respir Care Clin N Am*. 2005;11(2):201-224.

Simmons P, Simmons M. Informed nursing practice: the administration of oxygen to patients with COPD. *Medsurg Nurs*. 2004;13(2):82-85.

Siner JM, Manthous CA. Liberation from mechanical ventilation: what monitoring matters? *Crit Care Clin*. 2007;23(3):613-638.

St John RE, Malen JF. Contemporary issues in adult tracheostomy management. *Crit Care Nurs Clin North Am*. 2004;16(3):413-430.

St John RE, Seckel MA. Airway management. In: Burns SM, ed. *Care of Mechanically Ventilated Patients*. 2nd ed. Sudbury, MA: Jones and Bartlett; 2007.

Acute Respiratory Failure

Burns SM. The science of weaning: when and how? *Crit Care Nurs Clin North Am*. 2004;16(3): 379-386.

El-Masri MM, Williamson KM, Fox-Wasylyshyn SM. Severe acute respiratory syndrome: another challenge for critical care nurses. *AACN Clin Issues*. 2004;15(1):150-159.

Hill NS, Brennan J, Garpestad E, Nava S. Noninvasive ventilation in acute respiratory failure. *Crit Care Med*. 2007;35(10):2402-2407.

Keenan SP, Sinuff T, Cook DJ, et al. Does noninvasive positive pressure ventilation improve outcome in acute hypoxemic respiratory failure: a systematic review. *Crit Care Med*. 2004;32:2516-2523.

Markou NK, Myrianthefs PM, Baltopoulos GJ. Respiratory failure: an overview. *Crit Care Nurs Q*. 2004;27(4):353-379.

Ward NS, Dushay KM. Clinical concise review: mechanical ventilation of patients with chronic obstructive pulmonary disease. *Crit Care Med*. 2008;36(5):1614-1619.

Acute Lung Injury

Bream-Rouwenhorst HR, Beltz EA, Ross MB, Moores KG. Recent developments in the management of acute respiratory distress syndrome in adults. *Am J Health Syst Pharm*. 2008;65(1):29-36.

Cooper SJ. Methods to prevent ventilator-associated lung injury: a summary. *Intensive Crit Care Nurs*. 2004;20(6):358-365.

Dreyfuss D, Ricard JD. Acute lung injury and bacterial infection. *Clin Chest Med.* 2005;26(1):105-112.

George KJ. A systematic approach to care: adult respiratory distress syndrome. *J Trauma Nurs.* 2008;15(1):19-22.

Girard TD, Bernard GR. Mechanical ventilation in ARDS: a state-of-the-art review. *Chest.* 2007; 131(3):921-929.

Kane C, Galanes S. Adult respiratory distress syndrome. *Crit Care Nurs Q.* 2004;27(4):325-335.

Kleinman S, Gajic O, Nunes E, American Association of Blood Banks Transfusion-Related Acute Lung Injury Task Force. Promoting recognition and prevention of transfusion-related acute lung injury. *Crit Care Nurse.* 2007;27(4):49-53.

MacIntyre NR. Current issues in mechanical ventilation for respiratory failure. *Chest.* 2005;128 (5 Suppl 2):561S-567S.

Pruitt B. Take an evidence-based approach to treating acute lung injury. Recognize and promptly address ALI and ARDS to reduce substantial patient harm. *Nursing.* 2007;Spring Suppl:14-18.

Rance M. Kinetic therapy positively influences oxygenation in patients with ALI/ARDS. *Nurs Crit Care.* 2005;10(1):35-41.

Sevransky JE, Levy MM, Marini JJ. Mechanical ventilation in sepsis-induced acute lung injury/acute respiratory distress syndrome: an evidence-based review. *Crit Care Med.* 2004;32:S548-S553.

Taylor MM. ARDS diagnosis and management: implications for the critical care nurse. *Dimens Crit Care Nurs.* 2005;24(5):197-207.

Chronic Obstructive Pulmonary Disease

Ambrosino N, Simonds A. The clinical management in extremely severe COPD. *Respir Med.* 2007;101(8):1613-1624.

Andenaes R, Kalfoss MH, Wahl A. Psychological distress and quality of life in hospitalized patients with chronic obstructive pulmonary disease. *J Adv Nurs.* 2004;46(5):523-530.

Bellamy D, Bouchard J, Henrichsen S, et al. International Primary Care Respiratory Group (IPCRG) Guidelines: management of chronic obstructive pulmonary disease (COPD). *Prim Care Respir J.* 2006;15(1):48-57.

Booker R. Chronic obstructive pulmonary disease: non-pharmacological approaches. *Br J Nurs.* 2005;14(1):14-18.

Cazzola M, Donner CF, Hanania NA. One hundred years of chronic obstructive pulmonary disease (COPD). *Respir Med.* 2007;101(6):1049-1065.

Celli BR, MacNee W, ATS/ERS Task Force. Standards for the diagnosis and treatment of patients with COPD: a summary of the ATS/ERS position paper. *Eur Respir J.* 2004;23:932-946.

Donaldson GC, Wedzicha JA. COPD exacerbations. 1: Epidemiology. *Thorax.* 2006;61(2):164-168.

Fehrenbach C. Initiatives to improve outcomes for chronic obstructive pulmonary disease. *Prof Nurse.* 2005;20(6):43-45.

Frazier SC. Implications of the GOLD Report for chronic obstructive lung disease for the home care clinician. *Home Healthc Nurse.* 2005;23(2): 109-114.

Gronkiewicz C, Borkgren-Okonek M. Acute exacerbation of COPD: nursing application of evidence-based guidelines. *Crit Care Nurs Q.* 2004; 27(4):336-352.

Hockman RH. Pharmacologic therapy for acute exacerbations of chronic obstructive pulmonary disease: A review. *Crit Care Nurs Clin North Am.* 2004;16(3):293-310.

Hogg JC, Chu F, Utokaparch S, et al. The nature of small-airway obstruction in chronic obstructive pulmonary disease. *N Engl J Med.* 2004;350: 2645-2653.

Lomborg K, Bjorn A, Dahl R, et al. Body care experienced by people hospitalized with severe respiratory disease. *J Adv Nurs.* 2005;50(3):262-271.

Odencrants S, Ehnfors M, Ehrenberg A. Nutritional status and patient characteristics for hospitalised older patients with chronic obstructive pulmonary disease. *J Clin Nurs.* 2008;17(13):1771-1778.

O'Donnell DE, Parker CM. COPD exacerbations. 3: Pathophysiology. *Thorax.* 2006;61(4):354-361.

Sussman R. Part I: Identifying chronic obstructive pulmonary disease in patients with respiratory symptoms. *Curr Med Res Opin.* 2007;(Suppl 3): S5-S12.

Wise RA, Tashkin DP. Optimizing treatment of chronic obstructive pulmonary disease: an assessment of current therapies. *Am J Med.* 2007;120 (8 Suppl 1):S4-S13.

Asthma and Status Asthmaticus (Severe Asthmatic Attack)

Aldington S, Beasley R. Asthma exacerbations. 5: Assessment and management of severe asthma in adults in hospital. *Thorax.* 2007;62(5):447-458.

Balkissoon R. Asthma overview. *Prim Care.* 2008;35(1):41-60.

Bjermer L. Time for a paradigm shift in asthma treatment: from relieving bronchospasm to controlling systemic inflammation. *J Allergy Clin Immunol.* 2007;120(6):1269-1275.

Booker R. The effective assessment of acute breathlessness in a patient. *Nurs Times.* 2004;100(24): 61-63, 65, 67.

Braman SS, Hanania NA. Asthma in older adults. *Clin Chest Med.* 2007;28(4):685-702.

Corbridge SJ, Corbridge TC. Severe exacerbations of asthma. *Crit Care Nurs Q.* 2004;27:207-228.

Gordon BR. Asthma history and presentation. *Otolaryngol Clin North Am.* 2008;41(2):375-385.

Graham LM. Classifying asthma. *Chest.* 2006;130 (1 Suppl):13S-20S.

Hanania NA. Targeting airway inflammation in asthma: current and future therapies. *Chest.* 2008;133(4):989-998.

Mathur SK, Busse WW. Asthma: diagnosis and management. *Med Clin North Am.* 2006;90(1):39-60.

Moore WC, Peters SP. Severe asthma: an overview. *J Allergy Clin Immunol*. 2006;117(3):487-494.

National Asthma Education and Prevention Program Expert Panel Report. *Guidelines for the Diagnosis and Management of Asthma*. Washington, DC: US Department of Health and Human Services; 2002.

Peters SP, Ferguson G, Deniz Y, Reisner C. Uncontrolled asthma: a review of the prevalence, disease burden and options for treatment. *Respir Med*. 2006;100(7):1139-1151.

Pruitt B, Jacobs M. Caring for a patient with asthma. *Nursing*. 2005;35(2):48-51.

Spahn JD, Covar R. Clinical assessment of asthma progression in children and adults. *J Allergy Clin Immunol*. 2008;121(3):548-557.

Szefler SJ, Apter A. Advances in pediatric and adult asthma. *J Allergy Clin Immunol*. 2005;115(3):470-477.

Tilles SA. Differential diagnosis of adult asthma. *Med Clin North Am*. 2006;90(1):61-76.

Weir P. Quick asthma assessment: a stepwise approach to treatment. *Adv Nurse Pract*. 2004;12(1):53-56.

Wenzel S. Physiologic and pathologic abnormalities in severe asthma. *Clin Chest Med*. 2006;27(1):29-40.

Winters AC. Management of acute severe asthma. *Crit Care Nurs Clin North Am*. 2004;6(3):285-291.

Pulmonary Embolism

Anaya DA, Nathens AB. Thrombosis and coagulation: deep vein thrombosis and pulmonary embolism prophylaxis. *Surg Clin North Am*. 2005;85(6):1163-1177.

Carlbom DJ, Davidson BL. Pulmonary embolism in the critically ill. *Chest*. 2007;132(1):313-324.

Cloutier LM. Diagnosis of pulmonary embolism. *Clin J Oncol Nurs*. 2007;11(3):343-348.

Kluetz PG, White CS. Acute pulmonary embolism: imaging in the emergency department. *Radiol Clin North Am*. 2006;44(2):259-271.

Kucher N. Catheter embolectomy for acute pulmonary embolism. *Chest*. 2007;132(2):657-663.

Merli G. Diagnostic assessment of deep vein thrombosis and pulmonary embolism. *Am J Med*. 2005;118(Suppl 8A):3S-12S.

Merli GJ. Pathophysiology of venous thrombosis and the diagnosis of deep vein thrombosis-pulmonary embolism in the elderly. *Cardiol Clin*. 2008;26(2):203-219.

Nijkeuter M, Hovens MM, Davidson BL, Huisman MV. Resolution of thromboemboli in patients with acute pulmonary embolism: a systematic review. *Chest*. 2006;129(1):192-187.

Shaughnessy K. Massive pulmonary embolism. *Crit Care Nurse*. 2007;27(1):39-50.

Sims JM. An overview of pulmonary embolism. *Dimens Crit Care Nurs*. 2007;26(5):182-186.

Tran H, McRae S, Ginsberg J. Anticoagulant treatment of deep vein thrombosis and pulmonary embolism. *Clin Geriatr Med*. 2006;22(1):113-134.

Worster A, Smith C, Silver S, Brown MD. Evidence-based emergency medicine/critically appraised topic. Thrombolytic therapy for submassive pulmonary embolism? *Ann Emerg Med*. 2007;50(1):78-84.

Yang JC. Prevention and treatment of deep vein thrombosis and pulmonary embolism in critically ill patients. *Crit Care Nurs Q*. 2005;28(1):72-79.

Pneumothorax

Al-Qudah A. Treatment options of spontaneous pneumothorax. *Indian J Chest Dis Allied Sci*. 2006;48(3):191-200.

Baumann MH. Management of spontaneous pneumothorax. *Clin Chest Med*. 2006;27(2):369-381.

Currie GP, Alluri R, Christie GL, Legge JS. Pneumothorax: an update. *Postgrad Med J*. 2007;83(981):461-465.

Giacomini M, Iapichino G, Armani S, Cozzolino M, Brancaccio D, Gallieni M. How to avoid and manage a pneumothorax. *J Vasc Access*. 2006;7(1):7-14.

Henry M, Arnold T, Harvey J. Pleural Diseases Group, Standards of Care Committee, British Thoracic Society. BTS guidelines for the management of spontaneous pneumothorax. *Thorax*. 2003;58(Suppl 2):ii39-ii52.

Leigh-Smith S, Harris T. Tension pneumothorax—time for a re-think? *Emerg Med J*. 2005;22(1):8-16.

Reed MF, Lyons JM, Luchette FA, Neu JA, Howington JA. Preliminary report of a prospective, randomized trial of underwater seal for spontaneous and iatrogenic pneumothorax. *J Am Coll Surg*. 2007;204(1):84-90.

Runciman WB, Hibbert PD. Spontaneous ventilation pneumothorax. *Anaesth Intensive Care*. 2008;36(3):455-456.

Acute Pneumonia

Aarts MA, Hancock JN, Heyland D, McLeod RS, Marshall JC. Empiric antibiotic therapy for suspected ventilator-associated pneumonia: a systematic review and meta-analysis of randomized trials. *Crit Care Med*. 2008;36(1):108-117.

American Thoracic Society. Consensus statement: guidelines for the management of adults with hospital-acquired, ventilator-associated, and healthcare-associated pneumonia. *Am J Respir Crit Care Med*. 2005;171:388-416.

Carratalà J, Garcia-Vidal C. What is healthcare-associated pneumonia and how is it managed? *Curr Opin Infect Dis*. 2008;21(2):168-173.

Donowitz GR, Cox HL. Bacterial community-acquired pneumonia in older patients. *Clin Geriatr Med*. 2007;23(3):515-534.

Falsey AR. Community-acquired viral pneumonia. *Clin Geriatr Med*. 2007;23(3):535-552.

Goldhill DR, Imhoff M, McLean B, Waldmann C. Rotational bed therapy to prevent and treat respiratory complications: a review and meta-analysis. *Am J Crit Care*. 2007;16(1):50-61.

Goldrick BA. Infection in the older adult: long-term care poses particular risk. *Am J Nurs*. 2005;105(6):31, 33-34.

Hess DR. Patient positioning and ventilator-associated pneumonia. *Respir Care*. 2005;50(7):892-898.

Lindgren VA, Ames NJ. Caring for patients on mechanical ventilation: what research indicates is best practice. *Am J Nurs*. 2005;105(5):50-60.

Lutfiyya MN, Henley E, Chang LF, Reyburn SW. Diagnosis and treatment of community-acquired pneumonia. *Am Fam Physician*. 2006;73(3):442-450.

McQuillan DP, Duncan RA, Craven DE. Ventilator-associated pneumonia: emerging principles of management. *Infect Med*. 2005;22(3):104-118.

Moran GJ, Talan DA, Abrahamian FM. Diagnosis and management of pneumonia in the emergency department. *Infect Dis Clin North Am*. 2008;22(1):53-72.

Sarin J, Balasubramaniam R, Corcoran AM, Laudenbach JM, Stoopler ET. Reducing the risk of aspiration pneumonia among elderly patients in long-term care facilities through oral health interventions. *J Am Med Dir Assoc*. 2008;9(2):128-135.

Scannapieco FA. Pneumonia in nonambulatory patients. The role of oral bacteria and oral hygiene. *J Am Dent Assoc*. 2006;137(Suppl):21S-25S.

Tarver RD, Teague SD, Heitkamp DE, Conces DJ Jr. Radiology of community-acquired pneumonia. *Radiol Clin North Am*. 2005;43(3):497-512.

Pulmonary Aspiration

Bourgault AM, Ipe L, Weaver J, Swartz S, O'dea PJ. Development of evidence-based guidelines and critical care nurses' knowledge of enteral feeding. *Crit Care Nurse*. 2007;27(4):17-22, 25-29.

El Solh AA, Saliba R. Pharmacologic prevention of aspiration pneumonia: a systematic review. *Am J Geriatr Pharmacother*. 2007;5(4):352-362.

Janda M, Scheeren TW, Nöldge-Schomburg GF. Management of pulmonary aspiration. *Best Pract Res Clin Anaesthesiol*. 2006;20(3):409-427.

Kikawada M, Iwamoto T, Takasaki M. Aspiration and infection in the elderly: epidemiology, diagnosis and management. *Drugs Aging*. 2005;22(2):115-130.

Metheny NA, Clouse RE, Chang YH, Stewart BJ, Oliver DA, Kollef MH. Tracheobronchial aspiration of gastric contents in critically ill tube-fed patients: frequency, outcomes, and risk factors. *Crit Care Med*. 2006;34(4):1007-1015.

Petroianni A, Ceccarelli D, Conti V, Terzano C. Aspiration pneumonia. Pathophysiological aspects, prevention and management. A review. *Panminerva Med*. 2006;48(4):231-239.

Williams TA, Leslie GD. A review of the nursing care of enteral feeding tubes in critically ill adults: part I. *Intensive Crit Care Nurs*. 2004;20(6):330-343.

Williams TA, Leslie GD. A review of the nursing care of enteral feeding tubes in critically ill adults: part II. *Intensive Crit Care Nurs*. 2005;21(1):5-15.

Pulmonary Problems in Surgical Patients

★ Brooks JA. Postoperative nosocomial pneumonia: nurse-sensitive interventions. *AACN Clin Issues*. 2001;12:305-323.

Colice GL, Shafazand S, Griffin JP, Keenan R, Bolliger CT; American College of Chest Physicians. Physiologic evaluation of the patient with lung cancer being considered for resectional surgery: ACCP evidenced-based clinical practice guidelines (2nd ed). *Chest*. 2007;132(3 Suppl):161S-177S.

Fanning MF. Reducing postoperative pulmonary complications in cardiac surgery patients with the use of the best evidence. *J Nurs Care Qual*. 2004;19(2):95-99.

Gazarian PK. Identifying risk factors for postoperative pulmonary complications. *AORN J*. 2006;84(4):616-625.

Jensen L, Yang L. Risk factors for postoperative pulmonary complications in coronary artery bypass graft surgery patients. *Eur J Cardiovasc Nurs*. 2007;6(3):241-246.

McAlister FA, Bertsch K, Man J, Bradley J, Jacka M. Incidence of and risk factors for pulmonary complications after nonthoracic surgery. *Am J Respir Crit Care Med*. 2005;171(5):514-517.

Myatt RM. An introduction to thoracic surgery: assessment, diagnostics, treatment. *Br J Nurs*. 2006;15(17):944-947.

Wadlund DL. Prevention, recognition, and management of nursing complications in the intraoperative and postoperative surgical patient. *Nurs Clin North Am*. 2006;41(2):151-171.

Obstructive Sleep Apnea Syndrome

Colin W, Duval S. Surgical treatment of obstructive sleep apnea. *AORN J*. 2005;82(3):372-374, 377-378, 380.

Demko BG. Screening for obstructive sleep apnea in the dental office setting. *J Mass Dent Soc*. 2008;57(1):18-20.

Dodson KJ. Cardiovascular effects of sleep apnea. *JNP*. 2008;4(6):439-444.

Ecklund MM, Kurlak SA. Caring for the bariatric patient with obstructive sleep apnea. *Crit Care Nurs Clin North Am*. 2004;16(3):311-317.

Lee DS. Respiratory and cardiac manifestations of obstructive sleep apnea. *Nurs Clin North Am*. 2008;43(1):55-76.

Merritt SL, Berger BE. Obstructive sleep apnea-hypopnea syndrome. *Am J Nurs*. 2004;104(7):49-52.

Moos DD, Cuddeford JD. Implications of obstructive sleep apnea syndrome for the perianesthesia nurse. *J Perianesth Nurs*. 2006;(2):103-118.

The Cardiovascular System

SYSTEMWIDE ELEMENTS

Physiologic Anatomy

1. **Heart (Figures 3-1 and 3-2)**
   a. The heart lies in the mediastinum, on and to the left of the midline.
   b. Its long axis is oriented from the right shoulder blade to the left upper quadrant of the abdomen.
   c. The base (top wide area) of the heart (atria and great vessels) is located diagonally at the second intercostal space, right and left sternal borders.
   d. The apex, or tip, of the heart (junction of the ventricles and ventricular septum) is usually located at the fifth intercostal space, on the left midclavicular line.

2. **Cardiac wall structure**
   a. Pericardium: Fibrous sac surrounding the heart and containing small amounts (15 to 50 ml) of pericardial fluid. This lubricated space protects the heart from friction, allowing it to easily change volume and size during contractions. The pericardium also keeps heart muscle anchored within the mediastinum.
   b. Epicardium: Outer surface of the heart (includes epicardial coronary arteries, autonomic nerves, adipose tissue, lymphatics).
   c. Myocardium: Muscular, contractile portion of the heart. Muscle fibers wrap around the heart in multiple, interlacing layers.
   d. Endocardium: Inner surface of the heart.
   e. Papillary muscles: Myocardial structures extending into the ventricular chambers and attaching to the chordae tendineae.
   f. Chordae tendineae: Strong tendinous attachments from the papillary muscles to the tricuspid and mitral valves; prevent prolapse of the valves into the atria during systole.

3. **Chambers of the heart**
   a. Atria: Thin-walled, low-pressure chambers
      i. Right and left atria act as reservoirs of blood for their respective ventricles.
      ii. Right atrium (RA), located above and to the right of the right ventricle, receives systemic venous blood via the superior vena cava and inferior vena cava, and venous blood from the heart via the coronary sinus.
      iii. Left atrium (LA), superior and posterior to the other chambers, receives oxygenated blood returning to the heart from the lungs via the pulmonary veins.
      iv. When the mitral and tricuspid valves open, there is rapid filling of blood passively from atria into ventricles (about 80% to 85% of total filling).
      v. At the end of diastole, atrial contraction ("atrial kick") forcefully adds 15% to 20% more to the ventricular volume.

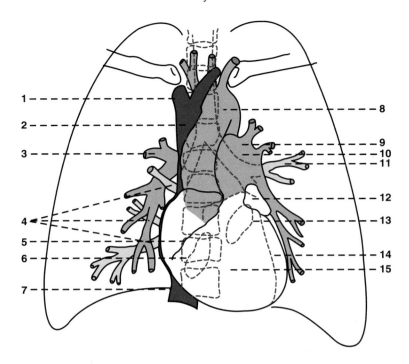

1. Right innominate vein
2. Superior vena cava
3. Right main branch of the pulmonary artery
4. Upper and lower lobe veins
5. Right atrium
6. Tricuspid valve
7. Inferior vena cava
8. Arch of the aorta
9. Left main branch of the pulmonary artery
10. Main pulmonary artery
11. Left upper lobe vein
12. Appendage of the left atrium
13. Mitral valve
14. Left ventricle
15. Right ventricle

FIGURE 3-1 ■ Cardiac silhouette, posteroanterior view. (From Gedgaudas E, Moller JH, Castaneda-Zuniga MD, et al. *Cardiovascular Radiology*. Philadelphia, PA: Saunders; 1985:38.)

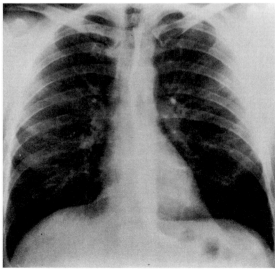

FIGURE 3-2 ■ Normal thoracicoroentgenogram, posteroanterior view. (From Gedgaudas E, Moller JH, Castaneda-Zuniga MD, et al. *Cardiovascular Radiology*. Philadelphia, PA: Saunders; 1985:38.)

    b. Ventricles: Major "pumps" of the heart

        i. Right ventricle (RV) is anterior under the sternum.

            (a) Thin-walled, low-pressure system

            (b) Contracts and propels deoxygenated blood into the pulmonary circulation via the pulmonary artery (the only artery in the body that carries deoxygenated blood)

        ii. Left ventricle (LV) is the main "pump": conical (ellipsoid) structure behind and to the left of the RV.

            (a) Thick-walled, high-pressure system

            (b) Squeezes and ejects blood into the systemic circulation via the aorta during ventricular systole

        iii. Interventricular septum is functionally more a part of the LV than of the RV. It forms the anterior wall of the LV. Its curved shape protrudes into the RV cavity.

4. Cardiac valves

    a. Atrioventricular (AV) valves

        i. Location and structure: Situated between the atria and the ventricles (tricuspid valve on the right, mitral valve on the left)

            (a) Tricuspid valve is composed of three leaflets: the large anterior leaflet and the two smaller posterior and septal leaflets.

            (b) Mitral valve is composed of two leaflets: the long, narrow posterior (mural) leaflet (like a toilet seat) and an oval anterior (aortic) leaflet (like a toilet lid).

        ii. Function: These are one-way "check" valves that permit unidirectional blood flow from the atria to the ventricles during ventricular diastole and prevent retrograde flow during ventricular systole

            (a) With ventricular diastole, the ventricles relax and the valve leaflets open.

            (b) With ventricular systole, the valve leaflets close completely.

            (c) First heart sound (S_1) is produced as the mitral (M_1) and tricuspid (T_1) valves close. M_1 is the initial and major component of S_1.

    b. Semilunar valves

        i. Location and structure

            (a) Pulmonary valve is situated between the RV and the pulmonary artery. It consists of three semilunar cusps that attach to the wall of the pulmonary trunk.

            (b) Aortic valve is situated between the LV and aorta. It consists of three slightly thicker valve cusps, the bases of which attach to a valve annulus (fibrous ring).

        ii. Function: Permit unidirectional blood flow from the outflow tract during ventricular systole and prevent retrograde blood flow during ventricular diastole

            (a) With ventricular systole, the valves open when the respective ventricle contracts and pressure is greater in the ventricle than in the artery.

            (b) After ventricular systole, pressure in the artery exceeds pressure in the ventricles. This and retrograde blood flow cause the valve to close.

            (c) Second heart sound (S_2) is produced when the aortic (A_2) and pulmonic (P_2) valves close. A_2 is normally the initial and major component of S_2.

5. Coronary vasculature (Figure 3-3)

    a. Arteries

        i. Two main arteries branch off at the base of the aorta, supplying blood to the heart.

        ii. Right coronary artery (RCA)

            (a) Originates behind the right coronary cusp of the aortic valve

            (b) Supplies

                 (1) RA and RV

                 (2) Sinoatrial (SA) node and AV node

                 (3) Inferior-posterior wall of the LV (in 90% of hearts)

                 (4) Inferior-posterior third of the interventricular septum

            (c) Main branches

                 (1) SA node in 55% of hearts

                 (2) RV branch

                 (3) AV node in 90% of hearts

                 (4) Posterior descending artery (supplying the inferior-posterior wall of the LV in 85% of hearts)

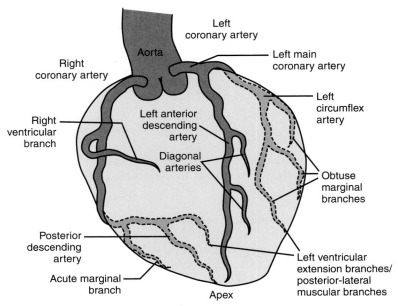

FIGURE 3-3 ■ Coronary artery anatomy.

    iii. Left coronary artery (LCA)

        (a) Left main coronary artery (LMCA): Branches into the left anterior descending and circumflex arteries

        (b) Left anterior descending (LAD) artery

            (1) Supplies the anterior two thirds of the interventricular septum and the anterior wall of the LV

            (2) Branches include diagonals (two to six other diagonals may be present), septal perforators (three to five other perforators may be present).

        (c) Left circumflex (LCX) artery: Also branches from the LMCA

            (1) LCX artery supplies

                a) SA node in 45% of hearts

                b) AV node in 10% of hearts

                c) Inferior-posterior LV in 10% of hearts

                d) Lateral posterior surface of the LV via the obtuse marginal branches (OMBs)

                e) Posterior descending artery arises from the LCX artery in 15% of hearts (see description under RCA)

            (2) Branches of the LCX include the OMBs (may be one to three), which supply the lateral wall of the LV and occasionally the posterior lateral muscular branch.

    iv. Coronary collaterals: Potential vascular connections between the RCA and LCA exist

        (a) They may open, if stenosis of one of the coronary arteries occurs, to supply blood from the other artery.

        (b) They cannot augment flow to meet acute requirements for increased flow.

  b. Cardiac veins

    i. Return deoxygenated blood to the RA, mostly through the coronary sinus

    ii. Follow paths similar to those of the arteries; have no valves

  c. Coronary blood flow

    i. Coronary vascular reserve: Coronary circulation has the ability to increase flow to meet added needs up to approximately six times normal

    ii. Coronary blood flow is about 70 to 90 ml/min.

    iii. The heart uses most of the oxygen available in the coronary circulation; little oxygen reserve exists.

      iv. Most of coronary blood flow is in diastole, because, in systole, coronary artery blood flow usually decreases as a result of ventricular compression and contraction.

      v. Coronary blood flow is reduced by

        (a) Hypotension

        (b) Tachycardia: Decreased LV diastolic filling times

        (c) Mechanical obstruction (coronary stenosis or spasm)

6. Neurologic control of the heart

  a. Autonomic nervous system: Influences contractility, depolarization-repolarization, and rate of conductivity

      i. Sympathetic stimulation: Norepinephrine release is the main impetus of stimulation to the heart; its two effects include the following:

        (a) α-Adrenergic: Causing peripheral arteriolar vasoconstriction

        (b) β-Adrenergic

          (1) Increases SA node discharge, increasing heart rate (positive chronotropy)

          (2) Increases the force of myocardial contraction (positive inotropy)

          (3) Accelerates AV conduction time

      ii. Parasympathetic stimulation: Occurs via the tenth cranial (vagus) nerve. Acetylcholine release is the main parasympathetic impetus to cardiac effects.

        (a) Decreases the rate of SA node discharge, slowing heart rate (negative chronotropy)

        (b) Slows conduction through AV tissue

      iii. Ventricles have mainly sympathetic innervation and only sparse vagal innervation.

      iv. Parasympathetic influences normally predominate in the conducting system (SA node, AV node).

  b. Chemoreceptors: Afferent receptors located in the carotid and aortic bodies. Sensitive to changes in partial pressure of oxygen, partial pressure of carbon dioxide, and pH, causing changes in heart rate and respiratory rate via stimulation of vasomotor center in the medulla.

  c. Baroreceptors: Stretch receptors in the heart and blood vessels that respond to pressure and volume changes.

7. Cardiac muscle microanatomy and contractile properties: See Box 3-1 for key elements

8. Anatomy of the cardiac conduction system (Figure 3-4)

▓ **BOX 3-1**
▓ **KEY ELEMENTS OF CARDIAC MUSCLE MICROANATOMY**

CARDIAC MUSCLE FIBERS

Two main contractile properties: Ability to shorten and to develop force

Syncytium: Fibers arranged in latticelike "network": When one fiber is stimulated, all fibers become stimulated

Sarcomere: Contractile unit composed of
- Contractile proteins: Myosin and actin (their interactions help to produce contraction, fiber shortening)
- Regulatory proteins: Troponin and tropomyosin (they inhibit myosin-actin interactions)

Intercalated disks:
- Interlock cardiac muscle fibers together at ends
- Provide quick transmission of electrical impulse

Myocardial working cells: Enable chemical energy to be transformed into mechanical actions (contraction and relaxation)

EXCITATION-CONTRACTION PROCESS

1. During excitation (depolarization), calcium enters working cell interior across sarcolemma.
2. Calcium binds with troponin, and myosin-actin inhibition is lost.
3. Actin and myosin may now interact, using adenosine triphosphate for energy.
4. Sarcomeres shorten, which results in muscle fiber shortening and subsequent cardiac muscle contraction.
5. Calcium is then pumped out of cell, allowing fiber to relax again until process repeats.

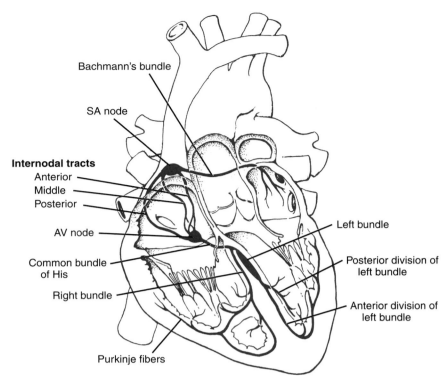

FIGURE 3-4 ■ Anatomy of the cardiac conduction system. *AV*, Atrioventricular; *SA*, sinoatrial.

  a. SA node
     i.   Normal pacemaker of the heart, possessing the fastest inherent rate of automaticity (approximately 70 beats/min)
     ii.   Located in the right superior wall of the RA at the junction of the superior vena cava and the RA
  b. Internodal atrial conduction
     i.   Impulse is conducted from the SA node through the RA and LA musculature to the AV node.
     ii.   Although the atria do not have specialized high-speed conduction tracts comparable to the ventricular bundles and fascicles, there are preferred conduction pathways (e.g., Bachmann's bundle, which conducts impulses from the SA node to the LA).
  c. AV node
     i.   Delays the impulse from the atria before it goes to the ventricles. This allows time for both ventricles to fill before ventricular systole.
     ii.   Inherent rate of automaticity is approximately 40 beats/min.
     iii. Located in the right interatrial septum, above the tricuspid valve's septal leaflet
  d. Bundle of His: Arises from the AV node and conducts the impulse to the bundle branch system. The bundle of His is close to the annulus of the tricuspid valve.
  e. Bundle branch system: Pathways that arise from the bundle of His and branch at the top of the interventricular septum
     i.   Right bundle branch is the smaller, direct continuation of the bundle of His. It transmits the impulse down the right side of the interventricular septum to the RV myocardium.
     ii.   Left bundle branch is the larger branch from the bundle of His. It transmits the impulse to the septum and the LV. The left bundle branch divides into three parts:
        (a) Left anterior fascicle: Transmits the impulse to the anterior and superior endocardial surfaces of the LV
        (b) Left posterior fascicle: Transmits the impulse over the posterior-inferior endocardial surface of the LV
        (c) Septal bundle

f. Purkinje system
  i.   Arises from the distal portion of the bundle branches, forming networks on the ventricle's endocardial surface
  ii. Transmits the impulse into the subendocardial and myocardial layers of both ventricles
  iii. Provides for depolarization of the myocardium (from endocardium to epicardium)
  iv. Ventricles have their own inherent rate of automaticity of approximately 20 to 30 beats/min.

9. Electrophysiology
  a. Electrophysiologic properties of cardiac muscle cells
   i.   Excitability: Ability to depolarize and form an action potential when sufficiently stimulated
   ii. Automaticity: Ability to generate an impulse without an outside stimulus
   iii. Conductivity: Ability to conduct an electrical impulse to neighboring cells, spreading the impulse throughout the heart to achieve total depolarization
   iv. Refractoriness: Temporary inability of the depolarized cell to become excited and generate another action potential
  b. Resting membrane potential (RMP): Electrical charge of cardiac muscle cell at rest. Cell ions consist primarily of sodium, potassium, and calcium.
   i.   Sodium ion concentration is greater outside the cell.
   ii. Potassium ion concentration is greater inside the cell.
   iii. Calcium ion concentration is greater outside the cell.
  c. Depolarization: Change in the electrical charge of a stimulated cell from negative to positive by the flow of ions across the cell membrane. Sodium moves into the cell, potassium moves out.
  d. Repolarization: Recovery or recharging of a cell's normal polarity. Sodium moves back out of the cell, potassium moves into the cell. The cell recovers its negative charge.
  e. Threshold potential: The electric voltage level at which cardiac cells become activated and produce an action potential, which leads to muscular contraction
  f. Stimulation of myocardial cells
   i.   Stimulus may be chemical, electrical, or mechanical.
   ii. When the cell is stimulated, the electrical charge inside the cell becomes less negative, and depolarization occurs.
   iii. When the threshold potential is reached, changes occur in the membrane.
   iv. SA and AV nodes achieve threshold potential first.
   v.   Cell membrane permeability is altered, and specialized channels in the membrane open, which allows the entry of sodium and calcium ions into the cell.
  g. Action potential: As cardiac cells reverse polarity, the electrical impulse generated during that event creates an energy stimulus that travels across the cell membrane—a high-speed, short-lived, self-reproducing current (heart only). This is represented on an action potential curve (Figure 3-5).
   i.   *Phase 0*—Depolarization: A quick upstroke (several milliseconds) representing the initial phase of excitation
   ii. *Phase 1*—Initial phase of repolarization
   iii. *Phase 2*—Plateau phase of repolarization: Slow inward current of calcium (and, to a lesser extent, sodium); potassium diffuses out of the cells
   iv. *Phase 3*—Last phase of repolarization: Outward current of potassium increases, and the slow, inward current of sodium and calcium decreases. Cells rapidly repolarize, returning to normal RMP.
   v.   *Phase 4*—Membrane at RMP
  h. Cardiac pacemaker cells (SA and AV nodes) action potential
   i.   Pacer cells, having increased automaticity, spontaneously depolarize in phase 4 without a stimulus. Other cells of the heart, having repolarized, require another stimulus to become depolarized.
     (a) Rate of automaticity may be altered by increasing or decreasing the slope of phase 4.
     (b) Increasing the slope speeds heart rate; decreasing the slope slows heart rate.

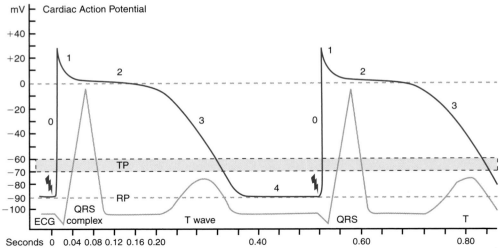

FIGURE 3-5 ■ Cardiac action potential of myocardial cells. *ECG*, Electrocardiogram; *RP*, resting membrane potential; *TP*, threshold membrane potential. (From Huszar RJ. *Basic Dysrhythmias: Interpretation and Management.* 3rd ed. Philadelphia, PA: Mosby; 2001:13.)

ii. Spontaneous depolarization of pacer cells is caused by a steady influx of sodium and efflux of potassium.

iii. SA node has the fastest rate of depolarization.

i. Refractoriness of heart muscle

    i. Absolute refractory period (effective refractory period): Another stimulus to the cell will not produce another action potential (phases 0, 1, and 2 and part of phase 3 of the action potential curve)

    ii. Relative refractory period: Only a very strong stimulus can initiate an action potential and cause depolarization (latter part of phase 3)

    iii. Supernormal period: Weak stimulus (one that would not normally elicit an action potential) can evoke an action potential and cause depolarization (at the end of phase 3)

10. **Events in the cardiac cycle (Figure 3-6)**

    a. Ventricular systole: Contraction and emptying of the ventricles

        i. QRS complex: Represents ventricular depolarization (an electrical event)

        ii. First phase of ventricular contraction (systole) is called isovolumetric contraction. Pressure increases, but no blood is ejected until LV pressure exceeds aortic pressure (and opens the aortic valve).

        iii. As pressure rises in the ventricles, the AV valves close, producing the first heart sound (S_1, composed of mitral [M_1] and tricuspid [T_1] components).

        iv. The "c" wave of the atrial pressure curve is produced when the AV valves are pushed backward toward the atria as ventricular pressure builds.

        v. When LV pressure exceeds the pressure in the aorta, the aortic valve opens (comparable events in the RV occur with the pulmonic valve).

        vi. Blood is rapidly ejected into the aorta (systolic ejection).

        vii. LV pressures decrease, falling below the pressure in the aorta, ventricular ejection stops, and the aortic valve closes. (Comparable events occur in the pulmonary artery, closing the pulmonic valve.)

        viii. Closing of the aortic and pulmonic valves produces the second heart sound (S_2, composed of aortic [A_2] and pulmonic [P_2] components).

        ix. Aortic valve closure is represented by the dicrotic notch in the aortic pressure waveform.

        x. Repolarization of the ventricles occurs at this time and produces the T wave on the electrocardiogram (ECG).

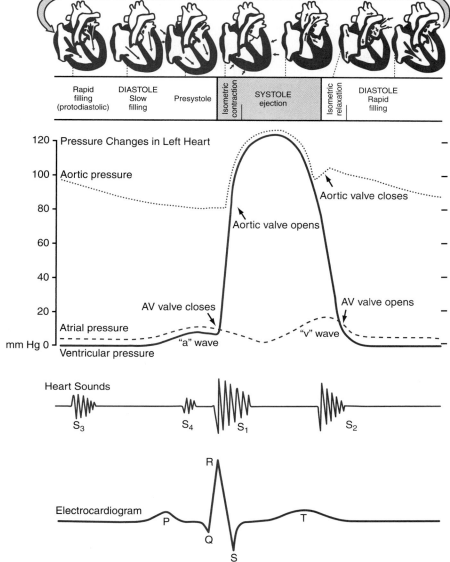

FIGURE 3-6 ■ Events in the cardiac cycle. *AV*, Atrioventricular. (Adapted from Jarvis C. *Physical Examination and Health Assessment*. 2nd ed. Philadelphia, PA: Saunders; 1996:518.)

    xi.   After the aortic valve closes, pressure in the LV falls rapidly (isovolumetric relaxation phase); no blood enters the ventricle.

   xii.   LA "v" wave is produced by rapid filling of the atria during ventricular systole, against closed AV valves. This marks the end of systole.

  b. Ventricular diastole: Filling phase of the ventricles

     i.   When pressure is lower in the ventricles than in the atria, the AV valves reopen, which initiates the early rapid filling phase of the ventricles during diastole. This marks the start of diastole.

    ii.   Pressure in the atria is higher than diastolic pressure in the ventricles, so blood flows from the atria into the ventricles.

   iii.   "a" wave: Atrial pressure rises with atrial contraction

    iv.   P wave (ECG): In late diastole, represents atrial depolarization (an electrical event)

11. Variables affecting LV function and cardiac output (CO)

   a. CO: Amount of blood ejected by the LV in 1 minute

      i.   CO is the product of stroke volume (SV) and heart rate (HR):

$$CO = SV \times HR$$

      ii.   SV is the amount of blood ejected by the LV with each contraction, or the difference between left ventricular end-diastolic volume (LVEDV) and left ventricular end-systolic volume (LVESV):

$$SV = LVEDV - LVESV \text{ (60 to 130 ml)}$$

      iii. Normal resting CO = 4 to 8 L/min.

      iv. CO is determined by preload, afterload, contractility, and heart rate.

   b. Preload: The degree to which muscle fibers are lengthened (stretched) before contraction

      i.   In the intact heart, preload is secondary to the volume (size) of the chamber. This is determined by the amount of blood filling the chamber.

      ii.   Increases in preload increase the CO as described by the Frank-Starling law of the heart.

      iii. Muscle fibers can reach a point of stretch beyond which contraction is no longer enhanced, and further increases in preload do not yield any further increase in CO.

      iv. Increased preload occurs with

         (a) Increased circulating volume

         (b) Venous constriction (decreases venous pooling and increases venous return to heart)

         (c) Drugs: Vasoconstrictors

      v.   Decreased preload occurs with

         (a) Hypovolemia

         (b) Mitral stenosis

         (c) Drugs: Vasodilators (e.g., nitrates), diuretics

         (d) Cardiac tamponade

         (e) Constrictive pericarditis

   c. Afterload: Initial resistance that must be overcome by the ventricles to develop force and contract, opening the semilunar valves and propelling blood into the systemic and pulmonary circulatory systems (systolic contraction)

      i.   Factors affecting afterload include arterial resistance (wall stress and thickness), aortic impedance, and blood viscosity.

      ii.   Systemic vascular resistance (SVR) is used as a rough estimate of afterload.

      iii. Normal SVR = 900 to 1400 dynes/sec/cm^{-5}.

      iv. Excessive afterload: Increases LV stroke work, decreases SV, increases myocardial oxygen demands, and may result in LV failure

      v.   Increased afterload is seen in

         (a) Aortic stenosis

         (b) Peripheral arteriolar vasoconstriction

         (c) Hypertension

         (d) Polycythemia

         (e) Use of arterial vasoconstrictor drugs

      vi. Decreased afterload is seen in

         (a) Hypovolemia

         (b) Sepsis

         (c) Use of arterial vasodilators

   d. Contractility (inotropic state): Heart's contractile strength

      i.   There is no way to measure contractility directly. Contractile state can be assessed indirectly through its effects on CO or with noninvasive imaging.

      ii.   Factors increasing the contractile state of the myocardium include

         (a) Use of positive inotropic drugs (e.g., digitalis, milrinone, epinephrine, dobutamine)

         (b) Increased heart rate (Bowditch's phenomenon)

         (c) Sympathetic stimulation (via β_1-receptors)

      iii. Factors decreasing the contractile state of the myocardium include
        (a) Negative inotropic drugs (e.g., type 1A antiarrhythmics, β-blockers, calcium channel blockers, barbiturates)
        (b) Hypoxia
        (c) Hypercapnia
        (d) Myocardial ischemia or infarction
        (e) Metabolic acidosis

e. Heart rate
    i. Influenced by many factors, including
      (a) Blood volume status
      (b) Sympathetic and parasympathetic tone
      (c) Drugs
      (d) Temperature
      (e) Respiration
      (f) Dysrhythmias
      (g) Peripheral vascular tone
      (h) Emotions
      (i) Metabolic status (increases with hyperthyroidism)
    ii. Determinant of myocardial oxygen supply and demand
      (a) Increased heart rates increase myocardial oxygen consumption.
      (b) Fast heart rates (above 150 beats/min) decrease diastolic coronary blood flow (shorter diastole).

f. Cardiac index (CI)
    i. CI is CO corrected for differences in body size (CO of 4 L/min may be adequate for a 100-lb woman but inadequate for a 200-lb man).
    ii. CI is based on body surface area (BSA) as estimated from a height and weight nomogram: CI = CO/BSA.
    iii. Normal CI is 2.5 to 4.0 L/min/m^2.

g. Ejection fraction (EF)
    i. Percentage of blood in the ventricle ejected with every beat
      (a) Normal LV EF = 50% to 75%.
      (b) Not clinically significant until less than 50%
    ii. Good reflection of LV performance

h. Ventricular function curve: Shows how to relate the contributions of preload, afterload, and contractility (but not heart rate) to ventricular function (Figure 3-7)

12. Systemic vasculature
    a. Major functions: Provides tissues with blood, nutrients, and hormones and removes metabolic wastes
    b. Resistance to flow: Depends on diameter of vessels (especially arterioles), viscosity of blood, and elastic recoil in vessel walls
    c. Circulating blood volume: There is approximately 5 L of total circulating blood volume in the adult body
    d. Major components of the vascular system
      i. Arteries
        (a) Strong, compliant, elastic-walled vessels that branch off the aorta, carry blood away from the heart, and distribute it to capillary beds throughout the body
        (b) A high-pressure circuit
        (c) Able to stretch during systole and recoil during diastole because of elastic fibers in the arterial wall
      ii. Arterioles
        (a) Control systemic vascular resistance and thus arterial pressure
        (b) Have strong smooth muscle walls innervated by the autonomic nervous system
        (c) Autonomic nervous system
          (1) Adrenergic (stimulatory) system: Releases two neurotransmitters (epinephrine, norepinephrine). Epinephrine stimulates β-receptors (increases heart

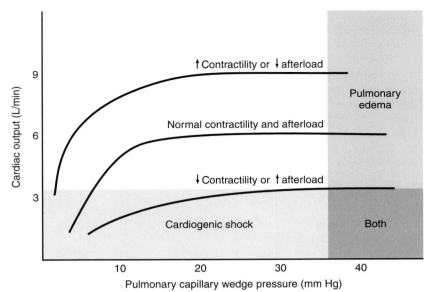

FIGURE 3-7 ■ Ventricular function curve. The ventricular function curve is not a Starling curve. It relates all the contributors to cardiac output, except heart rate, to ventricular function. It is an excellent framework for assessment and decision making.

rate, increases contractility, dilates arterioles). Norepinephrine stimulates α-receptors (vasoconstriction).
    (2) Cholinergic (inhibitory) system: Releases acetylcholine (decreases heart rate; releases nitric oxide, causing vasodilatation)
  (d) Lead directly into capillaries, supply tissue beds
  iii. Capillary system
    (a) Tissue bed exchange of oxygen and carbon dioxide and solutes between blood and tissues; site of fluid volume transfer between plasma and interstitium
    (b) Gas exchange caused by diffusion. Diffusion of a substance is from an area of high concentration to an area of low concentration until equilibrium is established.
    (c) Fluid homeostasis
      (1) Increased capillary hydrostatic pressure moves fluid from the vessel into the interstitium.
      (2) Greater capillary osmotic pressure moves fluid from the interstitium into the vessels.
      (3) Plasma protein concentration in the capillaries provides the osmotic gradient.
      (4) Retains fluid in the intravascular space
      (5) Prevents edema formation in the interstitium
      (6) Albumin accounts for 75% of total plasma osmotic pressure; fibrinogen accounts for a small amount.
      (7) Serum albumin level is a good indicator of a patient's colloid osmotic pressure.
    (d) Capillaries lack smooth muscle.
  iv. Venous system
    (a) Stores about 65% of total blood volume
    (b) Receives blood from capillaries
    (c) Conducts blood back to the heart within a low-pressure system
    (d) No muscle layer: Veins are compressed by the contraction of surrounding skeletal muscle
    (e) Valves in the veins prevent reverse blood flow.
    (f) Venous pressure in the lower extremities is normally 20 mm Hg or less.

13. **Control of peripheral blood flow**
    a. Autoregulation: Ability of the tissues to control their own blood flow (vasodilatation, vasoconstriction)
       i. Coronary blood flow remains fairly constant over a wide range of blood pressures.
       ii. As coronary perfusion pressure drops below 50 mm Hg, autoregulatory ability becomes impaired.
    b. Autonomic regulation of vessels
       i. Vasoconstriction occurs when norepinephrine is released by stimulation of the sympathetic nervous system (adrenergic effect).
       ii. Vasodilatation occurs when acetylcholine is released by stimulation of the parasympathetic nervous system (cholinergic effect) or by inhibition of vasoconstriction.
    c. Stretch receptors: Baroreceptors (pressoreceptors) keep mean arterial pressure (MAP) constant
       i. Receptor sites in the arteries (aortic arch, carotid sinus, pulmonary arteries, and atria)
       ii. Action with increased blood pressure
          (a) Respond to stretching of arterial walls
          (b) Impulse transmitted from the aortic arch via the vagus nerve to the medulla
          (c) Parasympathetic nervous system stimulated, sympathetic nervous system inhibited
          (d) Result: Decreased heart rate and contractility, dilation of peripheral vessels, decreased SVR, decreased blood pressure
       iii. Action with decreased blood pressure
          (a) Sympathetic nervous system stimulated, parasympathetic nervous system inhibited
          (b) Result: Increased heart rate and contractility, arterial and venous constriction (which preserves blood flow to the brain and heart), and increased blood pressure

14. **Arterial pressure**
    a. Neurohumoral regulation
       i. Renin-angiotensin-aldosterone system also helps control arterial pressure (see Chapter 5).
       ii. Renin is a protease secreted by the kidneys; converts angiotensinogen to angiotensin I.
       iii. Renin release from the kidneys is affected as follows:
          (a) Decreased blood pressure (i.e., hemorrhage, dehydration, diuretics, sodium depletion) → increases in renin secretion
          (b) Rise in sympathetic output β stimulation) → increases in renin secretion
          (c) Fall in sodium concentration → increases in renin secretion (decreased volume)
          (d) Increased blood pressure → decreases in renin secretion
       iv. Angiotensin I is converted to angiotensin II. (These effects are blocked by angiotensin-converting enzyme [ACE] inhibitors.)
       v. Angiotensin II, the most potent vasoconstrictor known, is produced when increased renin secretion stimulates its formation.
          (a) Effects of angiotensin II include the following:
             (1) Arteriolar constriction, which increases systolic and diastolic pressures
             (2) Stimulation of the adrenal cortex to secrete aldosterone, which causes sodium and water retention
             (3) Increase in extracellular fluid volume, which shuts off the stimulus that initiated renin secretion so that blood pressure is maintained at the normal level
          (b) Effects of angiotensin II are blocked at its receptors by angiotensin II receptor blockers (ARBs).
    b. Pulse pressure: Difference between systolic and diastolic pressures
       i. Function of SV and arterial capacitance
       ii. Normal pulse pressure: 30 to 40 mm Hg
       iii. Changes in SV (with exercise, shock, heart failure) are reflected in similar changes in pulse pressure.

    c. MAP: Average arterial pressure during the cardiac cycle; dependent on mean arterial blood volume and elasticity of the arterial wall

      i. $MAP = \dfrac{(Diastolic\,pressure \times 2) + Systolic\,pressure}{3}$

      ii. Example: Blood pressure of 120/60 mm Hg

$$MAP = [(60 \times 2) + 120]/3$$

$$MAP = (120 + 120)/3$$

$$MAP = 240/3 = 80$$

Patient Assessment

1. Nursing history
    a. Main complaint: Patient's explanation for seeking medical assistance
    b. History of present illness: Ascertain the following:
      i. Description of complaint
      ii. Onset: Date, time of day, duration, course, precipitating factors
      iii. Signs and symptoms: Exacerbations, remissions
        (a) Discomfort: Character, location, radiation, quality, duration, factors that aggravate or produce, factors that alleviate
        (b) Fatigue: With or without activity
        (c) Edema: Location, degree, duration
        (d) Syncope and presyncope: Onset (presyncopal warning or sudden event), time and circumstances of occurrence (postural, nonpostural, activity), provocative events (cough, micturition, head movement)
        (e) Dyspnea: Orthopnea, paroxysmal nocturnal dyspnea, dyspnea on exertion (determine how much exercise it takes to elicit in number of blocks, flights of stairs, etc.)
        (f) Palpitations: Nature, length, associated symptoms
        (g) Cough, hemoptysis
        (h) Claudication: Hip or calf? How many blocks can you walk?
        (i) Recent weight gain or loss
    c. Medical history: Identify all previous illnesses, injuries, and surgical procedures
      i. Patient's assessment of general health for last several years
      ii. Risk factors: Hypertension, hypercholesteremia, smoking, family history of cardiac disease, diabetes
      iii. Last medical examination, hospitalizations, prior relevant cardiac tests (e.g., echocardiography, catheterization)
      iv. Heart history: Coronary artery disease (CAD), angina, myocardial infarctions (MIs), hypertension, valvular disease, dysrhythmias, trauma, peripheral vascular disease, congenital heart defects, heart murmurs, rheumatic fever, cerebrovascular accident (CVA), transient ischemic attacks
    d. Family history: Identify
      i. State of health or cause of death and age at death of immediate family members
      ii. Hereditary, familial diseases pertaining to cardiovascular system
        (a) Diabetes mellitus
        (b) Hypertension
        (c) Cardiovascular disease
        (d) Sudden death or syncope
        (e) Lipid disorders
        (f) Stroke
        (g) Collagen vascular disease
    e. Social history: Identify
      i. Present and past work experiences
      ii. Level of activity, exercise

      iii. Smoking and drinking habits (present, past)

      iv. Daily living patterns

      v. Nutrition: Foods eaten, meals per day, who prepares meals

      vi. Support system: Relationship with significant others

      vii. Cultural issues and language barriers

  f. Medication history: Identify all prescribed or over-the-counter medications. Determine why and how often the patient is taking drug(s), dosages, any side effects, compliance issues.

  g. Allergies: Medications, foods (i.e., shellfish), environmental substances, iodine (potential reaction to contrast medium used during cardiac catheterization procedures)

2. Nursing examination of patient

  a. Physical examination data

      i. General overall appearance: Skin and mucous membranes

        (a) Color

        (b) Temperature

        (c) Moisture

        (d) Turgor

        (e) Edema: Found in dependent areas; pitting versus nonpitting (extremities and sacrum)

        (f) Nail bed: Color, refill

        (g) Angiomas

        (h) Petechiae

        (i) Cyanosis (circumoral, peripheral)

        (j) Clubbing of fingers or toes

      ii. Vital signs

        (a) Pulses: Palpate bilaterally

          (1) Check rate, rhythm, character, and volume

          (2) Describe pulses, using scale of 0 to 3

            a) 0 = absent pulses

            b) 1+ = palpable but thready, easily obliterated

            c) 2+ = normal, not easily obliterated

            d) 3+ = bounding, easily palpable, cannot obliterate

          (3) Common sites for palpation of arteries

            a) Radial

            b) Brachial

            c) Femoral

            d) Carotid

            e) Popliteal

            f) Dorsalis pedis

            g) Posterior tibialis

          (4) Describe pulse characteristics

            a) Normal pulse character: Smooth, rounded

            b) Pulse deficit: Inability to palpate all contractions of the heart

              1) Premature or rapid contractions may not generate a peripheral pulse.

              2) Determine by comparing radial pulse with auscultated apical pulse; record difference in rates.

            c) Pulsus alternans: Pulse waves alternate, every other beat is weaker; caused by impaired myocardium; noted in severe LV failure

            d) Water hammer (Corrigan's pulse)

              1) Abrupt, rapid upstroke followed by rapid downstroke

              2) Palpated in patients with aortic insufficiency, patent ductus arteriosus (PDA)

        (b) Blood pressure

          (1) Sphygmomanometer: Key points

            a) Width of cuff important

              1) Ideal width is 40% of the circumference of the arm.

              2) For obese patients, use a thigh cuff, 18 cm wide.

         b) Positioning of cuff: No less than 2.5 cm from the antecubital fossa

         c) Falsely low measurement: Cuff too large for arm, arm above heart level, inability to accurately hear first Korotkoff sound

         d) Falsely high measurement: Cuff too small for arm, loose cuff not centered over brachial artery, arm below heart level

      (2) Take blood pressure in both arms. More than a 10- to 15–mm Hg difference in systolic pressures indicates diminished arterial flow on the side with the lower reading (obstruction, dissection).

      (3) Orthostatic blood pressure drop: Assess at-risk patients

         a) Check blood pressure with patient supine, sitting, standing.

         b) Fall of more than 20 mm Hg of systolic pressure signifies orthostatic hypotension.

         c) Drop can be caused by vasodilating drugs, volume depletion.

      (4) Pulsus paradoxus: Exaggeration of the normal physiologic response to inspiration (blood pressure lower on inspiration than on expiration)

         a) Examine with the patient breathing normally.

         b) Inflate sphygmomanometer until no Korotkoff sounds are heard; slowly deflate cuff until Korotkoff sounds first heard on expiration; note pressure reading.

         c) Continue to deflate cuff until sounds heard during both expiration and inspiration; note reading.

         d) Subtract second reading from first to determine pulsus paradoxus.

         e) Normally, on inspiration, the difference between inspiration and expiration is less than 11 mm Hg. With pulsus paradoxus, fall in blood pressure on inspiration is 11 mm Hg or greater.

         f) Condition is seen in

            1) Cardiac tamponade

            2) Constrictive pericarditis

            3) Emphysema, asthma

            4) Hemorrhagic shock

  iii. Neck examination

    (a) Neck veins give important clues regarding fluid status.

      (1) Jugular veins reflect RA and RV filling pressures.

      (2) Internal jugular veins are harder to visualize than external jugular veins, but they more accurately reflect pressure and volume changes in the RA (central venous pressure).

      (3) Check for distention and pulsation.

         a) Elevate the head of the bed until jugular waves can be seen.

         b) Shine a bright light tangentially to illuminate vessels, if not obvious.

      (4) Determine jugular venous pressure.

         a) The sternal angle (angle of Louis) is roughly 5 cm above the atrium (when the patient is upright or lying down).

         b) Measure the distance in centimeters from the sternal notch to the top of the distended neck vein.

         c) The value obtained plus the 5 cm provides a rough estimate of central venous pressure.

    (b) Check for hepatojugular reflux.

      (1) Place the patient at a 45-degree angle.

      (2) Compress the upper right abdomen for 30 to 45 seconds (causes additional venous return from liver to heart).

      (3) If hepatojugular reflux is present, the jugular pulses become more pronounced, and the level of filling of neck veins will rise (signifies inability of the right side of the heart to deal with the added volume).

  iv. Chest examination

    (a) Shape and contour of the chest

    (b) Symmetry

    (c) Breathing pattern

v.   Cardiac examination
  (a) Palpate three areas: base, apex, and left sternal border; check for
    (1) Pulsations (e.g., the point of maximal intensity [PMI]; the patient must be supine)
    (2) Thrills (palpable vibrations, analogous to the sensation felt on the throat of a purring cat), which signify turbulence or murmur loud enough to feel (aortic stenosis, mitral stenosis, PDA, ventricular septal defect [VSD])
    (3) Left peristernal lift: Suggests RV dilatation
    (4) Apical impulse (PMI in the normal heart): Not always easy to palpate
      a) Normally located at the fifth left intercostal space, midclavicular line, and is approximately 2 cm in size
      b) PMI that can be palpated over two or more intercostal areas signifies diffuse PMI resulting from
        1) LV dilatation (LV volume overload)
        2) Aortic insufficiency, mitral regurgitation, dilated cardiomyopathy
      c) A forceful, sustained apical impulse indicates LV hypertrophy.
      d) Nonsustained but forceful apical impulses are created by high-output states (fever, anemia, anxiety, hyperthyroidism).
  (b) Auscultation of the heart
    (1) Use of the stethoscope
      a) Bell: Use to hear low-pitched sounds such as ventricular filling sounds (S_3 and S_4) and filling rumble of mitral and tricuspid stenosis
      b) When using the bell of the stethoscope, press only hard enough to create a seal; otherwise, underlying skin functions as a diaphragm and low-pitched sounds will not be heard.
      c) Diaphragm: Use to hear high-pitched sounds such as heart sounds S_1 and S_2, ejection clicks, opening snaps, and most murmurs
      d) Usual listening positions: Supine, left lateral decubitus position, sitting up, and leaning forward
      e) Main auscultation areas on the chest (Figure 3-8)
        1) Aortic area (second intercostal space, right sternal border)
        2) Pulmonic area (second intercostal space, left sternal border)
        3) Tricuspid area (fifth intercostal space, left sternal border)
        4) Mitral or apical area at the PMI (usually the fifth intercostal space, left midclavicular line)

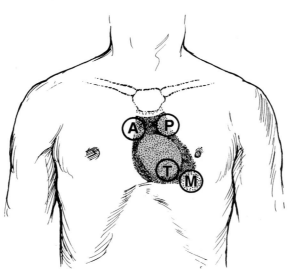

FIGURE 3-8 ■ Cardiac examination. Auscultation areas: Aortic *(A)*, pulmonic *(P)*, tricuspid *(T)*, and mitral *(M)*.

(2) Origin of heart sounds: Opening and closing of valves (see Figure 3-6) and rapid acceleration or deceleration of blood produce either low- or high-pitched sounds

(3) Normal heart sounds

    a) First heart sound (S_1): Produced by mitral and tricuspid valve closure

        1) Marks the onset of ventricular systole

        2) LV depolarizes and contracts before the RV.

        3) Best heard at the apex

        4) Component parts of S_1 may be split (mitral component [M_1] before tricuspid component [T_1]).

        5) Coincides with carotid artery pulse wave

    b) Second heart sound (S_2): Produced by aortic and pulmonic valve closure

        1) Listen with diaphragm at the pulmonic area.

        2) Both component parts of S_2 may be heard: Aortic component (A_2) before pulmonary component (P_2). Normal P_2 is heard only at pulmonic area.

    c) Fourth heart sound (S_4)

        1) Normal in many adults

        2) Audible only in sinus rhythms (requires atrial contraction)

    d) Physiologic (normal) split of S_2 (A_2P_2)

        1) P_2 is delayed on inspiration when the RV is slower to contract than the LV.

        2) Delay is due to increased volume loading of the RV in inspiration caused by increased venous return to the heart.

        3) RV ejection of blood is prolonged and delays pulmonic valve closure, prolonging the time from aortic closure (A_2) to pulmonic closure (P_2). A resulting split occurs between A_2 and P_2 during quiet inspiration.

        4) A_2 precedes P_2 and is generally louder.

        5) Split of S_2 is heard only over the pulmonic area.

        6) Split is best heard in quiet respiration when the patient is sitting or standing.

(4) Abnormal heart sounds: See Table 3-1

(5) Extracardiac sounds

    a) Ejection clicks: Sharp, high-pitched sounds just after S_1; caused by tensioning of the great vessels as they distend in early systole

    b) Pericardial friction rubs

        1) Are like leather rubbing or new snow crunching

        2) Should be heard with the diaphragm in full expiration (are loudest when the patient is leaning forward)

        3) Often have three components (ventricular systole, ventricular filling, and atrial systole)

    c) Opening snaps: Sounds produced by a stenotic mitral valve snapping into the open position

    d) Prosthetic valves: Crisp, sometimes metallic clicking, with both opening and closure heard

(6) Murmurs

    a) Sounds produced by turbulent blood flow (Box 3-2)

    b) Abnormal murmurs (hemodynamically significant): See Table 3-2

  vi. Abdominal examination: Note the following:

    (a) Aortic pulsations (expansile in abdominal aortic aneurysm)

    (b) Hepatomegaly

    (c) Ascites

  vii. Extremities examination: Note the following:

    (a) Edema: Indicates right-sided heart failure, venous stasis, venous insufficiency

    (b) Color, temperature changes: Indicate arterial insufficiency (especially if asymmetrically cool)

TABLE 3-1

Abnormal Heart Sounds

Abnormal Heart Sound	Cause/Circumstance	Seen In	Characteristics
Fixed splitting of S_2		Atrial septal defect	Does not change with expiration (no respiratory variation)
Persistent (wide) splitting of S_2	Occurs with any increase in RV volume or pressure, prolonged RV ejection and delayed pulmonary valve closure, or delay in RV systole (right bundle branch block)	Right bundle branch block Pulmonary hypertension of any cause Pulmonary stenosis Ventricular septal defect	Second heart sound is split on expiration and more widely split on inspiration
Paradoxical splitting (reversed splitting) of S_2 (e.g., P_2 earlier than A_2)	Occurs when LV ejection time is prolonged, resulting in delayed aortic closure; therefore, pulmonic valve closes first	Left bundle branch block Severe aortic stenosis Patent ductus arteriosus	Split widens on expiration and narrows on inspiration (P_2 precedes A_2)
Third heart sound (S_3): Ventricular gallop	Occurs during rapid phase of ventricular filling in early diastole; caused by resistance to ventricular filling, resulting from increased volume load or decreased ventricular compliance	Can normally be heard in children and young adults, and in women during the last trimester of pregnancy (physiologic S_3) Abnormal when heard in older age groups or in association with disease states (left-sided heart failure, ischemia, right-sided heart failure, fluid overload) Heard transiently in patients with ischemia	Sound is low pitched (heard best with bell) When originating in LV, heard best at the apex with patient in left lateral decubitus position When originating in RV, heard best along fourth intercostal space, left sternal border, in inspiration Sounds like cadence of "see" in "Tennessee"
Atrial gallop (presystolic or S_4)	Occurs during atrial contraction, just before S_1 during late phase of ventricular filling Occurs when there is volume overload of either ventricle or decreased ventricular compliance	Often a normal finding in adults Heard also in patients with myocardial ischemia or infarction, systemic and pulmonic hypertension, ventricular failure	Left-sided S_4 is usually heard best at the apex (does not change with respirations) Right-sided S_4 (less common) is usually louder on inspiration, over left lower sternal border Sounds like cadence of "a" in "appendix" or "Ken" in "Kentucky"
Summation gallop	Simultaneous occurrence of atrial (S_4) and ventricular (S_3) gallop	Heard with tachycardias (which cause shortening of diastole) and heart failure	

LV, Left ventricular; *RV*, right ventricular.

■ **BOX 3-2**
■ **EVALUATING MURMURS: SOUNDS PRODUCED BY TURBULENT BLOOD FLOW**

DETERMINE WHETHER MURMUR IS SYSTOLIC OR DIASTOLIC
- Concentrate first on systole (S1 to S2); listen at all areas, starting with the base and moving down to the apex.
- Listen to all areas in diastole (S2 to S1).
- Listen to all areas with the bell and diaphragm.

DETERMINE CHARACTERISTICS OF THE SOUND TO INCLUDE
- Site of maximal intensity
- Radiation of sound (murmurs radiate in the direction of blood flow)
- Timing, duration, and location
- Effect of respirations on murmur, whether increased or decreased with either inspiration or expiration
- Effect of patient position on the murmur's intensity

DESCRIBE PATTERNS, INTENSITY, AND QUALITY OF MURMURS
- Patterns
  Crescendo: Builds up in intensity
  Decrescendo: Decreases in intensity
  Crescendo-decrescendo: Peaks and then decreases in intensity
- Intensity: Based on a grade of I to VI; recorded with grade over VI to show scale used
  I/VI: Barely audible; the clinician can hear only after listening awhile
  II/VI: Easily audible
  III/VI: Loud; not associated with a thrill
  IV/VI: Loud and may be associated with a thrill
  V/VI: Very loud; can be heard with the stethoscope partly off the chest (tilted); associated with a thrill
  VI/VI: Very loud; can be heard with the stethoscope off the chest; associated with a thrill
- Quality: May be described as blowing, musical, rough, harsh, honking, vibratory, cooing
- Pitch: High pitched, low pitched

CHARACTERISTICS OF SPECIFIC HEART SOUNDS
- Ejection murmurs: Usually rough, extending into or through systole (e.g., aortic stenosis or sclerosis)
- Regurgitant murmurs: Are usually a more pure, uniform sound (e.g., mitral regurgitation)
- Pansystolic (holosystolic) murmurs: Heard from S_1 through S_2

COMMENTS ON FUNCTIONAL, INNOCENT MURMURS
- Hemodynamically insignificant, physiologic; usually ejection murmurs associated with either increased flow or volume
- Not associated with cardiovascular disease
- Common in children and pregnant women
- Heard in hyperthyroidism, anemia
- Diastolic murmurs are never functional or innocent.

    (c) Skin condition: Petechiae, jaundice
    (d) Hair loss: Indicates arterial disease
    (e) Ulcerations: Indicates stasis, ischemia
    (f) Peripheral pulses: Check for bruits
    (g) Motor and sensory function: Numbness, foot drop (in advanced peripheral ischemia)
    (h) Clubbing of nail beds: Cyanotic congenital heart defects
    (i) Varicosities
    (j) Gangrene

■ TABLE 3-2
■ ■ Abnormal Heart Murmurs: Main Characteristics

Abnormal Murmur	Location Where Heard Best	Characteristics	Comments
SYSTOLIC MURMURS			
Mitral insufficiency or regurgitation	Loudest at apex Radiates to left axilla	Blowing quality, high-pitched	Pansystolic—extends through A_2 May be rough and heard at base (mitral valve prolapse)
Tricuspid insufficiency or regurgitation	Loudest at lower left sternal border Radiates to right sternal border, liver	Blowing quality, low-pitched Variable in intensity (may increase with inspiration)	Pansystolic
Aortic stenosis	Maximal intensity at base of heart, usually at second intercostal space, right sternal border Radiates to neck and apex	Harsh in quality, medium or high-pitched May be crescendo–decrescendo murmur Intensity varies; no relation to severity of murmur	Systolic ejection murmur Extends to S_2 Thrill may be found at second intercostal space, right sternal border
Hypertrophic obstructive cardiomyopathy	Maximal intensity at second to fourth intercostal spaces, right sternal border May radiate to apex	Crescendo-decrescendo Decreases during expiration and squatting Increases with Valsalva maneuver	Ejection murmur Thrill may be found at lower left sternal border
Pulmonic stenosis	Maximal loudness at second intercostal space, left sternal border Louder when patient is supine and during inspiration	Harsh Usually grade III to IV intensity Persistent split of S_2; including expiration; the more severe the stenosis, the more pronounced the split	Pulmonary systolic ejection sound (click) Thrill may be felt at second intercostal space, left sternal border RV S_4 possible
Interventricular septal defect	Maximal loudness along lower sternal border Radiates widely	Harsh	Pansystolic or early systolic Thrill often present over left sternal border
Patent ductus arteriosus	Maximal intensity at second intercostal space, left sternal border	Machinery-like murmur	Continuous systolic and diastolic murmur Occasional thrill at second intercostal space, left sternal border
DIASTOLIC MURMURS			
Mitral stenosis	Maximal intensity at PMI May be heard only when patient lying on left side at the PMI with bell of stethoscope	Very low pitched Fading rumble Presystolic, crescendo if patient in normal sinus rhythm Intensity not affected by inspiration	Early diastolic and presystolic rumble (if in sinus rhythm) May be associated with an opening snap and accentuated S_1

Continued

■ TABLE 3-2
■ ■ **Abnormal Heart Murmurs: Main Characteristics—Cont'd**

Abnormal Murmur	Location Where Heard Best	Characteristics	Comments
Tricuspid stenosis	Maximal intensity at fourth intercostal space, left sternal border	Rumbling Low pitched Intensity should increase on inspiration, unless RV has failed	Early diastolic May have an opening snap
Aortic insufficiency or regurgitation	Maximal intensity at third to fourth intercostal space, left sternal border, and at apex Radiates to apex Heard best when patient is sitting up and leaning forward, during exhalation	Blowing quality High pitched Decrescendo Intensity varies with severity	Pandiastolic (unless acute, when it is short, early diastolic murmur)
Pulmonary insufficiency or regurgitation	Maximal loudness along second left intercostal space, left sternal border Radiates along left sternal border	Blowing quality High pitched Decrescendo	Sometimes increases with inspiration

PMI, Point of maximal intensity; *RV,* right ventricular.

    b. Monitoring data

        i. Complications of bedside hemodynamic monitoring

            (a) Dysrhythmias

            (b) Hemorrhage

            (c) Infection

            (d) Thrombi, emboli (air, blood)

            (e) Pneumothorax

            (f) Cardiac perforation

            (g) Pulmonary infarction (balloon left inflated)

            (h) Vascular occlusion or spasm

3. Appraisal of patient characteristics

    a. Resiliency

        i. Level 1—*Minimally resilient*: Mr. A., an 82-year-old man with severe aortic stenosis in rapid atrial fibrillation and recovering from a CVA

        ii. Level 3—*Moderately resilient*: Mrs. B., a 71-year-old woman with history of insulin-dependent diabetes and hypertension. She is admitted with a blood pressure of 195/110 mm Hg, sinus tachycardia, atypical chest pain, and abdominal discomfort.

        iii. Level 5—*Highly resilient*: Mr. C., a 45-year-old man with a history of hypertension, admitted complaining of left-sided chest and shoulder pain. Cardiac catheterization results are normal.

    b. Vulnerability

        i. Level 1—*Highly vulnerable*: Mr. A., whose family reports that he lost his wife (of 60 years) 4 days earlier when she suddenly collapsed at home. Results of his transesophageal echocardiography show several large clots in the LA.

        ii. Level 3—*Moderately vulnerable*: Mr. D., a 53-year-old man with a history of sudden cardiac death (requiring implantation of a cardiac defibrillator), ulcerative colitis, pericardial effusion, and steroid-induced diabetes. He is anemic, with tarry stools. His wife is also very anxious and requires a great deal of attention.

        iii. Level 5—*Minimally vulnerable*: Ms. E., a 48-year-old woman, admitted with acute pericarditis, responding well to an oral nonsteroidal anti-inflammatory drug (NSAID); her pain is resolving, and her condition is stable.

    c. Stability

        i. Level 1—*Minimally stable*: Mr. F., a 47-year-old man with history of scleroderma, Raynaud's disease, and severe pulmonary hypertension. He is presently receiving intravenous (IV) dobutamine. He has 2+ edema bilaterally in his lower extremities. His lungs have crackles in the bases. He is being evaluated for epoprostenol (Flolan) home therapy to assist in improving his quality of life. He is not eligible for heart transplantation.

        ii. Level 3—*Moderately stable*: Mrs. G., a 78-year-old woman with a history of ischemic cardiomyopathy, severe mitral regurgitation, hyperlipidemia, and three-vessel disease. Complained of chest pain at home, relieved with nitroglycerin.

        iii. Level 5—*Highly stable*: Mr. H., a 65-year-old man with a history of third-degree AV block, who received a permanent pacemaker 2 days earlier. His incision site is healing well, and he has minimal discomfort. The pacemaker is functioning appropriately.

    d. Complexity

        i. Level 1—*Highly complex*: Mr. S., a 63-year-old man with a history of open heart transplantation 10 years ago, hospitalized 1 month ago for endocarditis. Admitted from skilled care with an infected right Hickman catheter, an elevated temperature, and a heart rate of 105 beats/min with frequent premature ventricular contractions.

        ii. Level 3—*Moderately complex*: Ms. P., a 27-year-old woman with a history of open heart transplantation 7 years ago and MI 3 years ago. Has had numerous coronary interventions, including recent placements of stents to her LCA. She has a history of a permanent pacemaker, asthma, hypertension, heart failure, and chronic renal insufficiency. She is admitted with a large pericardial effusion.

      iii. Level 5—*Minimally complex*: Mrs. V., who had acute-onset atrial tachycardia and was given IV medications, after which her heart rhythm converted into sinus rhythm. She is up in her room ready for instructions before going home.

  e. Resource availability

      i. Level 1—*Few resources*: Ms. B., who lives alone and whose family is gone. It is physically hard for her to leave her apartment. She has a small income and cannot afford the combination of drugs prescribed for her hypertension, diabetes, and hyperlipidemia.

      ii. Level 3—*Moderate resources*: Mr. L., a 60-year-old man with a history of coronary artery bypass graft 3 years ago, who experienced chest discomfort while at his cardiac rehabilitation group. His wife and family are supportive and involved in his care.

      iii. Level 5—*Many resources*: Mrs. R., a 65-year-old woman with MI with ST-segment elevation, who had a percutaneous coronary intervention (PCI) and was given thrombolytics 90 minutes after the onset of symptoms. She is married to a staff physician, and her daughter is a nurse.

  f. Participation in care

      i. Level 1—*No participation*: Mrs. Q., a 68-year-old woman who experienced rapid atrial fibrillation on a medical floor and is transferred to the progressive care unit. She has a history of hypertension, renal failure, and dementia. She has a full code status.

      ii. Level 3—*Moderate level of participation*: Ms. P., who, although she is a patient with a highly complex condition, is very interested in her diagnosis, medication, and therapy. She attempts to watch her intake and diet. Her parents are also involved in all care aspects. They do, however, verbalize some inaccurate medical information leading to erroneous conclusions.

      iii. Level 5—*Full participation*: Ms. M., a 40-year-old woman with pulmonary hypertension who is awaiting heart transplantation. She is independent in her care activities. She and her husband take full advantage of educational resources and talk with transplant patients.

  g. Participation in decision making

      i. Level 1—*No participation*: Mr. T. is 68 years old and was admitted to the hospital for a total hip replacement. He had chest pain on postoperative day 1, ECG changes, and an elevation in cardiac enzyme levels. An urgent heart catheterization was done, with use of a radial approach.

      ii. Level 3—*Moderate level of participation*: Mr. O., a 60-year-old man admitted with chest pain due to a reoccluded coronary lesion, who decided he did not need to continue his clopidogrel after discharge from the hospital

      iii. Level 5—*Full participation*: Mr. F. (in a highly unstable condition), who with his family is actively involved in end-of-life decision making. In conferences with the physicians and nurses, he and his family have requested that he not be intubated or resuscitated if the situation presents. They want Mr. F. to have only comfort measures.

  h. Predictability

      i. Level 1—*Not predictable*: Mrs. G., who received an automatic implantable cardiac defibrillator during her hospitalization. The day after her discharge home, her defibrillator discharged eight times throughout the evening and night. She is readmitted to reevaluate medical therapy.

      ii. Level 3—*Moderately predictable*: Mr. H., a 49-year-old man, who was admitted for another MI (he had his first MI when he was 37 years old) and received brachytherapy and a stent to the circumflex artery. Eptifibatide (Integrilin) is infusing. Vital signs are stable.

      iii. Level 5—*Highly predictable*: Mr. X., who has a small VSD that does not require surgery. Staff stressed the importance of good dental care and prophylactic antibiotics because of the high risk of infectious endocarditis.

4. Diagnostic studies

  a. Laboratory

      i. Cardiac troponin T and troponin I: Group of compounds that bind to tropomyosin and help with excitation-contraction in muscle

         (a) Most sensitive cardiac markers; very specific, mark injury to myocytes (not just cell death)

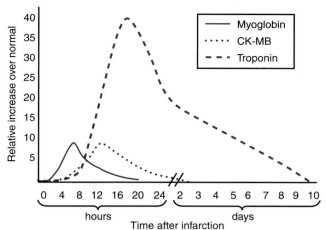

FIGURE 3-9 ■ Time course of the appearance of serum levels of creatine kinase MB isoenzyme *(CK-MB)*, myoglobin, and troponin in a patient with an ST-segment elevation myocardial infarction. (From Henry JB. *Clinical Diagnosis and Management by Laboratory Methods.* Philadelphia, PA: Saunders; 2001:297.)

  (b) Levels rise 4 to 6 hours after the onset of ischemic symptoms; peak at 18 to 24 hours after MI; fall slowly, over up to 2 weeks (Figure 3-9).
  (c) Cleared by kidneys, so levels are elevated in chronic renal failure
  (d) Rare for the value to be more than 0.1 ng/ml in a normal individual
  (e) Facilitate quicker decision making in identification, risk stratification, and treatment of patients
  (f) Predictor of high risk for subsequent cardiac events in acute coronary syndromes, postoperative vascular surgery; prognostic indicator for pulmonary embolus
 ii. Creatine kinase (CK): CK-MB isoenzyme
  (a) Enzyme associated with adenosine triphosphate conversion in contractile muscle tissue; found in the heart, brain, and skeletal tissues
  (b) MB isoenzyme levels very sensitive for cardiac tissue; not as sensitive in early MI less than 6 hours after onset
  (c) Level rises 4 to 8 hours after onset, peaks 12 to 24 hours after MI, returns to normal in approximately 24 to 48 hours.
  (d) CK-MB concentration of more than 5% of total CK indicates myocardial necrosis.
 iii. Myoglobin: Heme-containing protein
  (a) Very sensitive marker but not cardiac specific; can be elevated with cardiopulmonary resuscitation (CPR), falls, and injections
  (b) Level peaks 8 hours after infarct, then rapidly returns to normal in 18 to 24 hours.
  (c) Useful in the emergency department for early MI detection, ruling out of MI, reperfusion monitoring
 iv. Brain natriuretic peptide (BNP)
  (a) Released with myocardial stretch
  (b) Level correlates with LV dysfunction.
  (c) Used to evaluate heart failure (both LV and RV) and pulmonary emboli and to differentiate cardiac from pulmonary causes of pulmonary distress and dyspnea
  (d) Higher levels indicate poor prognosis.
  (e) Falsely low results can occur in obese patients because of clearance in adipose tissue (adipose tissue removes BNP from the circulation).
  (f) Falsely high results can occur in the elderly, hypertensive individuals, females, and patients being given nesiritide.
 v. C-reactive protein
  (a) Biomarker of inflammation

(b) Independent predictor of future cardiovascular risk

(c) Elevations may also indicate an acute infection, inflammatory disease processes, possible uremia.

vi. Clotting profile

(a) Partial thromboplastin time (PTT): Used for monitoring the effectiveness of heparin

(b) International normalized ratio (INR): Used for measuring the effectiveness of anticoagulant therapy

(1) For atrial fibrillation, therapeutic range for INR is 2.0 to 3.0.

(2) For prosthetic valves, therapeutic range for INR is 2.5 to 3.5.

(c) Activated clotting time (ACT): Bedside test done to measure the time required for blood coagulation. This test is also used to evaluate heparin effectiveness, usually at the bedside or in the catheterization laboratory to determine whether it is safe for vascular sheaths to be removed.

(d) Platelet count

vii. Complete blood cell count (CBC), hemoglobin (Hb) level, hematocrit (HCT)

viii. Electrolyte levels, blood urea nitrogen (BUN) level, creatinine level, glucose level

ix. Fasting serum lipid profile: Normal levels

(a) Total cholesterol level: Goal is less than 200 mg/dl

(b) High-density lipoprotein (HDL): Goal is HDL level above 40 mg/dl

(c) Low-density lipoprotein (LDL): Level of less than 100 mg/dl is optimal if CAD is present (otherwise, 130 mg/dl is the goal)

(d) Triglycerides: Desired level is less than 150 mg/dl; 150 to 199 mg/dl is borderline; 200 to 499 mg/dl is high; more than 500 mg/dl is very high

(e) Lipoprotein(a): Marker for CAD, not usually followed; levels of more than 30 mg/dl associated with CAD

x. Homocysteine level: To identify folic acid–responsive hyperlipidemia. Normal level is 5 to 15 μmol/L. Elevated levels considered an independent risk factor for CAD.

b. Imaging

i. Chest radiograph is used to visualize

(a) Cardiac size, position, chamber size

(b) Abnormalities of the heart, great vessels, lungs, pleura, and ribs

(c) Pulmonary vasculature

(d) Position of catheters, lines, and pacemaker leads

ii. Magnetic resonance imaging (MRI): Safe diagnostic technique involving no ionizing radiation. Used with contrast to produce a magnetic resonance angiogram (MRA).

(a) Provides a three-dimensional view of cardiovascular structure

(b) Creates a computer-assisted image, measures tissue proton density

(c) MRI is used to determine or identify

(1) Anatomy of the heart

(2) Congenital heart defects

(3) Masses in the myocardium or pericardium

(4) Ventricular aneurysm

(5) Aortic dissection

(6) Arterial disease (MRA)

(d) Safe alternative to radiography for children and pregnant women

(e) As a magnetic device, MRI machine interferes with pacemaker function

(f) Not used for patients with prosthetic metallic devices (valves, prosthetic joints). Can displace or damage such devices due to powerful magnet.

iii. Ultrafast (electron beam) computed tomography (EBCT): Form of computed tomography (CT) in which a rapid electron beam is used for high-speed imaging

(a) Provides two-dimensional image of cardiovascular structures

(b) Visualizes coronary calcium, silent atherosclerosis

(1) Amount of calcium can be predictive of multivessel CAD

(2) Not sufficiently specific

(c) Cost and specificity limit use at present.

iv. Myocardial imaging: Radioisotope is injected into a peripheral vein and its cardiac uptake can be imaged. Methods include
   (a) Multiple-gated acquisition (MUGA) scan
      (1) Used to measure the EF of the LV
      (2) Very accurate unless the patient has an irregular rhythm, because multiple images cannot be "gated" (superimposed) on ECG
   (b) Myocardial scintigraphy (perfusion imaging)
      (1) Involves the use of thallium-201 or technetium Tc 99m sestamibi to identify ischemia, infarct, and myocardial viability
      (2) Normal myocardium takes up the isotope from the blood.
      (3) Decreased myocardial perfusion results in decreased uptake; ischemic sites show normal uptake at rest and decreased uptake on exercise. Infarcted sites show no uptake at all.
      (4) Pharmacologic agents (dipyridamole, adenosine) are used to simulate the effects of exercise (potentially to induce ischemia) in patients who are unable to exercise.
      (5) Perfusion imaging is more sensitive and specific (80% to 85%) than exercise ECG–stress testing (70%).
   (c) Infarct-avid imaging (myocardial infarct indicators)
      (1) Technetium Tc 99m pyrophosphate is injected into a peripheral vein.
      (2) Infarcted areas of the heart show increased levels of radioactivity as "hot spots." These appear within 4 hours of infarction, may not peak until 12 to 24 hours later, and remain positive for 2 to 7 days.
      (3) Usefulness is limited in acute MI; useful when ECG changes are not definitive or when enzyme levels have already returned to normal.
   (d) Clinical uses of nuclear medicine: Evaluation of
      (1) Ischemic heart disease (including risk stratification)
      (2) LV function
v. Cardiac catheterization and angiography: High-quality coronary images produced by x-ray digital imaging. Radiopaque contrast medium is injected into the coronary arteries for visualization; recordings are made on digital media. Still photographs may be produced for patient records.
   (a) Patients selected include
      (1) Asymptomatic patients with
         a) Evidence of significant ischemia or severe LV dysfunction on noninvasive testing
         b) Survival after a sudden cardiac death event
         c) Valvular heart disease
      (2) Symptomatic patients with
         a) Angina—unstable or stable
         b) Atypical chest pain
         c) Recent MI
         d) Valvular disease
         e) Congenital heart defects
         f) Aortic disease
         g) LV failure
   (b) Technique
      (1) Right-sided heart catheterization performed via the right or left femoral or brachial vein with the catheter advanced into the RA and then past the tricuspid valve through the RV into the pulmonary artery to record pressures, perform angiography, determine CO and resistances, and define anatomy
      (2) Left-sided heart catheterization performed in a retrograde manner via the femoral or brachial artery (or transseptal approach through the RA and intraatrial septum); catheter is advanced into the LV to determine pressure
   (c) Left ventriculography

        (1) Technique: Radiopaque contrast medium is injected into the LV cavity

        (2) Purposes

            a) Evaluate ventricular wall motion and chamber size

                1) Identify akinetic areas and wall motion abnormalities

                2) Detect hypokinetic areas: Weaker than normal contractions in systole

                3) Detect dyskinetic areas: Areas bulge outward during systole instead of contracting

            b) Assess function, determining

                1) End-diastolic volume

                2) End-systolic volume

                3) Stroke volume

                4) EF

            c) Detect ventricular aneurysms

            d) Evaluate mitral, aortic valves

            e) Demonstrate ventricular-level left-to-right intracardiac shunts (VSD)

    (d) Aortography

        (1) Technique: Contrast injected into aortic root or descending aorta

        (2) Purpose: To assess

            a) Aortic valve insufficiency

            b) Aneurysms or dissections of ascending aorta

            c) Coarctation of the aorta

            d) Diseases of the aorta

            e) Presence of saphenous vein grafts

            f) Presence of PDA

    (e) Coronary arteriography

        (1) Radiopaque contrast material injected into the ostia of the LCA and RCA, allowing multiple views and recordings of coronary arterial circulation

        (2) Purpose

            a) To assess the extent of significant CAD by identifying the presence and severity of lesions

            b) To guide therapeutic options in ischemic heart disease

            c) To assess possible coronary arterial spasm

            d) To administer intracoronary thrombolytics and drugs

            e) To perform transcatheter interventional procedures: PCI, coronary stent placement, rotational atherectomy, and percutaneous transluminal coronary angioplasty (PTCA)

    (f) Complications of diagnostic cardiac catheterization

        (1) Death: Approximately 0.11% incidence (most frequently seen in left main disease)

        (2) MI: Approximately 0.05% incidence

        (3) Neurologic events (stroke): Approximately 0.07% incidence

        (4) Acute renal failure or oliguria caused by contrast medium and inadequate hydration

        (5) Transient cardiac dysrhythmias, bradycardia, conduction disturbances

        (6) Hemorrhage or hematoma at insertion site

        (7) Allergic reactions to contrast medium

        (8) Arterial perforation, thrombosis, embolus, and dissection

        (9) Hypovolemia (due to diuresis from contrast medium and nothing-by-mouth [NPO] status)

c. Other

    i. ECG: Records the electrical activity of the heart

        (a) Identifies

            (1) Dysrhythmias and conduction defects

            (2) Ischemia or infarction

            (3) Electrolyte abnormalities

            (4) Drug effects

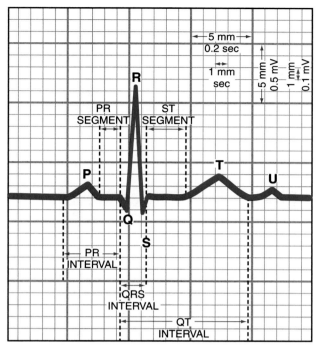

FIGURE 3-10 ■ Normal electrocardiogram complex

      (5) Hypertrophy of the ventricles and enlargement of the atria
      (6) Anatomic orientation of the heart
  (b) ECG paper (Figure 3-10)
      (1) Measures time along the horizontal axis
          a) Records P wave, QRS complex, and T wave (in time), as well as PR and QT intervals
          b) Each small box (1 mm) = 0.04 second
          c) Each large box (5 mm) = 0.20 second
          d) Normal speed of paper: 25 mm/sec
      (2) Measures voltage in the vertical direction
          a) Measures and records amplitude and voltage of P wave, QRS complex, and T wave
          b) Each small box (1 mm) = 0.1 mV
          c) Each large box (5 mm) = 0.5 mV
          d) Usual calibration standard is 10 mm = 1 mV
          e) Useful in detection of atrial and ventricular hypertrophy
  (c) Deflections: Waves of the ECG recording are either above or below the isoelectric line
      (1) Positive deflections occur when the heart's depolarization wave moves toward the positive electrode of the recording lead.
      (2) Negative deflections occur when the heart's depolarization wave moves away from the positive electrode of the recording lead.
      (3) Biphasic deflections occur when the heart's depolarization wave is moving both toward and away from the positive electrode. If the wave of depolarization is perpendicular to the positive electrode, waves may be small or absent.
  (d) ECG waves: Representation, measurement, abnormalities—see Table 3-3 and Figure 3-10
  (e) 12-Lead ECG (Box 3-3 and Figure 3-11)

■ **TABLE 3-3**
■ ■ **ECG Waves and Intervals: Description, Characteristics, and Abnormalities**

ECG	Description	Characteristics	Causes for Abnormalities
P wave	Represents atrial depolarization RA begins depolarization earlier than the LA	Normal duration: <0.10 sec Normal amplitude: ≤2.5 mm P waves >2.5 mm in amplitude in any lead are abnormal "2.5 × 2.5 rule" (handy rule of thumb): P wave should not be wider than 2.5 mm (LA enlargement) or taller than 2.5 mm (RA enlargement)	Atrial hypertrophy: Increased P amplitude or width RA hypertrophy: • Tall, peaked P waves in lead II, III, and aVF • May show tall or biphasic P waves in V_1 (>2.5 mm in amplitude) LA hypertrophy: • Wide, notched P waves in limb leads and V_4 to V_6 and/or P waves with broad negative deflection in lead V_1 (>1 mm); • P >2.5 mm in width
PR interval	Represents time required for conduction through AV node PR segment represents normal delay of impulse in AV node	Normal interval: 0.12-0.20 sec Measure from beginning of P wave to beginning of QRS complex	Prolonged delay (PR interval >0.20 sec) indicates diseased AV node, ischemia, drug effects, or increased vagal tone
QRS complex	Represents ventricular depolarization Atrial repolarization occurs during this time period but is obscured by QRS	Normal duration: 0.06-0.10 sec; borderline at 0.11 sec Measured from onset of Q wave (or R wave if no Q wave is present) to end of QRS	Abnormal if ≥0.12 sec; indicative of intraventricular conduction delay; seen in patients with bundle branch blocks (≥0.12), WPW syndrome, and hyperkalemia (sine wave)
Q wave	Present if the first deflection of the QRS is negative	Small physiologic Q waves are usually seen in leads I, aVL, V_5, and V_6, as well as in inferior leads II, III, and aVF	Q waves are pathologic when >0.04 sec wide (>0.03 sec in inferior leads II, III, and aVF) and >25% of R-wave amplitude Q waves in leads III, aVR, and V_1 are normal Pathologic Q waves result from myocardial infarction
R wave	First positive deflection occurring in the QRS complex		Prominent R waves may be seen with ventricular hypertrophy and in young adults, persons with thin chests, and patients with WPW syndrome
S wave	Negative deflection that follows an R wave		

ST segment	Represents initial ventricular repolarization	Measure immediately after QRS complex to beginning of T wave; normally isoelectric	Elevated ST segment is caused by pericarditis, injury, acute infarctions, LV aneurysms, and normal variation (early repolarization) Depressed ST segment may indicate subendocardial injury or ischemia, electrolyte disturbances, drug effect, or early repolarization, or it may be nonspecific
T wave	Represents ventricular repolarization		Inverted T waves may be associated with infarctions, ischemia, injury, or hypertrophy Tall, peaked T waves may be caused by hyperkalemia or acute injury or may be a normal variant
QT interval	Represents complete duration of ventricular depolarization and repolarization QT interval varies with heart rate, gender, and age	QTc takes heart rate into account and provides a normal range corrected for heart rate In general, QTc of ≥0.44 sec in males and ≥0.45 sec in females is considered abnormal Measure from the beginning of the Q wave to the end of the T wave	Causes of prolonged QTc: Ischemia, electrolyte imbalances (hypocalcemia), hypertrophy, antiarrhythmic drugs (procainamide, amiodarone), and congenital prolongation Prolonged QTc is associated with an increased incidence of polymorphic ventricular tachycardia (torsades de pointes) and, potentially, sudden death Causes of shortened QTc: Acute ischemia, hypercalcemia, and drugs (digitalis)

AV, Atrioventricular; *ECG,* electrocardiogram; *LA,* left atrium; *QTc,* corrected QT interval; *RA,* right atrium; *WPW,* Wolff-Parkinson-White.

▨ BOX 3-3
▨ TWELVE-LEAD ELECTROCARDIOGRAPH AND MCL₁ ELECTRODE PLACEMENT

Lead I: Right arm (negative electrode), left arm (positive electrode)
Lead II: Right arm (negative electrode), left leg (positive electrode)
Lead III: Left arm (negative electrode), left leg (positive electrode)
aVR: Right arm; normally a negative deflection
aVL: Left arm; usually a positive deflection
aVF: Left leg; usually a positive deflection
V_1: Fourth intercostal space, right sternal border
V_2: Fourth intercostal space, left sternal border
V_3: Halfway between V_2 and V_4
V_4: Fifth intercostal space, left midclavicular line
V_5: Level with V_4, left anterior axillary line
V_6: Level with V_4, left midaxillary line
V_4R: Fifth intercostal space, right midclavicular line
MCL₁ (monitoring lead used in a three-lead monitoring system): Fourth intercostal space, right sternal border (positive electrode); below left clavicle, midclavicular line (negative electrode); below right clavicle (ground)

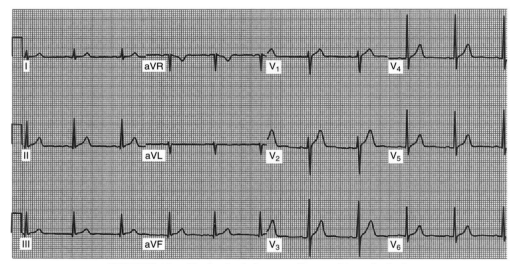

FIGURE 3-11 ■ Twelve-lead electrocardiogram (sinus rhythm).

(1) Standard limb leads: Two electrodes of opposing polarity (positive and negative) are used to record electrical activity. These bipolar electrodes are placed on the patient's arms and/or legs.

(2) Augmented limb leads: Electrical activity is recorded between one positive electrode (unipolar) and the electrical sum of other two standard limb electrodes. The wave's amplitude is augmented (enhanced voltage) for ease of visualization.

(3) Precordial (chest) V leads: Record electrical activity between one positive electrode (unipolar) and the electrical sum of the three standard limb electrodes

    a) R waves get progressively larger (normal R-wave progression) moving from V_1 toward V_5 (V_5 is higher than V_6)

    b) V_4R (analogous to V_4, only on right side): Used for RV infarcts

(f) See Box 3-4 for ECG and rhythm assessment checklist.

(g) See Table 3-4 for descriptions of cardiac dysrhythmias and conduction defects.

  ii. Echocardiography: One of the most important noninvasive tools

■ **BOX 3-4**
■ **CARDIAC RHYTHM ASSESSMENT CHECKLIST**

Analyze electrocardiogram rhythms systematically, including
- **Rates:** Atrial and ventricular
- **Rhythm:** Regular, irregular, pattern if irregular
- **P wave:** Identification
  1. Relation to QRS (before, after)
  2. Configuration or morphology
- **PR interval:** Measurement
- **QRS complex:** Measurement, configuration
- **ST segment:** Isoelectric, depressed, elevated
- **T wave:** Size, shape, direction
- **Dysrhythmia origin:** Identify if possible
- **Possible implications:** For patient and nursing care

(a) High-frequency ultrasonic vibrations are emitted via a transducer on the patient's chest or in the esophagus. The returning echo of sound waves is received. An image is created and recorded for interpretation.

(b) Provides information on
   (1) Chamber size and function, including
      a) LV systolic function: EF
      b) LV wall motion (shows areas of hypokinesis, akinesis, dyskinesis), wall thickness, cavity size
      c) LV diastolic function
      d) Chamber size
   (2) Valvular morphology and function
      a) Regurgitation
      b) Prosthetic valve function
      c) Stenotic valves
   (3) Intracardiac masses, including tumors, thrombi, and vegetations
   (4) Congenital defects and shunts
   (5) Pericardial disease
      a) Pericardial effusion
      b) Cardiac tamponade

(c) M-mode echocardiography is used to measure intracardiac dimensions; measures chamber size and wall thickness.

(d) Two-dimensional echocardiography provides real-time imagery of the heart and its structures by using a two-dimensional ultrasonic beam.

(e) Doppler echocardiography is used to demonstrate the velocity and direction of blood flow through the heart and great vessels.

(f) Color flow imaging: Doppler signals are processed to depict real-time velocities superimposed on a two-dimensional echocardiogram. Red represents flow toward the transducer; blue represents flow away from the transducer. Lighter shades mean higher velocity. Used to evaluate shunts, regurgitation, stenosis.

(g) Contrast echocardiography
   (1) Bubble echo (agitated saline): Used to detect congenital or acquired shunts, patent foramen ovale
   (2) Enhancing agents (e.g., Optison): Used to enhance the LV endocardial border and help identify myocardial infarct or ischemia

(h) Stress echocardiography: Images obtained before, during, and after exercise or pharmacologic stress (states of increased myocardial oxygen demand)
   (1) Methods used include treadmill (most common) and pharmacologic stressing (dobutamine, dipyridamole, adenosine).

Text continued on p. 177

■ TABLE 3-4
■ ■ **Cardiac Dysrhythmias and Conduction Defects**

Rhythm	Mechanism	Characteristics	Comments
SINUS RHYTHMS			
Sinus rhythm	Originates in SA node	Rate: 50-100 beats/min Rhythm: Regular P wave: • Normal and upright in leads II, III, aVF • Precede each QRS • Identical size and shape in any given lead • PR interval: 0.12-0.20 sec	Optimal cardiac rhythm **Sinus arrhythmia:** If rhythm varies (PP or RR interval varies >0.16 sec; usually related to respirations (RR intervals decrease with inspiration) Causes: Vagal responses (children, young adults), SA node disease (in elderly)
Sinus bradycardia		Rate: <50 beats/min PQRST: Complexes and intervals are normal	Causes: May be normal during sleep and in athletes and young hearts; seen in hypothermia, increased intracranial pressure, decreased sympathetic tone, increased parasympathetic tone, Valsalva maneuver, carotid massage, vomiting, drugs, hypothyroidism
Sinus tachycardia		Rate: 100-200 beats/min Rhythm: Regular PQRST: Complexes and intervals normal	Causes: Secondary to anxiety, exercise, pain, hyperthyroidism, shock, anemia, fever, hypoxia, hypercapnia, heat exposure, drugs, heart failure (early sign)

Sinus arrest or sinus pause	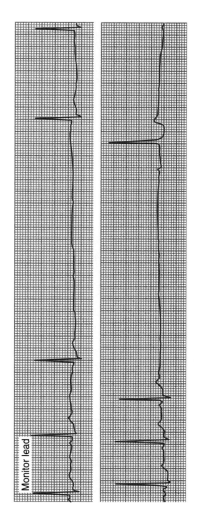	SA node fails, no impulse initiated, atrial standstill	PQRST complex: Not seen Sinus pause: If <3.0 sec Sinus arrest: If >3.0 sec Pause is usually greater than two regular RR intervals	Causes of sinus blocks and pauses: Increased vagal stimulation (i.e., by suctioning), MI, myocarditis, drug effects (e.g., from digitalis)

ATRIAL RHYTHMS

PAC	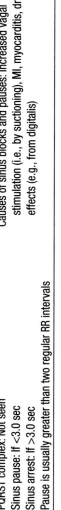 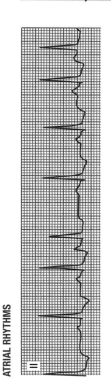 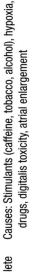	Early atrial impulse, interrupting the inherent regular rhythm	Normal QRS complex if ventricular repolarization was complete Abnormal QRS complex if conducted aberrantly (ventricle partially repolarized) No QRS complex if beat arrived too early during the ventricle's absolute refractory period (i.e., blocked PAC) Usually no compensatory pause, but may have a partial pause	Causes: Stimulants (caffeine, tobacco, alcohol), hypoxia, drugs, digitalis toxicity, atrial enlargement

Monitor lead

Continued

■ **TABLE 3-4**
■ ■ **Cardiac Dysrhythmias and Conduction Defects—Cont'd**

Rhythm	Mechanism	Characteristics	Comments
ATRIAL RHYTHMS—Cont'd			
Ectopic atrial tachycardia	Enhanced automaticity	Rates: 150-220 beats/min P wave: Different from sinus PR interval: Normal QRS complexes: Normal Speeds up, slows down	Brief runs Common in normal population May be seen in pneumonia, chronic obstructive pulmonary disease, MI, metabolic changes, alcohol use
Automatic atrial tachycardia	Triggered activity Intra-atrial reentry	Rates: 150-220 beats/min P wave: Different from sinus PR interval: Normal QRS: Normal Sudden start and stop	Seen in digoxin toxicity
Multifocal atrial tachycardia	Origin: Several ectopic foci in the atria that initiate impulses	Atrial rates: 100-200 beats/min Rhythm varies widely P wave shape: Changes often PR intervals: Vary	Often associated with chronic pulmonary disease

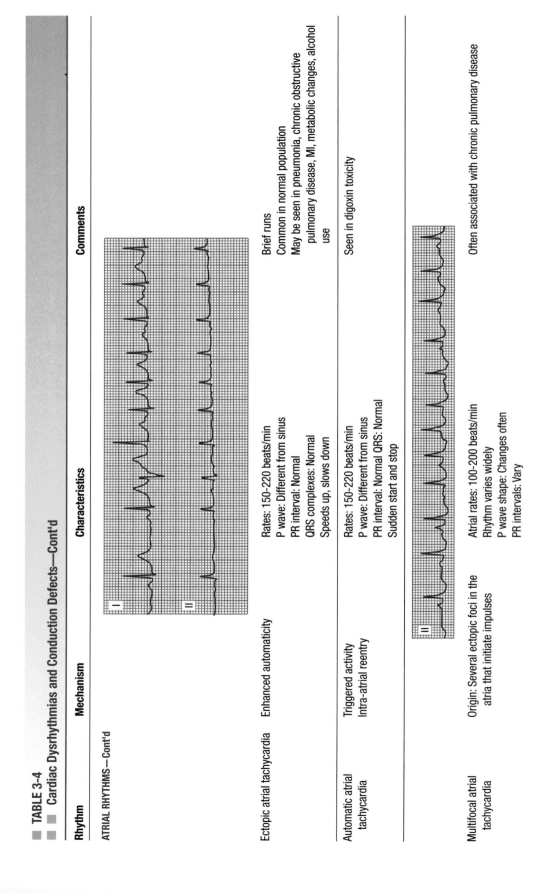

Atrial flutter

Origin: Reentry

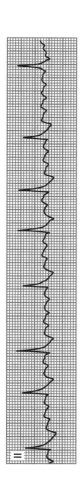

Atrial rates: 200-350 beats/min

Ventricular rates, along with rhythm, may be constant at 2:1, 3:1, 4:1 or may vary; if there is a variable AV conduction block

Flutter waves may appear as wide, sawtooth waves representing rapid atrial depolarization, persist through QRS complexes, and are best seen in leads II, III, and aVF

According to the "rule of 150," an SVT at a rate of 150 beats/min is usually atrial flutter with a 2:1 block

Atrial fibrillation

Chaotic, random, and rapid atrial activity

Atrial impulses are randomly conducted through the AV junction

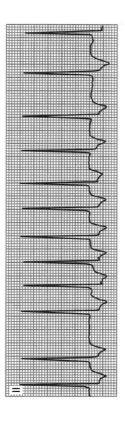

Atrial rates: 350-650 beats/min

Irregular fibrillatory waves of varying amplitude; best seen in V_1

P wave: Not seen

Ventricular rhythm is irregular

QRS complex: Often looks normal, but aberrantly conducted beats are often seen when a long RR interval is followed by a short RR interval, before ventricle is fully repolarized (Ashman's phenomenon)

Risk of atrial thrombi with atrial fibrillation

If ventricular rhythm becomes regular ("regularization of atrial fibrillation"), digitalis toxicity should be suspected

Continued

TABLE 3-4
Cardiac Dysrhythmias and Conduction Defects—Cont'd

Rhythm	Mechanism	Characteristics	Comments
JUNCTIONAL RHYTHMS			
AV junctional beats	Originate in AV junction, spreading both antegrade and retrograde	If conduction to atria and ventricles is simultaneous, P wave is buried in QRS complex (not visible) and QRS usually normal	AV junction includes cells in low atrium just above AV node, in AV node itself, and in bundle of His
With origin high in AV junction		Atria depolarize first (retrograde—producing inverted P wave), then ventricles depolarize; inverted P wave precedes QRS	
With origin low in AV junction		Ventricles depolarize first, producing QRS; inverted P wave follows QRS	
Premature junctional beats and premature junctional contractions	Early beat, disrupts rhythm and sinus pacing cadence	Same characteristics as AV junctional beats, except occur prematurely	PR interval is shortened (<0.12 sec)
Junctional escape rhythm	Origin: SA node automaticity is suppressed and next fastest pacemaker (AV node) takes over	Rate: 40-60 beats/min RR interval: Extremely regular P-wave morphology: See premature junctional beats QRS complex: Normal	Common causes: MI, ischemia, electrolyte imbalances, atrial myopathy, parasympathetic stimulation, effects of digitalis, other drugs

AV junctional tachycardia	An usurping rhythm	Rates: 60-120 beats/min Rhythm: Extremely regular P-wave morphology: See premature junctional beats QRS complex: Usually normal, narrow	Often caused by digitalis toxicity
AV nodal reentrant tachycardia, previously called paroxysmal supraventricular tachycardia or paroxysmal atrial tachycardia	Reentry Where two or more electrical pathways exist, circuit can be formed with rapid circular conduction until broken	Impulse often begins abruptly with a PAC Atrial and ventricular rates: 170-250 beats/min Rhythm: Regular P wave: Retrograde and buried in QRS complex, not visible (80%); seen just after QRS (10%); occur just before QRS (10%)	May have always been present
AVRT	Macroreentry rhythm using the AV node and an accessory pathway to complete a reentrant circuit		AVRT may or may not be associated with Wolff-Parkinson-White on baseline ECG (short P-R interval with a delta wave)
Orthodromic AVRT	Orthodromic circuit goes down the AV node and up the accessory pathway	Rates: 170-250 beats/min Rhythm: Regular P wave: Short R-P interval (<½ R-R interval) QRS: Narrow	Rx orthodromic AVRT with IV adenosine, cardioversion
Antidromic AVRT	Antidromic circuit goes down the AC and up the AV node	Rates: 170-250 beats/min Rhythm: Regular P wave: Short R-P interval (<½ R-R interval) QRS: Wide	Rx antidromic AVRT with IV procainamide, DC shock

Continued

■ TABLE 3-4
■ ■ Cardiac Dysrhythmias and Conduction Defects—Cont'd

Rhythm	Mechanism	Characteristics	Comments
VENTRICULAR RHYTHMS			
PVCS	Usurping, early beat originating in ventricles Conduction is slowed through muscle Retrograde conduction to atria may occur Interpolated PVCs occur early enough to allow ventricles to repolarize before the next beat and do not disrupt rhythm; no compensatory pause is seen	Wide, bizarre QRS complexes (>0.12 sec) Can have varying morphology Compensatory pause usually occurs SA node rate is not altered, so next occurring sinus beat is able to conduct through to ventricles and produces normal QRS complex on time In MCL$_1$ lead, QRS complex of a PVC originating in left ventricle is mostly positive deflection; PVC originating from right ventricle is mostly negative	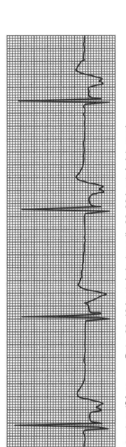A "full compensatory" pause: RR intervals surrounding the PVC are equal to two sinus-cycle intervals. To measure: 1. Mark off two normal RR intervals (three R waves) with calipers or paper 2. Place first mark on the QRS complex immediately preceding the PVC 3. Third mark should fall on QRS complex of the normal beat immediately following the PVC if fully compensated
Ventricular escape rhythm	Impulses from higher centers (SA or AV node) either are not generated or are blocked; ventricles initiate "escape" rhythm based on inherent automaticity of the ventricular tissue	Rate: 20-40 beats/min (usually 20-30 beats/min), rarely <20 beats/min Rhythm: Usually very regular QRS complex: Wide, bizarre No P-wave association with QRS complex	

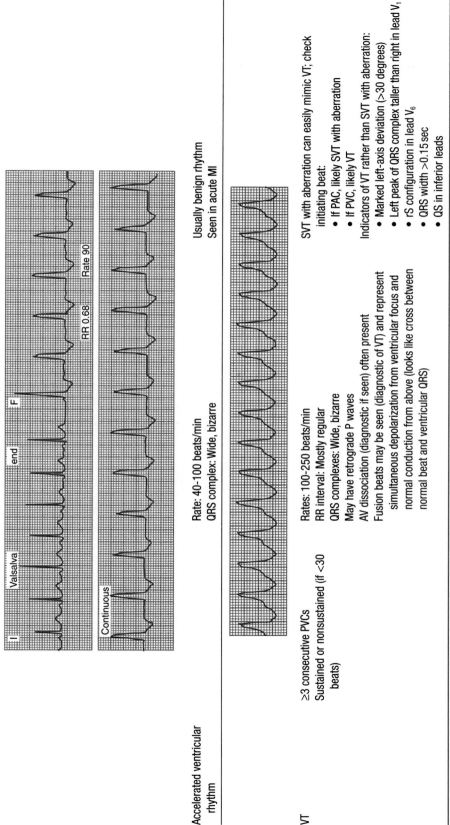

Accelerated ventricular rhythm	Rate: 40-100 beats/min QRS complex: Wide, bizarre	Usually benign rhythm Seen in acute MI
VT	Rates: 100-250 beats/min RR interval: Mostly regular QRS complexes: Wide, bizarre May have retrograde P waves AV dissociation (diagnostic if seen) often present Fusion beats may be seen (diagnostic of VT) and represent simultaneous depolarization from ventricular focus and normal conduction from above (looks like cross between normal beat and ventricular QRS)	SVT with aberration can easily mimic VT; check initiating beat: • If PAC, likely SVT with aberration • If PVC, likely VT Indicators of VT rather than SVT with aberration: • Marked left-axis deviation (>30 degrees) • Left peak of QRS complex taller than right in lead V_1 • rS configuration in lead V_6 • QRS width >0.15 sec • QS in inferior leads

≥3 consecutive PVCs
Sustained or nonsustained (if <30 beats)

Continued

TABLE 3-4
Cardiac Dysrhythmias and Conduction Defects—Cont'd

Rhythm	Mechanism	Characteristics	Comments
Torsades de pointes (twisting of points)	Form of VT (actually halfway between VT and ventricular fibrillation)	Rate: 150-250 beats/min Irregular and wide QRS complexes undulate and twist on isoelectric axis Associated with a prolonged QT interval (QTc >0.46 sec)	Usually terminates spontaneously after 5-30 sec but may continue and degenerate into ventricular fibrillation Seen with electrolyte imbalances (hypomagnesemia, hypokalemia), or in association with antiarrhythmic drug therapy and tricyclic antidepressant use
VF	Uncoordinated chaotic activity of ventricles	Erratic waveforms with no discernible PQRST complexes Coarse VF: Obvious coarse baseline Fine VF: Small or barely discernible waveforms, may be mistaken for asystole	
Ventricular asystole (standstill)	No ventricular activity	QRS complex: Not seen P wave: Seen if sinus rhythm is maintained	

AV CONDUCTION DEFECTS

| First-degree AV block | Impulse is delayed at AV junction | PR interval: >0.20 sec
Every sinus beat is conducted to the ventricles, producing normal QRS complex for every P wave | |

Second-degree AV block

Impulses are not all conducted through AV node

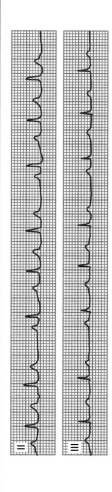

II

III

Mobitz type I or Wenckebach

Progressive delay in conduction through AV node until a QRS complex is dropped

PR interval: Gradually increases until impulse fails to conduct through AV junctional tissue; produces dropped QRS at varying or constant intervals

PR interval: Shortest after each dropped beat

PP interval: Constant if in sinus rhythm (untrue, if sinus dysrhythmia)

RR interval: Progressively shortens

P waves and QRS: Normal

Related to infarction, drug effect, or vagal effect

Continued

TABLE 3-4
Cardiac Dysrhythmias and Conduction Defects—Cont'd

Rhythm	Mechanism	Characteristics	Comments
Mobitz type II	SA node discharges regularly Produces constant PP interval one or more atrial impulses fails to conduct to ventricles (no QRS complex seen)	PR intervals: Constant with conducted beats (unlike those in type I) RR interval: Fixed Ratio of P waves to QRS may vary: 2:1, 3:1, 4:1	Second-degree AV block with 2:1 conduction may be either Mobitz I or II. • Narrow QRS suggests Wenckebach (type I) • Wider QRS (i.e., bundle branch block, LV conduction delay) suggests Mobitz type II Mobitz II is less common, but more serious

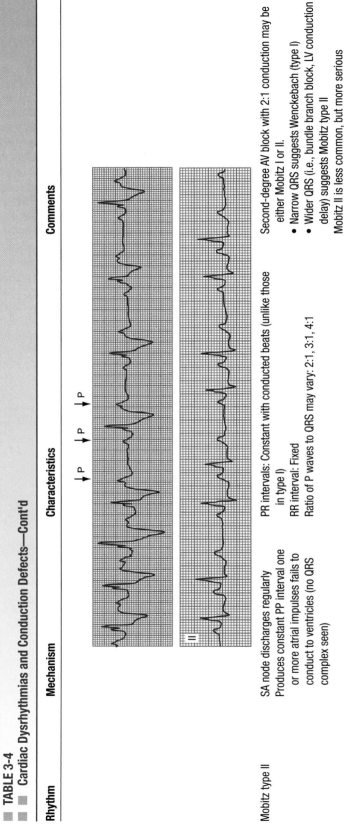

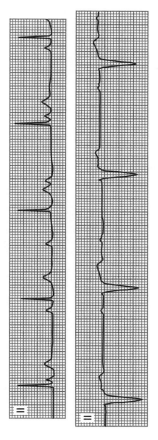

Third-degree (complete) AV block

Occurs anywhere in AV node or bundle of His: No conduction of sinus impulses

Two pacemakers become apparent

Upper: SA node fires normally

Lower: Ventricles respond to an escape pacemaker

Two independent rhythms

P waves, QRS complexes not associated

PP interval: Regular

Rate: 60-100 beats/min, if sinus rhythm

RR interval: Usually very regular, ventricular rate depends on site and inherent rate of escape pacemaker

Continued

■ **TABLE 3-4**
■ ■ **Cardiac Dysrhythmias and Conduction Defects—Cont'd**

Rhythm	Mechanism	Characteristics	Comments
ECG CHANGES WITH ELECTROLYTE IMBALANCES			
POTASSIUM IMBALANCES			
Hypokalemia		Prominent U wave T-wave amplitude decreased ST segment depressed P wave may be prominent PR interval may be prolonged Prolonged QTc interval (actually QT-U)	When U-wave height is same as T-wave height, potassium level is usually ≤3.0 mEq/L

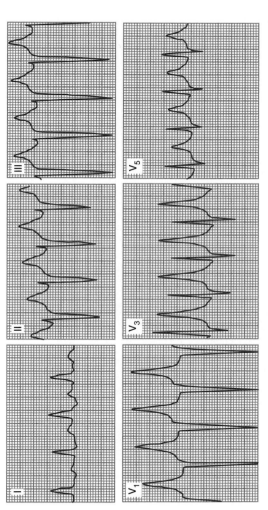

Hyperkalemia

Tall T waves
P wave may disappear

Serum levels >5.5 mEq/L: T wave symmetrically peaked, narrowed, and elevated
At ≥6.5 mEq/L: PR interval increases, P wave gets smaller or disappears

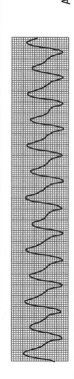

At ≥7.5 mEq/L: QRS pattern widens to sine wave

Continued

■ TABLE 3-4
■ ■ Cardiac Dysrhythmias and Conduction Defects—Cont'd

Rhythm	Mechanism	Characteristics	Comments
CALCIUM IMBALANCES			
Hypocalcemia		Prolonged QTc interval and prolonged isoelectric ST segment	
Hypercalcemia		Shortened QTc interval ST segment is shortened or absent T waves are generally unchanged	

Figures from Chou T, Knilans TK. *Electrocardiography in Clinical Practice.* 4th ed. Philadelphia, PA: Saunders; 1996.
AV, Atrioventricular; *AVRT,* atrioventricular reciprocating tachycardia; *ECG,* electrocardiogram; *MI,* myocardial infarction; *PAC,* premature atrial contraction; *PVC,* premature ventricular contraction; *SA,* sinoatrial; *SVT,* supraventricular tachycardia; *VF,* ventricular fibrillation; *VT,* ventricular tachycardia.

(2) Ischemia results in a region of hypokinesis (decreased wall motion).

(3) Evaluates extent and location of CAD and ischemic mitral regurgitation

(i) Transesophageal echocardiography (TEE): Transducer is placed in the esophagus

(1) Capable of exquisite definition of cardiac structure and function because of the proximity of the transducer to the heart

(2) Used in the operating room when the adequacy of valvular repair is to be evaluated and when more detail is needed (in cases of prosthetic valves or suspected patent foramen ovale, LA thrombus, or aortic dissection; in patients with poor acoustic penetration of the ultrasonic signal from the chest, such as patients with chronic obstructive pulmonary disease or a heavy build)

iii. Intravascular ultrasonography (IVUS): A small ultrasonic transducer attached to a catheter tip is threaded into the coronary artery over a guidewire. It provides high-resolution images of the inside of the artery. Invaluable in the catheterization laboratory for interventional procedures. Assesses the following:

(a) Size of the lumen, degree of stenosis

(b) Structure of the arterial wall

(c) Proper coronary stent placement

iv. Exercise electrocardiography (exercise stress testing)

(a) ECG is taken during exercise.

(b) Indications for exercise testing include the following:

(1) To identify suspected CAD

(2) To rule out ischemia

(3) To perform a functional assessment in patients known to have CAD (such as patients who have had an MI or angioplasty or are undergoing coronary bypass surgery) to assess risk, severity, and prognosis

(4) To evaluate the effectiveness of revascularization or medical therapy for CAD

(5) To evaluate dysrhythmias, especially exercise-induced ventricular tachycardia (VT)

(6) To evaluate patients with rate-responsive pacemakers

(7) To screen persons entering physical fitness programs or high-risk professions (e.g., airline pilots) for CAD

(c) Contraindications to exercise testing include the following:

(1) Acute MI

(2) Unstable (preinfarction) angina (at rest)

(3) Uncompensated heart failure (HF)

(4) Severe aortic stenosis

(5) Uncontrolled, severe hypertension

(6) Severe illness such as fulminant infection, asthma, renal failure

(7) Acute pericarditis or myocarditis

(d) Limitations

(1) Patient must be able to exercise to at least 85% of the maximum predicted heart rate to have a successful test.

(2) Resting ECG must have normal ST segments at baseline.

(3) Test is insensitive to single-vessel disease (will miss 40% of such cases, giving a false-negative result).

(4) False-positive results are frequent in patients at low risk for CAD, patients taking digoxin, and patients with LV hypertrophy.

v. Long-term ambulatory monitoring

(a) Types

(1) Holter monitor: ECG continuously recorded over a 24- to 48-hour period. Tape scanned and analyzed.

(2) Cardiac event monitors (e.g., King of Hearts monitor): Looping event recorder kept with the patient for up to 30 days. Patient records ECG tracings when symptoms occur, then transmits over telephone. ECG then forwarded and evaluated by the physician.

(3) Implanted loop recorders: Cardiac monitors implanted in the patient to identify suspected rhythms that have not otherwise been seen
(b) Used in documenting the following:
(1) Dysrhythmias not demonstrated by resting or exercise ECG, especially with symptoms of palpitations, syncope
(2) Efficacy of surgical and medical therapy for dysrhythmias
(3) Pacemaker function
(4) Silent ischemia (if proper recording equipment is used)
(c) Records at least two leads: I and V_5 simultaneously
(d) Diary is kept by the patient to note symptoms (chest pain, palpitations, syncope) and activities during recording to correlate with rhythm.
vi. Electrophysiologic studies (EPS): Series of programmed electrical stimuli is applied within the heart to the endothelium through electrodes in the cardiac chambers, under fluoroscopic guidance. Used to induce cardiac dysrhythmias.
(a) Purpose: To reproduce dysrhythmias in a controlled environment to assess the best mode of therapy for their control (e.g., medications, pacemaker, ablation)
(b) Patients selected include
(1) Patients with ventricular or supraventricular tachydysrhythmias
(2) Patients at high risk for sudden cardiac death
(3) Patients with unexplained recurrent syncopal episodes with suspected cardiac cause
(4) Patients who have survived a cardiac arrest without identified cause
(5) Candidates for an implantable defibrillator
(6) Candidates for ablation therapy

Patient Care

1. **Decreased CO**
   a. Description of problem: Decreased CO can be due to either mechanical or electrical cardiac dysfunction. Findings can include the following:
   i. Changes in the patient's hemodynamics: Blood pressure, heart rate, CO
   ii. ECG changes or dysrhythmias
   iii. Chest pain
   iv. Weakness, fatigue, dizziness
   v. Shortness of breath, dyspnea, crackles
   vi. Cold and clammy skin, cyanosis, pallor
   vii. Decreased peripheral pulses
   viii. Decreased or absent urinary output (oliguria, anuria)
   ix. Diminished mentation or loss of consciousness
   x. Jugular vein distention
   b. Goals of care
   i. Work of the heart is decreased by decreasing myocardial oxygen demands.
   ii. Myocardial oxygen supply is increased (minimizing ischemia, size of infarct).
   iii. Hemodynamics are normal: CO is adequate.
   iv. Heart rate is controlled, and dysrhythmias are eliminated.
   v. Patient is free of chest pain.
   vi. Patient has normal urinary output.
   c. Collaborating professionals on health care team: Nurse, physician, pharmacist, and physical therapist
   d. Interventions
   i. Monitor heart rate, rhythm, and patient responses (e.g., blood pressure, mental status, diaphoresis, pain, shortness of breath).
   ii. Assess blood pressure at regular intervals and with changes in the patient's condition. Discuss with the physician what drug is to be administered for significant changes in blood pressure.
   iii. Watch the patient's oxygenation by frequently checking pulse oximetry readings and assessing breath sounds, respirations, and circulation. Administer oxygen as needed.

iv.   Assess changes in the patient's neurologic status. Observe for central nervous system disturbances (confusion, restlessness, agitation, dizziness).

v.   Administer fluids as ordered to maintain blood pressure.

vi.   Monitor for heart failure.

vii.   Monitor intake and output (urine output should average at least 30 ml/hr), daily weights.

viii.   Check presence and quality of peripheral pulses.

ix.   Check for other signs of perfusion deficits: cool skin, sluggish capillary refilling.

x.   Have the patient notify the nurse immediately at the onset of chest discomfort and other associated symptoms of distress. Place the patient in a semi-Fowler position or position of comfort. Stress the importance of early recognition and treatment of problems.

xi.   Watch for and identify any ECG changes.

(a)   Document the rhythm strip (at least once a shift).

(b)   Obtain a 12-lead ECG if a new dysrhythmia is noted.

(c)   Determine the patient's response to dysrhythmia, verbally and through vital signs.

(d)   Administer appropriate emergency drugs if the patient's cardiac rhythm becomes significantly bradycardic or tachycardic, per unit protocols.

(e)   Have emergency equipment readily available and fully stocked.

(f)   Be knowledgeable about and prepared to use emergency equipment (defibrillator, transcutaneous pacer, transvenous pacer).

(g)   Administer CPR and call code if the patient is pulseless, in ventricular fibrillation (VF), or in asystole.

e.   Evaluation of patient care

i.   Blood pressure, heart rate, and hemodynamics are within normal limits or those set for the patient.

ii.   Sinus rhythm is normal on ECG.

iii.   Patient is alert and oriented.

iv.   Patient is comfortable and pain free.

v.   Skin is warm and dry.

vi.   Urinary output is adequate.

2. **Acute chest pain**

a. Description of problem: Acute pain due to ischemia. Findings can include the following:

i.   Patient communication of discomfort: Description of quality (on a scale of 1 to 10, with 10 being the worst), intensity, location, radiation, timing, and aggravating and alleviating factors (movement, deep inspiration, positioning)

ii.   Anxiety

iii.   Diaphoresis

iv.   Changes in blood pressure, heart rate, respiratory rate

v.   Nausea, vomiting

vi.   ECG changes (ST segment, T waves) or dysrhythmias

b. Goals of care

i.   Pain or discomfort is relieved completely.

ii.   Vital signs are stable and within normal limits.

c. Collaborating professionals on health care team: Nurse, physician, physician assistant, advanced registered nurse practitioner, pharmacist, occupational and physical therapists, dietitian, social worker, home health aide

d. Interventions

i.   Have the patient notify the nurse immediately at the onset of chest discomfort and other associated symptoms of distress. Stress the importance of early recognition and treatment of chest discomfort.

ii.   Administer oxygen per unit protocol.

iii.   Check vital signs, monitor ECG.

iv.   Do a 12-lead ECG immediately.

v.   Ensure that the patient has a patent IV line.

vi.   Administer and titrate medications to alleviate angina.

      vii. Notify the physician.

     viii. Collaborate with the physician on medication needs (types, dosages, frequency, route) and titrations and adjustments of medications, depending on the patient response.

      ix. Monitor the patient's pain.

        (a) Assess quality, duration, intensity, frequency of the pain.

        (b) Assess the effectiveness of medications.

        (c) Look for trends and drug interactions, and identify other possible comfort measures.

      x. Provide other comfort interventions as appropriate (e.g., back rub, repositioning, special mattresses).

      xi. Alert the physician if pain continues so that further actions can be determined. Cardiac pain means the myocardium is in jeopardy, and immediate interventions are needed.

  e. Evaluation of patient care

      i. Patient is pain free and comfortable (with or without analgesia).

     ii. Vital signs are stable.

    iii. Patient reports pain or discomfort, when it occurs, immediately and clearly to the nurse.

3. Activity intolerance

  a. Description of problem: Because of cardiac dysfunction, the patient may exhibit the following clinical findings, reflecting a decreased tolerance for the activities of daily living:

      i. Fatigue, weakness

     ii. Dyspnea with progressively less exertion

    iii. Leg cramps

    iv. Discomfort in chest, neck, jaw, shoulder, arm

     v. Increased heart rate and/or blood pressure

    vi. Dysrhythmias

    vii. ST-segment and T-wave changes signifying ischemia

  b. Goals of care

      i. Cause is identified and treated.

     ii. Patient engages in progressive ambulation.

    iii. No complications of bed rest are present (skin intact, breath sounds clear, no signs of deep venous thromboembolism).

    iv. Patient is educated regarding the need for routine exercise and weight control (as needed).

  c. Collaborating professionals on health care team: Physical and occupational therapists; cardiac rehabilitation nurse for activity plans in hospital and after discharge; social worker to assist with home equipment acquisition, home visits, nursing home placement (temporary or permanent); dietitian

  d. Interventions

      i. Assess and document the patient's response to progressive ambulation, including monitoring of heart rate and rhythm, respiration, and blood pressure.

     ii. Assist the patient with initial increases in ambulation.

    iii. Administer pain medication, as needed, before planned ambulation (if the patient is pain free, progression in ambulation will be more successful).

    iv. Plan rest periods between various treatments, visits, and ambulation.

     v. Teach the patient how to progress safely: Instruct in correct positioning and efficient use of body for each step.

        (a) Active range-of-motion exercises

        (b) Dangling

        (c) Transfers from bed to chair or bedside commode

        (d) Ambulation in room and hallway

    vi. Ensure that the patient is instructed with regard to the availability and use of special equipment to assist in ambulation (walkers, canes, wheelchairs), if needed.

    vii. If the patient's condition becomes unstable (ischemic pain, vital signs beyond set limits, dysrhythmias), help the patient back to bed and immediately evaluate the need for oxygen, medications (e.g., nitrates, antiarrhythmics), ECG, notification of the physician, emergency equipment.

viii. Arrange consultations with other health professionals, as appropriate.

ix. Encourage the patient and family to openly ventilate feelings and ask questions regarding the ability to ambulate and lifestyle resumption and changes.

e. Evaluation of patient care

   i. Patient has verbalized and demonstrated an understanding of activity capacity and limitations.

   ii. Exercise program is incorporated into the patient's lifestyle. Weight control goals are met, if appropriate.

   iii. Activity plan includes a support system and community services, as needed, to achieve the desired lifestyle.

4. Inadequate knowledge of cardiac diagnosis, medications, or treatment

  a. Description of problem

   i. Patient and/or family verbalizations indicate a lack of knowledge or inappropriate or incorrect information.

   ii. Patient may have been noncompliant with the recommended regimen, which resulted in incorrect or inappropriate care at home.

   iii. Patient is easily agitated, hostile, worried, suspicious (because of misinformation, misunderstanding, or misinterpretation).

   iv. Patient and/or family is unable to plan realistic goals or home care.

  b. Goals of care

   i. Patient (and family) verbalizes an understanding of the diagnosis, medications, treatment, and follow-up care.

   ii. Patient demonstrates proper home care techniques.

  c. Collaborating professionals on health care team: See Acute Chest Pain

  d. Interventions

   i. Identify learning needs.

   ii. Assess readiness to learn (the patient is alert, pain free, not sleep deprived; information is not given immediately after sedatives are administered).

   iii. Determine the best methods for the patient to learn (group, one to one, videos).

   iv. Reinforce learning with the use of printed materials related to the disease, discharge instructions, procedures, and medications.

   v. Instruction sheets should be available in languages other than English.

   vi. Arrange for an interpreter if the patient does not understand English (staff, family member, interpretation services). Caution is used if instructions are given to a family member.

   vii. Document teaching and the patient's response.

   viii. Arrange appropriate consults: cardiac rehabilitation; dietary, occupational, and physical therapy; home health; social work.

   ix. Schedule practice and return demonstrations of psychomotor skills.

  e. Evaluation of patient care

   i. Patient or significant other verbalizes an understanding of the medical condition, medications, necessary home care, follow-up, and diet and any other lifestyle changes.

   ii. Patient or significant other knows where to seek assistance for information and help.

   iii. Patient or significant other demonstrates proper techniques for various applicable home self-care procedures (low–molecular-weight heparin injections, pulse monitoring, wound care, IV therapy).

SPECIFIC PATIENT HEALTH PROBLEMS

Coronary Artery Disease

CAD is a progressive disorder in which the coronary arteries become occluded as a result of atherosclerosis.

1. Pathophysiology

  a. Injury (due to LDL cholesterol, toxins, infections, or mechanical causes) occurs to the endothelial cells in the intima of the coronary arteries, altering cell structure.

   b. Platelets adhere and aggregate at the site of injury, and macrophages migrate to the area as a result of injury. Smooth muscle cells and macrophage foam cells enter the intimal layer. These accumulations promote the development over time of a fatty fibrous plaque, or "fatty streak." Migration of LDL into the subintimal space results in "lipid core."
   c. This plaque is a pearly white accumulation in the intimal lining, consisting mostly of smooth muscle cells but also collagen-producing fibroblasts and macrophages. These deposits protrude into the lumen, obstructing blood flow.
   d. Progressive narrowing of the vessel occurs.
   e. This process tends to occur at vessel bifurcations and at the proximal end of the artery.
   f. The fatty fibrous plaque can rupture and form either a mural thrombus or an occlusive thrombus.
      i. A mural thrombus can partially or totally obstruct the artery. The disrupted plaque and mural thrombus can develop into a more fibrotic, stenotic lesion, which changes the plaque's geometry.
      ii. An acute, labile, occlusive thrombus can totally obstruct the artery and create clinical complications (MI, unstable angina, sudden cardiac death).
      iii. The ruptured plaque, caused by endothelial injury and exposure to blood flow, activates platelet and fibrin formation, enhancing thrombus formation.
   g. Coronary blood flow may be further diminished by vasoconstriction (resulting from the release of vasoactive agents [thromboxane A_2, angiotensin II], impaired vasodilatation, and platelet activation).
   h. Atherosclerotic process causes
      i. Decreases in blood flow and oxygen supply to the myocardium
      ii. An imbalance between myocardial oxygen supply and demand, which results in myocardial ischemia
2. **Etiology and risk factors**
   a. Heredity: Familial component for premature heart disease; MI or sudden cardiac death in father, mother, or siblings
   b. Age: CAD is more prevalent among middle-aged and older persons (men older than 45 years; women older than 55 years)
   c. Gender: CAD is more prevalent among men
      i. Before age 55 years, prevalence is three to four times higher among men than among women (before menopause).
      ii. After age 55 years, prevalence rates slowly equalize for both sexes; at age 75 years, rates are close to equal.
   d. Smoking
      i. Enhances atherogenic progression; decreases HDL cholesterol level; influences thrombus formation, plaque instability, dysrhythmias
      ii. Dose and duration dependent: Risk of death from CAD is two to six times higher among smokers than among nonsmokers
   e. Hyperlipidemia: High levels of triglycerides, LDL, and very-low-density lipoproteins are associated with an increased risk of CAD
      i. Triglycerides: Higher than 200 mg/dl
      ii. LDL: Higher than 130 mg/dl
      iii. HDL: Lower than 40 mg/dl (HDL level higher than 60 mg/dl is a negative risk factor)
   f. Hypertension
      i. Contributes to direct vascular injury, along with the effects of increased wall stress and oxygen demands
      ii. Approximately 30% of American adults have hypertension (the rate is up to three times higher in African Americans than in the general population). Women have a higher incidence of hypertensive heart disease.
      iii. Defined as systolic blood pressure higher than 140 and/or diastolic pressure higher than 90 mm Hg (Chobanian, Bakris, Black, et al, 2003)
   g. LV hypertrophy: Heart's response to chronic pressure overloads; associated with increased risk for cardiovascular events

   h. Thrombogenic risk factors: Deficiencies in serum coagulation inhibitors (antithrombin III, protein C, and protein S), elevated plasma fibrinogen level, enhanced platelet aggregation
   i. Diabetes mellitus: In patients with diabetes mellitus CAD is twice as likely to develop as in persons without diabetes
   j. Obesity: Positively associated with an increased rate of CAD; also contributes to the development of hypertension and diabetes
    i. Fat distribution plays a role (abdominal or central obesity carries a higher risk).
    ii. Metabolic syndrome: Recognized syndrome (also referred to as insulin resistance syndrome) associated with higher risk and identified by the presence of three or more of the following:
        (a) Abdominal obesity: Waist circumference greater than 40 inches in men and greater than 35 inches in women
        (b) Triglyceride level higher than 150 mg/dl
        (c) HDL level lower than 40 mg/dl in men and 50 mg/dl in women
        (d) Blood pressure higher than 130/85 mm Hg
        (e) Glucose level (fasting) higher than 110 mg/dl
   k. Sedentary lifestyle; studies show a positive relationship between inactivity and CAD, mainly resulting from its aggravation of other risk factors
3. Signs and symptoms
   a. History
    i. Assessment of the aforementioned risk factors
    ii. Possible sequelae of CAD include the following:
        (a) Angina pectoris
        (b) MI
        (c) Ventricular aneurysm or rupture
        (d) Heart failure, cardiogenic shock
        (e) Dysrhythmias, sudden cardiac death
        (f) Cardiomyopathy
        (g) Mitral insufficiency
   b. Physical examination (see Patient Assessment section): CAD may be asymptomatic and may be diagnosed because of abnormal findings on tests (stress testing, echocardiography)
4. Diagnostic study findings
   a. Laboratory
    i. Fasting lipid profile: Total cholesterol, HDL, LDL, triglyceride levels
    ii. Fasting serum glucose levels
   b. Exercise ECG stress testing: Used to rule out ischemia, to evaluate chest pain symptoms, to stratify the risk of known CAD, to detect dysrhythmias, and to assess the efficacy of treatment
   c. Myocardial perfusion imaging (with exercise or pharmacologic stress): Used to detect inadequate myocardial perfusion (ischemia) or the absence of perfusion (infarction) by assessing the degree of uptake in the myocardium of a radioactive tracer
   d. Echocardiography
    i. Exercise stress echocardiography: Ultrasound images taken during or after treadmill or bicycle exercise
    ii. Pharmacologic stress echocardiography: Dobutamine or adenosine is used to increase myocardial oxygen requirements (similar to exercise demands)
   e. Cardiac catheterization and coronary angiography: Used to define cardiac function and coronary anatomy to guide therapy
   f. IVUS: Catheter-tipped two-dimensional ultrasonic probe is used to define intracoronary anatomy
5. Goals of care
   a. Modifiable risk factors are under control and/or improved.
   b. Risk factor modification is incorporated into the patient's lifestyle.
   c. Goals of the treatment program are met.
6. Collaborating professionals on health care team: Physician, nurse, dietitian, pharmacist, community service worker (i.e., smoking cessation programs)

7. Management of patient care
  a. Anticipated patient trajectory: Primary prevention is the key to decreasing the morbidity and mortality of CAD
   i. Nutrition
      (a) Nutritional status, dietary habits should be assessed.
      (b) Education should be provided on the rationale for compliance with a cholesterol-controlled diet if lipid levels are above the goals.
      (c) Information should be provided to the patient and family on low-fat, low-cholesterol foods. Referrals should be given to hospital and community resources for follow-up and reinforcement.
      (d) Diet should include the use of monounsaturated and polyunsaturated fats (olive, sunflower, and corn oils; soft oleomargarine) and avoidance of trans-fatty acids, which should be less than 7% of total calories. Other dietary additions can include fish and omega-3 fatty acids, fiber, and flaxseed.
      (e) Goals for weight should be discussed. Weight and height should be measured. Body mass index (BMI) should be determined.

$$BMI = \frac{\text{Weight in pounds}}{(\text{Height in inches})^2} \times 703$$

         (1) Desirable waist circumference: Less than 41 inches in males and less than 36 inches in females
         (2) BMI: Desired = 18 to 24.9 (25 to 30 indicates overweight; more than 30 indicates obesity)
   ii. Pharmacology
      (a) Antiplatelet agents (such as aspirin [acetylsalicylic acid], 81 mg/day) should be included in the patient's health regimen, if not contraindicated.
      (b) Lipid-lowering agents will often be necessary; the patient should be aware of their uses and side effects, and follow-up requirements.
      (c) Antihypertensive agents may be necessary (diuretics, ACE inhibitors, β-blockers).
   iii. Psychosocial issues
      (a) An adequate support system to assist in changing to heart-healthy behaviors and lifestyle is important.
      (b) Complementary and alternative medical methods to assist with stress reduction include massage therapy, yoga, regular exercise, postural therapy, and acupuncture.
   iv. Treatments
      (a) Provide the patient with information regarding the risk factors for CAD.
      (b) Encourage the patient and significant others to quit smoking; provide information and help regarding risks, methods for stopping, and nicotine replacement.
      (c) Provide information on lipid-lowering diets that have 30% or less fat, with less than 7% saturated fat.
      (d) Goals for lipid management include the following:
         (1) LDL level of less than 130 mg/dl (less than 100 mg/dl if CAD is present)
         (2) HDL level of more than 40 mg/dl
         (3) Triglyceride level of less than 200 mg/dl
      (e) If the patient is hypertensive
         (1) Blood pressure goal is 140/90 mm Hg or lower
         (2) Modifications include weight control, routine exercise, moderate alcohol consumption, and sodium restriction
      (f) Weight control should be discussed with the patient and a plan for weight loss developed (especially for patients who are more than 120% of their ideal weight for height). Hypertensive patients and/or patients with elevated glucose or triglyceride levels should receive information on achieving ideal body weight.
      (g) Encourage exercise and physical activity (after risks are assessed, often after exercise testing in patients over 40 years of age).
         (1) Goal is 30 minutes, three to four times weekly (minimum); preferably 30 to 60 minutes of moderate exercise, including walking, cycling, jogging, swimming.

(2) Other opportunities for increased physical activity should be explored.
    (h) Increased emphasis is being placed on education regarding women and cardio-vascular disease and on more aggressive medical management for women along with the inclusion of more female patients in clinical trials.
  b. Potential complications: See the following sections for each of the possible sequelae of CAD
8. Evaluation of patient care
  a. Patient verbalizes an understanding of how to manage or modify the risk factors contributing to CAD progression.
  b. Patient and family have educational resources (i.e., smoking cessation program, medication information sheets, follow-up plan) to assist in implementing new health practices.

Chronic Stable Angina Pectoris

1. Pathophysiology
  a. Myocardial oxygen demand outstrips oxygen supply.
  b. Progressive coronary atherosclerosis increasingly limits coronary blood flow and myocardial perfusion.
2. Etiology and risk factors
  a. Precipitating factors
    i. Increased myocardial oxygen demand owing to
      (a) Increased heart rate resulting from exertion, tachydysrhythmia, anemia, fever, anxiety, pain, thyrotoxicosis, drugs, digestion, hyperadrenergic states
      (b) Increased contractility resulting from exercise, tachycardia, anxiety, drugs, hyperadrenergic states
      (c) Increased afterload resulting from hypertension, aortic stenosis, drugs (pressors)
      (d) Increased preload resulting from volume overload, drugs
    ii. Decreased oxygen supply due to
      (a) CAD (fixed narrowing of coronary arteries)
      (b) Coronary artery spasm (cocaine abuse, cold air, drugs [ergots])
      (c) Circulatory diversion (digestion, coronary artery steal)
      (d) Anemia
      (e) Hypoxemia
      (f) Hypovolemia
      (g) Shock
      (h) Heart failure
  b. Risk factors: The common risk factors of CAD
3. Signs and symptoms
  a. Subjective findings: Anginal discomfort is any exertional, rest-relieved symptom and may be described as burning, squeezing, aching, heaviness, pressure sensation, smothering, indigestion-like, or a "band across the chest." It may occur anywhere between the ears and the umbilicus.
    i. Etiologic or precipitating factors: Elicit pertinent information from the patient
    ii. Characterize the patient's symptoms.
      (a) Duration of discomfort: Chest pain from acute coronary syndromes generally lasts more than 20 minutes
      (b) Location and radiation of discomfort: Can include the chest, neck, jaws, arms, back, epigastrium
      (c) Discomfort level: Patient is asked to quantify the discomfort by using a scale from 1 (the least) to 10 (the worst pain ever experienced by the patient)
      (d) Associated symptoms: May include nausea, diaphoresis, palpitations, shortness of breath, syncope, and presyncope
      (e) Effect of exertion and rest: The timing of the discomfort is crucial. Was it with activity, in bed at rest, postprandial? With what kind of activity? How often does it recur? What starts it? What relieves it?
      (f) Effect of nitrates (if the patient has CAD, nitrates should decrease or abolish the discomfort in 1 to 2 minutes, not 15 to 20 minutes)

    b. Objective findings

        i.   Determine the type or form of discomfort.

            (a) Unstable angina: New-onset angina or angina that has changed in frequency, severity, or duration or occurs with less exertion or at rest. Duration of pain is usually more than 20 minutes (see Acute Coronary Syndromes).

            (b) Chronic, stable angina: Angina that has not increased in frequency or severity over time. Caused primarily by obstructive, fixed atheromatous coronary lesions.

            (c) Prinzmetal's (variant) angina: Resting angina caused by coronary artery spasm, associated with transient ST-segment elevation

        ii.   Other important aspects of the history include the following:

            (a) Presence of risk factors for CAD

            (b) Cardiac review of systems

            (c) Medication history (including use of illicit drugs)

            (d) History of tests, interventions; coronary artery bypass graft (CABG), PTCA

            (e) Allergies to shellfish, iodine (contrast dye)

            (f) If the patient underwent intervention (PCI, CABG), try to elicit the patient's anginal history before the intervention.

4. Diagnostic study findings

    a. Laboratory: Levels of troponins or CK-MB isoenzymes are not elevated with stable angina

    b. ECG: May be normal or show nonspecific ST or T-wave changes or evidence of prior infarction

    c. Echocardiography: May or may not show transient abnormal wall motion, valve dysfunction, hypertrophy

    d. Treadmill stress testing: Results may or may not be positive for CAD. Very sensitive for left main artery or three-vessel disease but can miss up to 40% of single-vessel disease. Used in low-risk patients who are pain free for 12 to 24 hours and without symptoms of heart failure.

    e. Dobutamine or exercise stress echocardiography: Can demonstrate ischemia (stress-induced wall motion abnormalities), ventricular dysfunction, and ischemic mitral regurgitation

    f. Myocardial scintigraphy (thallium, Tc 99m sestamibi) with exercise or pharmacologic stress (adenosine, dipyridamole): May demonstrate ischemia, infarction, and LV dysfunction

    g. Coronary catheterization: Used to assess the extent and severity of CAD, as well as to assess valvular and ventricular function. It facilitates risk assessment and guides therapy (medical or interventional).

5. Goals of care

    a. Ischemia, MI, and death are prevented by

        i.   Decreasing myocardial oxygen demand (β-blockers, calcium channel blockers, nitrates)

        ii.   Improving myocardial oxygen supply (nitrates)

    b. Disease process is modified.

        i.   Antiplatelet and antithrombin therapy

        ii.   Lifestyle modifications (i.e., smoking cessation, diet, blood pressure control, diabetes control)

6. Collaborating professionals on health care team: Physician (cardiologist, cardiac surgeon), nurse, physical and occupational therapists, social worker, cardiac rehabilitation team, dietitian, pharmacist

7. Management of patient care

    a. Anticipated patient trajectory: Prognosis varies widely depending on LV function, the severity of CAD and associated risk factors. Prompt diagnosis and treatment enable elimination of symptoms and improved longevity.

        i.   Discharge planning

            (a) Risk factor modification teaching

               (1) Smoking cessation to reduce recurrence of cardiac events

               (2) Weight control

               (3) Exercise: Daily routine important

(4) Blood pressure: Less than 130/85 mm Hg
(5) Diabetes: Tight glucose control
(6) Lipid control: If LDL level is higher than 100 mg/dl; discuss lipid target levels, diet, medications

(b) For PCI: Teach discharge activities, symptoms to report (e.g., masses, bleeding, increased localized pain and bruising at the site of insertion, tingling or numbness, extremity weakness, shortness of breath, chest discomfort), medications, diet, risk factors, and actions to take:
(1) Call physician and apply pressure for bleeding or swelling at catheter site.
(2) Limit activities for 2 days. Do not lift more than 10 lb.
(3) Do not drive for 1 day.
(4) Recognize the importance of following the medication plan (e.g., antiplatelet therapy).
(5) Follow discharge follow-up schedule.

(c) Give the patient a stent information packet and an identification stent card and ensure that questions regarding care are answered.
(d) Provide clear instructions regarding all medications (types, rationales, dosages, side effects) to the patient and significant others.

ii. Pharmacology
(a) Nitroglycerin (NTG): To relieve angina
(b) Aspirin: 81 mg daily (clopidogrel given if unable to take aspirin)
(c) β-Blockers: Given unless contraindications exist
(d) Calcium antagonists and/or long-acting nitrates: If β-blockers are unsuccessful or contraindicated
(e) ACE inhibitors: For patients with diabetes, LV systolic dysfunction
(f) Lipid-lowering agents: Statins

iii. Psychosocial issues: Aggressive risk factor modification and lifestyle changes are necessary. Barriers and challenges to these goals need to be identified. Reduction of emotional stressors may improve long-term prognosis.

iv. Treatments
(a) PCIs: Used to increase the luminal diameter of coronary arteries that have been stenosed by CAD and to increase coronary blood flow with use of PTCA, coronary stent placement, and atherectomy (Figures 3-12 and 3-13)

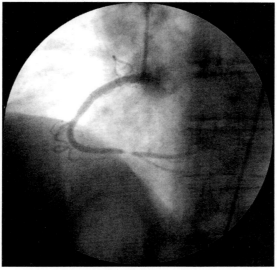

FIGURE 3-12 ■ Stenosis of the right coronary artery before percutaneous coronary intervention. (Courtesy Dr. Steve Ramee, Ochsner Clinic Foundation.)

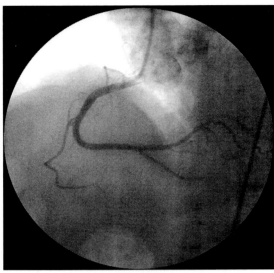

FIGURE 3-13 ■ Right coronary artery revascularization after percutaneous coronary intervention with a coronary stent procedure. (Courtesy Dr. Steve Ramee, Ochsner Clinic Foundation.)

(1) PTCA
   a) Balloon catheter is placed across stenosis and inflated.
   b) Enlarges lumen diameter by mechanically compressing and splitting plaque
(2) Coronary stent placement
   a) Devices are placed intraluminally to achieve maximal lumen size and maintain the patency of the vessel's lumen. Majority of PCI procedures now include some form of stenting with PTCA.
      1) Stents are made from various metals; some stents are "bare metal," and others are drug eluding.
      2) Drug-eluding stents: Made of synthetic materials with the ability to deliver drugs to almost eliminate the restenosis of stents
   b) Indications
      1) Primary stenting to restore the normal luminal diameter
      2) Restenosis: After PCI
      3) Intimal tears: After PCI
(3) Coronary atherectomy: Removal of atheromatous material from the artery (debulking). Procedure is now used less because of improved stenting procedures.
   a) Directional coronary atherectomy: Plaque is cut by a catheter with a rotating cutter and trapped in its chamber for removal
   b) Transluminal extraction atherectomy: Slower rotating cutter is used with vacuum suction to withdraw atheromatous debris
   c) Rotational atherectomy: High-speed, rotating burr grinds atheromatous material into microdebris in the bloodstream
(4) Brachytherapy: Intracoronary radiation procedure to treat and prevent in-stent restenosis
(5) Key points for nursing care after PCI procedure: See Box 3-5
(b) CABG: Surgical revascularization of the myocardium with bypass grafting
   (1) Saphenous vein graft: Reversed saphenous vein from leg used to create a conduit. One end of the graft is sewn onto the aorta and the other end is sewn onto the affected coronary artery distal to the obstruction

■ **BOX 3-5**
■ **KEY POINTS IN NURSING CARE AFTER PERCUTANEOUS CORONARY INTERVENTION PROCEDURES**

GENERAL NURSING CARE
1. Observe for complications.
2. Maintain the patient on bed rest for 2 to 6 hours with progressive elevation of head of bed (initially, less than 30 degrees). Time of restrictions depends on method of postprocedure closure: Manual pressure, mechanical closure (e.g., FemoStop), collagen closure plugs (e.g., Angio-Seal), percutaneous suture devices (e.g., Perclose).
3. Affected limb should be kept straight, immobile; soft leg restraint may be used.
4. Patient may be positioned in reverse Trendelenburg's position to facilitate eating and comfort, and repositioned on side by log rolling, if procedure site is not bleeding.
5. Take electrocardiogram on return from procedure and if chest discomfort is present.
6. Ensure that blood work is done for serial measurement of cardiac markers.
7. Monitor vital signs closely.
8. Monitor pulses, warmth, sensation of affected limb; assess for bleeding and hematoma at femoral site.
9. If there is bleeding or hematoma, hold direct pressure until bleeding has stopped.
10. Mark hematoma and closely watch for signs of increased size. Inflatable femoral compression systems may be applied to maintain hemostasis.
11. Finger foods are easier for patient while head-of-bed elevation is restricted.
12. Assess need for medication for back and groin discomfort.
13. Maintain intravenous (IV) fluids as ordered and encourage drinking of fluids (to facilitate excretion of catheterization dye by kidneys).
14. Ensure adequate output. Foley catheter may be necessary for patients who cannot void (within 2 to 4 hours), for patients who are unable to void in bed at required position, or for patients who are at high risk for bleeding.
15. Patient may be on heparin drip after percutaneous coronary intervention: Monitor partial thromboplastin time for adequate anticoagulation (ordered parameters). Perform other monitoring to detect bleeding problems (check urine, vomit, stools; watch for nosebleeds; monitor neurologic status). Heparin should be stopped 1 to 4 hours before sheath removal.
16. Check activated coagulation time if sheath is to come out (if <150 seconds, sheath may be removed if patient is stable and without ischemic pain).
17. Various closure devices are used, each with its own postcatheter protocol.

POSTPROCEDURE NURSING CARE DURING SHEATH REMOVAL
1. Thoroughly explain removal process to patient.
2. Medicate patient before removal to diminish discomfort. Medications include morphine or other fast-acting analgesics along with local anesthesia to site.
3. Have normal saline bolus and atropine (0.5 mg IV) readily available at bedside for vasovagal reactions (hypotension, bradycardia, diaphoresis, nausea).
4. Gather all other equipment for removal: suture removal kit; syringes; gloves, goggles, and gown; dressings; Doppler device, compression devices, if used.
5. Aspirating 5 to 10 ml of blood from each sheath (both venous and arterial lines) ensures that there are no clots on the tip of the sheath to embolize on withdrawal and that any heparin is removed from the patient's system.
6. Locate arterial pulse. Apply manual, direct pressure just above puncture site (and over arterial pulse) for a minimum of 20 minutes after sheath removal until hemostasis is complete. Pulling the arterial sheath first and then the venous sheath after hemostasis avoids potential risk of arteriovenous fistula.
7. If using a compression device, follow protocols for safe use during and after sheath removal.

POSTPROCEDURE NURSING CARE AFTER SHEATH REMOVAL
1. After sheath removal check vital signs every 15 minutes four times, every 30 minutes four times, and then every hour.
2. Continue to monitor and document pulses and assess for bleeding or hematoma; promptly treat with direct pressure until hemostasis is complete. Notify physician if bleeding recurs.
3. Maintain bed rest for 2 to 6 hours after sheath removal per protocol for closure method and procedure site (i.e., radial, femoral). Elevate head of bed progressively (initially less than 30 degrees), with affected limb immobilized.

Continued

4. Continue to medicate for discomfort from bed rest.
5. Auscultate for systolic bruit at site of sheath insertion at least every 8 hours: Positive bruit along with localized pain and pulsatile mass suggests possible pseudoaneurysm; notify physician immediately. Surgery or ultrasonographically guided compression is necessary for closure. Patients at high risk for pseudoaneurysm include the following:
   - Obese patients (difficult to apply direct pressure)
   - Patients in whom sheath size larger than No. 8 French was used (larger injury to artery)
   - Patients receiving postprocedure anticoagulants (hemostasis problem)
   - Elderly patients (artery wall changes with age)
   - Females (fat distribution, smaller arteries, potential for multiple punctures during catheterization procedure)

(2) Internal mammary artery bypass
    a) Proximal artery remains attached to the subclavian artery from which it arises, and the distal end is dissected from the anterior chest wall and sewn onto the coronary artery distal to the obstruction.
    b) Long-term patency rate is better (more than 90% at 10 years) than with saphenous vein graft (40%).
    c) Avoids need for leg incisions if only one or two vessels require bypass
(3) Complications during surgery
    a) MI: 2% to 7%
    b) Intraoperative stroke: 1% to 2%
    c) Death: 1% to 2%
(4) Immediately postoperative complications
    a) Low CO, hypotension: Due to inadequate volume replacement, fluid shifts (third spacing), hemorrhage. Can decrease systemic perfusion, affecting the kidneys, brain, and heart.
    b) Hemorrhage
    c) Hypertension (increased afterload decreases CO)
    d) Cardiac tamponade: Suspect if decreased CO and hypotension are present with increased central venous pressure (CVP) (unless hypovolemic), narrowed pulse pressure, distended jugular veins, pulsus paradoxus, distant heart sounds
    e) Dysrhythmias: Caused by electrolyte imbalances, hypoxemia, drug toxicity, hypothermia, anesthesia, pulmonary artery catheters. Atrial fibrillation is common (approximately 25% of patients).
    f) Respiratory failure: Associated with hypoxemia, alveolar hypoventilation
    g) Prerenal azotemia: Caused by decreased CO, hypovolemia
    h) Electrolyte imbalances: Hypokalemia, hypocalcemia, hypomagnesemia (common)
    i) Graft closure: The risk of graft closure can be reduced by antiplatelet aggregation therapy with risk factor modification
(5) Agents commonly used after CABG
    a) Volume support (albumin, hetastarch, and/or whole and packed red blood cells): To increase the preload, elevate CVP, increase systolic blood pressure if it falls below predetermined parameters, and increase the HCT
    b) Drugs for acute management: See Heart Failure
    c) Antiarrhythmic agents often administered prophylactically to decrease the incidence of atrial fibrillation
  (c) Ventricular assist device (VAD): See Heart Failure

   b. Potential complications of PCIs
      i. Recurrent pain: Restenosis
         (a) Mechanism of restenosis: Results from intimal hyperplasia during healing. Factors associated with increased risk of restenosis include multivessel CAD, proximal LAD stenosis, diabetes, final lumen diameter of less than 100%.
         (b) Management: Follow interventions for acute chest pain (see earlier Acute Chest Pain under Patient Care). PCI or CABG may be indicated.
      ii. Iodine contrast reaction
         (a) Mechanism: Allergic reaction (itching, rash, laryngospasm, swelling, or anaphylaxis)
         (b) Management: Treat with diphenhydramine (Benadryl) 25 to 50 mg orally, epinephrine 0.5 to 1 ml (1:1000 IV), IV steroids
      iii. Acute coronary occlusion
         (a) Mechanism: Results from dissection
         (b) Management: Emergency CABG in fewer than 0.5% of cases
      iv. MI: See ST-Segment Elevation Myocardial Infarction
  8. Evaluation of patient care
    a. Patient is free from cardiac pain.
    b. Patient has no complications associated with the various angina therapies received.
    c. Patient and significant others have received education and written handouts and demonstrate understanding regarding the disease process, the rationale for therapy (medications, procedures), symptoms to report, applicable risk factors to modify and a plan for accomplishment, and follow-up care.

Acute Coronary Syndromes: Unstable Angina Pectoris and Non–ST-Segment Elevation Myocardial Infarction

Unstable angina and non–ST-segment elevation myocardial infarction (NSTEMI) have similar pathophysiology, presentations, and therapy. Unstable angina is not, however, associated with elevations in the levels of cardiac biomarkers (troponins).

  1. Pathophysiology: Whereas chronic stable angina (ischemia) results when myocardial oxygen demand outstrips supply, acute coronary syndromes result from abrupt, nonexertional plaque rupture, thrombosis, vasoconstriction, or arterial occlusion, often with subsequent reperfusion
    a. Coronary occlusion
      i. Plaque rupture
      ii. Platelet-mediated thrombosis
      iii. Vasoconstriction
      iv. Arterial occlusion (subtotal or total)
    b. Coronary spasm (Prinzmetal's angina) can temporarily occlude coronary artery flow.
    c. Restenosis after PCI can create an obstruction to blood flow without spasm or thrombus.
    d. Severity and number of obstructions, availability of collateral circulation, and amount of thrombus all factor into the clinical presentation.
  2. Etiology and risk factors
    a. Precipitating factor: Atherosclerotic plaque
    b. Risk factors: The common risk factors of CAD
    c. Identifiers of patients at high risk
      i. Prolonged pain (particularly at rest)
      ii. Dysrhythmias: Bradycardias, tachycardias
      iii. Hypotension
      iv. Transient ST changes during pain
      v. New mitral regurgitation murmur, S_3, crackles
      vi. New bundle branch block (BBB)
  3. Signs and symptoms
    a. Subjective and objective findings: Same as for chronic stable angina, except for the following:

      i.   Symptoms occur at rest.

      ii. Symptoms usually last longer than 20 minutes.

   b. Physical findings

      i.   Fear

      ii. Minimal movement

      iii. Possible clutching of chest

      iv. Tachycardia (increased sympathetic tone)

      v. Transient mitral regurgitation—new murmur

      vi. Transient rales—new symptom

      vii. Transient S_3, S_4

      viii. Hypotension

4. Diagnostic study findings

   a. Laboratory

      i.   Levels of troponins or CK-MB isoenzymes are not elevated in unstable angina. Levels of troponins (cardiac troponin T and troponin I) are more than 0.1 ng/ml for troponin T and more than 0.4 ng/ml for troponin I in NSTEMI.

         (a) Elevations noticeable 4 to 12 hours after onset of symptoms

         (b) Follow-up sampling needed at 8 to 12 hours

         (c) Elevations in troponin levels: Strong prognostic indicators of mortality risk

      ii. CBC: Check for cause of anemia (decreased oxygen supply)

      iii. Creatinine, BUN levels: Assess renal function (for dye administration, heparinization)

      iv. C-reactive protein (inflammatory marker) and BNP (indicates ventricular dilatation, pressure overload): Markers used to evaluate risk for future events

   b. ECG: May or may not show evidence of myocardial injury or ischemia (see ST-Segment Elevation Myocardial Infarction)

      i.   Transient ST changes with pain: Occurrence of ST changes with symptoms and at rest are highly suggestive of ischemia and probably severe CAD

      ii. ST depression

      iii. Inverted T-wave changes

      iv. New BBB

      v. Sustained VT

   c. Echocardiography: May or may not show transient abnormal wall motion, valve dysfunction, hypertrophy. Identifies LV dysfunction.

   d. Dobutamine stress echocardiography: Demonstrates ischemia, stress-induced wall motion abnormalities, ventricular dysfunction, ischemic mitral regurgitation

   e. Myocardial scintigraphy (thallium, Tc 99m sestamibi) with pharmacologic stress (adenosine, dipyridamole) may demonstrate ischemia, infarction, and LV dysfunction

   f. Coronary catheterization

5. Goals of care

   a. Ischemia, MI, and death are prevented by

      i.   Decreasing myocardial oxygen demand

      ii. Improving myocardial oxygen supply

   b. Disease process is modified.

      i.   Antiplatelet and antithrombin therapy

      ii. Lifestyle modifications (smoking cessation; diet; weight, blood pressure, and glucose control)

6. Collaborating professionals on health care team: See Chronic Stable Angina

7. Management of patient care

   a. Anticipated patient trajectory: Therapy with effective antiplatelet agents and prompt angiography have resulted in significant gains in infarct prevention and myocardial preservation

      i.   Positioning: See Chronic Stable Angina

      ii. Nutrition: Low-fat, low-sodium diet

      iii. Discharge planning: See Chronic Stable Angina

      iv. Pharmacology: Pain and ischemia management

         (a) NTG: Rapid-acting nitrate

          (1) Actions
             a) Dilates veins and arteries
             b) Decreases venous return by systemic pooling of blood: Decreases preload
             c) Reduces myocardial oxygen demand and consumption
             d) Relieves coronary artery spasm
          (2) Dosages
             a) Sublingually 0.4 mg every 5 minutes; up to three doses
             b) IV drip started at 5 to 10 mcg/min. Titrate until pain is relieved or adverse side effects occur (hypotension).
          (3) Side effects include hypotension, headache, sweating, nausea, tachycardia, bradycardia.
          (4) If IV NTG results in decreased blood pressure, give fluid bolus and place patient with the feet elevated.
          (5) Patients often develop tolerance of NTG's hemodynamic effects after 12 to 24 hours of administration. Infusion rate may need to be adjusted with continued use. If an NTG patch is used, it may be discontinued for 8 to 12 hours each day (usually at nighttime).
          (6) NTG should not be taken within 24 hours of taking phosphodiesterase inhibitors such as sildenafil (Viagra) because severe hypotension may result from the drugs' combined vasodilatory effects.
      (b) Morphine sulfate: Analgesic, anxiolytic
          (1) Used when NTG is ineffective for pain relief or symptoms of pulmonary edema are present
          (2) Doses of 1 to 5 mg IV
      (c) β-Blockers (e.g., atenolol, metoprolol)
          (1) Action
             a) Decrease angina
             b) Decrease heart rate and contractility
             c) Decrease myocardial oxygen demand
             d) Increase diastolic filling time
             e) Increase exercise tolerance
          (2) IV administration initially is used for continued chest pain.
          (3) Contraindications: Bronchial asthma, heart failure (unless caused by ischemia), AV blocks, hypotension
          (4) Side effects: Hypoglycemia, dysrhythmias (including conduction blocks), central nervous system effects (decreased energy, decreased libido, nightmares, confusion), gastrointestinal effects (diarrhea, nausea, constipation)
          (5) Sudden withdrawal of the drug can have rebound effects (including angina, hypertension, MI). Gradual withdrawal or adjustment should be made, unless an emergency (e.g., bradycardia) mandates immediate discontinuation.
      (d) Calcium channel antagonists: Nondihydropyridines (e.g., verapamil or diltiazem)
          (1) Actions
             a) Negative inotropic; negative chronotropic effects on SA and AV conductive tissue
             b) Increase angina threshold, reduce ischemia, increase exercise tolerance, decrease afterload
             c) Vasodilators help to improve myocardial blood supply.
          (2) Use cautiously in combination with β-blockers because of possible adverse effect on heart rate and LV function suppression.
          (3) Contraindications: Aortic valve disease, severe anemia, AV blocks, Wolff-Parkinson-White (WPW) syndrome (verapamil)
      (e) ACE inhibitors: Used if hypertension continues in a patient receiving NTG, β-blockers, especially when caused by LV dysfunction or heart failure symptoms
v. Pharmacology: Antiplatelet and antithrombotic combination therapy (Table 3-5)
      (a) Aspirin: Blocks only one pathway to platelet aggregation

■ TABLE 3-5
■ Pharmacologic Antiplatelet and Antithrombotic Combination Therapy

Drug	Actions	Administration	Comments
Aspirin	Platelet inhibition and antiinflammatory properties	Initial dosing of 325 mg, non-enteric coated, taken as soon as possible after symptom onset Daily doses of 75-160 mg	Adverse side effects of bleeding, GI distress are minimized with lower dosages
Adenosine diphosphate antagonist (e.g., clopidogrel, ticlopidine)	Interferes early in process of platelet thrombus development, inhibits and diminishes platelet aggregation	Clopidogrel • Acts rapidly (therapeutic levels within 2 hr) when loading dose of 300-600 mg given • Daily dose of 75 mg is given for up to 1 yr after PCI • Ticlopidine • Requires several days of therapy before reaching maximum effectiveness • Loading dose is 500 mg • Daily dose of 250 mg bid	If patient needs coronary artery bypass graft, clopidogrel ideally should be withheld for 5-7 days before surgery to minimize bleeding complications Used also if patient is intolerant to aspirin (allergy, GI disturbances, bleeding disorders) Routine blood monitoring (platelet and white blood cell counts) required when taking drug to identify neutropenia (occurs in 2% of patients), thrombotic thrombocytopenic purpura (occurs in 0.03%, more fatal)
Heparin: UFH	Anticoagulant agents	For UFH a weight-based dose is given, 60-70 units/kg IV bolus (maximum 5000 units) • Initially 12-15 units/kg/hr (maximum 1000 units/hr) to reach activated PTT goal of 1.5-2 times control	Close blood monitoring required routinely (every 6 hr until therapeutic level reached and with dosage changes) to ensure tight PTT goal maintenance control Given in conjunction with aspirin (unless contraindicated) Monitor for heparin-induced thrombocytopenia
Heparin: LMWH		LMWH (e.g., enoxaparin) is administered 1 mg/kg subcutaneously every 12 hr	Advantages: Avoidance of need for close blood monitoring, less likely to induce thrombocytopenia Disadvantages: More frequent minor bleeding events are seen with its use

Drug	Action	Dosage	Considerations
Glycoprotein IIb/IIIa blockers and receptor inhibitors (e.g., eptifibatide, tirofiban, abciximab)	Prevent binding of von Willebrand factor and fibrinogen, combating platelet aggregation. Significantly reduce death or myocardial infarction in short term. Used with aspirin and heparin for patients who undergo early PCI, or are at high risk for intervention	Administered IV only for set time periods and at set dosages (before, during, and after PCI). Present dosing regimens: Eptifibatide: 180 mcg/kg bolus, then 2 mcg/kg/min for 72-96 hr. Tirofiban: 0.4 mcg/kg/min for 30 min, then 0.1 mcg/kg/min for 48-96 hr. Abciximab: 0.25 mcg/kg bolus, then 0.125 mcg/kg/min (maximum 10 mcg/min) for 12-24 hr	Oral glycoprotein IIb/IIIa receptor inhibitors have not proven effective or safe to date
Thrombolytics	Not appropriate and harmful in this setting		May increase risk of myocardial infarction

GI, Gastrointestinal; IV, intravenous; LMWH, low–molecular-weight heparin; PCI, percutaneous coronary intervention; PTT, partial thromboplastin time; UFH, unfractionated heparin.

(b) Glycoprotein IIb/IIIa (GPIIb/IIIa) receptor blockers
    (1) Block the final common pathway of platelet aggregation
    (2) Therefore, may be ideal in treating acute coronary syndromes
vi. Psychosocial issues: See Chronic Stable Angina
vii. Treatments (See also Chronic Stable Angina)
    (a) PCI: Early invasive strategy is recommended for patients with the following:
        (1) Angina or ischemia recurring at rest or with minimal activity with aggressive medical therapy
        (2) Angina or ischemia recurring with symptoms of heart failure (S_3, pulmonary edema, increased crackles, new or worse mitral regurgitation)
        (3) EF of less than 40%
        (4) Hemodynamic instability, hypotension with angina at rest
        (5) PCI within previous 6 months
        (6) Prior CABG
        (7) Sustained VT
    (b) CABG: See Chronic Stable Angina
    (c) VAD: See Heart Failure
b. Potential complications: See Chronic Stable Angina
8. Evaluation of patient care: See Chronic Stable Angina

ST-Segment Elevation Myocardial Infarction

ST-elevation myocardial infarction (STEMI) is characterized by the necrosis of myocardial tissue due to the interruption of coronary perfusion to the myocardium.

1. Pathophysiology (see also Coronary Artery Disease)
  a. Blood flow may be obstructed acutely by a thrombus in the coronary artery.
  b. Site and amount of necrosis depend on the location of the arterial occlusion, on collateral circulation, and on the previous occurrence of any infarctions or disease.
  c. Extent of necrosis
    i. Transmural: Full thickness (endocardium to epicardium) STEMI
    ii. Nontransmural: Non–Q wave (subendocardial)
  d. See also Acute Coronary Syndromes

2. Etiology and risk factors
  a. Atherosclerotic CAD (see also Coronary Artery Disease): Slow, progressive coronary artery narrowing with an acute ruptured plaque that develops into an occlusive thrombotic lesion. Most prevalent cause of MI.
  b. Coronary artery spasm
  c. Severe anemia (decreased oxygen supply)
  d. Severe aortic stenosis
  e. Other causes include hyperthyroidism, emboli (endocarditis, atrial fibrillation), trauma, dissection, drugs (cocaine)
  f. Other precipitating factors include acute hypotension, tachydysrhythmias
  g. Risk factors: See Coronary Artery Disease

3. Signs and symptoms
  a. Patient history alone continues to be sufficient to rule in MI, even in the absence of ECG changes; 10% of patients with acute MI have normal ECG initially.
  b. Discomfort in the chest that has lasted longer than 20 to 30 minutes and is unrelieved by rest or nitrates. May radiate to neck, jaw, arms, and back. These areas may be the only locations of discomfort. Similar to angina in the character of the discomfort, but usually more intense and longer in duration (see Chronic Stable Angina for a description).
  c. Other findings vary with the size and extent of the infarction, the patient's status, and the history of previous MI.
    i. Pallid, diaphoretic, cool, clammy skin
    ii. Weakness, light-headedness
    iii. Vagal effects (bradycardia, nausea, and vomiting)
    iv. Dyspnea (most common presentation in the elderly)
    v. Dysrhythmias

      vi. Low, normal, or high blood pressure

     vii. Irregular, slow, fast, and/or thready pulse

    viii. Apprehension, physical "stillness"

      ix. S$_3$: Diastolic (ventricular) gallop (in acute LV failure)

      x. Ankle edema

     xi. Crackles in acute LV failure

    xii. Murmurs

   xiii. Pericardial friction rub

4. Diagnostic study findings

  a. Laboratory

    i. Troponins

      (a) Troponin I level: Diagnostic of MI (false elevations in renal insufficiency)

      (b) Troponin T level: Can be elevated in skeletal muscle injury

      (c) Remain elevated for 14 to 21 days

    ii. CK-MB isoenzyme levels elevated within 6 hours. May be dissipated if 24 hours since the onset of symptoms. CK-MB levels have dramatic elevation with reperfusion therapy and decrease quickly.

    iii. Leukocytosis (large MI) due to stress and tissue necrosis; peaks 2 to 4 days after the infarction

  b. ECG: Most important diagnostic tool; changes on ECG correlate with the location of the necrosis (as opposed to ST changes) (Table 3-6)

    i. ECG signs of MI: Necrosis (cell death)

      (a) Acute ST elevation

      (b) Abnormal Q wave

TABLE 3-6

Acute Myocardial Infarction: Infarct Area, Electrocardiographic (ECG) Evidence, Associated Coronary Arteries, and Potential Complications

Area of Infarct	ECG Evidence		Associated Coronary Artery	Potential Complications
	Leads Reflecting Infarct Area Directly	Leads Reflecting Reciprocal Changes		
LEFT VENTRICLE				
Lateral wall, high	I, aVL	II, III, aVF	Left circumflex	Pump failure, conduction disturbances
Inferior wall	II, III, aVF	I, aVL, V$_5$, V$_6$	Right coronary, possibly left circumflex	Sinoatrial and atrioventricular nodal conduction disturbances; valve dysfunction
Septal wall	V$_1$-V$_2$	II, III, aVF	Left anterior descending	Pump failure, conduction disturbance
Anterior wall	V$_2$-V$_4$	II, III, aVF	Left anterior descending	Pump failure, conduction disturbance
Lateral wall, low (apical area)	V$_5$-V$_6$	II, III, aVF	Left anterior descending	Pump failure, conduction disturbance
Posterior	V$_7$-V$_9$*	V$_1$-V$_3$	Posterior descending, right coronary, or left circumflex	Atrioventricular nodal conduction disturbance
RIGHT VENTRICLE†	V$_4$R	—	Right coronary	Atrioventricular nodal disturbance, valve dysfunction, hypotension

From Bucher L, Melander S. *Critical Care Nursing.* Philadelphia, PA: Saunders; 1999:230.

*Leads are placed on the left posterior chest wall at the fifth intercostal space, beginning at the left posterior axillary line.

†Right ventricular infarction is present in approximately one third of patients with inferior myocardial infarctions, and assessment of this lead should be performed routinely in all patients diagnosed with an acute inferior myocardial infarction.

(1) More than 0.04 seconds in duration (0.03 seconds for inferior MI)

(2) Appears within hours of transmural MI

ii.   Other causes of Q waves

(a) Normal Q waves; small Q wave in leads I, aVL, V$_5$, V$_6$, aVR

(b) Normal Q wave in lead III: Less than 0.03 seconds, decreased with inspiration

(c) Left BBB

(d) Myocarditis, cardiomyopathy

iii. Determination of the age of the infarction (Table 3-7)

iv.   Serial ECGs essential, along with those done during ischemic pain

c. Echocardiography: Assesses LV function, wall motion abnormalities, and complications such as VSD, thrombi, aneurysms, mitral regurgitation, pericardial effusions

d. Coronary catheterization

5. **Goals of care**

a. Patient has no pain.

b. Patient has limited myocardial injury due to reperfusion (through thrombolysis or PCI).

c. Patient has adequate hemodynamic parameters.

d. Dysrhythmias are absent or controlled.

6. **Collaborating professionals on health care team: See Chronic Stable Angina**

7. **Management of patient care**

a. Anticipated patient trajectory: Minimizing time to thrombolytic or PCI therapy increases survival and preservation of myocardial function

i.   Positioning

(a) Maintain bed rest for the first 12 hours, with use of a bedside commode.

(b) Postprocedure issues include leg or arm immobilization, head of bed lower than 15 degrees (dependent on closure protocols).

(c) Early immobilization is important: use of a chair or bedside commode in the first 24 hours (improves well-being, lowers risk of pulmonary embolus).

(d) Increase ambulation in room as tolerated during the first 48 hours.

ii. Pain management

(a) Relieve discomfort with analgesics.

(1) Relief of pain decreases elevated sympathetic response and myocardial workload (lowering heart rate and blood pressure) and counters the arrhythmic effect of circulating catecholamines.

(2) Morphine: 2 to 4 mg IV every 5 minutes to relieve pain

a) Decrease dosages in the elderly and in patients with respiratory disease.

b) Respiratory depression with morphine sulfate usually peaks 7 minutes after IV injection and is dose related (not usually a problem in patients with MI).

c) Orthostatic hypotension can result from volume depletion: Provide volume support and keep the patient in Trendelenburg's position.

d) Naloxone, 0.4 mg IV (repeated up to three times at 3-minute intervals), may be given to counteract narcotic-induced depressed respirations and hypotension.

(3) Remind the patient to notify the nurse immediately if discomfort recurs.

(b) Antiemetics may be necessary because of the high degree of acute vagal tone with MI and the emetic side effects of opiate analgesia.

(c) Anxiolytics (e.g., benzodiazepines, haloperidol) may be used if the patient is agitated, delirious, or very anxious, experiences sleep deprivation, or has intensive care unit psychosis.

iii. Nutrition

(a) Keep the patient on NPO status until the discomfort or pain is gone, then give clear liquids and progress the diet.

(b) Feed a low-fat, low-sodium diet.

(c) Earlier "coronary precautions" have now been abandoned (e.g., restriction of hot and cold fluids, avoidance of caffeine; regular caffeine drinkers develop tolerance and can experience withdrawal symptoms of increased heart rate or headaches; several cups of coffee have no ill effects).

TABLE 3-7

Changes in the Facing Electrocardiographic (ECG) Leads During the Four Phases of a Transmural, Q-Wave Myocardial Infarction

Phase of Infarction	Q Waves	R Waves	ST Segments	T Waves	ECG
Phase 1 (0-2 hr): Onset of extensive ischemia occurs immediately, subendocardial injury occurs within 20-40 min, and subendocardial necrosis occurs in about 30 min; necrosis extends to about half of the myocardial wall by 2 hr	Unchanged	Unchanged or abnormally tall	Onset of elevation	Amplitude increases; peaking may occur	
Phase 2 (2-24 hr): Transmural infarction is considered complete by 6 hr as necrosis involves about 90% of the myocardial wall; the rest of the necrosis occurs by the end of phase 2	Width and depth begin to increase	Amplitude begins to decrease	Maximum elevation	Amplitude and peaking lessen; T waves still positive	
Phase 3 (24-72 hr): Little or no ischemia or injury remains as healing begins	Reach maximum size	Absent	Return to baseline	Become maximally inverted	
Phase 4 (2-8 wk): Necrotic tissue is replaced by fibrous tissue	Q waves persist	May return partially	Usually normal	Slight inversion	

From Huszar RJ. *Basic Dysrhythmias: Interpretation and Management.* 3rd ed. St Louis, MO: Mosby; 2002:330.

iv. Discharge planning
   (a) Teaching issues include the rationales for and descriptions of therapy, methods for treating discomfort or pain at home.
   (b) Stress smoking cessation after MI. Patient may need nicotine replacement if he or she is a heavy smoker or has withdrawal symptoms.
v. Pharmacology
   (a) Oxygen: 2 to 4 L/min to keep oxygen saturation above 90%. Hypoxemia is due to ventilation-perfusion mismatch and LV failure.
   (b) NTG: Sublingual, IV infusions (see Acute Coronary Syndromes)
   (c) β-Blockers: Reduce myocardial ischemia and increase hospital survival rates. Usually IV β-blockers (e.g., metoprolol, 10 mg IV; atenolol, 5 mg IV) given initially to ensure rapid lowering of heart rate, blood pressure.
   (d) ACE inhibitors: For patients with anterior MI, pulmonary congestion, LV EF of less than 40% (unless systolic blood pressure is less than 100 mm Hg). Contraindicated in renal failure.
   (e) ARBs: For patients intolerant of ACE inhibitors
   (f) Antiplatelet-antithrombotic therapy
      (1) Aspirin given immediately. Usually 325 mg, chewed. Daily dose of 81 mg.
      (2) Clopidogrel used if the patient cannot take aspirin and after PCI
      (3) Heparin (low molecular weight): See Table 3-5
      (4) GPIIb/IIIa receptor blockers if direct PCI planned
   (g) Thrombolytics
   (h) Stool softeners
   (i) Statins: Lipid-lowering therapy. Goal is LDL level of less than 100 mg/dl (the lower, the better).
vi. Psychosocial issues
   (a) Denial is an emotion many patients exhibit, both before admission and during hospitalization.
   (b) Flexible visiting hours can assist in relieving anxiety and other stress that can create a situation promoting pain occurrence (depending on the patient's status, need for rest, procedures, and family dynamics).
vii. Treatments
   (a) Place the patient on a monitor. Watch closely for dysrhythmias, because VF is common in the early hours of MI.
   (b) Ensure that the patient has at least two good IV sites for administration of drugs, volume support, reperfusion therapy.
   (c) RV MI: Preload is vital for maintaining forward output in RV MI. Ensure that the patient has sufficient volume before giving NTG because of the high risk of hypotension. Goal: CVP of 15 to 20 mm Hg.
   (d) Primary PCI: PCI with stenting to open the occluded artery and limit myocardial necrosis. Indicated if
      (1) Available
      (2) Door to PCI is less than 1 hour
      (3) Emergency medical service (EMS) to stent is less than 90 minutes
      (4) Pain is present less than 3 hours
   (e) Thrombolysis (see Box 3-6): IV thrombolytic as soon as possible (in the emergency department, EMS, critical care unit)
      (1) If PCI not available
      (2) If door to PCI is more than 1 hour
      (3) If EMS to PCI is more than 90 minutes
      (4) There is no difference between tissue plasminogen activator (t-PA) and streptokinase if used early (within the first hour).
   (f) If the patient presents with or develops severe hypotension, the patient may require transfer to intensive care and the utilization of an intra-aortic balloon pump (IABP) (see Heart Failure). IABP is used during MI for the following:

(1) Acute mitral regurgitation
(2) Refractory ventricular dysrhythmias
(3) Post-MI angina
(4) As a bridge to revascularization
b. Potential complications
i. Postinfarction pain (persistent, recurrent)
(a) Mechanism: Common causes are ischemia, reinfarction, pericarditis (Dressler's syndrome). Pericarditis does not occur in the first 24 hours.
(b) Management
(1) When pain is present, obtain an ECG and compare with previous ECGs.
(2) Pain recurring after MI suggests ongoing ischemia and should be treated promptly.
ii. Cardiogenic shock
(a) Mechanism: Seen in the first 48 hours, especially with large anterior MI, due to ischemia or with severe mitral regurgitation
(b) Management: See Heart Failure and Shock
iii. Dysrhythmias: Atrial fibrillation, VT, VF, bradydysrhythmias
(a) Mechanism: See Basic Dysrhythmias for Progressive Care
(b) Management
(1) Monitor the patient's ECG and watch for hypotension and bradycardia.
(2) Watch for reperfusion dysrhythmias. In the initial period after coronary blood flow is restored, ventricular dysrhythmias frequently occur.

BOX 3-6
CONTRAINDICATIONS AND CAUTIONS FOR THE USE OF FIBRINOLYSIS IN ST-SEGMENT ELEVATION MYOCARDIAL INFARCTION*

ABSOLUTE CONTRADICTIONS
- Any prior intracranial hemorrhage
- Known structural cerebral vascular lesion (e.g., arteriovenous malformation)
- Known malignant intracranial neoplasm (primary or metastatic)
- Ischemic stroke within 3 months except acute ischemic stroke within 3 hours
- Suspected aortic dissection
- Active bleeding or bleeding diathesis (excluding menses)
- Significant closed head or facial trauma within 3 months

RELATIVE CONTRAINDICATIONS
- History of chronic, severe, poorly controlled hypertension
- Severe uncontrolled hypertension on presentation (systolic blood pressure higher than 180 mm Hg or diastolic blood pressure higher than 110 mm Hg)†
- History of prior ischemic stroke longer than 3 months ago, dementia, or known intracranial pathology not covered in contraindications
- Traumatic or prolonged (longer than 10 minutes) cardiopulmonary resuscitation or major surgery (less than 3 weeks ago)
- Recent (within 2 to 4 weeks) internal bleeding
- Noncompressible vascular punctures
- For streptokinase or anistreplase: Prior exposure (more than 5 days ago) or prior allergic reaction to these agents
- Pregnancy
- Active peptic ulcer
- Current use of anticoagulants: The higher the international normalized ratio, the higher the risk of bleeding

From Antman DM, Anbe DT, Armstrong PW, et al. ACC/AHA guidelines for the management of patients with ST-elevation myocardial infarction: executive summary: a report of the ACC/AHA Task Force on Practice Guidelines (Committee to Revise the 1999 Guidelines on the Management of Patients with Acute Myocardial Infarction). *J Am Coll Cardiol.* 2004;44(3):671-719.
*Viewed as advisory for clinical decision making and may not be all-inclusive or definitive.
†Could be an absolute contraindication in low-risk patients with ST-segment elevation myocardial infarction (see Section 6.3.1.6.3.2 of the full-text ACC/AHA guidelines).

(3) AV sequential pacing may be required for increasing CO (blocks are common).
(4) Instruct the patient to avoid Valsalva maneuvers: may result in dramatic changes in heart rate and blood pressure (ventricular filling) and can cause dysrhythmias (especially in patients younger than 45 years of age).
   iv. Other complications
      (a) Reocclusion: Symptoms include ST-segment changes, chest discomfort, dysrhythmias, hypotension
      (b) LV thrombus: More likely with a CK rise of more than 3200 IU/L. Treatment includes anticoagulation for 3 to 6 months.
      (c) VSDs: Surgical repair is needed immediately if the patient has unstable hemodynamics or if CO is low (IABP, inotropic drugs, vasodilators, surgical or catheter-based closure)
      (d) LV aneurysm: Surgical repair is often combined with CABG, valve repair
      (e) Severe acute mitral regurgitation: IABP, inotropic drugs, catheterization, surgery
      (f) Rupture of LV free wall or papillary muscle rupture: Volume support, IABP, vasoactive medications, surgery. Majority of patients with free wall rupture do not survive.
8. **Evaluation of patient care**
   a. Patient has no pain.
   b. Coronary artery flow is restored within 30 to 90 minutes.
   c. Patient has adequate hemodynamic parameters (CO) without mechanical support (e.g., IABP, VAD).
   d. Dysrhythmias are controlled or absent.
   e. Peripheral pulses are present, and circulation is good.
   f. Patient verbalizes knowledge of home care and follow-up requirements.

Heart Failure

Heart failure is a clinical presentation of impaired cardiac function in which one or both ventricles are unable to maintain an output adequate to meet the metabolic demands of the body. Heart failure can occur on either the right or the left side of the heart and is due to systolic dysfunction (poor contraction), diastolic dysfunction (impaired filling), increased afterload (increased resistance), or alterations in heart rate (too fast, too slow).
1. **Pathophysiology**
   a. Left-sided heart failure, systolic dysfunction
      i. Impaired forward output caused by decreased LV contractility (e.g., CAD, cardiomyopathies) in which the EF is reduced to below normal
      ii. To compensate, the LV dilates and the heart rate increases in an attempt to maintain a normal output. This increase in the SV and heart rate may return the CO toward normal despite a poor EF.
      iii. LV filling pressures rise because of increased preload or decreased LV compliance (producing LV diastolic dysfunction).
      iv. LA and pulmonary venous pressures rise, producing pulmonary congestion and edema.
         (a) When pulmonary capillary oncotic pressure (30 mm Hg) is exceeded, fluid leaks into the pulmonary interstitial space, creating pulmonary edema.
         (b) Decreased oxygenation of the blood occurs as oxygen exchange is impeded by the presence of fluid.
      v. Right-sided heart pressure increases as a result of increased pressure in the pulmonary system.
      vi. Right-sided heart failure may then occur because of the pulmonary hypertension, resulting in peripheral and organ edema.
   b. Left-sided heart failure, diastolic dysfunction
      i. A noncompliant, stiff LV (due to hypertrophy, ischemia, infiltration, scarring) has less ability to relax, which interferes with adequate filling and results in rising diastolic (filling) pressures.
      ii. As a consequence, LA, pulmonary venous, and pulmonary capillary pressures increase.
      iii. Pulmonary artery and right-sided heart pressures rise if the condition is untreated.

iv.   Systolic function is often normal and accounts for the fact that up to 30% to 50% of patients with "heart failure" have normal LV systolic function.

c. Right-sided heart failure, systolic dysfunction
i.   The right side of the heart is unable to pump blood forward adequately, which results in a drop in CO.
ii.   Causes include pulmonary hypertension (most common), as well as RV MI.
iii.   RV dilatation and elevation of filling pressure develop, which results in peripheral edema.

d. Right-sided heart failure, diastolic dysfunction: Can occur with RV hypertrophy and cardiomyopathies; analogous to left-sided heart diastolic dysfunction, except the consequence is peripheral edema rather than pulmonary edema, associated with elevated right-sided heart filling pressures (increased jugular venous pressures)

e. Four stages of heart failure progression
i.   Stage A: High risk of heart failure, no cardiac structural disorders
ii.   Stage B: Structural defect or disorder of the heart, no symptoms of heart failure
iii.   Stage C: Structural defect or disorder of the heart, present or past symptoms of heart failure
iv.   Stage D: End-stage cardiac disease; the patient needs continuous therapy (inotropic drugs, mechanical supports, transplantation, hospice care)

2. **Etiology and risk factors: See Table 3-8 for factors related to left- and right-sided heart failure**

▓ TABLE 3-8
▓ ▓ Etiologic or Precipitating Factors in Heart Failure

| Left-Sided Heart Failure | | Right-Sided Heart Failure | Both Sides |
Systolic	Diastolic		
Ischemic heart disease (50% of all cases)	Coronary artery disease	Left-sided heart failure	Patient noncompliant regarding
Myocardial infarction	Myocardial ischemia	Atherosclerotic heart disease	• Medications
Myocardial stunning, hibernation	Left ventricular hypertrophy	Acute right ventricular myocardial infarction	• Dietary restrictions
Coronary artery disease	Cardiomyopathy: hypertrophic, restrictive,	Pulmonary embolism	• Alcohol use
Idiopathic dilated cardiomyopathy	dilated	Fluid overload, excess sodium intake	Medications
Myocardial contusion	Increased circulating volume	Myocardial contusion	• Negative inotropic agents
Aortic insufficiency	Cardiac tamponade	Cardiomyopathy	• Causing sodium retention
Dysrhythmias: Ventricular tachycardia, atrial fibrillation	Constrictive pericarditis	Valvular heart disease	
Postpump syndrome	Left ventricular hypertrophy	Atrial or ventricular septal defect	
Myocarditis	Mitral stenosis or insufficiency	Pulmonary outflow stenosis	
Infectious: Viral, bacterial, fungal	Aortic stenosis or insufficiency	Chronic obstructive pulmonary disease	
Acute rheumatic fever	Age (decreased compliance of	Pulmonary hypertension (cor pulmonale)	
Drug abuse: Heroin, alcohol, cocaine	heart muscle)	Sleep apnea	
Nutrition deficits: Protein, thiamine	Diabetes mellitus		
Electrolyte disorders: Decrease in calcium, sodium, potassium, phosphate	Intracardiac shunts		
Diabetes, thyroid disease			
Drugs suppressing contractility (negative inotropic)			

3. **Signs and symptoms: Patients generally have asymptomatic heart failure for an uncertain time before the recognition of symptoms. Decrease in activity tolerance and/or fluid retention is generally the first complaint identified**.
   a. History: See Table 3-9 for clinical findings in left- and right-sided heart failure
   b. Physical examination of patient
      i. See Table 3-9
      ii. Functional therapeutic classification of patients with heart failure
         (a) I: Symptoms occur with strong exertion
         (b) II: Symptoms occur with normal exertion
         (c) III: Symptoms occur with minimal exertion
         (d) IV: Symptoms occur at rest
4. **Diagnostic study findings**
   a. Laboratory
      i. BNP level: Elevations reflect myocyte stretch and increased ventricular pressures; prognostic indicator
      ii. C-reactive protein level: May be elevated
      iii. HCT, Hb level: Assess for anemia
      iv. Electrolyte levels: Imbalances due to diuresis
      v. Thyroid-stimulating hormone level: Hypothyroidism, hyperthyroidism causes
      vi. Renal function tests: BUN, creatinine levels
      vii. Liver function tests (right-sided failure)
      viii. Cardiac troponin, enzyme levels (if potential acute MI)
      ix. Human immunodeficiency virus (HIV) testing: If the patient is at high risk for this cause

TABLE 3-9
Clinical Findings in Heart Failure

| Left-Sided Heart Failure | | Right-Sided Heart Failure |
Systolic	Diastolic	
Anxiety	Exercise intolerance	Increased fatigue
Sudden light-headedness	Orthopnea	Hepatomegaly
Fatigue, weakness, lethargy	Dyspnea, dyspnea on exertion, paroxysmal nocturnal dyspnea	Splenomegaly
Orthopnea	Cough with frothy white or pink sputum (in pulmonary edema)	Dependent pitting edema
Dyspnea, dyspnea on exertion, paroxysmal nocturnal dyspnea	Tachypnea (on exertion)	Ascites
Tachypnea (on exertion)	Basilar crackles, rhonchi, wheezes	Cachexia
Cheyne-Stokes respirations (if severe)	Pulmonary edema	Abdominal pain (from congested liver)
Diaphoresis	Symptoms of right-sided heart failure	Anorexia, nausea, emesis
Palpitations	Hypoxia, respiratory acidosis	Weight gain
Sacral edema, pitting of extremities	Elevated pulmonary artery diastolic pressure, pulmonary capillary wedge pressure	Low blood pressure
Basilar rales, rhonchi, crackles, wheezes	S_3, S_4 heart sounds	Oliguria, nocturia (increased renal perfusion, blood volume when lying in bed)
Cool, moist, cyanotic skin	Holosystolic murmur (if tricuspid, mitral regurgitation)	Venous distention
Hypoxia, respiratory acidosis		Hepatojugular reflux
Elevated pulmonary artery diastolic pressure, pulmonary capillary wedge pressure		Fatigue, weakness
Nocturia		Kussmaul's sign (if constriction)
Mental confusion		Murmur of tricuspid insufficiency
Decreased pulse pressure		S_3, S_4 heart sounds (right-sided)
Pulsus alternans		Elevated central venous pressure and right atrial and right ventricular pressures
Lateral displacement of point of maximal impulse		
S_3, S_4 heart sounds		
Murmur of mitral insufficiency		

    b. Radiologic: Results often normal

        i. Pulmonary vasculature: Edema, congestion

        ii. Cardiac silhouette: May show cardiac chamber enlargement

        iii. Pleural effusion (left-sided failure)

        iv. Valve calcifications

    c. ECG

        i. Nonspecific changes

        ii. Dysrhythmias, ischemic disease, conduction abnormalities, drug and electrolyte effects

    d. Echocardiogram: To assess

        i. Chamber size, wall thickness

        ii. Systolic and diastolic function

        iii. Thrombus formation

        iv. Valvular function

        v. Pericardial disease

    e. Radionuclide imaging

        i. Assessment of chamber function and volume

        ii. Myocardial perfusion imaging for ischemia, infarction

    f. Ultrafast CT and MRI: To assess structural abnormalities, tumors, vascular anomalies, pericardial disease

    g. Cardiac catheterization with arteriography: To assess

        i. Coronary anatomy (two thirds of patients have CAD as a contributing cause)

        ii. Pressures in right and left chambers

            (a) High filling pressures represent diastolic dysfunction.

            (b) Diuretic and IV NTG use can create a false-negative result by artificially normalizing the filling pressures.

        iii. Ventricular contractility

        iv. Valvular function, cardiac defects

5. Goals of care

    a. Symptoms are relieved.

    b. Hemodynamics are stabilized rapidly (by using diuretics, vasodilators, inotropic agents).

    c. Excess fluid is removed and edema is corrected.

    d. Complications from dysrhythmias are prevented.

6. Collaborating professionals on health care team: See Chronic Stable Angina; also electrophysiologist, psychologist, home health aide, financial aid counselor

7. Management of patient care

    a. Anticipated patient trajectory: A common clinical cardiology problem with a poor prognosis. Quality of life and longevity can be improved dramatically with available medications and therapy.

        i. Positioning

            (a) Placement in reverse Trendelenburg's position and/or use of extra pillows may increase ease of breathing.

            (b) Prevent complications of deep venous thrombosis by range-of-motion exercises, use of thromboembolic disease hose, pneumatic antiembolic stockings.

        ii. Skin care: If the patient is on prolonged bed rest, institute measures to prevent the hazards of immobility

        iii. Pain management: Administer medications to alleviate discomfort, as ordered

        iv. Nutrition

            (a) Monitor intake and output closely.

            (b) Closely observe restrictions on fluid (1000 to 1500 ml/day) and sodium.

            (c) Weigh patient daily.

        v. Discharge planning: Before discharge, the patient and/or significant others should be able to do the following:

            (a) Explain heart failure and its prognosis.

            (b) List symptoms that indicate a worsening of the condition, whether from heart failure or from drug side effects. Patient should know when to call for medical advice to prevent rehospitalizations and complications.

(c) Describe each current medication: name, purpose, dosage, frequency, side effects, and benefits of compliance.

(d) Identify the lifestyle changes necessary to prevent recurrence.

(1) Diet and weight control

a) Sodium restriction (diet, drugs)

b) Fluid restrictions, as ordered

c) Foods rich in potassium (important for patients taking loop diuretics)

d) Daily weight monitoring

(2) Cessation of high-risk activities: Smoking, alcohol, and/or drug use

(3) Routine exercise: Increases exercise tolerance, decreases symptoms

(e) Identify the rationale for the control of blood pressure, lipid levels, diabetes.

(f) Demonstrate how to take the pulse; recognize the need to have blood pressure taken routinely.

(g) Verbalize the importance of follow-up care.

vi. Pharmacology

(a) See Table 3-10 for drugs commonly used in the treatment of heart failure.

(b) Avoid drugs that decrease myocardial contractility (except β-blockers).

(1) Antiarrhythmic drugs (except amiodarone)

(2) Calcium channel blocking agents (except for amlodipine, felodipine)

(3) NSAIDs: Cause sodium retention, renal insufficiency

(4) Chemotherapeutic drugs (e.g., daunorubicin, doxorubicin)

vii. Psychosocial issues

(a) Patient will likely need help at home (help arrange home services).

(b) Noncompliance with the prescribed diet, weight, fluid intake, and medications can be devastating with this disorder. Patient and significant others need education, support, and close follow-up.

(c) Coping with a long-standing, progressive disease becomes a strain on both patient and caregivers. Assess for signs of depression.

(d) High costs of medications, hospitalizations, interventions create additional strains.

viii. Treatments

(a) Biventricular pacing: Cardiac resynchronization therapy (CRT) has been shown to increase LV systolic function by synchronizing ventricular contraction so that the right and left ventricles, along with the septum, contract simultaneously, which results in increased CO and improved remodeling. Pacemaker education (procedure, rationales, incision care, follow-up) is needed.

(b) IABP placement: May be necessary to stabilize the patient as a bridge to other interventions. Patient and significant others should be prepared for this procedure.

(c) VAD, implanted device (in either or both ventricles) that bypasses the affected ventricle: Takes over its pumping action, and allows the heart to rest and recover, thus preventing end-organ failure

(d) Mechanical ventilation: Used in patients with hypoventilation and severe hypoxia

(e) Surgery

(1) Revascularization for ischemic heart failure

(2) Valvular repair or replacement

(3) Transplantation

b. Potential complication: Death

8. Evaluation of patient care

a. Patient is hemodynamically stable: CO and tissue perfusion are adequate.

b. Decrease in edema and return to normal weight are achieved.

c. Lungs are clear, according to auscultation and radiography.

d. Intake and output are balanced.

e. Dysrhythmias are controlled or absent.

TABLE 3-10

Drugs Commonly Used to Treat Heart Failure in the Progressive Care Setting

Agent	Action/Indications	Administration	Comments
Nesiritide (BNP)	Causes vasodilatation, ↑ renal blood flow, ↑ urinary output, and improved hemodynamics	Dosage: 2 mcg/kg IV bolus, then infusion starting at 0.01 mcg/kg/min (titrated up to 0.03 mcg/kg/min for maximum of 48 hr)	Drug is expensive at present, used if patient does not respond to first-line drugs ↑ BNP levels (false-positive BNP test result)
INOTROPIC AGENTS			
Phosphodiesterase inhibitors (milrinone)	↑ Myocardial contractility without increasing HR Relaxes vascular (arterial and venous) smooth muscle, producing peripheral vasodilatation (↓ afterload and preload)	Half-life: 20-45 min Dosage: 50 mcg/kg undiluted is administered over 10 min (loading dose), followed by a 0.375- to 0.75-mcg/kg/min infusion	Untoward effects include tachycardia, dysrhythmias, hypotension (to correct hypovolemia)
Dobutamine (Dobutrex)	↑ Myocardial contractility ↑ Stroke volume and CO ↓ SVR No beneficial renal effects	Dosage: Infused at an IV rate of 2.5-15 mcg/kg/min Contraindications: Hypertrophic cardiomyopathy, severe AS	Monitor for tachydysrhythmias, (ventricular ectopy) Can ↓ BP in low dosages (usually associated with volume depletion, excessive diuresis, IV nitroglycerin); check for volume depletion before administering drug
VASOPRESSORS			
Dopamine (Intropin)	Used to support BP	Dosages of 2-10 mcg/kg/min (β-adrenergic effects) ↑ BP, cerebral and renal perfusion Dosages of >10 mcg/kg/min (α-adrenergic effects) cause peripheral vasoconstriction, ↑ SVR, ↑ afterload and BP (possible ↓ CO)	May cause tachycardia Check skin color, temperature, capillary refill; α-adrenergic stimulation causes peripheral venoconstriction. Infuse in central or large vein. Extravasation causes tissue necrosis and sloughing. If this occurs: stop infusion and immediately inject phentolamine (Regitine), 5-10 mg diluted in 10-15 ml of saline solution, around site to lessen deleterious effects of infiltrated dopamine.
Other vasoactive drugs, including vasopressin (antidiuretic hormone), norepinephrine (Levophed)			Monitor hemodynamic parameters closely, especially when using vasoactive drugs (monitor arterial and hemodynamic pressures often with noninvasive BP monitoring, arterial lines, and pulmonary artery catheter)

Continued

TABLE 3-10
Drugs Commonly Used to Treat Heart Failure in the Progressive Care Setting—Cont'd

Agent	Action/Indications	Administration	Comments
AFTERLOAD REDUCTION			
ACE inhibitor (e.g., captopril, enalapril)	Used for afterload and preload reduction ↑ Heart function and exercise capacity ↓ Mortality risk Contraindicated in shock, hyperkalemia (K^+ >5.5 mEq/L)	Angiotensin II receptor blockers may be used in patients who are unable to tolerate ACE inhibitors, usually due to cough	Monitor for • Symptomatic hypotension • ↑ K^+ (increases retention) • ↑ Creatinine (decreased renal function)
PRELOAD REDUCTION			
IV nitroglycerin	Improves left ventricular function by lowering preload via vasodilatation, to relieve discomfort		Evaluate for patient response: ↑ Urinary output, ↓ edema, improved lung sounds and breathing; ↓ central venous pressure and PCWP Monitor for complications: • Electrolyte imbalances (↓ Na^+, ↓ K^+, ↓ Mg^{++}) • Impaired renal function (↑ creatinine) • Hypovolemia • Other symptoms: Fatigue, nausea, vomiting, headache, dry mouth, muscle cramps, wooziness
Diuretics (i.e., torsemide, furosemide, bumetanide)	↓ Intravascular and extravascular fluid volume, and subsequently ↓ preload		
β-Blockers	Beneficial in decreasing symptoms of heart failure, increasing patient well-being	Watch for fluid retention, fatigue, hypotension, increased symptoms	Carvedilol combines β-blockade with vasodilatation properties

Drug	Effects/Uses	Dosage	Notes
Digoxin (Lanoxin)	Beneficial in decreasing symptoms, improving exercise tolerance, especially in combination therapy Also used for rate control of atrial fibrillation, atrial flutter		
Spironolactone (Aldactone)	Antagonist to aldosterone ↓ Mortality, hospitalization	Dosages: 12.5-25 mg/day	Watch K$^+$ retention Not used in renal insufficiency
Anticoagulation (warfarin)	Used for atrial fibrillation, thromboembolism risk		
Morphine	↓ Preload ↓ Venous return to heart (↑ capacitance) ↓ Pain, anxiety ↓ Myocardial oxygen consumption	3-5 mg IV	

ACE, Angiotensin-converting enzyme; AS, aortic stenosis; BNP, brain natriuretic peptide; BP, blood pressure; CO, cardiac output; HR, heart rate; IV, intravenous; PCWP, pulmonary capillary wedge pressure; SV, stroke volume; SVR, systemic vascular resistance.

Pericardial Disease

1. **Pathophysiology**
   a. Pericarditis
      i. Inflammation of the pericardium with a wide variety of causes
      ii. May be acute or chronic
      iii. Acute pericarditis most commonly of viral or idiopathic origin
         (a) Produces acute illness characterized by fever, chest pain (characteristically relieved by sitting up or leaning forward), pericardial friction rub, global ST elevation, little to no pericardial effusion
         (b) Is usually self-limited and responds to NSAIDs
         (c) May be recurrent with relapses
   b. Pericardial effusion
      i. Abnormal amount of pericardial fluid can result when pericardial fluid is produced too rapidly to be reabsorbed.
      ii. If pericardial fluid accumulates slowly, the pericardium stretches with little increase in intrapericardial pressure. Cardiac filling and function are not disturbed. If effusion accumulates rapidly, intrapericardial pressure rises, and tamponade may result.
      iii. Huge effusions (several liters) may develop slowly without tamponade (especially in uremic pericarditis).
      iv. Same causes as for pericarditis
   c. Cardiac tamponade
      i. Common causes are few: aortic dissection, MI with myocardial rupture, trauma (catheter or pacemaker perforation, contusion during CPR), laceration during pericardiocentesis (postoperative bleeding).
      ii. Results when pericardial fluid accumulates too rapidly to allow the pericardium to stretch. Can occur with small amounts of fluid or blood (approximately 150 ml) in the pericardial space.
      iii. Intrapericardial pressure rises dramatically.
      iv. Increased intrapericardial pressure exceeds the filling pressures of the right side (pretamponade) and then of both sides, impairing ventricular filling and output.
      v. CVP and jugular venous pressures rise (may not be seen in marked hypovolemia).
      vi. Pulsus paradoxus develops.
      vii. CO falls dramatically.
      viii. Compensatory tachycardia develops.
      ix. Hypotension and death result in minutes.
   d. Constrictive pericarditis
      i. Results from chronic scarring and thickening of the pericardium after pericarditis of any cause
      ii. Most common causes are posttraumatic, postpericardiotomy, and postradiation factors; neoplasm; and tuberculosis.
      iii. Epicardium becomes thickened with tough and rigid fibrous tissue that calcifies.
      iv. This interferes with filling (especially of the right side of the heart) in mid- to late diastole, which results in decreased CO and increased jugular venous filling pressures.
      v. Syndrome of right-sided heart failure with decreased output develops.
      vi. Pulmonary edema is not seen.
      vii. Death is the usual outcome, unless life-saving but high-risk (5% to 15% mortality) pericardiectomy is performed.
2. **Etiology and risk factors for pericarditis**
   a. Idiopathic, acute, or nonspecific (most common)
   b. Infection
      i. Viral: Echovirus and coxsackievirus B (the two most common causes of acute pericarditis); adenovirus, enterovirus, and influenza, mumps, measles, smallpox, and chickenpox viruses
      ii. Bacterial: Pneumococci, staphylococci, *Mycobacterium tuberculosis*, streptococci, *Pseudomonas* species
      iii. Fungal: *Histoplasma, Aspergillus, Candida*

        iv. Rickettsial, spirochetal (Lyme disease, due to *Borrelia burgdorferi*)

        v. HIV infection and acquired immunodeficiency syndrome: Becoming a prevalent cause worldwide

  c. Neoplasms (especially metastatic tumors from the lung and breast; melanomas; lymphomas)

  d. Connective tissue diseases: Systemic lupus erythematosus, rheumatoid arthritis, polyarteritis nodosa, and scleroderma

  e. Radiation therapy to the thorax: Treatments for Hodgkin's disease, breast or lung cancer

  f. Acute MI: Early inflammatory process (24 to 72 hours after) or delayed immunologic response (Dressler's syndrome). Dressler's syndrome (occurring weeks or months after MI) has decreased in incidence due to advanced MI therapy (use of thrombolytics).

  g. Postcardiotomy or postthoracotomy syndrome (occurs 2 to 10 days after surgery). Pericardial effusions are common. In heart transplant patients, effusions are associated with a higher incidence of acute rejection.

  h. Chest trauma, penetrating (stabbing, rib fractures) or nonpenetrating, including surgical procedures such as pacemaker insertion

  i. Dissecting aortic aneurysm

  j. Systemic disease: Uremia, myxedema, sarcoidosis, severe hypothyroidism (pericardial effusions)

  k. Immunologic or hypersensitivity reactions: Drug reactions (e.g., to hydralazine, procainamide, penicillin, phenytoin, isoniazid)

3. Signs and symptoms

  a. Subjective and objective findings

        i. Sharp or stabbing precordial pain, increased with inspiration, lying down, swallowing or belching, or turning of thorax; may be relieved by sitting up and/or leaning forward. Pain may also be dull (hard to distinguish from MI pain).

        ii. Associated trapezius ridge pain (specific for pericarditis)

        iii. Nonspecific influenza-like complaints such as low-grade fever, joint discomfort, fatigue, weight loss, night sweats

        iv. Weakness, exercise intolerance

        v. History of any of the etiologic findings

        vi. Recent history of taking immunosuppressive drugs (e.g., corticosteroids)

        vii. Weight loss

  b. Pulsus paradoxus: In cardiac tamponade, pulsus paradoxus is the result of the influence of respiration on the beat-to-beat filling of the LV by flow from the pulmonary veins

        i. During inspiration, there is less pulmonary venous return to the left side of the heart; this is exaggerated by impaired filling caused by high intrapericardiac pressure.

        ii. Result is decreased left-sided heart output and decreased blood pressure during inspiration.

        iii. Pulsus paradoxus is an inspiratory decrease in blood pressure of 11 mm Hg or greater.

        iv. Condition may not be seen in states in which LV filling is not solely dependent on pulmonary venous return (aortic insufficiency, VSD).

  c. Pericardial friction rub

        i. Has two or three components with scratchy or squeaky sounds. May be very transient. Absence of a rub does not rule out pericarditis.

        ii. Heard best with the stethoscope diaphragm pressed firmly

        iii. Loudest over the left mid-lower sternal border when the patient is sitting up and leaning forward

        iv. Having the patient hold the breath will help differentiate from pleural friction rub

  d. Other physical findings: Depending on the severity, any or all of the following symptoms may be observed:

        i. Dyspnea with or without pain, orthopnea

        ii. Cough, hemoptysis

        iii. Tachycardia

        iv. Fever

        v. Anxiety, confusion, restlessness

        vi. Pallor

       vii. Anorexia

      viii. Jugular venous distention

      ix. Kussmaul's sign (rise in CVP on inspiration): Seen in patients with constrictive pericarditis

      x. Flushing, sweating

      xi. Peripheral edema, abdominal swelling or discomfort (constrictive pericarditis)

      xii. Increased cardiac dullness in large effusions

      xiii. Hepatojugular reflux

      xiv. Heart sounds often normal except muffled and distant sounding with effusion

      xv. Pericardial "knock" in constriction

4. Diagnostic study findings

    a. Laboratory

      i. Troponin: Elevated levels mark myocardial injury

      ii. Moderate leukocytosis, increased sedimentation rate in acute or chronic pericarditis

      iii. C-reactive protein: Elevated levels

      iv. Blood cultures: To identify causative organisms and their sensitivity to antibiotics

      v. Antinuclear antibody test: Results positive in connective tissue diseases

      vi. BUN level: Renal status evaluation

      vii. Purified protein derivative testing: Tuberculosis

      viii. Pericardiocentesis, especially pericardial biopsy and drainage, may be helpful diagnostically

    b. ECG

      i. In acute pericarditis

        (a) Diffuse ST-segment elevation in most leads

        (b) PR segment may be depressed

        (c) ST segment reverts to normal and T wave inverts after several days

      ii. Dysrhythmias: Bradycardias, tachycardia (sinus or atrial dysrhythmias, atrial fibrillation)

    c. Radiologic: Normal or shows cardiac enlargement resulting from pericardial effusion

    d. Echocardiography: To identify and quantify pericardial effusions, wall motion abnormalities, RA and RV diastolic collapse (pretamponade)

      i. Results usually normal in acute pericarditis unless effusions present

      ii. In tamponade: Identifies pericardial effusions, LA compression, and respiratory variation in LV inflow of more than 25% (tamponade)

      iii. Restriction in ventricular filling (constriction)

    e. MRI, CT: To detect thickening of the pericardium, calcifications

    f. Right-sided heart catheterization: Used to

      i. Evaluate and monitor hemodynamics

      ii. Evaluate the severity of constriction

      iii. Assess the need for pericardiotomy

      iv. Assist in the differential diagnosis of constriction and restrictive cardiomyopathy

      v. Identify increased RV and LV filling pressures with equalization (constriction)

5. Goals of care

    a. Treatment is directed toward the underlying disease.

    b. Patient is comfortable, pain free, and without symptoms.

    c. Hemodynamics, vital signs, and ECG are within normal limits.

    d. Patient is free from complications (heart failure, tamponade).

    e. Laboratory values and clinical findings return to normal.

6. Collaborating professionals on health care team: See Chronic Stable Angina; also infectious disease specialist

7. Management of patient care

    a. Anticipated patient trajectory: Cardiac tamponade is a life-threatening condition, and the patient will die if emergent pericardiocentesis is not performed. Constrictive pericarditis is lethal and requires pericardiectomy. Pericarditis is generally self-limited.

      i. Positioning: Position the patient for comfort; sitting up and leaning forward will help to increase comfort

ii. Pain management
   (a) Frequently ask the patient about pain and discomfort; if present, assess characteristics.
   (b) Give medications to relieve pain caused by the inflammatory process (acetaminophen, aspirin, anti-inflammatory agents). Pain is often gone or diminished significantly in 24 to 48 hours but may last weeks. Corticosteroids are given for recurring, severe pain.
   (c) Reassure the patient regarding the nonischemic cause of the pain.
iii. Pharmacology
   (a) Antimicrobial agents: If culture or serologic evidence of a susceptible etiologic agent is present
   (b) NSAIDs: For pericarditis, pleural effusions. Use caution in patients with renal disease.
   (c) Corticosteroids: If unresponsive to NSAIDs after 48 hours. Used cautiously for short term and tapered quickly. They can contribute to recurrences due to viral proliferation.
   (d) Colchicine: May help prevent recurrences
   (e) Anticoagulants: Withheld with pericardial effusions to lower risk of tamponade. Heparin can be used, if necessary, because of its shorter half-life and reversibility.
   (f) Volume support (IV fluids) and/or inotropic agents (e.g., dobutamine): Used as a temporizing agent to improve CO during tamponade
iv. Treatments
   (a) Nursing care for cardiac tamponade
      (1) If tamponade occurs, place the patient in Trendelenburg's position, notify the physician.
      (2) Administer oxygen as ordered.
      (3) Prepare the patient for pericardiocentesis.
      (4) Emergency pericardiocentesis is life saving. Removal of 50 to 100 ml of fluid can bring major hemodynamic improvement.
      (5) If a pericardial catheter is present, aspirate pericardial fluid, per orders.
      (6) Give fluids to increase preload.
      (7) Discontinue agents that decrease preload (diuretics, nitrates, morphine).
   (b) Pericardiocentesis: For persistent effusions, tamponade, purulent pericarditis
      (1) Echocardiographic guidance of the procedure improves safety.
      (2) Sclerosing agents may be infiltrated intrapericardially for chronic effusions.
   (c) Pericardiotomy procedures for effusions and diagnostic biopsy, subxiphoid pericardiotomy, pericardial window surgery
   (d) Pericardiectomy: Treatment for constrictive pericarditis. Higher-risk surgery (10% to 25% mortality) in severe or chronic disease.
b. Potential complications
   i. Cardiac tamponade: Complication of pericarditis (see Treatments earlier)
   ii. Recurrent pericarditis
      (a) Mechanism
         (1) Probable autoimmune response, may reoccur numerous times, over years
         (2) Can be related to tapering or stopping of anti-inflammatory agents
      (b) Management
         (1) Corticosteroids often needed to stop painful symptoms. Steroid dependency and adverse side effects are major concerns. Nonsteroidal agents (e.g., colchicine, azathioprine) can be used to help avoid recurrence.
         (2) Pericardiectomy is considered when medical therapy is unsuccessful.

8. Evaluation of patient care
   a. Patient states that pain is reduced or alleviated.
   b. Laboratory values show that antimicrobial therapy is effective (e.g., leukocyte count and CBC returning to normal or within normal limits; blood culture results are negative).

Myocarditis

Myocarditis is an inflammation of the myocardium caused by various microorganisms, drugs, or chemicals. Can be acute or chronic (subacute) and focal or diffuse. It may mimic MI. There may be complete recovery, or it can lead to severe cardiovascular compromise and death from dilated cardiomyopathy.

1. **Pathophysiology**
   a. Myocardial damage occurs due to infection or injury.
   b. Interstitial infiltrates develop. Immune responses to inflammation ensue, and myocardial fibers become injured, hypertrophy, and begin to die.
   c. Necrosis of the myofibers may be global or spotty.
   d. Vascular responses to inflammation include vasculitis and spasm, which contribute to myocardial fibrosis and necrosis.
   e. Pericardial involvement often occurs at the same time.
   f. Contractility and CO decrease.
   g. LV function may be sufficiently impaired to cause heart failure.
   h. Myocardial injury can continue after active infection as a result of persistent immune and autoimmune responses.
2. **Etiology and risk factors**
   a. Causes can include viral, bacterial, rickettsial, parasitic, or mycotic organisms. There are also noninfectious causes, which include autoimmune disorders, drugs, and cardiac toxins.
   b. In Europe and North America, viral infection (in particular, infection with coxsackievirus B) is the most common cause of myocarditis.
   c. Viral
      i. Most common types include coxsackievirus A and B, adenovirus, and echovirus.
      ii. Others include influenza virus, cytomegalovirus, HIV, hepatitis B virus, and mumps and rubella viruses.
   d. Bacterial
      i. Infection with *Salmonella typhi, Coxiella burnetii*
      ii. Diphtheria: Most common cause of death
      iii. Tuberculosis
      iv. Streptococci, meningococci, clostridia, staphylococci
   e. Rickettsial
   f. Fungal: Aspergillosis
   g. Protozoal: Chagas' disease (*Trypanosoma cruzi*), seen in patients traveling to or living in Central and South America; malaria
   h. Autoimmune disorders: Systemic lupus erythematosus, Wegener's granulomatosis
   i. Cardiac toxins (e.g., cocaine, catecholamines)
   j. Drugs: Doxorubicin (Adriamycin), amitriptyline (Elavil)
3. **Signs and symptoms: Viral myocarditis is a diagnosis of exclusion. The responsible virus is very difficult to identify.**
   a. Clinical manifestations of viral myocarditis
      i. Patient may have complaints of a "common cold," fever, chills, sore throat, abdominal pain, nausea, vomiting, diarrhea, arthralgia, and myalgia up to 6 weeks before overt symptoms of heart failure appear.
      ii. Chest pain (two thirds of patients) with no evidence of pericarditis or ischemia. Pain may be pleuritic, precordial, or associated with sweating, nausea, or vomiting. Chest pain can imitate ischemic pain.
      iii. Dyspnea: Dyspnea at rest, exertional dyspnea, paroxysmal nocturnal dyspnea, orthopnea
      iv. Palpitations
      v. Fatigue, weakness
   b. Physical findings
      i. Tachycardia
      ii. Symptoms of heart failure (rapid, fulminant)
      iii. Increased jugular venous pressure

        iv. Enlarged lymph nodes: Seen with sarcoidosis

        v. Pruritic rash (maculopapular): Drug reaction

        vi. Pulsus alternans (extreme heart failure)

        vii. Narrow pulse pressure

        viii. Hypotension

        ix. S_1 diminished (decreased contractility)

        x. S_3 gallop: Common

        xi. Murmurs: Mitral or tricuspid regurgitation (if ventricular dilatation is present)

        xii. Pericardial friction rub: Uncommon

4. Diagnostic study findings

    a. Laboratory

        i. Cultures (blood, throat, urine, stool specimens): To rule out bacterial and fungal causes

        ii. Cardiac enzyme levels

        iii. CBC: Slight to moderate leukocytosis

        iv. Erythrocyte sedimentation rate: Elevated

        v. Titers for *Rickettsia*, virus, fungus

        vi. Skin test for tuberculosis

    b. Radiologic: Findings may be normal or

        i. Pulmonary congestion

        ii. Cardiomegaly

    c. ECG

        i. Sinus tachycardia

        ii. ST segment can be elevated, T waves inverted; nonspecific ST, T-wave changes.

        iii. QTc interval is prolonged.

        iv. ST returns to baseline in several days.

        v. T-wave changes may last weeks or months (with severe myocarditis).

        vi. Dysrhythmias are seen in one third of patients.

            (a) VT, supraventricular tachycardia (SVT), premature ventricular contractions

            (b) Atrial fibrillation

            (c) AV blocks

    d. Echocardiography: Used to rule out other causes of heart failure and evaluate LV function

        i. Diffuse hypocontractility

        ii. Pericardial effusions

        iii. Valvular dysfunction

        iv. Chamber enlargement

        v. Ventricular thrombi

    e. Endocardial biopsy: Although myocarditis is a nonspecific histologic diagnosis, routine biopsy has no proven utility, because of the high level of insensitivity and numerous false-negative results (up to 55% when only five specimens are obtained)

    f. Right-sided heart catheterization: To evaluate hemodynamic measurement such as CO, CI, SVR, pulmonary vascular resistance (PVR) for LV function

    g. Coronary angiography: To exclude other causes of heart failure; CAD, valvular disease, congenital disorders

    h. EPS: If history of sudden death, VF, and/or VT

5. Goals of care

    a. CO, hemodynamics, and vital signs are within normal limits.

    b. Patient has no dysrhythmias.

    c. Patient has no signs or symptoms of heart failure.

    d. Plan is developed for progressive activities and exercise.

    e. Patient shows a progressive (slow) increase in activity tolerance.

6. Collaborating professionals on health care team: See Chronic Stable Angina; also infectious disease specialist

7. Management of patient care

    a. Anticipated patient trajectory: Usually a mild disease; bed rest is important, along with management of symptoms. Patient is often in a stepdown unit, unless symptoms of heart failure, heart block, or other complications arise.

    i.   Positioning
- (a) Maintain bed rest at first (the patient needs activities restricted); exception would be use of a bedside commode, if tolerated.
- (b) Allow patient to slowly ambulate with assistance.
- (c) Monitor heart, respiratory rates, blood pressure, and oxygen saturation with activity.

    ii.   Pain management: Relieve chest pain promptly

    iii.   Nutrition: Low-sodium diet, fluid restriction, if signs of heart failure are present

    iv.   Discharge planning
- (a) Instruct the patient about the need for a progressive increase in ambulation over the next 2 months.
- (b) Teach the patient which symptoms to look for and report regarding activity tolerance. Patient should be able to monitor his or her pulse.
- (c) Facilitate and assist with the development of an activity and exercise program for the patient, both in the hospital and at home.

    v.   Pharmacology
- (a) Oxygen: Ensure adequate oxygenation; check pulse oximetry results, maintain oxygen saturations at over 92%. Hypoxia is common with myocarditis.
- (b) Afterload reduction agents (ACE inhibitors, ARBs, diuretics): For cardiac failure
- (c) IV pressors and inotropic agents: If hemodynamic support is needed
- (d) Antiarrhythmics: As needed; monitor closely for dysrhythmias—high risk for sudden death
- (e) Antiviral therapy (pleconaril): Used for enteroviruses
- (f) β-Blockers : To decrease heart rate, dysrhythmias
- (g) Immunosuppressive therapy: Has not proved beneficial for preservation of LV function or survival (except in a small number of patients)
- (h) NSAIDs: Ineffective; may facilitate disease process, increase mortality

    vi.   Treatments: Focused on managing symptoms
- (a) Treat causative agent if known.
- (b) Temporary transvenous pacemaker for AV blocks
- (c) Temporary left ventricular assist devices (LVADs) may be required: IABP, LVAD to assist in CO and as a bridge to transplantation.
- (d) Heart transplantation

b. Potential complications

    i.   Dysrhythmias
- (a) Mechanism: Myocardial injury, infection
- (b) Management
  - (1) SVTs: Cardioversion
  - (2) Heart blocks: Temporary transvenous pacemaker (transient condition usually not requiring permanent pacemaker)

    ii.   Dilated cardiomyopathy, heart failure
- (a) Mechanism: Can develop slowly over time
- (b) Management: Patient with myocarditis routinely followed to evaluate LV function

8. Evaluation of patient care

  a. Plan of care is consistent with the patient's responses to activity, and appropriate limits are set.

  b. Support services and significant others are actively involved in the patient's rehabilitation.

Infective Endocarditis

Infective endocarditis (IE) is an acute or a chronic infection of the heart's endocardial surface, including valves, chordae tendineae, septum, and mural endothelium. Median age of affected patients has increased to 50 years, because of the decrease in rheumatic heart disease, increase in longevity, and emergence of nosocomial causes. Disease frequency is 2.5 times greater in men than in women.

1. **Pathophysiology**
   a. Infecting organisms may be present in the bloodstream (may be a very transient invasion).
   b. Valves and endothelial surface of the heart can be predisposed to injury. Infecting organisms have an affinity for traumatized areas and preexisting defects such as with valvular disease, prosthetic valves, septal defects, or local trauma (from indwelling catheters).
   c. When traumatic injury from abnormal hemodynamic or endothelial stress has occurred, deposits of platelets and fibrin form microscopic thrombotic lesions.
   d. Affected areas are then amenable to colonization by microorganisms. Bacteria and organisms from other infections in the body (skin, genitourinary tract, lungs, mouth) attach to the valves and to these thrombotic lesions.
   e. As the microorganisms colonize, they cause the deposition of platelets, leukocytes, erythrocytes, and fibrin, forming vegetations. Eventually, valvular tissue is destroyed by the infection, and the valve leaflets may become incompetent, ulcerate, rupture, abscess (ring or annular), or perforate.
   f. Valves on the left side of the heart are more often affected (85% of cases). Mitral valve is most commonly affected. Right-sided IE is predominantly caused by IV drug use and generally involves the tricuspid and pulmonic valves.
   g. The bacteria and other microorganisms from the vegetations are circulated systemically, which causes bacteremia.
   h. Antibody formation increases the levels of immune complexes in the blood, which causes hypersensitivity reactions (allergic vasculitis) in peripheral parts of the body involving the arterioles, vessel walls, and cutaneous tissue.
   i. Embolization of infective material may occur throughout body (left-sided vegetation causes systemic emboli; tricuspid valve vegetation causes pulmonary emboli).
2. **Etiology and risk factors**
   a. A wide variety of microorganisms cause endocarditis. Common organisms include the following:
      i. *Streptococcus* types (50% to 60%)
         (a) *Streptococcus viridans*: Had been the most prevalent causative organism in subacute cases (now involved in only approximately one third of cases)
         (b) Group B, D, or G streptococci
         (c) Enterococci: Often a nosocomial cause; resistant to medical therapy
      ii. *Staphylococcus* types (15% to 40%)
         (a) *Staphylococcus aureus*: Most prevalent causative organism in acute and nosocomial cases (i.e., methicillin-resistant strains)
         (b) Coagulase-negative species: Often the cause of prosthetic valve endocarditis
      iii. Gram-negative rods (HACEK organisms [*Haemophilus* species, *Actinobacillus actinomycetemcomitans, Cardiobacterium hominis, Eikenella corrodens, Kingella kingae*])
      iv. Enterobacteriaceae: *Pseudomonas aeruginosa*
      v. Fungi: *Candida albicans, Aspergillus fumigatus*
      vi. Viruses: Coxsackievirus, adenovirus
   b. Surgery or procedures predisposing to IE bacteremia risk
      i. Dental procedures (extractions, surgery, cleaning) that cause mucosal or gingival bleeding: Cause 20% of cases of bacteremia
      ii. Tonsillectomy, adenoidectomy
      iii. Bowel surgeries, esophageal procedures
      iv. Genitourinary surgery, biopsies
   c. Other therapies and procedures predisposing patients to IE bacteremia risk
      i. Invasive tests and monitoring (pulmonary artery catheters)
      ii. Prolonged IV therapy (hyperalimentation)
      iii. Immunosuppressive therapy
      iv. Hemodialysis
   d. Medical conditions that predispose to IE
      i. Prosthetic valve
      ii. Rheumatic valvular disease: Previously most common predisposing condition (accounts for 7% to 18% of cases)

       iii.   Previous IE episode

       iv.   Congenital heart defect (e.g., PDA, coarctation of the aorta, VSD): About 14% of cases

       v.   Degenerative valve disease: About 9% of cases

       vi.   Mitral valve prolapse

       vii.   Hypertrophic, obstructive cardiomyopathy

       viii.   Abscesses on skin

       ix.   Inflammatory gastrointestinal disease, gastrointestinal tumors

   e. Other factors: IV drug abuse, unidentified causes of IE bacteremia (30% to 40% of IE cases)

3. **Signs and symptoms**

   a. Subjective findings: Patient may complain of nonspecific, vague symptoms

       i.   Fever (prolonged, unknown source, sudden onset)

       ii.   Chills, night sweats

       iii.   Fatigue, malaise

       iv.   Neurologic dysfunctions: Headache, vision loss, stroke, confusion

       v.   Nausea, vomiting, anorexia, weight loss

       vi.   Arthralgias, myalgias

       vii.   Back pain (cause unknown)

       viii. Dyspnea

   b. Physical findings: Depend on the presence of a systemic versus a local infection, the presence of systemic emboli, immune responses, and the duration of infection

       i.   Fever: Temperature higher than 100.4° F (38° C)

       ii.   Signs and symptoms of heart failure

       iii.   Petechiae (caused by emboli or allergic vasculitis): Seen in 20% to 40% of patients on the conjunctivae, neck, chest, abdomen, and mucosa of the mouth (usually a sign of a long-standing infection)

       iv.   Osler's nodes (resulting from immunologically mediated vasculitis): Small, very tender, reddened, raised nodules on fingers and toe pads

       v.   Roth's spots (resulting from emboli or allergic vasculitis): Round or oval white spots on the retina

       vi.   Purpuric pustular skin lesions (caused by emboli)

       vii.   Janeway lesions (caused by septic emboli or allergic vasculitis): Large, nontender nodules on the palms of the hands, toes, and soles of the feet

       viii.   Splinter hemorrhages of the nails (resulting from emboli or allergic vasculitis)

       ix.   Conduction disturbances seen on ECG

       x.   Central nervous system disturbances (e.g., hemiplegia, confusion, headache, seizures, transient ischemic attacks, aphasia, ataxia, changes in the level of consciousness, psychiatric symptoms) if embolization to the brain has occurred

       xi.   Hematuria, oliguria, flank pain, hypertension, if the kidney is infarcted or abscessed from emboli. Glomerulonephritis frequently caused by allergic or immunologic reactions; kidney involvement is common.

       xii.   Tachypnea, dyspnea, hemoptysis, sudden pain in the chest or shoulder, cyanosis, and restlessness if the lung is infarcted

       xiii.   Abdominal pain (caused by mesenteric emboli)

       xiv.   Decreased or no pulses in cold limbs (emboli)

       xv.   Splenomegaly or pain caused by splenic infarction

       xvi.   If heart failure present, possible hepatojugular reflux, jugular venous distention, or peripheral edema

       xvii.   New murmurs of valvular insufficiency. Murmurs may also develop later, with therapy, and may change character.

       xviii. Decreased or absent breath sounds or adventitious breath sounds if the lungs are infarcted

4. **Diagnostic study findings**

   a. Laboratory data

       i.   Positive blood culture results (minimum of two separate sample sets initially, drawn 12 hours apart). Negative blood culture results do not necessarily rule out IE.

        ii.   Other associated findings
- (a) Elevated sedimentation rate and C-reactive protein level (immune response)
- (b) Anemia (common in subacute endocarditis)
- (c) Leukocytosis, thrombocytopenia (associated with splenomegaly)
- (d) Proteinuria, microscopic hematuria, pyuria
- (e) Rheumatoid factor levels may be elevated, as may circulating immune complex levels
- (f) Hyperglobulinemia (common)
- (g) Abnormal laboratory values associated with affected organs (kidneys, lungs, heart)

   b. ECG
- **i.** Signs of ischemia or infarction if coronary artery emboli have occurred
- **ii.** New AV blocks, BBB

   c. Chest radiograph: Occasional pleural effusion; multiple, patchy pulmonary infiltrates

   d. Transthoracic echocardiography: Presence of vegetations on any of the valves; assesses degree of valvular dysfunction and complications (e.g., ruptured chordae tendineae, perforated valve cusps)

   e. MRI or CT of head: With neurologic symptoms, to evaluate for infarction, abscess, or bleeding

   f. TEE: Better sensitivity for vegetations, recommended for prosthetic valves
- **i.** Excellent views of prosthetic valves, mitral valve, aortic valve, ring abscesses
- **ii.** Evaluation of ventricular function
- **iii.** Assessment of the severity of mitral regurgitation
- **iv.** Negative TEE results do not exclude IE.

   g. Catheterization: Preoperative evaluation, if valve replacement planned. Assesses the following:
- **i.** Valve dysfunction
- **ii.** Aneurysms, intracardiac shunts
- **iii.** Underlying CAD

5. Goals of care
- **a.** Patient is afebrile.
- **b.** Patient has negative blood culture results.
- **c.** Patient is well hydrated, as evidenced by normal skin turgor, balanced intake and output, and moist mucosa.

6. Collaborating professionals on health care team: See Chronic Stable Angina; also infectious disease specialist, home health nurse (IV therapy)

7. Management of patient care
- **a.** Anticipated patient trajectory: Prompt diagnosis is difficult but important for successful treatment. Prognosis is good with effective antibiotic therapy; however, mortality remains approximately 20%. Elderly patients with symptoms of heart failure, renal insufficiency, or systemic embolization have a worse prognosis.
  - **i.** Skin care: Monitor for problems in skin integrity resulting from fever and sweating. Ensure that the patient is turning or turned often while on bed rest.
  - **ii.** Nutrition
    - (a) Assess the patient for signs of dehydration.
    - (b) Monitor caloric and fluid intake and output. Weigh patient daily.
  - **iii.** Infection control
    - (a) Monitor vital signs, especially temperature. Persistent or recurring fevers can indicate failure of or hypersensitivity to antimicrobial therapy, nosocomial infections, emboli, abscesses, thrombophlebitis, or drug reaction.
    - (b) Assist in reduction of fever (e.g., administer antimicrobials, antipyretics, and cooling measures, as ordered; encourage fluid intake, if no evidence of heart failure).
    - (c) Draw several blood culture samples initially and if temperature spikes (proper technique for drawing blood samples for culture is vital because of the difficulty in choosing antibiotics to adequately treat microorganisms).

      (d) Ensure that proper preventive measures are taken against nosocomial causes: provide meticulous monitoring and care of indwelling catheters (change dressings and tubing; limit the duration of site use).

  iv. Discharge planning

      (a) Preventive teaching includes the following:

          (1) Discussion of the use of prophylactic antibiotics (for predisposing procedures, e.g., dental, bowel, bladder surgery). Provision of written material on high-risk procedures and recommended IE prophylaxis.

          (2) Stress good oral hygiene to decrease the frequency of bacteremia.

             a) Stress the importance of close monitoring (physician appointments, laboratory work) during therapy and for several months afterward. Patient needs to be aware of the symptoms (i.e., fever, rash) to report promptly. Relapses generally occur within 2 months after therapy has been completed.

             b) If the patient is to go home with continued outpatient IV antimicrobial therapy, then a demonstrated knowledge of drugs, indwelling catheter care, and home health services is necessary.

  v. Pharmacology

      (a) Antimicrobial-antibiotic therapy

          (1) Initiate as soon as possible after initial blood culture results (to halt continued valvular damage and abscess formation). Patient will likely receive prolonged IV antibiotic therapy.

          (2) Check antimicrobial peak and trough serum levels to monitor therapeutic effects and prevent toxicity.

          (3) Assess for musculoskeletal involvement (arthralgias, back pain, and myalgia are common symptoms). Antibiotic therapy usually helps decrease symptoms.

          (4) Fever usually stops after 3 days of therapy. If fever persists longer than 14 days, secondary infection or antibiotic resistance should be suspected.

          (5) If the patient is responding and stable, home outpatient IV therapy may be considered to finish the course of drug therapy.

      (b) Anticoagulants: Do not prevent IE emboli and may increase bleeding risks

  vi. Treatments

      (a) Prolonged IV administration of appropriate antimicrobials

      (b) Valve replacement surgery indicated (30% to 50% of cases) if the patient has significant damage to the valves (prosthetic valves), ring or annular abscesses, heart failure, or refractory bacteremia

          (1) With aortic valve IE, valve replacement is imperative.

          (2) In mitral or tricuspid valve IE, repair of valve is possible.

b. Potential complications

  i. Heart failure

      (a) Mechanism: Main cause of death from IE. Occurs when aortic and/or mitral valve becomes incompetent or regurgitant, or chordae tendineae rupture. May be progressive or acute (more often caused with aortic regurgitation).

      (b) Management

          (1) Assess the patient for signs and symptoms of heart failure.

          (2) Monitor for new murmurs during hospitalization. Murmurs may change or appear during the course of the illness.

          (3) Valve replacement surgery: Immediate surgery is generally required

  ii. Embolization

      (a) Mechanism: Occurs from vegetations on the valves. May be the presenting symptom; can happen at any time, and numerous events may occur. Seen in 20% to 50% of cases of IE. Often affects the central nervous system and the lower extremities, kidney, spleen, and bone.

      (b) Management

          (1) Assess the patient for signs and symptoms of systemic embolization.

(2) Monitor level of consciousness: Check for signs of cerebral emboli (e.g., headache, numbness, weakness, tingling, paralysis, ataxia, sudden blindness, or sudden hemiplegia).

(3) Check for petechiae on neck, upper trunk, eyes, and lower extremities.

(4) Observe the extremities for painful nodes, swelling, erythema, decreased or absent pulses, coolness, decreased capillary refill.

(5) Assess the patient for signs and symptoms of MI; monitor the ECG.

(6) Arrange for guaiac test of stools, tests for blood in urine and nasogastric aspirations.

(7) If pulmonary, myocardial, or cerebral embolism occurs, administer oxygen therapy, position the patient for comfort and ease of breathing, and give pain medications as ordered.

(8) Ultrasonography, CT, and/or MRI used in diagnosis

(9) This type of embolization is not treated with anticoagulants unless the patient has a previous indication for their use (such as a prosthetic valve). Anticoagulants have not proved to be beneficial in therapy and may result in the complication of intracranial hemorrhage.

(10) Treatment is aimed at the infection, and antimicrobials are given.

(11) Surgery for valve replacement is considered if embolization occurs more than once, if infection is uncontrolled, or if there is persistent heart failure.

   iii. Abscess

     (a) Mechanism: Occurs from contaminants, bacteremia

      (1) Cardiac valve ring abscess: Occurs with prosthetic valve endocarditis. Infection at the suture site of the valve can cause valve incompetency and dehiscence.

      (2) Extracardiac abscess: Often involves the spleen

     (b) Management: Splenectomy is the main therapy if the spleen is involved

   iv. Neurologic complications

     (a) Mechanism: Due to emboli and subsequent cerebral infarction, hemorrhage, cerebral abscesses, mycotic aneurysms (late complication). Neurologic complications are seen in 30% to 40% of IE patients and are associated with a high (40%) mortality rate.

     (b) Management: Watch for the development of headaches, seizures. See Chapter 4.

   v. Renal insufficiency

     (a) Mechanism: Caused by immune-response glomerulonephritis, renal embolic infarcts. Azotemia develops.

     (b) Management: Usually improves with antimicrobial therapy

   vi. Conduction defects

     (a) Mechanism: Due to infectious process at the aortic valve; affects the AV node or bundle of His and includes all AV blocks, BBB

     (b) Management: Surgical intervention generally required

8. Evaluation of patient care

  a. Patient's temperature returns to normal.

  b. Blood culture results are negative; there are no signs of active infection.

  c. Skin has normal turgor, and mucous membranes are moist; intake equals output.

  d. Cardiac function is normal.

  e. Patient has no evidence of systemic embolization, heart failure, or other complications.

Cardiomyopathy

Cardiomyopathy is a chronic or acute disorder of the heart muscle. The three classifications include dilated, hypertrophic, and restrictive cardiomyopathy.

1. Pathophysiology

  a. Dilated cardiomyopathy (DCM; most common type in the United States): Disorder is 2.5 times more common in males

    i. Myocardial fibers degenerate, and fibrotic changes occur.

    ii. Severe dilatation of the heart occurs; includes atrial and ventricular dilatation, which creates global enlargement.

      iii. Systolic and diastolic dysfunction occur and contractility decreases, which results in decreased SV, decreased EF, low CO, and compensatory increase in heart rate.

      iv. Mitral annular dilatation is secondary to LV dilatation and results in mitral insufficiency.

      v. Heart failure develops, is often refractory to treatment, and is accompanied by malignant ventricular dysrhythmias (often the cause of death).

  b. Hypertrophic cardiomyopathy (HCM)

      i. Increased mass and thickening of the heart muscle, which results in diastolic dysfunction

      ii. Myocytes become abnormal: lose their geometric parallel arrangement and become fibrotic.

      iii. Ventricles become rigid and stiff, restricting filling. Filling volumes decrease, and thus SV decreases.

      iv. LV chamber becomes very small (hypertrophy occurs inwardly at the expense of the LV chamber).

      v. LA becomes dilated.

      vi. Contractility may be normal or increased.

      vii. Obstructive form of HCM can occur: Often associated with an LV outflow tract dynamic obstruction that may be caused by concentric hypertrophy or localized hypertrophy. This obstructive form is referred to as *hypertrophic obstructive cardiomyopathy* (HOCM).

      viii. These processes may continue for years with no obvious problems and delayed onset of symptoms, or they may end with sudden cardiac death as a first sign of the disease process, due to malignant ventricular dysrhythmias (VF, VT).

      ix. Men and women are equally affected.

  c. Restrictive cardiomyopathy (least common)

      i. Restricted filling of ventricles

      ii. Usually caused by an infiltrative process, most often amyloidosis in adults

      iii. Heart loses its compliance, grows stiff, and cannot distend well in diastole or contract well in systole.

      iv. Left ventricular end-diastolic pressure (LVEDP) increases; contractility decreases, which results in low CO, heart failure, and death.

2. Etiology and risk factors

  a. DCM

      i. Idiopathic

      ii. Familial: 25% to 30% of cases

      iii. Infection (autoimmune reaction): Bacterial, parasitic, fungal, protozoal

      iv. Metabolic disorders: Chronic hypophosphatemia, thiamine deficiency, protein deficiency

      v. Toxins: Alcohol, lead, arsenic, uremic substances

      vi. Connective tissue disorders: Lupus erythematosus, rheumatoid disease, polyarteritis, scleroderma

      vii. Viral myocarditis

      viii. Drugs: Amitriptyline, doxorubicin, cocaine

      ix. Ischemia

      x. Pregnancy (third trimester) or the postpartum period (common in multiparous women who are older than 30 years or have a history of toxemia)

      xi. Neuromuscular disorders: Muscular dystrophy, myotonic dystrophy

      xii. Infiltrative disorders: Sarcoidosis, amyloidosis

      xiii. Beriberi

  b. Hypertrophic cardiomyopathy

      i. Strong familial component (60% to 70% of cases)

      ii. Idiopathic

      iii. Neuromuscular disorders: Friedreich's ataxia

      iv. Metabolic: Hypoparathyroidism

      v. Hypertension

c. Restrictive cardiomyopathy
   i.   Idiopathic
   ii. Infiltrative: Amyloidosis, sarcoidosis, hemochromatosis, neoplasms
   iii. Endomyocardial fibroelastosis in children
   iv. Glycogen and mucopolysaccharide deposition
   v.   Radiation
3. **Signs and symptoms: See Table 3-11 for physical findings associated with DCM, HCM, and restrictive cardiomyopathy. HCM may present at any age, may remain asymptomatic**.
   a. Ascertain the patient's chief complaint and the history of the present illness.
   b. Patient may complain of angina, syncope, palpitations, exertional dyspnea, orthopnea, fatigue.
   c. Determine whether there is a familial component (family history of cardiomyopathy or sudden death in young adults).
   d. Rule out other disease processes, such as hypertension, ischemic heart disease, amyloidosis, and toxemia.
   e. Identify potential etiologic factors such as recent infections, history of alcohol use, current use of medications, use of cocaine, pregnancy, and any endocrine disorders.
4. **Diagnostic study findings**
   a. Laboratory
      i.   Arterial blood gas (ABG) levels: Check for hypoxemia
      ii. Electrolyte levels: Decreased potassium, decreased magnesium
      iii. Cardiac enzyme levels: Infarct
      iv. Renal function: BUN, creatinine levels

■ **TABLE 3-11**
■ ■ **Physical Findings Associated with Dilated, Hypertrophic, and Restrictive Cardiomyopathy**

Cardiomyopathy	Patient Complaint	Inspection	Palpation	Percussion	Auscultation
Dilated	Dyspnea on exertion, orthopnea, fatigue, palpitations	Clinical manifestations of HF, dysrhythmias on monitor, conduction defects	Narrow pulse pressure, pulsus alternans, cool skin, JVD, PMI laterally displaced, left ventricular heave, peripheral edema, hepatomegaly	Cardiac enlargement, dullness in bases of lungs	Irregular heart beat, third and fourth heart sounds, mitral and tricuspid insufficiency, pulmonary rales
Hypertrophic	Dyspnea on exertion, orthopnea, PND, angina, syncope, palpitations	Dyspnea, orthopnea	Forceful and laterally displaced apical impulse, systolic thrill (in HOCM)		Fourth heart sound, a third heart sound may be heard, split-second heart sound, systolic ejection murmur
Restrictive	Fatigue, weakness, dyspnea on exertion, anorexia, poor exercise tolerance	Dysrhythmias, distended neck veins, Kussmaul's sign	Edema, ascites, HJR, right upper quadrant pain	Cardiac enlargement, pulmonary congestion	Third and fourth heart sounds, mitral and tricuspid insufficiency

HF, Heart failure; *HJR*, hepatojugular reflux; *HOCM*, hypertrophic obstructive cardiomyopathy; *JVD*, jugular venous distention; *PMI*, point of maximal impulse; *PND*, paroxysmal nocturnal dyspnea.

   b. Radiologic
      i.   Heart normal or enlarged
      ii. Pulmonary congestion
   c. ECG
      i.   Dysrhythmias or conduction defects (e.g., sinus tachycardia, atrial fibrillation, ventricular ectopy, BBBs)
      ii. Atrial fibrillation: High incidence (70% to 80%)
      iii. Evidence of both LA and LV enlargement: Increased QRS voltage
      iv. Abnormal Q waves
      v.   VT
      vi. Prolonged QTc interval
   d. Transthoracic echocardiography
      i.   LV systolic function: EF of 15% to 30% in DCM
      ii. Valvular dysfunction
      iii. LV hypertrophy (in HCM)
      iv. Marked asymmetric septal hypertrophy (in HCM, HOCM) and LV outflow tract pressure gradient (in HOCM)
      v.   LA enlargement
   e. Radionuclide tests: May reveal increased ventricular volumes, decreased EF in DCM, increased uptake in patients with amyloidosis, defects in cardiac wall in patients with neoplasms or sarcoidosis
   f. TEE: To evaluate anatomy and rule out thrombosis
   g. Right-sided heart catheterization: To determine hemodynamic measurements such as CO/CI, pulmonary artery pressures, PAOP (pulmonary artery occlusion pressure)
   h. Left-sided heart catheterization, angiogram, arteriogram
      i.   Rule out CAD
      ii. Mitral regurgitation
      iii. LV outflow tract gradient in HOCM
   i. EPS and Holter study: To identify VF and VT and to guide therapy
   j. Endomyocardial biopsy: To identify the cause of restrictive cardiomyopathy

5. Goals of care
   a. Symptoms of heart failure are relieved.
   b. Cause (especially if toxin) is determined and removed or treated.
   c. Sinus rhythm is maintained, if possible. Atrial fibrillation or other dysrhythmias are treated promptly.
   d. High risk of sudden death is reduced.

6. Collaborating professionals on health care team: See Chronic Stable Angina

7. Management of patient care
   a. Anticipated patient trajectory: In most patients, cardiomyopathy may be stabilized or actually improved with medical management. A few patients will succumb to progressive heart failure unless transplantation is possible.
      i.   Positioning: Use preventive measures, especially for patients at high risk
          (a) Assist with passive and active exercises while the patient is confined to bed.
          (b) Apply antiembolism stockings.
          (c) Encourage ambulation as tolerated.
          (d) Position the patient so that angulation at the groin and knees is avoided. Elevate the patient's legs when the patient is out of bed. Patient should be instructed not to cross the legs or ankles. Avoid using the knee joint on a Gatch bed.
          (e) Instruct the patient to avoid activities that may cause straining or increase the obstruction, such as strenuous exercise, Valsalva maneuvers, and sitting or standing suddenly.
      ii. Pain management: Administer supportive measures as the situation dictates (e.g., oxygen therapy, pain medications, sedatives, emotional support)
      iii. Nutrition: Sodium-restricted diet, weight control
      iv. Infection control: IE prophylactic therapy

v. Discharge planning: Patient education regarding the following:
  (a) Activities that aggravate symptoms
  (b) Benefits of weight reduction, sodium restriction, smoking and/or alcohol use cessation, exercise
  (c) Blood pressure control
  (d) Follow-up evaluations
  (e) Screening of family members (physical examination, laboratory tests, ECG, echocardiography) starting at age 12 years
vi. Pharmacology
  (a) ACE inhibitors: Used to decrease afterload and remodeling, improve LV EF
  (b) β-Blockers (e.g., metoprolol, atenolol)
     (1) Function by slowing or reversing the progression of LV dysfunction (due to hyperadrenergic tone)
     (2) Increase LV EF
     (3) Decrease heart rate, increase ventricular filling time
     (4) Decrease hospitalization for heart failure
  (c) Antiarrhythmic agents (atrial fibrillation, VT)
  (d) Anticoagulants: For atrial fibrillation (monitor INR, PTT; observe for bleeding)
  (e) Antibiotics: Because the patient is at risk for IE, instruct the patient to notify the dentist before any dental or surgical procedures (for prophylactic antibiotics)
  (f) Treatment specific to DCM
     (1) Inotropic agents to improve myocardial contractility and decrease heart failure
     (2) Diuretics to relieve pulmonary congestion; monitor volume status
     (3) Afterload- and preload-reducing agents such as ACE inhibitors and ARBs to decrease myocardial workload, improve CO, and decrease pulmonary venous pressure
     (4) Spironolactone: Helpful in decreasing mortality in heart failure
  (g) Treatment specific to HOCM
     (1) Goal is to administer medications to reduce outflow tract obstruction to relieve syncope, angina, dyspnea, and dysrhythmias, and prevent sudden cardiac death. β-Blockers (i.e., propranolol), calcium channel blockers (verapamil), or a type IA antiarrhythmic (i.e., disopyramide) are used.
     (2) Avoid agents that decrease preload (nitrates, diuretics, or morphine). Hypovolemia can be very detrimental because the LV is very preload dependent for adequate CO.
     (3) Avoid administering isoproterenol, dopamine, or digitalis preparations because they increase contractility and hence worsen the obstruction.
  (h) Treatment specific to restrictive cardiomyopathy: Avoid digoxin in patients with cardiac amyloidosis, because it concentrates in the amyloid fibrils and can result in digitalis toxicity
vii. Psychosocial issues
  (a) Help the patient identify stressors and teach methods of stress reduction.
  (b) Counseling may be needed for the patient and family members if alcohol or cocaine use is present and is suspected as a cause.
viii. Treatments
  (a) Closely monitor vital signs, ECG, intake and output, hemodynamics, laboratory values.
  (b) For HOCM patients
     (1) Surgical septal myectomy: Septal muscle creating obstruction is surgically excised. Hypertrophied muscle does not regenerate. Many patients can return to their normal lifestyles.
     (2) Septal ablation (alternative to surgery): Alcohol is injected, via a percutaneous transluminal catheter, into the small coronary artery supplying the obstructive area; muscle is destroyed and shrinks, which lessens the obstruction. Potential complications include heart blocks, dysrhythmias, VSD, and MI.

(c) Biventricular synchronized pacemaker used to help improve CO in DCM and HOCM
  (1) Patients with an LV EF of less than 35%, QRS of more than 0.12 mm. Used in older patients.
  (2) Can decrease obstruction. Increases activity tolerance and quality of life, used as a bridge.
  (3) Prepare the patient for this procedure. Be knowledgeable about the pacemaker procedure, equipment, protocols.
(d) Automatic implantable cardiac defibrillator (AICD): The following patients are candidates:
  (1) Patients who have experienced sudden cardiac death
  (2) Patients with impaired systolic function
(e) Patients with end-stage disease may be candidates for cardiac transplantation (see End-Stage Heart Disease).

b. Potential complications
  i. Heart failure, LV failure (see Heart Failure)
  ii. Dysrhythmias, particularly atrial and ventricular, on ECG: Atrial fibrillation, ventricular dysrhythmias (see Basic Dysrhythmias for Progressive Care). Dysrhythmias attributed to HCM are a common cause of sudden cardiac death in young adults.
    (a) With atrial fibrillation: Rate and rhythm control by cardioversion, drugs (e.g., amiodarone)
    (b) Patients at high risk for sudden cardiac death evaluated for AICD
    (c) Bradycardias, AV conduction defects may require permanent pacemakers.
  iii. IE: See Infective Endocarditis section
  iv. Embolism
    (a) Mechanism: Stasis of blood can cause deep venous thrombosis, pulmonary embolism
      (1) Patients at risk are the elderly and immobile patients on bed rest; patients who are in heart failure or atrial fibrillation, or who have a dilated myocardium.
      (2) Yearly risk of systemic embolization and stroke with HOCM and atrial fibrillation is 20%.
    (b) Management: Long-term anticoagulation, use of supportive stockings, performance of range-of-motion exercises

8. Evaluation of patient care
  a. Patient is hemodynamically stable; vital signs are within set parameters for the patient.
  b. Patient is alert and oriented.
  c. Sinus rhythm is maintained, atrial fibrillation is rate controlled.
  d. Lungs are clear on auscultation.
  e. Patient has no embolic episodes or pulmonary congestion. Sequelae of cardiomyopathy are minimized or absent.
  f. Patient can identify and recognize the need for management measures such as prevention of endocarditis, anticoagulation therapy and monitoring of parameters, and follow-up.

End-Stage Heart Disease

In end-stage heart disease, the disease has advanced to a point at which all possible medical or surgical interventions have been exhausted. Life expectancy is less than 24 months. Patient is free of other life-threatening disease; dysfunction of other organ systems is reversible.

1. Pathophysiology
  a. Severe LV dysfunction with CO; EF is less than 25%
  b. See Pathophysiology subsection under Heart Failure

2. Etiology and risk factors
  a. Ischemic heart disease and CAD
  b. DCM: Idiopathic or secondary to pregnancy or viral infections
  c. Valvular disease
  d. Drug-related myocardial injury

e. Congenital heart disease

f. Infection (Chagas' disease)

3. Signs and symptoms: The number of candidates for transplantation far exceeds the number of donor hearts. Careful assessment and selection are necessary to determine who can potentially return to a functional life after transplantation, as well as to ensure that all conventional remedies have been exhausted.

a. Subjective findings: Complaints of dyspnea, angina, low exercise tolerance (bed-to-chair existence, bedridden)

b. Physical findings

   i. Severe heart failure necessitating frequent "tune-ups" and hospitalizations

   ii. Cardiac cachexia: Anorexia, weight loss

   iii. Life-threatening dysrhythmias

4. Diagnostic study findings

a. See Heart Failure. Follow-up studies to evaluate disease progression and treatment effectiveness and to prevent complications.

b. Right-sided heart catheterization: Used to guide therapy

   i. Assess PVR

     (a) Irreversible pulmonary hypertension is a cause of perioperative mortality.

     (b) Donor heart cannot generate pressure high enough to maintain a sufficient pulmonary flow.

     (c) Patients with irreversible pulmonary hypertension may be candidates for heart-lung transplantation.

     (d) Pharmacologic agents (e.g., sildenafil) may be used to evaluate the potential for reversibility of increased PVR.

c. Cardiac arteriography: Pretransplantation to ascertain the degree of CAD and the potential for revascularization

d. Cardiac biopsy: To rule out amyloidosis and identify patients with sarcoidosis or myocarditis for possible immunosuppressive therapy

e. EPS: To assess the effectiveness of antiarrhythmic therapy

5. Goals of care

a. Balanced fluid status, intake, and output are maintained.

b. Patient and family participate in identifying lifestyle changes and support required in coping with transplantation.

c. Patient tolerates the new heart (successful transplantation).

6. Collaborating professionals on health care team: See Chronic Stable Angina; also electrophysiologist, transplant coordinator, psychologist, home health aide, financial services counselor

7. Management of patient care

a. Anticipated patient trajectory: Heart transplantation is the standard of care and is performed in patients of all ages from newborn to 65 years. Mortality rate is as low as 4% from heart transplantation; average survival time is longer than 5 years.

   i. Positioning: Head of bed elevated for patient comfort and breathing ease

   ii. Nutrition

     (a) Assess nutritional status: To optimize the potential for posttransplantation success and facilitate the healing process

     (b) Restrict diet to less than 2 g sodium, 1000 to 1500 ml fluid

   iii. Infection control

     (a) Observe for and prevent infections (from IV drips, central lines, immunosuppressive therapies). Screen visitors for communicable illnesses because of the patient's suppressed immune system. (Have visitors use masks, wash hands, limit contact.)

     (b) Administer antimicrobial prophylaxis used to prevent nosocomial infections.

   iv. Discharge planning

     (a) Discuss with the patient and family the following aspects of the transplantation process:

       (1) Body image changes with the new heart

   (2) Importance of family support

   (3) Unknown waiting period

   (4) Cost: Huge financial burden; insurance coverage

   (5) Frequency of checkups, tests; stress need for regular examinations

   (6) Possibility of failure to be accepted as a transplantation candidate

   (7) Possibility of rejection reaction after transplantation

   (8) Dependency issues

   (9) Arrange for the patient and family to talk with transplantation survivors.

  (b) Home oxygen: May be required for dyspnea, pulmonary congestion

  (c) Home health care: Includes IV therapy

  (d) Information on the use of indwelling catheters: For home-based IV therapy to reduce infection risks

  (e) Hospitalizations: Patient and significant others need to be instructed with regard to the following:

   (1) Possible need for frequent hospital visits for "tune-ups," medication changes, close observation

   (2) Need for high-dose medications

   (3) Use of mechanical assists: IABP, VAD, ventilators

v. Pharmacology: See also Heart Failure

  (a) Preload reduction: Diuretics, nitrates

  (b) IV inotropic drugs (e.g., milrinone, dobutamine to increase CO, improve renal perfusion)

  (c) Afterload reduction

  (d) Antiarrhythmic therapy

  (e) Anticoagulation: For risk of thromboembolism

  (f) Immunosuppressive protocols (e.g., cyclosporine, tacrolimus, steroids)

  (g) Statin therapy: Lowering lipid levels shows positive effects on cardiac allograft rejection; immunosuppressive drugs can cause hyperlipidemia

  (h) Antibiotic prophylaxis

vi. Psychosocial issues

  (a) Prepare the patient for the rigors of waiting for transplantation and the care before and after.

  (b) Assess emotional status: psychiatric history, motivational issues. Transplantation is a major stressful undertaking.

  (c) Assess the support system: strong family, friends, and medical support are needed.

  (d) Assess financial issues: insurance coverage for costly procedure, drugs, follow-up care.

  (e) Determine alcohol and drug use history.

  (f) Assess the ability to comply with a complex lifelong medical regimen: frequent follow-up examinations (include endomyocardial biopsies, strict medication protocols, rejection issues). Transplantation requires active patient participation.

  (g) Determine dependency issues. Formulate a plan with the patient and significant others.

   (1) Allow the patient to do what he or she can.

   (2) Family is included in care in the hospital.

   (3) Home services are arranged.

   (4) Need for immediate readiness is emphasized. When a donor heart becomes available, ischemic time (time from cross-clamp [donor] to cross-clamp [recipient]) must be less than 5 hours (or the heart is not usable); therefore, the patient must not travel.

vii. Treatments

  (a) Patient refractory to IV inotropic therapy should be transported to a facility with a cardiac transplantation program.

  (b) AICD may need to be placed to prevent sudden death.

(c) Extracorporeal devices (e.g., LVAD) are used as a bridge to transplantation or therapy for patients (see Heart Failure).

(d) Evaluate the potential for posttransplantation success.

(1) In patients with insulin-dependent diabetes, steroid therapy after transplantation can increase blood glucose levels.

(2) In patients with renal disease, cyclosporine therapy is nephrotoxic.

(e) Teaching points for immediately postoperative cardiac transplantation care are similar to those for CABG care.

b. Potential complications

i. Related to ventricular dysfunction: Dysrhythmias, heart failure, cardiomyopathy

ii. Postoperative CABG complications and additional transplantation complications, which include the following:

(a) Allograft rejection

(b) RV failure from high pulmonary vascular resistance

(c) Bradycardia: Pacemaker may be needed; isoproterenol may be used. Atropine will not help denervated transplanted heart.

(d) Immunosuppressive therapy complications

(1) Increased susceptibility to infection

(2) Adverse effects that can include nephrotoxicity, hypertension, hyperlipidemia, seizures

8. Evaluation of patient care

a. Balanced fluid status (intake and output) is maintained.

b. Patient and family actively participate in the plan of care.

c. Transplantation process is successful. Patient is tolerating the new heart without signs of infection or rejection.

d. Patient demonstrates an understanding of the information and skills required for complex home management.

Basic Dysrhythmias for Progressive Care

Life-threatening cardiac rhythms are divided into dysrhythmias that are either too slow, too fast, or unable to generate an adequate pulse.

Symptomatic Bradycardia: Bradycardias, Conduction Defects, and Slow Escape Rhythms

1. Pathophysiology

a. Dysfunction of the SA node: Result of ischemia, infarction, disease, degeneration, defects, or drug effects (SA exit blocks, severe sinus bradycardia, sinus pause, sinus arrest, sick sinus syndrome)

b. Dysfunction of the AV node: Result of ischemia, infarction, disease, defects, degeneration, or drug effects; leads to AV conduction defects—second-degree, types I and II, third-degree (complete) heart block

i. AV nodal tissue slows or fails to propagate electrical impulses to the ventricles.

ii. Slower pacemaker cells in lower sites (junctional, bundle of His, ventricular) escape and take over as the cardiac pacemaker in third-degree blocks.

iii. In acute anterior MI, complete heart block develops in 6% to 10% of patients.

iv. In inferior MI, ischemia or infarction of the AV node may create a temporary conduction defect, which usually resolves in less than a week.

c. Hypersensitivity of the carotid sinus: Exaggerated response to vagal stimulation causes slowing of the heart rate and conductivity and lowering of the blood pressure

2. Etiology and risk factors

a. Parasympathetic or vagal stimulation: Valsalva maneuver, nausea, vomiting, suctioning

b. Aging: Structural degeneration of the conductive system

c. MI, ischemic heart disease

d. Drugs: Calcium channel blockers (verapamil, diltiazem); cardiac glycosides (digoxin); β-blockers (propranolol)

e. Infectious process: Endocarditis, myocarditis, typhoid fever, rheumatic fever, Chagas' disease

    f. Metabolic disorders: Myxedema, hypothermia, hypercalcemia

    g. Aortic stenosis

    h. Tumors

    i. Trauma (post–cardiac surgery)

    j. Connective tissue disease (sarcoidosis, amyloidosis, systemic lupus erythematous, thyroid disease)

    k. Dive reflex (immersion in cold water)

3. Signs and symptoms

    a. Syncope or presyncope

    b. Wooziness, light-headedness

    c. Fatigue, weakness

    d. Shortness of breath

    e. Angina

    f. Pauses in pulse longer than 3 seconds

    g. Heart rates lower than 40 beats/min

    h. Hypotension

    i. Signs of heart failure, cardiogenic shock

    j. Dyspnea

    k. Exercise intolerance

    l. Decreased CO, CI

4. Diagnostic study findings

    a. ECG: See Table 3-4 for dysrhythmia features

        i. Correlation of symptoms with documented ECG is main diagnostic tool.

        ii. Pauses more than 3 seconds in duration

        iii. Third-degree heart block with inferior MI: Usually narrow QRS complex accompanies bradycardia (higher escape pacemaker)

        iv. Third-degree heart block with anterior MI: Wide QRS complex may be observed (lower escape pacemaker)

    b. Holter monitoring: To identify dysrhythmias not documented elsewhere and correlate with symptoms

    c. EPS: To test SA and AV node function, confirm need for permanent pacemaker

5. Goals of care

    a. Hemodynamics are improved via improved heart rate.

    b. Symptoms from bradycardia are decreased or absent.

6. Collaborating professionals on health care team: See Chronic Stable Angina; also electrophysiologist

7. Management of patient care

    a. Anticipated patient trajectory: Marked bradycardia results in diminished CO, poor tissue perfusion, hypotension, and potentially loss of consciousness and death

        i. Infection control: Proper wound care and site observation (for drainage, redness, tenderness) is necessary to decrease the potential for infection from pacemakers. Monitor temperature, laboratory results (white blood cell count).

        ii. Discharge planning: Patient education regarding the following:

            (a) Rationales, procedure, and wound care for pacer placement

            (b) Daily pulse checks at home (permanent pacemaker)

            (c) Symptoms to report: Wooziness, fainting, prolonged weakness, fatigue, palpitations, chest pain, difficulty breathing, fever, redness, drainage or swelling at surgical site, prolonged hiccups, electrical shocks

            (d) Follow-up care: To assess pacemaker function, adjust pacemaker parameters

            (e) Hazards or interference to avoid: Digital pagers, cellular phones, microwaves less than 1 ft away

            (f) Identification bracelet (medical alert)

            (g) Home (telephonic) pacemaker monitoring

        iii. Pharmacology

            (a) If the patient is symptomatic, administer atropine, 0.5 to 1.0 mg IV.

                (1) Given every 3 to 5 minutes IV; total IV dosage of up to 0.04 mg/kg

   (2) Effective for marked sinus bradycardia, second-degree and some third-degree blocks

   (3) Dose of less than 0.5 mg IV can cause paradoxical bradycardia.

  (b) Other potential medications include dopamine, epinephrine, isoproterenol.

  (c) Isoproterenol is used for heart transplant patients; because of vagal denervation, these patients will not respond to atropine.

 iv. Treatments

  (a) If the patient is in stable condition or asymptomatic: Monitor closely, notify the physician, determine possible causes, have medications and transcutaneous pacemaker equipment readily available (especially if the patient is in third-degree block or second-degree AV block type II)

  (b) Ensure adequate oxygenation: Oxygen saturations of 92% or higher

  (c) IV lines: Check patency

  (d) Pacemakers: If the patient is unable to maintain adequate CO, use of a temporary or permanent pacemaker is indicated

   (1) Purpose: To provide an extrinsic electrical impulse so that depolarization and subsequent contraction occur

   (2) Modes of pacing (see Figure 3-14)

    a) Fixed rate (asynchronous): Impulses are delivered at a predetermined rate, irrespective of any intrinsic electrical activity

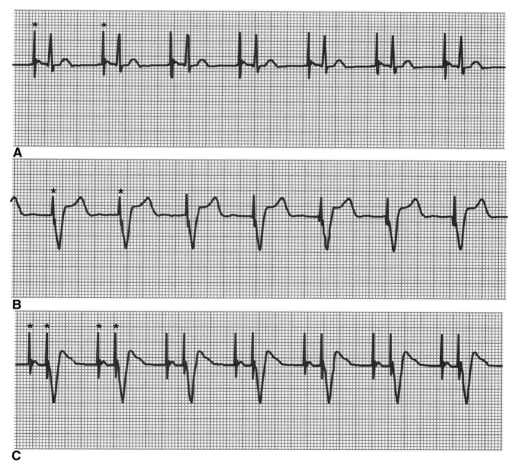

FIGURE 3-14 ■ Pacing examples. **A,** Atrial pacing. **B,** Ventricular pacing. **C,** Dual-chamber pacing. The asterisk indicates the pacemaker impulse. (From Urden LD, Stacy KM, Lough ME. *Thelan's Critical Care Nursing: Diagnosis and Management.* Philadelphia, PA: Mosby; 2002:378.)

b) Demand (synchronous): Impulses are delivered at a predetermined rate only if the patient's own heart rate is less than the pacemaker's set rate

c) Dual chamber: Pacemakers that can sense electrical activity in and pace either or both chambers to provide the normal sequence of atrial and ventricular contraction (AV sequential pacing) are the most common

d) Rate responsive: Pacemakers increase the heart rate to meet the demands of increased activity

(3) Components of all pacemakers

a) Battery

1) In temporary pacers, battery longevity depends on use and capabilities. Batteries should be checked routinely and changed per unit standards.

2) Permanent pacemaker batteries last 7 to 10 years (varies with the degree of the patient's pacemaker dependency).

b) Lead system: Transmission of electrical impulse as follows:

1) Unipolar electrode systems: One pole is the pacing lead tip and the other pole is the pacemaker generator; produce large pacing spikes, easily seen on monitors and ECGs

2) Bipolar electrode systems (most common): Both negative and positive electrode poles are at the distal end of the pacing lead; produce small pacing spikes, often not seen on monitors and ECGs

c) Pulse generator; pacemaker's control box

(4) Capture threshold level: Minimum pacemaker output setting required to pace the heart 100%

a) Factors increasing the threshold: Hyperkalemia, hypoxia, drugs (β-blockers, type I antiarrhythmics)

b) Factors decreasing the threshold: Increased catecholamine levels, digitalis toxicity, corticosteroids

(e) Transcutaneous pacemaker: Emergency therapy used until a transvenous pacer can be inserted. Many have monitoring, defibrillation, and pacing capabilities.

(1) One large anterior pacing electrode is ideally placed over the heart, and the other is placed directly posterior on the back. Other models have sternal-apex electrodes.

(2) Pacemaker electrodes are attached to an output cable attached to a pacing unit. Pacing unit is generally part of a portable defibrillator unit.

(3) Pacing rate and output are then set. Rate initially is set at 80 beats/min. Output is gradually increased until a pacer spike with a depolarization (pacer-generated QRS) is seen.

(f) Transvenous pacemaker: Pacing catheter is placed via the percutaneous route to the RA, RV, or both for pacing. The proximal end of the catheter is attached to a pacing generator.

(1) Initial rate usually set at 60 to 80 beats/min.

(2) Output is set to an intermediate level (approximately 5 mA) and decreased until capture is lost (usually at less than 2 mA).

(3) Pacing output is then set to two to three times the level required for capture.

(g) Epicardial transthoracic pacing: Electrode wires are attached to the epicardium (RA, RV, or both). Used during cardiac surgery in anticipation of conduction defects or dysrhythmias. Proximal ends exit through the chest wall for attachment to the pulse generator.

(1) Electrode wires need to be insulated when not in use.

(2) May have one or two RA and one or two RV wires and a ground wire

(h) Permanent pacemaker: Leads placed in contact with the endocardium. Generator is implanted in a subcutaneous, subclavicular, or abdominal pocket. Capabilities can include sequential pacing of the RA, RV, or both; programmability and rate responsiveness to allow for heart rate increases during exercise.

(i) Key points for nursing care of patients with pacemakers: See Box 3-7

▓ **BOX 3-7**
▓ **KEY POINTS IN THE NURSING CARE OF PATIENTS WITH PACEMAKERS**

TRANSCUTANEOUS PACEMAKERS
- Patient will need sedation and analgesia because of increased output requirements (50 to 200 mV) for transcutaneous route.
- Cardiopulmonary resuscitation may be performed safely over pacing electrodes, if needed.
- Frequent inspection of skin is needed to prevent potential burns, if pacing is prolonged.

EPICARDIAL TRANSTHORACIC PACEMAKER
- Electrode wires need to be insulated when not in use.

PERMANENT PACEMAKER
- Keep defibrillator paddles 1 to 2 inches away from permanent pacemaker site on chest.
- Ensure pacer is interrogated after defibrillation or code is over.
- Have magnet (doughnut) available: Used over pacer to program to asynchronous mode if pacemaker-mediated tachycardia is suspected or if electrocautery is to be used.

  b. Potential complications
     i.   Monitor for complications of pacemaker insertion.
        (a) Pneumothorax
        (b) Myocardial perforation: Can lead to hypotension, tamponade
        (c) Hematoma
        (d) Dysrhythmias (premature ventricular contractions)
        (e) Infections (systemic or local)
        (f) Hiccups, muscle twitches (from stimulation of the diaphragm, abdomen)
     ii. Monitor for pacemaker malfunctions (Box 3-8 and Figures 3-15 and 3-16).
8. Evaluation of patient care
  a. Heart rate is sufficient to maintain stable vital signs and CO.
  b. Dysrhythmias are controlled or absent.
  c. Pacemaker functions properly with no signs of failure to pace, capture, or sense.
  d. Patient or significant other verbalizes an understanding of the rationale, procedure, and follow-up for pacemaker use.

Symptomatic Tachycardia

Rhythms in this section include SVTs or VTs that cause symptoms necessitating immediate conversion or control.

1. Pathophysiology
  a. With increased heart rate at rest, diastolic filling period shortens and CO falls because of decreased ventricular filling.
  b. Eventually, blood pressure drops.
  c. Pulmonary venous pressures increase, causing shortness of breath and dyspnea as the result of pulmonary congestion.
  d. Heart rate at which CO declines is variable and depends on the patient's substrate cardiac function.
  e. Myocardial oxygen demands increase and myocardial oxygen supply decreases due to diminished coronary perfusion at rapid heart rates; subendocardial ischemia can result.
  f. Loss of atrial systole (kick) decreases the ventricular diastolic filling volume; SV and CO fall 10% to 15% in rhythms without a normal atrial-ventricular sequence of contraction.
  g. Decreased output can result in end-organ dysfunction (e.g., syncope, presyncope, oliguria, ischemia).
2. Etiology and risk factors
  a. SVTs
     i.   Acute MI
     ii. Ischemia

▨ **BOX 3-8**
▨ **COMPLICATIONS ASSOCIATED WITH PACEMAKER FUNCTIONING**

FAILURE TO PACE
No pacer spike seen at appropriate times
Caused by
- Battery failure
- Lead dislodgment
- Wire fracture
- Disconnection of wire or cable
- Generator failure
- Oversensing: No impulse generated because some other activity (often muscular) has been sensed and misinterpreted as a QRS complex

FAILURE TO CAPTURE
Pacer-generated QRS not seen
Caused by
- Lead dislodgment or malposition
- Battery failure
- Pacing at voltage below capture threshold
- Faulty connections
- Lead fracture
- Ventricular perforation

FAILURE TO SENSE
Pacemaker may compete with patient's own intrinsic rhythm
Caused by
- Sensitivity setting that is too high
- Battery failure
- Malposition of catheter lead
- Lead fracture
- Pulse generator failure
- Lead insulation break

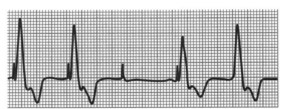

FIGURE 3-15 ▪ Failure of the pulse generator to capture. (From Phillips RE, Feeney MR. *The Cardiac Rhythms.* 2nd ed. Philadelphia, PA: Saunders; 1980:347.)

    iii. Reentry (most common cause of paroxysmal SVT)
    iv. Valvular heart disease
    v. Use of stimulants: Alcohol, coffee, tobacco
    vi. Congenital heart disease
    vii. Pulmonary disease
    viii. Drug toxicity: Digitalis, antidepressants
    ix. WPW syndrome (accessory pathway)
    x. Cardiomyopathies

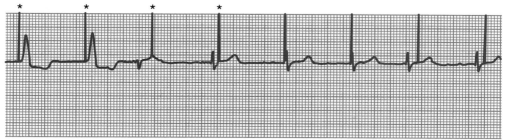

FIGURE 3-16 ■ Pacemaker malfunction: Undersensing. Notice that after the first two paced beats, a series of intrinsic beats occurs; the pacemaker unit fails to sense these intrinsic QRS complexes. These spikes do not capture the ventricle because they occur during the refractory period of the cardiac cycle. The asterisk indicates the pacemaker impulse. (From Urden LD, Stacy KM, Lough ME. *Thelan's Critical Care Nursing: Diagnosis and Management.* Philadelphia, PA: Mosby; 2002:447.)

    b. VT: Sustained (>30 seconds)
- **i.** Acute MI
- **ii.** Ischemia
- **iii.** Cardiomyopathies
- **iv.** Tetralogy of Fallot
- **v.** Drugs: Digitalis, antiarrhythmic agents
- **vi.** Electrolyte imbalances: Low potassium, magnesium
- **vii.** Hypoxia
- **viii.** LV aneurysms
- **ix.** Congenital long QT syndromes
- **x.** Valvular heart disease

3. Signs and symptoms
- **a.** Dyspnea
- **b.** Palpitations
- **c.** Shortness of breath
- **d.** Angina
- **e.** Syncope
- **f.** Weakness, exercise intolerance
- **g.** Anxiety
- **h.** Mentation changes
- **i.** Heart rate exceeding 100 beats/min
- **j.** Jugular venous distention
- **k.** Polyuria, oliguria
- **l.** Hypotension
- **m.** Unconsciousness
- **n.** Rapid, thready pulse or pulse deficit

4. Diagnostic study findings
- **a.** Laboratory: To ascertain
  - **i.** Imbalances of electrolytes, include magnesium
  - **ii.** ABG levels: Hypoxia, acidosis
  - **iii.** CBC: To rule out hemorrhage, infection
- **b.** ECG
  - **i.** See ECG features for VT (see Table 3-4)
  - **ii.** See ECG features for SVTs (see Table 3-4)
- **c.** Electrophysiology study, after the patient's condition is stabilized

5. Goals of care
- **a.** Rapid rhythm is terminated or rate is controlled to maintain adequate CO and tissue perfusion.
- **b.** Patient has relief of symptoms related to the rapid rhythm.

6. Collaborating professionals on health care team: See Chronic Stable Angina; also electro-physiologist, anticoagulation clinic or nurse
7. Management of patient care
    a. Anticipated patient trajectory: Marked tachycardia results in diminished CO, poor tissue perfusion, hypotension, and potentially loss of consciousness and death
        i. Pharmacology
            (a) Stable narrow QRS supraventricular rhythms
                (1) Adenosine may be administered, 6 mg IV, injected over 3 seconds or less, followed by a dose of 12 mg 1 to 2 minutes later.
                    a) Adenosine often terminates AV nodal reentry and sinus nodal reentrant tachycardia.
                    b) Not used for atrial fibrillation or flutter
                (2) Atrial fibrillation: Most frequently seen supraventricular tachydysrhythmia
                    a) Main goals are to lower ventricular response rate, decrease symptoms, and convert to sinus rhythm if and when possible.
                    b) If the duration of atrial fibrillation is longer than 48 hours (or if unknown), anticoagulation is necessary to decrease the risk of atrial thrombi and CVA. INR of 2 to 3 (for at least 1 month) is necessary before elective direct current (DC) cardioversion. IV heparin is initiated and continued until the treatment plan is determined.
                    c) If the duration is less than 48 hours, diltiazem, digoxin, or β-blockers are used for rate control.
                    d) If the duration is less than 48 hours, amiodarone may be used to convert the rhythm before elective cardioversion.
                    e) If the duration is longer than 48 hours, antiarrhythmic drugs (amiodarone, procainamide) are not used, because they could convert the rhythm and place the patient at risk for a thrombotic event before adequate anticoagulation.
                    f) Rate control of chronic atrial fibrillation has better long-term outcomes than attempts to maintain sinus rhythm with antiarrhythmics.
                (3) Atrial flutter: Rate control with β-blockers. Calcium channel blockers and digoxin are given before DC cardioversion or radiofrequency ablation.
                (4) Automatic atrial tachycardia (produced by enhanced automaticity in atrial tissue): β-blockers, propafenone (amiodarone, if poor LV function)
                (5) Multifocal atrial tachycardia (MAT): Metoprolol, verapamil, magnesium
                    a) Correct the underlying cause.
                    b) MAT is unresponsive to cardioversion.
                    c) Theophylline levels should be checked (toxicity can cause MAT): MAT is often seen in respiratory failure.
                (6) AV nodal reentrant tachycardia (AVNRT), atrioventricular reciprocating tachycardia (AVRT), orthodromic (WPW syndrome): Adenosine
            (b) Stable wide QRS dysrhythmias
                (1) VT
                    a) Amiodarone, 150 mg IV over 10 minutes, followed by 1 mg/min infusion for 6 hours, then maintenance infusion of 0.5 mg/min for 18 hours
                        1) Drug of choice with known LV dysfunction in both supraventricular and ventricular dysrhythmias
                        2) Adverse effects: Hypotension, QT interval prolongation
                    b) Lidocaine, 0.5 to 0.75 mg/kg IV push, given every 5 to 10 minutes to a total of 3 mg/kg if desired; maintenance infusion is 1 to 4 mg/min IV
                    c) Procainamide, if LV function is known to be good (EF of more than 40%)
                        1) 20 to 30 mg/min IV, injected slowly
                        2) Maximum dose: 17 mg/kg
                        3) End points for therapy: Dysrhythmia termination; hypotension; widening of QRS by more than 50%
                        4) If procainamide is successful at terminating VT, infusion is started at 1 to 4 mg/min.

d) Treatment includes correcting the underlying cause. Choice of antiarrhythmic agent, when the patient is in stable condition, is guided by EPS or some other documented test of efficacy (e.g., serial Holter monitoring).

e) Adenosine is no longer recommended to be used with wide QRS tachycardias as a diagnostic tool.

(2) Torsades de pointes (a polymorphic form of VT)

a) Often seen as a proarrhythmic dysrhythmia as a result of antiarrhythmic drug therapy

b) Responds to measures that shorten the QT interval (isoproterenol, phenytoin, magnesium, overdrive pacing)

c) If the patient's condition is unstable, cardioversion is performed immediately per the advanced cardiac life support (ACLS) standards for VT.

ii. Treatments

(a) Evaluate stability by rapid assessment of vital signs, level of consciousness, related symptoms.

(b) Ensure adequate airway, breathing, circulation.

(c) Administer oxygen as needed to provide for oxygen saturations exceeding 92%.

(d) DC cardioversion: If the patient is symptomatic and unstable (heart rate above 150 beats/min), prepare for immediate cardioversion

(1) Cardioversion is delivery (to the patient) of a selected amount of electrical energy synchronized with the R wave of the patient's intrinsic rhythm.

(2) Amount of energy required to convert tachydysrhythmias varies from 50 J to 360 J for a monophasic defibrillator and from 30 J to 200 J for a biphasic defibrillator.

(3) Explain the entire procedure to the patient and significant others, including the risks.

(4) Obtain a consent form, if conditions are not deteriorating too rapidly.

(5) Sedative and anesthetic drugs are given to the patient before the procedure, if the patient is conscious (an anesthesiologist is often used for elective procedures).

(6) Attach the defibrillator monitor leads to the patient; these leads can be piggybacked to many bedside monitors for quick ECG access.

(7) Make sure the monitor is synchronized to the patient's rhythm: the "Sync" button should be on, and spikes indicating the recognition of R waves should be seen on the monitor. If spikes are not seen, check the gain on the machine, try another lead, and/or adjust the electrodes.

(8) Code cart and suction equipment should be at bedside. Knowledge of the safe use of the defibrillator is vital.

(9) Place the defibrillator on the left side of the bed if possible, to prevent the operator from leaning over the bed while cardioverting the patient.

(10) If the patient goes into VF, deliver immediate defibrillation; turn off the Sync button, if necessary (most machines default to defibrillation mode after a cardioversion attempt). Remember to turn the Sync button back on each time, if repeated cardioversion is necessary.

(e) Vagal maneuvers (gagging, cold water immersion of the face) often terminate AVNRT. These are more successful when performed as soon after onset as possible. Patient should be instructed as to a safe procedure for home use.

(f) Radiofrequency ablation: Patient may need to be prepared for radiofrequency catheter ablation of accessory pathways

(1) In the procedure, done in the EPS laboratory, a catheter is used to deliver low-voltage, high-frequency, alternating current that selectively damages myocardial tissue.

(2) Ablation stops the conduction of electrical impulses and disrupts the reentry circuit.

(3) Uses include the following:

a) Accessory pathways: WPW syndrome

b) Symptomatic SVT: AVNRT, AVRT with an accessory pathway, rapid AV conduction of atrial fibrillation, sinus node reentrant tachycardias

c) Junctional tachycardia: Caused by enhanced automaticity; seen in infants and children after surgery for congenital heart defects and in digitalis toxicity

d) Atrial flutter (treatment of choice)

e) VT with bundle branch reentry, refractory VT

(4) Complications of radiofrequency ablation include the following:

a) Bleeding at the catheter site

b) Deep venous thrombosis

c) Cardiac tamponade

d) Myocardial perforation

e) Infection

f) Ischemia

g) Stroke

h) Complete AV block

i) Pulmonary embolism

j) Pneumothorax

(5) Patient education issues are as follows:

a) Procedure description, rationale

b) Procedure length (2 to 4 hours average, up to 10 hours)

c) Possible need for a permanent pacemaker

d) Recurrence rate for tachydysrhythmias: 8% to 12%

e) Monitoring of the patient and site (see Box 3-5)

(g) Atrial or transesophageal pacing (antitachycardia) may also be considered for termination of persistent stable tachycardias (atrial fibrillation, AVNRT, atrial tachycardia, AVRT in selected patients).

(h) Surgical endocardial or epicardial techniques for ablation of pathways are used in cases in which radiofrequency catheter ablation is not possible and the patient's symptoms are hindering quality of life. The surgical maze procedure is very successful in abolishing atrial fibrillation.

(i) AICD

(1) Device is implanted into the patient with sensing leads and defibrillator patches attached to the endocardium and to a pulse generator. This is done by transvenous approach or a thoracotomy.

(2) Capabilities include the following:

a) Bradycardia pacing

b) Overdrive pacing

c) Cardioversion: At 25 J

d) Defibrillation

e) ECG measurement with storage and event logs

f) Dual-chamber pacing

(3) Indications: Recurrent VT, VF; sudden cardiac death; or decreased LV EF of less than 30% (MADIT II trials; Moss et al, 1999)

(4) Important issues to understand and teach to the patient and significant others:

a) If the AICD discharges, it is not dangerous to the staff or family.

b) Incidence of spontaneous (appropriate or inappropriate) discharge is 75% the first year.

c) Concurrent use of antiarrhythmic agents is still necessary to decrease the frequency of events.

d) Interrogator units can analyze the history of shocks, battery life, and heart rhythm at the time of shock.

8. **Evaluation of patient care**

a. Signs of adequate CO are present.

b. Tachycardia is controlled and terminated.

Absent or Ineffective Pulse

All cases of absent or ineffective pulse are life threatening and necessitate immediate intervention, usually CPR.

1. **Pathophysiology**
   a. No CO and, subsequently, no tissue perfusion
   b. Respirations cease. Patient is clinically dead.
   c. Rapid cell death. Brain cells start to die after 4 to 6 minutes of circulatory collapse. After 10 minutes, some degree of brain death is inevitable.
   d. VF: Inability to generate an organized impulse for muscular contraction
   e. Asystole: No electrical activity initiated
   f. Pulseless electrical activity (PEA): Electrical activity and conduction occur, with the absence of a palpable pulse and blood pressure. Rhythms seen are any rhythm except VF or VT.
      i. Caused by lack of ventricular filling volume (hypovolemia, fluid losses, saddle emboli, tamponade)
      ii. Caused by the myocardium's inability to contract effectively: Lack of oxygen, acidotic states, electrolyte disturbances (elevated or decreased potassium levels), physical impairment to contraction (tension pneumothorax, tamponade, pericardial effusion), muscular dysfunction from necrosis (MI), thrombosis, hypothermia, drug overdose

2. **Etiology and risk factors**
   a. Causes of VF or pulseless VT
      i. MI
      ii. Ischemia
      iii. Myocardial disease: Cardiomyopathies, myocarditis
      iv. Anoxia: Smoke inhalation, drowning, respiratory failure, airway obstruction
   b. Causes of asystole
      i. Hypokalemia
      ii. Hyperkalemia
      iii. Hypothermia
      iv. Acidosis
   c. Causes of PEA
      i. Hypovolemia: Most common cause
      ii. Hypoxia
      iii. Tension pneumothorax
      iv. Acidosis
      v. Acute MI
      vi. Pulmonary embolism
      vii. Hyperkalemia
      viii. Tamponade
      ix. Drug overdose: Calcium channel blockers, digitalis, tricyclic antidepressants, β-blockers
      x. Hypothermia

3. **Signs and symptoms**
   a. History
      i. History taking is often deferred or performed in conjunction with emergency, life-preserving measures.
      ii. Determine whether the patient has a history of any of the aforementioned causes.
   b. Physical examination
      i. No pulse
      ii. Unconsciousness or rapidly deteriorating level of consciousness
      iii. No respiration

4. **Diagnostic study findings**
   a. ABG levels: Measured after immediate actions taken, to check oxygenation, acidosis
   b. Electrolyte levels
   c. ECG or monitor
      i. In PEA, there is organized electrical activity but no significant CO.
      ii. VF (coarse versus fine)

         iii. Pulseless VT (very rapid)

    d. No invasive studies are performed until the patient's condition is stabilized.

5. Goals of care
    a. Life is preserved.
    b. CO and tissue perfusion are restored rapidly without brain death.

6. Collaborating professionals on health care team: Physician, nurse, pharmacist, respiratory therapist, chaplain

7. Management of patient care
    a. Anticipated patient trajectory: Patient "clinically dead." Preservation of life and avoidance of brain death require prompt action.

        i. Positioning: Lay patient flat, with a board under the back for support during CPR

        ii. Pharmacology

            (a) Emergency medications for VF and pulseless VT: See the current ACLS standards of the American Heart Association for detailed descriptions, algorithms

                (1) 100% oxygen

                (2) Epinephrine, 1 mg IV push, every 3 to 5 minutes during arrest; start after initial defibrillation

                (3) Vasopressin, 40 units IV, one time, as an alternative drug; half-life is 10 to 20 minutes

                (4) After epinephrine or vasopressin administration, and repeated defibrillation attempts, antiarrhythmic drugs are considered.

                    a) Amiodarone: Dose is 300 mg IV, diluted in 20 to 30 ml dextrose 5% in water, infused rapidly; dose of 150 mg IV × 1 dose given for recurrent VF

                    b) Other antiarrhythmics used include lidocaine, 1 to 1.5 mg/kg IV (up to 3 mg/kg total); procainamide; and magnesium, 1 to 2 g IV (if polymorphic VT, hypomagnesemia).

            (b) Medications for asystole and PEA

                (1) Emergency medications given in boluses

                (2) Epinephrine, 1 mg IV push, every 3 to 5 minutes during arrest

                (3) Atropine, 1 mg IV, every 3 to 5 minutes (up to a total of 0.04 mg/kg maximum vagolytic dose)

                (4) Vasopressin is not recommended for PEA or asystole.

                (5) Sodium bicarbonate, 1 mEq/kg, is used if the patient had prearrest hyperkalemia or drug overdose (i.e., tricyclic antidepressants).

                (6) Defibrillation is reattempted after each drug intervention.

                (7) If hypokalemia: Potassium and magnesium are given

                (8) If hyperkalemia: Sodium bicarbonate, glucose and insulin, Kayexalate, digitalis, albuterol may be given

                (9) Thrombolytic agents may be given for massive pulmonary embolism.

            (c) IV infusions are not hung during immediate arrest; they can be hung only after the patient's heart rate and rhythm have been restored.

        iii. Psychosocial issues: Family needs support during this time. Chaplain, social worker, nursing supervisor, and charge nurse can assist with comforting and communicating with significant others.

        iv. Treatments

            (a) Immediately call cardiac arrest code team.

            (b) Assess airway, breathing, and circulation (ABC); perform CPR.

            (c) Ensure that crash cart and emergency equipment are at bedside.

            (d) Defibrillate as soon as equipment is available, without delay if the patient is in VF, pulseless VT, or asystole (could be fine VF).

                (1) Use 200, 300, and 360 J per ACLS standards.

                (2) Be familiar with the safe use of the defibrillator. Always treat it as if it is a weapon and visually ensure that everyone at the bedside is clear from the bed before defibrillating (each time).

                (3) If the monitor shows a flat line, check the power (cables connected?), check the gain (too low?), check the other leads (activity may be seen in a different axis or defibrillator may be set to monitor through defibrillation pads).

        (e) Ensure that CPR is resumed promptly after defibrillation or any assessments.

        (f) Automatic external defibrillator may be the only defibrillator available in some areas of the hospital.

           (1) Fully or semiautomatic models

           (2) Cables attach to two adhesive conductive pads.

           (3) Machine records rhythm, analyzes data, states command to "Clear," and delivers electrical shocks.

           (4) CPR must be stopped for the machine to analyze the rhythm (takes 15 to 20 seconds), then it will deliver shocks.

           (5) Most problems result from operator difficulties (learn to use the equipment properly).

        (g) Transcutaneous pacemakers for asystole: If considered, should be used early in arrest (less than 5 min after onset) for the best chance of success. May be temporizing, to help the heart pace while the causes are identified and treated.

        (h) Induced hypothermia may be used to improve neurologic outcome after sudden cardiac death survival.

        (i) AICD is often used if the patient survives arrest.

        (j) Promptly assess and treat for the common causes of PEA.

           (1) Administer immediate volume replacement. Can lift legs for immediate autoinfusion.

           (2) Listen for breath sounds; check for pneumothorax.

           (3) Ensure proper oxygenation.

           (4) Hyperventilate the patient: respiratory acidosis usually occurs in arrest as a result of inadequate ventilation.

           (5) Check ABG results for acidosis.

           (6) Assist the physician with pericardiocentesis for tamponade, needle decompression of pneumothorax.

           (7) Draw blood for measurement of electrolyte levels, drug screens.

   v. Ethical issues

        (a) Health care professionals should be aware of the patient's wishes regarding CPR before emergencies occur. Advance directives should be identified at admission and "Do not attempt resuscitation" orders initiated and communicated to all appropriate staff. Patient and family need to understand that outpatient directives must be reinstituted as a medical order when the patient is hospitalized in order to be valid.

        (b) Duration of resuscitative efforts depends on many factors (i.e., age, medical condition).

  8. Evaluation of patient care

    a. Signs of life are present: Adequate airway, breathing, circulation, and CO, and good mentation

    b. Dysrhythmia is controlled and terminated.

    c. Cause of arrest is identified and treated.

    d. Patient's advance directive is respected by initiating a "Do not attempt resuscitation" order as appropriate.

Mitral Regurgitation

In mitral regurgitation, blood is partially regurgitated into the LA during ventricular systole because of an incompetent mitral valve. This may happen acutely or develop as a chronic condition.

  1. Pathophysiology

    a. With the failure of the mitral valve to close completely during ventricular contraction, some fraction of the LV output is ejected backwards into the LA.

    b. Pressures in the LA and pulmonary veins rise (dramatically if the onset is acute), and pulmonary congestion and/or edema results in dyspnea.

    c. Reduced forward output results in chronic fatigue (or hypotension if acute).

    d. The pathophysiology and clinical course vary dramatically, depending on whether the onset is acute or chronic.

    e. Acute onset

      i.   Pressures within the LA and pulmonary vasculature dramatically increase.

      ii.   LA has no time to compensate and initially remains small and noncompliant (which creates high pressures).

      iii. Forward output falls dramatically, and cardiogenic shock develops.

      iv. Pulmonary congestion may develop as a result of high pressures within the pulmonary vascular bed, and pulmonary edema rapidly ensues.

  f. Chronic process

      i.   LA has time (often years) to enlarge and develop compliance to keep pressures at near-normal levels.

      ii.   Pulmonary artery pressures remain relatively normal.

      iii. Eventually the degree of mitral regurgitation may exceed the capacity of the LA to compensate, and pulmonary congestion and dyspnea may develop.

      iv. LV compensates for chronic volume overload by dilating in an attempt to maintain normal forward output, while emptying a large volume of its output backward into the LA.

      v.   LV can dilate to the extent that it is unable to recover, even after surgical correction of mitral regurgitation.

      vi. As pressures within the pulmonary vein and left ventricle increase, pulmonary hypertension may develop.

      vii. Atrial fibrillation often is seen and occurs secondary to LA enlargement.

      viii. RV also will progressively hypertrophy, and right-sided heart failure may follow.

2. Etiology and risk factors

  a. Acute causes

      i.   Acute rupture of the chordae tendineae as a result of endocarditis or chronic strain on the mitral valve apparatus by mitral valve prolapse, rheumatic heart disease

      ii.   Papillary muscle dysfunction or rupture secondary to acute MI

      iii. Trauma

  b. Chronic causes

      i.   Rheumatic heart disease

      ii.   Congenital malformations of the mitral valve, chordae tendineae, or mitral annuli

      iii. Mitral valve prolapse

      iv. LV dilatation from other causes

      v.   Connective tissue disease (e.g., Marfan's syndrome)

      vi. IE

      vii. Calcified mitral annulus

3. Signs and symptoms

  a. Subjective findings: Patient complains of

      i.   Shortness of breath

      ii.   Orthopnea

      iii. Paroxysmal nocturnal dyspnea

      iv. Weakness or becoming easily fatigued

      v.   Palpitations

      vi. Symptoms of RV failure

  b. Objective findings: History of past rheumatic fever, streptococcal infection, endocarditis, ischemia, trauma, mitral valve prolapse

  c. Physical findings

      i.   If the patient is in heart failure, the following may be seen:

          (a) Tachypnea

          (b) Anxiety

          (c) Diaphoresis

          (d) Cyanosis

          (e) Confusion

          (f) Edema

          (g) Jugular venous distention (right-sided heart failure)

          (h) Signs of pulmonary edema (frothy, pink sputum)

      ii.   Other findings include the following:

(a) Apical impulse (PMI) is laterally displaced, diffuse, and hyperdynamic (in chronic mitral regurgitation).

(b) Apical systolic thrill may be felt.

(c) Pulse may be irregular if in atrial fibrillation.

(d) Hepatomegaly (late sign)

iii. Auscultation

(a) High-pitched, blowing holosystolic murmur

(1) Heard best at apex with radiation to axilla

(2) Begins at S_1 and extends through S_2 (aortic closure)

(b) Rales if pulmonary congestion or edema present

(c) S_2 may be widely split or accentuated (P_2) as a result of early closure of the aortic valve, because LV ejection time is shortened; pulmonic closure delayed because of right-sided heart pressure overload

(d) Possible RV lift secondary to RV pressure overload

4. **Diagnostic study findings**

   a. Radiologic

   i. LA and LV enlargement in chronic mitral regurgitation

   ii. No enlargement of LA with acute onset

   iii. Calcification of mitral valve

   iv. Pulmonary edema

   b. ECG: Atrial fibrillation

   c. Echocardiography: Helps determine the cause, LV function and dimensions, indications for surgery

   i. Degree of insufficiency

   ii. LA and LV enlargement in chronic mitral insufficiency

   iii. Mitral valve prolapse, mitral annular calcification, flail leaflet, vegetations, rheumatic heart disease

   iv. Abnormal regional wall motion if papillary muscle dysfunction is the cause

   d. TEE: Used in guiding mitral valve reconstructive surgery; superior to transthoracic echocardiography in visualizing the mitral valve leaflets

   e. Cardiac catheterization

   i. Documents the severity of mitral regurgitation

   ii. Screens for CAD

   iii. Documents pulmonary capillary wedge pressure (PCWP) and right-sided heart pressures

5. **Goals of care**

   a. Patient is hemodynamically stable and in sinus rhythm.

   b. Symptoms of reduced CO are identified and treated promptly.

   c. Patient receives appropriate teaching regarding surgical interventions, medications, and discharge care.

6. **Collaborating professionals on health care team: See Chronic Stable Angina**

7. **Management of patient care**

   a. Anticipated patient trajectory: Severe mitral regurgitation must be corrected, or progressive left-sided heart failure and early death occur

   i. Discharge planning

   (a) Instructions include the usual postoperative instructions for any heart surgery.

   (b) If the valve is replaced, the importance of endocarditis prophylaxis and chronic anticoagulation is stressed (if the patient does not comply with the follow-up medication regimen, stroke and possibly death are highly likely).

   ii. Pharmacology

   (a) Treat atrial fibrillation: Slow the ventricular response, increase exercise capacity with digitalis, β-blockers, calcium antagonists

   (b) Antibiotics: For prophylaxis of recurrent rheumatic heart disease, prophylaxis for IE during dental procedures

   (c) Acute mitral regurgitation may respond to administration of vasodilators to decrease afterload (e.g., nitroprusside) or as a prelude to valve surgery

(d) Diuretics, nitrates: To lower pulmonary congestion; use carefully, may lower CO

(e) Anticoagulants: Prevent embolization if atrial fibrillation is present. Goal is an INR of 2 to 3.

   iii. Treatments

(a) In severe cases, the use of an IABP may be required.

(b) If the valve is to be surgically reconstructed (surgical mitral valvuloplasty) or replaced, the patient and family must be counseled with regard to the surgery.

(1) Explain the disease process, preoperative routines, surgical procedure (including the replacement valve to be used), and expectations during the immediate postoperative period.

(2) Mitral valve reconstruction is shown to yield improved rest and exercise EFs after surgery (benefits are partly the result of preserved chordae tendineae, papillary muscles, valve shape) and decreased mortality.

(3) Chronic anticoagulant use is not necessary with reconstruction if the patient is in sinus rhythm.

(4) Postoperative general care for valve repair is similar to postoperative care for most cardiac surgical operations.

  b. Potential complications

    i. Systemic emboli with atrial fibrillation requiring anticoagulation

    ii. IE: IE prophylaxis needed (see Infective Endocarditis)

8. Evaluation of patient care

  a. Hemodynamic stability is evidenced by normal vital signs and lack of, or control of, dysrhythmias.

  b. After surgery, no complications are noted.

  c. On discharge, the patient and significant others relate an understanding of all postoperative care measures (e.g., wound care, sternal precautions), the need for antibiotic prophylaxis when the patient undergoes future surgical or dental procedures, and, if necessary, chronic anticoagulant therapy.

Mitral Stenosis

Mitral stenosis is a progressive narrowing of the mitral orifice that impedes the flow of blood from the LA to the LV during ventricular diastole.

1. Pathophysiology

  a. Progressive fibrosis, scarring, and thickening of the valve leaflets develop, usually from rheumatic valvular disease.

  b. Extensive fusion of the leaflets and chordae tendineae develops.

  c. Area of a normal adult's mitral valve orifice is 4 to 6 cm^2. In mild mitral stenosis, it is 2 cm^2 (symptoms may be experienced only with exercise, atrial fibrillation). In severe mitral stenosis, it is 1 cm^2, with symptoms apparent even at rest.

  d. Elevation of LA pressures results from the obstruction to the flow from the LA to the LV. As the valve continues to narrow, the LA slowly dilates and hypertrophies.

  e. Intractable atrial fibrillation usually results.

  f. As atrial pressures elevate, pulmonary capillary hydrostatic pressure rises above the plasma oncotic pressure, and fluid escapes into the pulmonary interstitium and alveoli.

  g. As the valve orifice narrows to smaller than 1 cm^2, pulmonary hypertension occurs and RV pressures increase, with eventual hypertrophy and dilatation. RV failure frequently follows.

  h. Stenotic obstruction impedes forward blood flow and alone is often enough to decrease SV and CO. Loss of atrial kick resulting from atrial fibrillation or tachycardia compounds the problem, decreasing LV filling time and further decreasing CO.

  i. Atrial thrombi form in the LA appendage, and systemic or cerebral emboli may ensue.

2. Etiology and risk factors: Incidence has decreased in the United States

  a. Rheumatic heart disease (most common cause)

  b. Congenital mitral valve disease (uncommon)

  c. Tumors of the LA (atrial myxoma)

  d. Risk factor: Pregnant women with mitral stenosis often have cardiac decompensation in the third trimester

3. **Signs and symptoms**
   a. History
      i.   Gradual decline in physical activity over the years
      ii.   Palpitations (frequent complaint): Possibly from frequent premature atrial contractions, paroxysmal atrial fibrillation
      iii. Shortness of breath, dyspnea on exertion
      iv.   Paroxysmal nocturnal dyspnea
      v.   Cough (bronchial irritability), hoarseness
      vi.   Orthopnea
      vii. Fatigue
      viii. Hemoptysis (ruptured bronchial vessels)
      ix.   Symptoms of right-sided heart failure (occur later)
      x.   Dysphagia (enlarged atrium displaces the esophagus)
      xi.   History of systemic emboli, rheumatic heart disease
   b. Objective findings: Signs and symptoms of right-sided heart failure occur as late signs (See Heart Failure)
   c. Physical examination: Findings depend on the degree of heart failure present
      i.   Inspection
           (a) Any of the signs of heart failure
           (b) Jugular venous distention
      ii. Palpation
           (a) May feel the RV lift if pulmonary hypertension is present; an LV "tap" may be present
           (b) Diastolic thrill may be present at the apex (with the patient in the left lateral recumbent position).
      iii. Auscultation
           (a) Pronounced S_1
           (b) Low-pitched apical diastolic murmur (best heard at the apex, radiates to the left sternal border)
           (c) Associated murmur of tricuspid insufficiency may be present if RV failure exists. Listen at the left lower parasternal area.
           (d) Pulmonary component, S_2, later and louder if pulmonary hypertension exists
           (e) Mitral opening snap present just after pulmonic component of S_2

4. **Diagnostic study findings**
   a. Radiologic: Chest radiograph reveals the following:
      i.   LA and RV hypertrophy
      ii. Interstitial edema, pulmonary vascular redistribution to the upper lobes of the lungs
   b. ECG
      i.   If in sinus rhythm, broad P waves: Notched in lead I, biphasic in V_1
      ii. Atrial fibrillation
      iii. RV hypertrophy pattern (with pulmonary hypertension)
   c. Transthoracic echocardiography with Doppler
      i.   Reveals thickened, tethered, and doming (stuck together) anterior and posterior mitral valve leaflets
      ii. Calculates mitral valve area
      iii. Shows enlarged LA
      iv. Shows enlarged RV
      v.   Assess the degree of pulmonary hypertension and mitral regurgitation, and the function of the other valves.
   d. TEE: For identification of an LA appendage thrombus (seen in 20% of cases of atrial fibrillation)
   e. Cardiac catheterization: Used if the echocardiographic results are confusing or questionable given the patient presentation
      i.   To assess CO and hemodynamic parameters
      ii. Coronary arteriography: Used to assess the function of the other valves and rule out CAD

5. **Goals of care**
   a. Hemodynamics improve.
   b. Complications (including atrial fibrillation, recurrent infections, atrial thrombus) are treated and/or prevented.
6. **Collaborating professionals on health care team: See Chronic Stable Angina**
7. **Management of patient care**
   a. Anticipated patient trajectory: Patient with mitral stenosis will gradually develop limiting symptoms and heart failure, with the likelihood of stroke and early death
      i. Nutrition: Restricted sodium intake
      ii. Infection control: IE prophylactic therapy
      iii. Discharge planning: Patient education regarding the following:
         (a) Activity limitations
         (b) Medications
         (c) Anticoagulation and follow-up requirements
      iv. Pharmacology
         (a) Diuretics, nitrates: To lower pulmonary congestion; use carefully, may lower CO
         (b) Digitalis, β-blockers, calcium antagonists: To treat atrial fibrillation, slow ventricular response, and increase exercise capacity
         (c) β-Blocking agents may increase exercise tolerance by slowing the heart rate and lengthening the diastolic filling period. Use carefully in patients with impaired LV function.
         (d) Anticoagulants: Prevent embolization. Goal is an INR of 2 to 3.
         (e) Antibiotics: Prophylaxis for recurrent rheumatic heart disease; prophylaxis for IE during dental procedures
      v. Treatments
         (a) Medical management is palliative; mechanical correction is eventually required to improve CO and decrease atrial and pulmonary pressures.
         (b) Current treatment options include surgical mitral valve replacement, open surgical commissurotomy, percutaneous balloon mitral valvuloplasty.
         (c) Cardioversion, if atrial fibrillation is present.
   b. Potential complications
      i. Systemic or pulmonary emboli from atrial thrombus
         (a) Mechanism: High risk for thrombus formation during atrial fibrillation or heart failure
            (1) Central nervous system embolism: Symptoms of stroke (e.g., paralysis, weakness, dysphasia, confusion)
            (2) Pulmonary embolism: Symptoms of tachycardia, tachypnea, hypoxia, dyspnea, cough, hemoptysis, elevated PAP, hypotension, chest pain, abnormal ABG values, cyanosis, positive lung scan results
            (3) Renal embolism: Hematuria, oliguria, back pain, rising BUN level
            (4) Splenic embolism: Left upper quadrant pain with radiation to the left shoulder
            (5) Mesenteric embolism: Pain in the lower abdomen, bloody diarrhea, elevated leukocyte count, and elevated erythrocyte sedimentation rate
         (b) Management: Dependent on type, anticoagulation
      ii. Other complications: Heart failure, infection
8. **Evaluation of patient care**
   a. Systemic or pulmonary emboli are absent or resolved.
   b. Patient is hemodynamically stable.

Aortic Regurgitation

In aortic regurgitation (AR), an incompetent aortic valve causes the backward flow of blood from the aorta to the LV during ventricular diastole.
1. **Pathophysiology**
   a. Aortic valve can become incompetent as a result of destruction of the cusps (endocarditis), degeneration of the cusps, unhinging of the valvular apparatus (dissection), rheumatic disease, connective tissue disease, congenital heart disease, trauma, or degenerative change.

    b. Acute onset

        i. Increased regurgitation into the LV produces volume overload, markedly increasing the LVEDP.

        ii. CO falls and hypotension develops.

        iii. There is a drop in the aortic diastolic pressure that diminishes the coronary blood flow.

        iv. The compensatory increase in heart rate adds to the already elevated myocardial oxygen demand.

        v. Patient comes for treatment with pulmonary edema, cardiogenic shock. Ischemia and sudden cardiac death may occur.

    c. Chronic process

        i. LV compensates by dilating to increase its SV to maintain an adequate forward output. This gradually increases myocardial oxygen demands.

        ii. The LV myocardial fibers stretch and hypertrophy. Preload and EF, at this point, remain relatively normal.

        iii. As the disease progresses, the LV fails and decompensates; SV and EF decrease. LV systolic and diastolic pressures increase.

        iv. Wide pulse pressure develops as a result of low aortic diastolic pressures.

        v. Decreased blood flow to the coronary arteries during diastole results in myocardial ischemia.

2. Etiology and risk factors

    a. Acute causes

        i. IE (most common cause of acute AR): Can also be a chronic cause

        ii. Aortic dissection

        iii. Blunt trauma, causing valve rupture (e.g., motor vehicle collision)

        iv. Prosthetic valve dysfunction

    b. Chronic causes

        i. Idiopathic calcification of the valve

        ii. Congenital malformations (bicuspid aortic valve)

        iii. Hypertension

        iv. Rheumatic disease

        v. Aortic aneurysms (e.g., Marfan's syndrome)

        vi. Diseases of the aortic valve and root

        vii. Systemic lupus erythematosus

        viii. Drugs: Appetite suppressants

        ix. Syphilis (rare)

3. Signs and symptoms: Can be well tolerated. Symptoms often do not become evident to the patient until the disease is fairly well advanced.

    a. Subjective findings

        i. Dyspnea (most common symptom)

        ii. Angina pectoris

        iii. Paroxysmal nocturnal dyspnea

        iv. Orthopnea

        v. Presyncope and syncope

    b. Physical examination: Many of physical findings are absent in acute AR. Widening pulse pressure of chronic disease creates these findings. Acute disease has a narrow pulse pressure.

        i. Inspection

            (a) Signs and symptoms of left-sided heart failure

            (b) Distinct carotid artery pulsations

            (c) De Musset's sign (nodding of the head with each beat of the heart)

            (d) Flushed appearance

        ii. Palpation

            (a) Diffuse apical impulse, displaced laterally and downward (in chronic forms); the apical impulse does not change with acute onset

            (b) Water-hammer pulse: Bounding, abrupt rise and fall in the carotid arteries and other peripheral pulses

(c) Positive Quincke's sign: When the fingertip is pressed, capillary pulsation of the nail beds is visible
   iii. Auscultation
     (a) High-pitched, blowing, decrescendo diastolic murmur
      (1) Loudest at lower left sternal border, third-fourth intercostal space
      (2) Starts immediately after S_2
      (3) Short (early diastole) with acute aortic insufficiency
      (4) Long (through diastole) if chronic
      (5) If hard to hear, have the patient sit up and lean forward. Press firmly with the bell.
     (b) S_3 common
     (c) S_4 heard in more severe disease (abnormal LV compliance)
     (d) Rales at the bases, if the onset is acute

4. Diagnostic study findings
  a. Radiologic: Chest radiograph reveals the following:
    i. LV enlargement (normal with acute aortic insufficiency)
    ii. Wide mediastinum (if due to aortic dissection)
    iii. Possible aortic valve calcification
    iv. Possible interstitial pulmonary edema
  b. ECG: Often normal in mild to moderate AR
    i. LV hypertrophy: Increased amplitude of QRS
    ii. As disease progresses, ST segment and T waves invert.
    iii. Sinus tachycardia (acutely)
  c. Echocardiography: Very important tool, particularly in the diagnosis of acute cases
    i. Identifies cause and severity of AR
    ii. Shows LV cavity dilatation with chronic cases
    iii. Reveals vegetations
  d. MRI or CT scan: To exclude aortic dissection
  e. Radionuclide imaging: Used to evaluate the severity of AR and LV function
  f. TEE: To assess the ascending and descending thoracic aorta for aneurysms, dissection, and the cause and severity of aortic insufficiency
  g. Cardiac catheterization
    i. Evaluates hemodynamics
     (a) CO assessment
     (b) Increased LA pressure
     (c) Increased right-sided heart pressures (late)
    ii. Quantifies the degree of insufficiency
    iii. Assesses LV function and EF, reveals other abnormalities
    iv. Reveals coronary anatomy
    v. Evaluates for aortic dissection

5. Goals of care
  a. Stable hemodynamics are maintained.
  b. Afterload is reduced.
  c. Pulmonary congestion, if evident, is decreased.

6. Collaborating professionals on health care team: See Chronic Stable Angina; also electrophysiologist, infectious disease specialist

7. Management of patient care
  a. Anticipated patient trajectory: When severe, AR will ultimately result in irreversible heart failure and early death if not recognized and corrected with aortic valve replacement before LV dysfunction
    i. Positioning: Head of bed elevated, if signs of heart failure are present
    ii. Infection control: Prophylaxis for IE risk
    iii. Discharge planning
     (a) Teach the patient about the need for adherence to the medication regimen and follow-up evaluations.
     (b) Prophylactic antibiotics will be used to prevent IE. Patient should understand what types of procedures require antibiotic prophylaxis.

    iv. Pharmacology
        (a) Inotropic agents (dopamine, dobutamine): To increase CO in acute AR (before surgery)
        (b) ACE inhibitors: To decrease LV remodeling and hypertrophy, reduce afterload (if necessary)
        (c) Diuretics, nitrates: With symptoms of heart failure, to decrease pulmonary congestion
        (d) Antibiotics: IE prophylaxis
        (e) β-Blockers: Avoided in acute AR; used very cautiously because the patient often needs sinus tachycardia to support output
    v. Treatments
        (a) Cardiac surgery
            (1) If the patient is symptomatic or asymptomatic with LV dysfunction or significant dilatation, valve replacement is the main treatment for the incompetent valve.
            (2) AR caused by IE: Does not require a delay in surgery, if the patient is symptomatic
        (b) In severe cases, possible institution of hemodynamic monitoring
        (c) EPS study: If VT is present, AICD implantation because of the high risk of sudden cardiac death
        (d) Atrial pacing: May be needed to increase the heart rate, decrease regurgitation
        (e) IABP contraindicated
  b. Potential complications
    i. IE: Most significant complication to prevent
    ii. Dysrhythmias: Ventricular, heart blocks, electromechanical dissociation
    iii. Heart failure, cardiogenic shock, death

8. Evaluation of patient care
  a. Patient is free of signs and symptoms and has improved hemodynamics.
  b. Symptoms are improved or relieved if the patient underwent surgical replacement of the aortic valve.
  c. Patient demonstrates a knowledge of IE prophylaxis, exercise guidelines, requirements for follow-up care, medications.
  d. Patient verbalizes an understanding of anticoagulation therapy (if needed) and has received written guidelines regarding dietary interactions with medication, laboratory testing and anticoagulation follow-ups, and activity.

Aortic Stenosis

Aortic stenosis is shown in Figure 3-17. Ejection from the LV during systole is impaired because of an obstructive narrowing. Stenosis may be supravalvular, subvalvular, or valvular. Obstructions above the valve are rare and are usually congenital. Obstructions below the valve are associated with hypertrophic cardiomyopathy. Obstructions at the valve itself are the most common cause.

1. Pathophysiology
  a. Valve becomes thickened and calcified, with a progressive fusing of the cusps. LV afterload gradually increases. Aortic insufficiency often develops.
  b. Systolic pressure gradient develops between the LV and the aorta.
  c. To maintain SV and adequate CO, the LV hypertrophies in a concentric manner.
  d. LV becomes stiff and noncompliant; the LVEDP increases.
  e. LA pressures increase, which increases the pulmonary vascular pressures. Pulmonary congestion develops and eventually increases the pressures in the right chambers.
  f. Because the left side of the heart has to pump against increased afterload, myocardial oxygen demand is greatly increased.
  g. LV hypertrophy and increased LVEDP cause a decrease in subendocardial coronary perfusion, and ischemia can result in angina and dysrhythmias.
  h. Because forward CO cannot be augmented to meet requirements, exertional syncope may result.

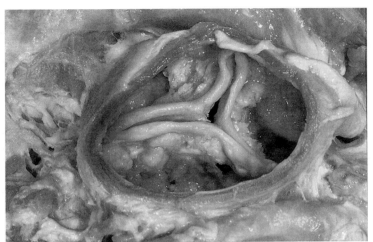

FIGURE 3-17 ■ Gross pathology of degenerative aortic stenosis. (From Crawford MH, DiMarco JP, Paulus WJ, eds. *Cardiology*. 2nd ed. Philadelphia, PA: Mosby; 2004:1122.)

2. **Etiology and risk factors**
   a. Most common cause: Calcific or degenerative process (progressive disease in patients older than 65 years)
   b. Congenital heart defects: Bicuspid valve (symptoms usually seen in patients in their fifties and sixties); associated with other defects, especially coarctation of the aorta. Most common cause in younger adults.
   c. Rheumatic valvular heart disease (the commissure fuses, leaflets thicken and fibrose; symptoms often seen in patients in their thirties and forties), associated with mitral valve disease
   d. Prevalence of aortic stenosis: Increases with age
3. **Signs and symptoms**
   a. Dyspnea on exertion (pulmonary congestion)
   b. Syncope on exertion (transient dysrhythmias, decreased cardiac and cerebral perfusion) or presyncope
   c. Angina (caused by LV hypertrophy, increased myocardial demands, lowered coronary blood flow)
   d. Symptoms of LV failure
   e. Palpitations
   f. Fatigue or weakness
   g. History of a gradual decrease in physical activity to avoid dyspnea
   h. Inspection
      i. Anxiety
      ii. Labored respiration, tachypnea
      iii. Jugular veins: Presence of an "a" wave (if right-sided heart failure is present and the patient is in sinus rhythm)
   i. Palpation
      i. Forceful, sustained apical impulse
      ii. Systolic thrill felt rarely in the second or third right intercostal space
      iii. Pulsus parvus and tardus (small carotid upstroke and delayed peak) is variably present.
   j. Auscultation
      i. Harsh, loud systolic ejection murmur, crescendo-decrescendo, loudest at the second right intercostal space, radiating up to the base of the neck and at apex
      ii. Paradoxical split S_2
      iii. S_3 (in severe LV dysfunction)
      iv. S_4 (with LV hypertrophy)
      v. Rales (LV failure)

4. **Diagnostic study findings**
   a. Radiologic: Studies may be normal in significant stenosis
      i. Cardiac enlargement in late stages
      ii. Pulmonary vascular congestion
      iii. Calcified aortic valve
      iv. Dilated ascending aorta
   b. ECG: Normal in 20% to 30% of patients
      i. LV hypertrophy and strain pattern (increased QRS voltage, ST changes)
      ii. Conduction defects: Left BBB, occasional heart block
      iii. Left axis deviation
      iv. Atrial fibrillation in late stages
   c. Echocardiography: For diagnosis, follow-up
      i. Presence and severity of aortic stenosis
      ii. LV hypertrophy (concentric), impaired LV diastolic function
      iii. LA enlargement
      iv. Other valvular disease
   d. Exercise treadmill study: Unsafe unless aortic stenosis is mild
   e. Cardiac catheterization: Used to assess the following:
      i. CAD: 50% of patients have coexisting CAD
      ii. Hemodynamics
         (a) Increased LV systolic pressure and LVEDP
         (b) Pressure gradient between the LV and the aorta usually more than 50 mm Hg
         (c) Calculation of the aortic valve area
5. **Goals of care**
   a. Patient is free of the signs and symptoms of complications (i.e., heart failure, dysrhythmias, emboli).
   b. Patient demonstrates a knowledge of the disease progress, medications, and therapies to allow active participation in decision making regarding surgical interventions.
6. **Collaborating professionals on health care team: See Chronic Stable Angina; also infectious disease specialist, electrophysiologist, stroke team**
7. **Management of patient care**
   a. Anticipated patient trajectory: Aortic stenosis threatens the patient with limiting angina, heart failure, and death and can be surgically corrected at any age
      i. Nutrition: Diet should be low in sodium
      ii. Infection control: IE prophylaxis
      iii. Discharge planning
         (a) Teach the patient about the symptoms to report promptly and disease progression: the patient is at increased risk for sudden cardiac death.
         (b) Activity restrictions: Moderate aortic stenosis—avoid competition sports. Severe aortic stenosis—low-level activity only.
      iv. Pharmacology: Medical management is palliative. Treatment is based on symptom presentation.
         (a) Antibiotics: To prevent IE
         (b) Antihypertensives: To control hypertension
         (c) Antiarrhythmics: To prevent and control rhythm disturbances (e.g., digoxin, amiodarone for atrial fibrillation)
         (d) If signs of heart failure, pulmonary congestion are present: Digitalis, diuretics, ACE inhibitors. Watch preload. These drugs can lower CO, because the LV is very dependent on preload.
         (e) Vasodilators: Should be avoided; can cause profound hypotension
         (f) Statins: Therapy slows rate of progression of aortic stenosis
      v. Psychosocial issues: Patient's goals and wishes are important because of the high risk of mortality. Activity limitations have a major impact on home life, finances, and morale.
      vi. Treatments
         (a) Surgery is the only effective therapy for critical aortic stenosis.

(1) Valve replacement is performed with stented bioprosthetic mechanical valves or pulmonic autograft (Ross procedure).

(2) Lifelong anticoagulant therapy is necessary when prosthetic mechanical valves are used.

(b) Aortic percutaneous balloon valvuloplasty and débridement are not an alternative to surgery.

(1) Used as a bridge to surgery in patients with pulmonary edema or cardiogenic shock, to improve hemodynamics

(2) Used for patients who are not surgical candidates to improve symptoms

(3) Does not improve survival

(4) Benefits last only a few months

b. Potential complications

i. Sudden cardiac death

(a) Mechanism: High incidence after the patient becomes symptomatic, often resulting from ventricular dysrhythmias

(b) Management: AICD may be required

ii. Other complications (see also applicable sections)

(a) LV failure (diastolic dysfunction)

(b) Conduction defects: Heart blocks (especially in degenerative disease)

(c) IE (more common in younger patients)

(d) Emboli: Stroke, vision problems

8. **Evaluation of patient care**

a. Patient is free of signs and symptoms of heart failure.

b. Symptoms are improved or relieved if the patient underwent surgical repair or replacement of the aortic valve.

c. Patient verbalizes an understanding of anticoagulation therapy (if needed) and the importance of IE prophylaxis.

d. Written guidelines are given regarding dietary interactions with medication, laboratory testing and anticoagulation clinic follow-ups, and exercise.

e. Patient can summarize the symptoms to report promptly and disease progression.

Atrial Septal Defect

Atrial septal defect (ASD) is a defect in the interatrial septum that allows free communication between the right and left sides of the heart at the atrial level. Found in 7% to 10% of patients with congenital heart defects. Can result in shortened life span and morbidity as a result of dyspnea and right-sided heart failure. Paradoxical emboli (right-to-left circulation) can result after the right side of the heart fails.

1. **Pathophysiology**

a. Common types of ASD include the following:

i. Secundum defect (fossa ovalis): Located in the middle of the septum in the area of the foramen ovale. This is the most common type (70%).

ii. Primum defect (often associated with endocardial cushion defects): Located at the lower end of the septum, superior to the interventricular septum (20%)

iii. Sinus venosus defect: Located high in the septum at the junction of the RA and superior vena cava. Frequently associated with partial anomalous pulmonary venous return of the right upper lobe vein to the superior vena cava. Least common type (5% to 10%).

iv. Patent foramen ovale: Open congenital "hole" defect found in up to 27% of adults. Large patent foramina ovales and/or defects with right-to-left shunting are associated with cryptogenic strokes (focal neurologic deficits owing to focal ischemia).

b. As a result of the defects, flow is from the normally higher-pressure LA to the RA, which creates a left-to-right shunt.

c. Right-side heart and pulmonary artery flow increase because these structures handle both the normal systemic venous return from the body and the left-to-right shunt flow through the ASD.

d. This results in volume overload of the right chambers.

e. RA, RV, and pulmonary artery dilate.

    f. Systolic murmur of an ASD results from increased flow across the normal pulmonic valve (flow murmur). Diastolic rumble can occur from increased flow across the tricuspid valve.

    g. Spontaneous closure rarely occurs after 2 years of age.

    h. Pulmonary hypertension and pulmonary vascular disease may develop over time (seen in 15% to 20% of adults with this defect). In extreme cases, the shunt may reverse, becoming right to left and irreversible (Eisenmenger's syndrome).

    i. RV dilatation, hypertrophy, and failure can result.

    j. Atrial fibrillation is often seen.

    k. Mitral valve anomalies (with cleft leaflets) often occur in endocardial cushion defects (associated with ostium primum defects), resulting in mitral insufficiency.

2. Etiology and risk factors

    a. Occurs twice as often among females

    b. Exact cause unknown; may be due to

        i. Genetic factors

        ii. Maternal and fetal infection during the first trimester of pregnancy (e.g., rubella)

        iii. Effects of drugs or medications

        iv. Dietary deficiencies during fetal development

3. Signs and symptoms: Symptoms often develop in the fourth to sixth decades of life. Presentations vary, depending on the direction of the shunt. When the shunt reverses to right to left, signs and symptoms of severe heart failure with cyanosis will be present.

    a. Patient may complain of

        i. Mild fatigue

        ii. Exertional dyspnea

        iii. Palpitations

    b. Appearance is generally normal.

    c. Symptoms of heart failure may be seen in older patients.

    d. Cyanosis, clubbing of the fingers and toes (with right-to-left shunts) occur.

    e. Palpation: Systolic, hyperdynamic lift along the left sternal border, caused by enlarged RV

    f. Auscultation

        i. Systolic ejection murmur: Heard best in the second left intercostal space; caused by increased flow across the pulmonic valve

        ii. Fixed, widely split S_2

        iii. Early, low-pitched diastolic murmur may be heard best at the lower left sternal border or xiphoid area; caused by increased blood flow across the tricuspid valve if shunt flow is large

4. Diagnostic study findings

    a. Radiologic: Chest radiograph may be normal or may reveal the following:

        i. Mild to moderate enlargement of the RA, RV, pulmonary artery

        ii. Increased pulmonary vascular markings

    b. ECG

        i. Atrial fibrillation and/or atrial flutter

        ii. PR prolongation

        iii. Incomplete right BBB

        iv. Left axis deviation in ostium primum defects

    c. Echocardiography

        i. RV enlargement

        ii. Actual defect is occasionally seen with two-dimensional echocardiography, color-flow Doppler studies.

        iii. IV injection of contrast medium demonstrates the shunt by the early appearance of contrast medium in the left heart chambers.

    d. TEE: Used to evaluate the mitral valve

    e. Cardiac catheterization: Used predominantly to evaluate CAD, hemodynamics, associated heart disease. Can be used for quantifying shunt.

        i. Characteristic finding is an increase (step-up) in oxygen concentration in the RA.

        ii. Increased pulmonary artery pressures may be documented.

5. **Goals of care**
   a. Prompt aggressive treatment of heart failure symptoms is provided.
   b. Elective repair of the defect is accomplished as soon as possible.
6. **Collaborating professionals on health care team: See Chronic Unstable Angina; also pediatrician**
7. **Management of patient care**
   a. Anticipated patient trajectory: ASD can rob people of two decades of life and should be corrected as soon as recognized
      i. Pharmacology
         (a) Antibiotics to prevent endocarditis
         (b) Medical management of heart failure
      ii. Treatments
         (a) Surgical repair is the standard treatment for a significant ASD.
            (1) Prepare the patient and family (parents, if the patient is a child) for the possibility of surgical repair, including providing an explanation of the disease process, preoperative routines, the surgical procedure, expectations for the postoperative period.
            (2) Using a median sternotomy or right thoracotomy, the surgeon closes the defect with a pericardial or Dacron patch or suture.
            (3) Early defect repair is recommended to prevent pulmonary hypertension, heart failure, and early death.
            (4) Repair may be deferred in children but should be performed before they enter school (2 to 5 years of age).
            (5) In older children and young adults, the repair should be performed before pulmonary hypertension develops; pathophysiologic changes may be irreversible if the defect is not repaired.
            (6) Postoperative care for ASD repairs is similar to postoperative care for most cardiac operations; stress the importance of preventing potential complications (atrial fibrillation, embolization).
         (b) Transcatheter closure of an ASD and patent foramen ovale is now being used in suitable patients.
         (c) Heart-lung transplantation becomes the only available option if the disease has progressed to include irreversible pulmonary hypertension and pulmonary vascular disease.
   b. Potential complications
      i. Transient heart block
         (a) Mechanism: Most common complication after closure of a septum primum defect because of edema or injury to the AV node
         (b) Management: Temporary pacing may be required. Occasionally, heart block is permanent.
      ii. Other complications include
         (a) Dysrhythmias: Watch for atrial fibrillation, flutter, AV blocks (more frequent in older patients). SVTs may continue after surgery.
         (b) Heart failure (left side and right side), pulmonary hypertension
         (c) Pulmonary embolism or thrombosis, stroke
         (d) Brain abscess
8. **Evaluation of patient care**
   a. Patient is free from associated complications from the interventions.
   b. If complications occur, they are promptly identified and treated.

Ventricular Septal Defect

VSD is an abnormal opening between the ventricles occurring in the membranous or muscular portion of the ventricular septum. Constitutes 25% of all defects and is frequently associated with other defects.
1. **Pathophysiology**
   a. Common types of this defect include the following:
      i. Perimembranous defects

             (a) Occur in approximately 80% of patients with VSD

             (b) Located at the base of the septum under the aortic valve

             (c) Aortic insufficiency can result if the valve cusp is poorly supported.

      ii. Muscular defects

             (a) Occur in 5% to 20%

             (b) Occasionally multiple defects

  b. Small defects

      i. 75% close spontaneously before the affected individuals are age 20 years (50% by age 4 years).

      ii. Generally create no hemodynamic disturbance or pulmonary hypertension in adults; low risk of IE

      iii. Small left-to-right shunt with high pressure gradient between the LV and RV causes a high-velocity jet and a loud (usually grade IV/VI) murmur.

  c. Large defects

      i. Left-to-right shunting through the defect as a result of the higher LV pressures

      ii. Increased RV pressures and PAP occur.

      iii. Increased pulmonary blood flow results in increased pulmonary venous return to the LA. LA pressures, along with the LVEDP, increase. The left heart chambers are volume overloaded, which leads to dilatation, failure, and pulmonary edema.

      iv. Over time, the pulmonary hypertension can become irreversible, often exceeding systemic pressures. The shunt then reverses, becoming right to left, with resulting cyanosis (Eisenmenger's syndrome).

2. Etiology and risk factors

  a. Precise cause of the congenital defect unknown

  b. Associated with coarctation of the aorta, PDA

  c. Factors contributing to congenital defects

      i. Genetic abnormalities

      ii. Chromosomal abnormalities (e.g., Down syndrome)

      iii. Maternal and fetal infections during the first trimester of pregnancy (e.g., rubella)

      iv. Effects of drugs and medications (e.g., cocaine use) during fetal development

      v. Dietary deficiencies during fetal development

      vi. Effects of maternal smoking and/or alcohol intake during pregnancy

      vii. High altitudes

  d. Acute MI: VSD is a serious but infrequent complication of MI and rapidly leads to heart failure, shock, and death

3. Signs and symptoms: Effects of large defects often become evident at 3 to 12 weeks of age. Symptoms depend on defect size and the patient's age.

  a. Subjective findings

      i. Small defects: Patients are usually asymptomatic

      ii. Large defects

             (a) Fatigue, exercise intolerance

             (b) Exertional dyspnea

             (c) Angina-like symptoms (caused by pulmonary hypertension)

             (d) Eisenmenger's syndrome

  b. Objective findings

      i. Frequently normal growth and development

      ii. Possible difficulty in feeding

      iii. May have a history of slow weight gain, small size

      iv. History of endocarditis

      v. History of frequent respiratory infections, often with bronchopneumonia

      vi. History of heart murmurs from birth

      vii. Family history of heart defects

      viii. Maternal exposure to infectious process or poor nutrition, drugs, and medications in the first trimester

  c. Physical examination of the patient: Signs vary, depending on shunt direction and size. Right-to-left shunts produce signs and symptoms of severe heart failure and cyanosis.

       i.   Inspection
- (a) Restlessness, irritability
- (b) Frail appearance, thinness, paleness, waxen complexion
- (c) Tachypnea, air hunger, grunting respirations
- (d) Excessive sweating
- (e) Hemoptysis
- (f) Symptoms of heart failure, cyanosis
- (g) Prominent sternum: From large RV while growing

     ii.   Palpation
- (a) Systolic thrill over lower left sternal border, fourth intercostal space
- (b) PMI may be displaced laterally in larger defects.
- (c) Lift may be felt over the left sternal border.
- (d) Peripheral pulses: Rapid, thready

   iii.   Auscultation
- (a) Harsh, loud, high-pitched holosystolic murmur (even with a small VSD)
  - (1) Loudest at the left sternum, third to fifth intercostal space
  - (2) The louder the murmur, the smaller the defect
  - (3) Nonradiating murmur
- (b) Loud S_2, split but not fixed (may be single in Eisenmenger's syndrome)
- (c) Mitral diastolic rumble at the apex (from increased flow through the mitral valve) indicates a large defect.
- (d) Aortic insufficiency murmurs (associated with membranous defects) may be heard.
- (e) Patient with Eisenmenger's syndrome may not have a murmur (with equalization of right- and left-sided heart pressures).
- (f) Rales with failure

4. Diagnostic study findings
  a. Radiologic (findings may be normal for small VSDs)
- i. LA and LV enlargement
- ii. RA and RV enlargement in the presence of pulmonary artery hypertension
- iii. Increased pulmonary vascular markings
- iv. Pulmonary artery dilatation

  b. ECG
- i. Small defects produce a normal ECG.
- ii. Large defects
  - (a) LA enlargement and LV hypertrophy
  - (b) RV hypertrophy

  c. Echocardiography
- i. Distinguishes shunt flow, increased pulmonary flow, aortic insufficiency; checks prosthetic patches (postoperatively), aneurysms (after closure complication)
- ii. Reveals chamber enlargement
- iii. Demonstrates shunting by the use of echocardiographic contrast material and color-flow Doppler studies

  d. TEE: Identifies residual shunt flow (intraoperatively)
  e. Cardiac catheterization: Can confirm and quantify shunt; assesses hemodynamics; documents the degree of pulmonary hypertension and associated disease (pulmonary stenosis, AR, CAD)

5. Goals of care
  a. Patient's response to the VSD is evaluated to identify the need for interventions.
  b. If symptoms or complications occur, they are promptly identified and treated.
  c. Patient is taught about infection risks, follow-up care.

6. Collaborating professionals on health care team: See Chronic Stable Angina; also pediatrician, dentist

7. Management of patient care
  a. Anticipated patient trajectory: Most VSDs close within the first 2 years of life, but the remainder put patients at risk of endocarditis, limitations due to dyspnea, heart failure, and early death if not corrected

    i. Nutrition: Diet high in calories to assist with infant growth; nasogastric tube may be required

    ii. Infection control: IE prophylaxis

    iii. Discharge planning

       (a) Teach the patient the importance of good dental hygiene.

       (b) Instruct regarding the need for antibiotic prophylaxis to prevent IE (if a small, residual VSD).

    iv. Pharmacology

       (a) Antibiotics: For IE prophylaxis

       (b) Diuretics (i.e., furosemide, chlorothiazide): To treat pulmonary edema, lower intravascular volumes. Electrolytes and renal function need monitoring.

       (c) Afterload reduction

    v. Treatments: Depend on defect size

       (a) Asymptomatic patients who have no pathologic changes do not require surgery. Small defects may close spontaneously over time.

       (b) Plasma exchange transfusions (if HCT higher than 65%) for severe polycythemia

       (c) Catheter closure of VSDs now being done with occlusive devices especially for muscular VSDs

       (d) Patients require surgery when

          (1) Patient is symptomatic with heart failure

          (2) Patient is asymptomatic with a ratio of pulmonary to systemic blood flow in the shunt of 1.5:1 or higher

          (3) Patient shows failure to thrive (at 6 months, the prospect of spontaneous closure has diminished considerably)

          (4) Patient experiences repeated, severe respiratory infections or recurrent endocarditis

b. Potential complications (see specific sections in chapter)

    i. Heart failure (causes 11% of deaths from VSD)

    ii. IE: 4% to 10% risk

    iii. Dysrhythmias, sudden cardiac death: Frequently seen with Eisenmenger's syndrome

8. Evaluation of patient care

  a. Patient is free of associated complications from the interventions.

  b. Complications are promptly identified and treated.

  c. Patient complies with the need for IE prophylaxis and good oral hygiene.

Patent Ductus Arteriosus

PDA is a persistent patency of the fetal circulation between the aorta and the pulmonary artery that failed to close after birth, seen in 2% of adults.

1. Pathophysiology

  a. During fetal circulation: Blood from the pulmonary artery flows through the ductus into the descending aorta to bypass collapsed lungs. Ductus functionally closes within 24 to 48 hours after birth but may remain open up to 8 weeks.

  b. Ductus closure: Contraction of smooth muscles in the ductus wall results from increased arterial oxygen tension. If the smooth muscles do not contract, the ductus remains open (i.e., hypoxia at birth). Prostaglandin inhibitors can stimulate closure.

  c. If the ductus has not closed spontaneously by 3 months of age, it probably will not.

  d. Because the aorta has higher pressures, blood flows back through the patent ductus into the lower-pressure pulmonary artery in a left-to-right shunt, and oxygenated blood is recirculated to the lungs.

  e. Resistance in the ductus to the shunting of blood is caused not only by the diameter of the defect but also by its length.

  f. Small PDAs may have no hemodynamic effects and calcify with aging.

  g. With larger PDAs, LV workload increases (handles both normal CO and shunt flow), but right-sided heart flow is not increased.

    i. Increased blood return to the LA and LV overloads the left side of the heart. LV compensates by enlarging, and symptoms of left-sided heart failure develop.

    ii.   Pulmonary hypertension may develop over time.

  h. Large shunts can result in equal pressure in the systemic and pulmonary systems (Eisenmenger's syndrome with irreversible pulmonary hypertension).

  i. Increased pulmonary pressures then lead to increased work for the RV (which enlarges and fails).

  j. If obstructive pulmonary vascular lesions develop, pulmonary artery pressure will rise above aortic pressure and the shunt will reverse, becoming right to left. Cyanosis and right-sided heart failure result. Deoxygenated blood is distributed to the left arm and the lower body below the ductus (causing cyanosis and clubbing of the toes), whereas the upper body receives oxygenated blood with no abnormalities.

  k. All patients with PDAs are at risk for heart failure and IE. Vegetations may embolize to the lungs, which leads to infarctions and death.

2. Etiology and risk factors

  a. Failure of the ductus to close at birth.

  b. Associated anomalies: ASDs and VSDs

  c. Individuals at risk

    i.   Infants with congenital rubella (acquired in first trimester)

    ii.   Infants with birth hypoxia or respiratory distress, lung disease

    iii. Premature infants (weighing less than 1000 g)

    iv. Infants born at high altitudes (chronic hypoxia)

    v.   Females (twice as common as among males)

3. Signs and symptoms: Shunt size and PVR determine the hemodynamic effects. Asymptomatic in 50% of cases. Moderate-sized PDA may not become symptomatic until LV failure and pulmonary hypertension develop.

  a. Child

    i.   Easy fatigability, irritability, poor feeding that results in poor weight gain

    ii.   History of maternal rubella during first trimester

    iii. History of hypoxia at birth

    iv. Failure to thrive; growth and developmental problems

    v.   High number of respiratory tract infections

  b. Physical findings can include

    i.   Dyspnea on exertion, tachypnea, hemoptysis

    ii.   Angina-like pain, tachycardia, syncope, signs and symptoms of heart failure

    iii. Deafness, cataracts

    iv. Hoarseness (compression of the laryngeal nerve)

    v.   Clubbing, mild cyanosis possible in the left fingers (because of the entry of unsaturated blood into the left subclavian artery); cyanosis in the lower parts of the body and clubbing of the toes (if right-to left shunting); leg fatigue

    vi. Palpation

      (a) Hyperdynamic precordium: Distinct LV impulse (overload)

      (b) Bounding, brisk peripheral pulses (especially with large defects)

      (c) Prominent apical impulse

      (d) Possible systolic thrill in the second left intercostal space

    vii. Auscultation

      (a) Loud, rough, continuous machinery-like murmur is indicative of a PDA; peaks at S_2, heard in more than 50% of patients

        (1) Is loudest high, at left upper sternal border (pulmonic area), left infraclavicular area

        (2) Caused by pressure gradient between the aorta and the pulmonary artery

        (3) Possible mitral flow rumble at the apex

      (b) Wide pulse pressure

4. Diagnostic study findings

  a. Radiologic: Chest radiograph

    i.   LA and LV enlargement (in large left-to-right shunts)

    ii.   Increased pulmonary vascular markings, pulmonary edema in failure

    iii. Enlarged aorta; prominent ascending aorta and aortic knob

       iv. Central pulmonary artery enlarged

  b. ECG (normal in small- and medium-sized PDAs)

       i. LV hypertrophy with left axis deviation

       ii. LA enlargement

  c. Transthoracic echocardiography: Detects the PDA, reveals enlarged chambers, shows flow from the aorta to the pulmonary system in diastole. Color-flow Doppler study helps visualize small shunts and associated congenital defects

  d. TEE: To delineate the PDA

  e. Cardiac catheterization: Not usually necessary

       i. Establishes the aortopulmonary communication and shunt size and direction

       ii. Assesses pulmonary pressures and resistance

       iii. Increased pressures will be evident in the pulmonary artery with right-to-left shunts.

5. Goals of care

  a. Duct is closed by transcatheter or surgical techniques.

  b. Prompt, aggressive treatment is provided for symptoms of heart failure.

  c. IE is prevented.

6. Collaborating professionals on health care team: See Chronic Stable Angina; also pediatrician, obstetrician-gynecologist

7. Management of patient care

  a. Anticipated patient trajectory: Patients with PDA are at risk of endocarditis, heart failure, and possibly shortened life span unless the congenital defect is closed

       i. Infection control: Antibiotic prophylaxis for IE or endarteritis until surgical repair, generally not needed after closure

       ii. Nutrition: Control of fluid and sodium intake, if heart failure symptoms are present

       iii. Discharge planning: IE prophylaxis, follow-up care and evaluation

       iv. Pharmacology

          (a) Patients usually are asymptomatic and do not require medication (except IE prophylaxis) until PDA closure.

          (b) Treatment of heart failure

       v. Treatments

          (a) Pharmacologic closure of PDA with prostaglandin inhibitors such as indomethacin (effective only in infancy). Complications of the use of indomethacin are increased bleeding risks due to platelet dysfunction, necrotizing enterocolitis.

          (b) Transcatheter closure with a detachable coil closure device deployed in the duct to occlude the shunt is being used for older children and adults.

          (c) Surgical ligation of the PDA is the alternative and long-standing treatment. It is primarily performed on large ducts and in young infants.

             (1) Surgery is performed through a small left thoracotomy incision.

             (2) In adults, calcification and rigidity of the ductus make closure much more difficult. A patch may be needed.

             (3) Video-assisted thoracoscopic surgery and robotic techniques are also used.

             (4) Postoperative nursing care involves the same basic care as for thoracotomy.

          (d) Heart-lung transplantation may be indicated in cases of fixed pulmonary hypertension and right-to-left shunting.

  b. Potential complications (see also applicable sections)

       i. IE

       ii. LV heart failure

       iii. Pulmonary hypertension and Eisenmenger's syndrome

       iv. Postoperative complications: Uncommon, include recurrent nerve injury, infections, bleeding, possible hemothorax, pneumothorax, or chylothorax

       v. Complications of the surgical procedures: Failure to close, emboli, vascular complications

8. Evaluation of patient care

  a. Patient is free of associated complications from the interventions and heart failure.

  b. Complications are promptly identified and treated.

Coarctation of the Aorta

Coarctation of the aorta is a congenital deformity of the aorta that creates a narrowing of the lumen and, subsequently, decreased flow. Usually located just beyond the left subclavian artery or just distal to the ligamentum arteriosum. Can be associated with other congenital defects of the heart (e.g., bicuspid aortic valve, VSD).

1. **Pathophysiology**
   a. In the fetus, the smooth muscle of the ductus arteriosus extends into the aorta. After birth, tissue contracts to close the duct, the aorta is pulled inward, and abnormal infolding or narrowing occurs.
   b. Thickening of the aortic medial tissue can form a ridge projecting into the lumen of the aorta, obstructing aortic flow.
   c. Fetal development of the aortic arch may also be abnormal, in conjunction with the formation of other cardiac defects (VSD, mitral valve defects, bicuspid aortic valve).
   d. Pressure gradient develops: pressures proximal to the coarctation are increased and pressures distal are decreased.
   e. LV pressures increase, as do pressures in all aortic arch vessels.
   f. Progressively, the LV dilates, hypertrophies, and can fail because of increased afterload.
   g. Cerebral and upper extremity systemic hypertension results from the mechanical obstruction and stimulation of the renin-angiotensin system due to decreased renal blood flow.
   h. Collateral circulation develops and supports the lower body and extremities, compensating for the decreased blood flow through the aorta. Collaterals involved include the internal mammary, internal thoracic, scapular, epigastric, intercostal, lumbar, and thyrocervical arteries.
   i. If the coarctation is left untreated, death is caused by the consequences of the prolonged hypertension (e.g., strokes, CAD, heart failure, aortic rupture, or dissection). Other complications include IE, cerebral hemorrhage.

2. **Etiology and risk factors**
   a. Incidence higher in males
   b. Associated with the following disorders: VSD, Turner's syndrome, cerebral aneurysms (circle of Willis)
   c. Average life expectancy of an untreated patient with significant coarctation is less than 30 years.

3. **Signs and symptoms: Usually diagnosed in childhood. Newborns may have heart failure and require intervention. After infancy, many patients are asymptomatic until after age 20 to 30 years. Coarctation is often discovered on routine examinations as a result of hypertension or murmur (i.e., during school physicals for sports).**
   a. Subjective findings: Patient may complain of headaches, visual disturbances, epistaxis, leg cramps or fatigue (with exercise), dizziness, dysphagia
   b. Objective findings: Unremarkable in an asymptomatic patient
      i. Cyanosis in preductal coarctation, more noticeable in the fingers than in the toes
      ii. Possible irritability, poor feeding, tachypnea in a critically ill infant
      iii. Oliguria
      iv. Metabolic acidosis
      v. Hypotension
   c. Physical examination
      i. Inspection
         (a) Forceful thrust may be seen at the apex as a result of LV hypertrophy.
         (b) Infants may have lower-extremity cyanosis.
         (c) Rarely, the upper body may be more developed (athletic) than the lower body, which may be underdeveloped (thin legs, narrow hips).
      ii. Palpation
         (a) Check radial and femoral pulses simultaneously for pulse lag (forceful upper extremity pulses, typically weak and delayed or absent lower extremity pulses). Femoral pulses are absent in about 40% of affected patients (the result of narrow pulse pressure, not of absent flow).

(b) Blood pressure in the lower extremities is less than that in the upper extremities (often by more 20 mm Hg). Systolic hypertension seen in the upper extremities.

(c) Blood pressure may vary in the arms, especially if the coarctation is proximal to the left subclavian artery.

(d) Suprasternal notch thrill

(e) Apical thrust

iii. Auscultation

(a) Systolic ejection murmur, heard best at the right upper sternal border

(b) Loud S_2 (aortic component)

(c) S_4 present with left hypertrophy

4. **Diagnostic study findings**

a. Radiologic: Chest radiograph may be the first means of discovery

i. Enlarged LV

ii. Notching of ribs (inferior margins of the third through eighth ribs), caused by the collateral circulation of the intercostal arteries

iii. "3" sign: Dilated ascending aorta followed by the constricted area, followed by the poststenotic dilatation

b. ECG: LV hypertrophy pattern

c. Echocardiography: LV hypertrophy—screen for other associated aortic stenoses, VSDs

d. MRI, CT: Confirms the diagnosis safely in pregnant patients (MRI), provides good images of the thoracic aorta and the site of coarctation

e. Cardiac catheterization: Used to exclude CAD in adults preoperatively. Aortogram shows the location, degree, and character of the aortic lumen narrowing.

5. **Goals of care**

a. Prompt, aggressive treatment is provided for symptoms of heart failure.

b. Hypertension is controlled.

6. **Collaborating professionals on health care team: See Chronic Stable Angina; also pediatrician, obstetrician-gynecologist**

7. **Management of patient care**

a. Anticipated patient trajectory: Patients with unrecognized coarctation of the aorta will be exposed to severe hypertension and acceleration of atherosclerosis, which can result in heart failure, stroke, MI, and early death if the defect is not repaired

i. Infection control: IE antibiotic prophylaxis

ii. Discharge planning

(a) Lifelong monitoring for recoarctation, stenosis, hypertension, valvular disease

(b) Genetic counseling for female patients considering pregnancy

(c) Pregnancy should be avoided until the repair is accomplished. Close supervision for hypertension issues is necessary.

iii. Pharmacology: Antihypertensives for blood pressure control with close follow-up monitoring

iv. Psychosocial issues: Issues regarding contraceptive use and pregnancy are sensitive matters and can cause anxiety and stress in younger patients

v. Treatments

(a) Coarctation is relieved by surgery

(1) If the patient is asymptomatic, surgery is usually delayed until age 1 to 5 years but should be performed as soon as possible to avoid hypertension.

(2) The older the patient, the higher the risk of death is from surgery.

(3) Surgical correction decreases the hypertension and reverses LV failure.

(b) When surgery is undertaken, a left thoracotomy incision is performed.

(1) Postoperative nursing involves the basic care for a thoracotomy patient.

(2) Record blood pressure in both arms.

(3) Assess brachial and femoral pulses simultaneously.

(c) Percutaneous transluminal angioplasty, with or without balloon-expandable endovascular stents, is employed more often, especially with recoarctation.

  b. Potential complications
    i.   IE
    ii.   Common causes of death from coarctation in older patients are spontaneous aortic rupture, heart failure, IE, and cerebral hemorrhage.
    iii. Postoperative complications are recoarctation, paradoxical or persistent systemic hypertension, aortic dissection or rupture, heart failure, and stroke; 20% of patients have transient postoperative abdominal pain and/or distention (probably due to restoration of normal pulsatile blood flow and pressure).
    iv.   Paradoxical systolic hypertension may occur for the first 24 to 36 hours after surgery; caused by increased levels of circulating catecholamines; treated with sodium nitroprusside, β-blockers, ARBs.
    v.   Complications after percutaneous transluminal angioplasty for restenosis include aneurysms, rupture, recoarctation, stroke.
    vi.   Pregnancy: Increased risk of aortic dissection
 8. Evaluation of patient care
  a. Blood pressure is controlled per predetermined parameters.
  b. Patient is free of associated complications from surgery. Any complications are promptly identified and treated.
  c. Patient and significant others discuss the need for follow-up.

Hypertensive Crisis

Hypertensive crisis is a life-threatening elevation in blood pressure necessitating emergency treatment (within 1 hour) to prevent severe end-organ damage and death.
 1. Pathophysiology
  a. Hypertensive pathophysiology and its effects on the heart, brain, and kidneys: See Table 3-12
  b. Hypertensive encephalopathy: Sudden, excessive elevation of the blood pressure (higher than 250/150 mm Hg) → dysfunction of cerebral autoregulation → vasospasm → ischemia → increased capillary pressure and permeability → cerebral edema, hemorrhage
 2. Etiology and risk factors
  a. Untreated or uncontrolled hypertension
  b. Poor compliance with antihypertensive medication regimen
  c. Renal dysfunction (acute glomerulonephritis, acute or chronic renal failure, renal tumors, renovascular hypertension caused by acute renal artery occlusion)
  d. Preeclampsia of pregnancy

■ **TABLE 3-12**
■ ■ **Sequelae of Hypertension: Its Effects on End Organs That May Lead to Hypertensive Crisis**

HYPERTENSION
Enhanced sympathetic stimulation
Effects of renin-angiotensin system (increased fluid retention, increased systemic vasoconstriction)
Necrosis of arterioles
Decreased blood flow to end organs

Heart	Brain	Kidney
Tachycardia	Loss of autoregulatory mechanisms	↓ Renal perfusion
↑ Cardiac output	Arterial spasm and ischemia → TIAs	↓ Ability to concentrate urine
↓ Perfusion → angina → MI	Weakened vessels → aneurysms → hemorrhage → CVA	↑ BUN, creatinine levels
CAD		↑ Proteinuria
LV hypertrophy		Kidney failure
LV failure		Uremia
Angina		

→, Leading to; *BUN*, blood urea nitrogen; *CAD*, coronary artery disease; *CVA*, cerebrovascular accident; *LV*, left ventricular; *MI*, myocardial infarction; *TIA*, transient ischemic attack.

   e. Adrenergic crisis: Seen with a sharp rise in catecholamine levels caused by drug reactions (monoamine oxidase inhibitor interactions, β-adrenergic agonist ingestion, abrupt withdrawal from antihypertensive therapy), pheochromocytoma
   f. Postoperative complications: CABG surgery, renal transplantation, peripheral vascular surgery
   g. Pituitary tumors
   h. Adrenocortical hyperfunction
   i. Severe burns
   j. Risk factors: Diabetes, obesity, smoking, hyperlipidemia, oral contraceptives, history of hypertension with pregnancy, alcohol abuse
3. Signs and symptoms: Patient may be unable to respond to questions; significant other may need to answer history inquiries (e.g., complaints of severe headache, epistaxis) (Figure 3-18)
   a. History
      i.   Chronic hypertension
      ii. Positive family history of hypertension
      iii. Medication history positive for monoamine oxidase inhibitors, oral contraceptives, appetite suppressants, pressor agents, street drugs

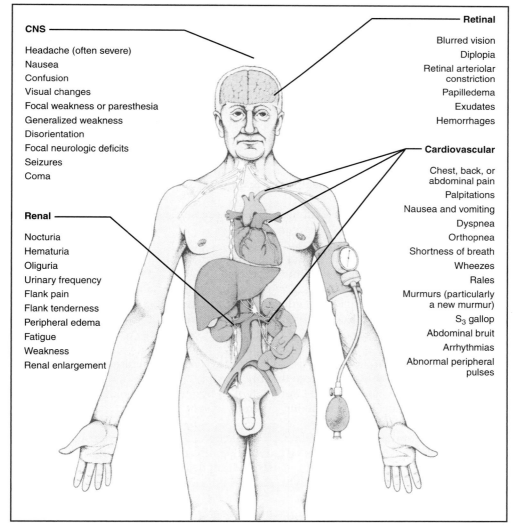

CNS

Headache (often severe)
Nausea
Confusion
Visual changes
Focal weakness or paresthesia
Generalized weakness
Disorientation
Focal neurologic deficits
Seizures
Coma

Renal

Nocturia
Hematuria
Oliguria
Urinary frequency
Flank pain
Flank tenderness
Peripheral edema
Fatigue
Weakness
Renal enlargement

Retinal

Blurred vision
Diplopia
Retinal arteriolar constriction
Papilledema
Exudates
Hemorrhages

Cardiovascular

Chest, back, or abdominal pain
Palpitations
Nausea and vomiting
Dyspnea
Orthopnea
Shortness of breath
Wheezes
Rales
Murmurs (particularly a new murmur)
S_3 gallop
Abdominal bruit
Arrhythmias
Abnormal peripheral pulses

FIGURE 3-18 ■ Symptoms and signs associated with target-organ damage in hypertensive crisis. *CNS*, Central nervous system. (From Antman EM, ed. *Cardiovascular Therapeutics: A Companion to Braunwald's Heart Disease.* Philadelphia, PA: Saunders; 2002:821.)

        iv.   History of any etiologic factor mentioned

        v.   History of CAD, renal dysfunction

   b. Clinical picture in hypertensive encephalopathy

        i.   Blood pressure exceeding 250/150 mm Hg

        ii.   Retinopathy

        iii.   Papilledema of the optic disc

        iv.   Severe headache

        v.   Vomiting

        vi.   Altered level of consciousness (obtunded, comatose)

        vii.   Transitory focal neurologic signs (e.g., nystagmus)

        viii. Seizures

        ix.   Signs and symptoms of heart failure

        x.   Increased MAP

4. Diagnostic study findings

   a. Laboratory

        i.   BUN and creatinine values elevated in patients with renal disease

        ii.   Electrolyte levels: Hypocalcemia, hyponatremia, hypokalemia

        iii.   Enzyme levels for MI

   b. Radiologic: Chest radiograph may show LV enlargement

   c. ECG: LV hypertrophy may be seen

   d. Echocardiogram: Impairment of diastolic function, LV hypertrophy, wall motion abnormalities

   e. MRI or CT: To exclude stroke or hemorrhage when neurologic symptoms present. Shows diffuse brain edema with hypertensive crisis.

   f. Renal ultrasonography: To identify renal artery stenosis

5. Goals of care

   a. Rapid, life-preserving treatment of elevated blood pressure is provided.

   b. MAP is lowered no more than 25% in the first 2 hours, or to 160/100 mm Hg.

   c. Blood pressure is lowered in small decrements to avoid causing hypotension, oliguria, and/or mental changes from renal, coronary, or cerebral ischemia.

   d. Cause of the hypertension is identified and treated.

6. Collaborating professionals on health care team: See Chronic Stable Angina

7. Management of patient care

   a. Anticipated patient trajectory: Immediate blood pressure reduction is essential for the prevention or minimization of end-organ damage

        i.   Nutrition

            (a) Obtain accurate intake and output measurements, along with daily weights

            (b) NPO initially, later a sodium-restricted diet

            (c) Dietary consult: For education on weight control, sodium restriction

        ii.   Discharge planning: Patient education regarding the following:

            (a) Importance of blood pressure control: High risk for renal, cerebral, coronary problems with uncontrolled hypertension. Compliance with medication regimen essential.

            (b) Need for follow-up to assess the effectiveness of medications and to check for potential side effects from therapy

            (c) Lifestyle modification: Limitation of sodium intake, smoking cessation, moderation in alcohol use, walking program, weight control

        iii.   Pharmacology

            (a) Nitroprusside: "Gold standard" for acute malignant hypertensive therapy. Drug of choice for hypertensive encephalopathy, cerebral infarction or bleeding, dissecting aortic aneurysm. Contraindicated in pregnancy (can cause fetal renal impairment). A patient who receives Nipride should be transferred to an intensive care unit.

            (b) Fenoldopam (selective dopamine receptor agonist): Very potent vasodilator; as effective as nitroprusside in lowering blood pressure. A patient who receives fenoldopam should be transferred to an intensive care unit.

            (c) Sympathetic blocking agents

(1) Labetalol (drug of choice for intracranial hemorrhage)

(2) Dosage: 20-mg IV bolus, then 20 to 80 mg every 10 minutes or IV infusion

(3) An α- and β-adrenergic blocking agent, used especially for adrenergic crisis. Does not increase heart rate (good in CAD).

(d) ACE inhibitors

(1) Drug of choice for LV failure and pulmonary edema

(2) Enalapril: 1.25 to 5 mg IV every 6 hours

(3) Onset of action: 10 to 15 minutes

(e) β-Blockers: Block the effects of increased adrenergic tone, reduce mortality and morbidity

(1) Metoprolol: 5 mg IV every 5 minutes up to 15 mg total

(2) Esmolol: 500 mg/kg/min for 4 minutes, then 50 to 300 mg/kg/min IV

(f) IV NTG for hypotension due to cardiac causes (acute MI, failure)

(g) Loop diuretics (torsemide, furosemide, ethacrynic acid) for LV failure, pulmonary edema. Watch for volume depletion.

iv. Psychosocial issues

(a) Reassure the patient and family.

(b) Create a calm, quiet atmosphere, conducive to ample rest for the patient.

(c) If the patient has been noncompliant with the medication regimen and has not addressed known risk factors, explore the reasons for noncompliance.

(1) Make sure the patient knows the rationales for medications and the consequences of inaction.

(2) Blood pressure medications are expensive. Help the patient find resources—financial services, drug programs for the indigent, use of pill splitters (buying larger doses and splitting the pills may be more economical), purchase of generics.

v. Treatments

(a) Ensure that the patient has adequate IV access; prepare for central line insertion, if needed.

(b) Patient should undergo continuous arterial monitoring while drugs are being titrated and the condition is unstable.

(c) Adjust antihypertensive IV medications promptly by titration, depending on the patient's response. Watch for side effects of medications.

(d) Accurately monitor fluid and electrolyte status. Observe for abnormalities in laboratory test results (i.e., electrolyte levels).

(e) If symptoms of tissue ischemia develop, reduce the speed with which blood pressure is lowered. Note: Most problems that occur in hypertensive crisis occur when treatment is too aggressive for the patient to tolerate.

b. Potential complications (see also Figure 3-18)

i. Cerebral dysfunction: Hypertensive encephalopathy, intracerebral or subarachnoid hemorrhage, head injuries, intracranial masses, embolic brain infarction

(a) Mechanism: Increased intracranial pressure (from cerebral edema)

(b) Management: Watch for changes in mentation or vision, headaches, nausea, vomiting. Intracranial pressure monitoring may be needed.

ii. Cardiac or vascular dysfunction

(a) Mechanism: Caused by LV failure, dissecting aortic aneurysm, acute MI, unstable angina, coarctation of the aorta, dysrhythmias

(b) Management: Monitor the ECG, observe for T-wave inversions that occur with rapid blood pressure reductions; ischemia is rare. Sudden chest pain may indicate aortic dissection.

iii. Renal failure

(a) Mechanism: Can be a cause or a result of severely elevated blood pressure

(b) Management: Close monitoring, blood pressure control; dialysis may be required

8. Evaluation of patient care

a. Blood pressure is within set parameters.

b. No side effects of medications are evident.

    c. Electrolyte levels are normal.

    d. No signs of cerebral dysfunction or increased intracranial pressure are noted.

    e. ECG is in sinus rhythm.

    f. CO is adequate as evidenced by hemodynamic assessments, urinary output, adequate circulation.

Aortic and Peripheral Arterial Disease

Diseases of the aorta, cerebral arteries, and peripheral arteries have consequences that include aneurysm formation, dissection, or ischemia in their respective perfusion beds (Figures 3-19 and 3-20).

  1. Pathophysiology

    a. Aortic aneurysm

      i. Focal or diffuse weakness of the aortic wall

      ii. Atherosclerosis is the most common cause.

      iii. Dilatation, increased pressures, and thinning of the wall all increase wall stress, further weakening and dilating the vessel and producing an aneurysm.

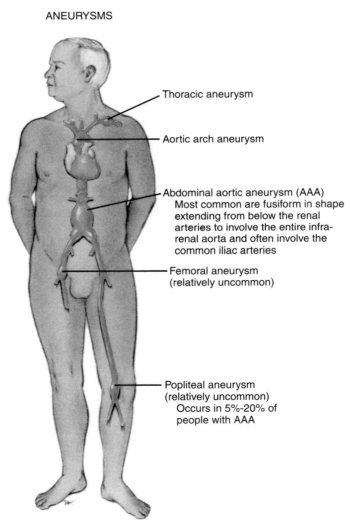

ANEURYSMS

Thoracic aneurysm

Aortic arch aneurysm

Abdominal aortic aneurysm (AAA)
Most common are fusiform in shape extending from below the renal arteries to involve the entire infra-renal aorta and often involve the common iliac arteries

Femoral aneurysm (relatively uncommon)

Popliteal aneurysm (relatively uncommon) Occurs in 5%-20% of people with AAA

FIGURE 3-19 ■ Peripheral artery disease: Aneurysms. (From Jarvis C. *Physical Examination and Health Assessment.* 2nd ed. Philadelphia, PA: Saunders; 1996:597.)

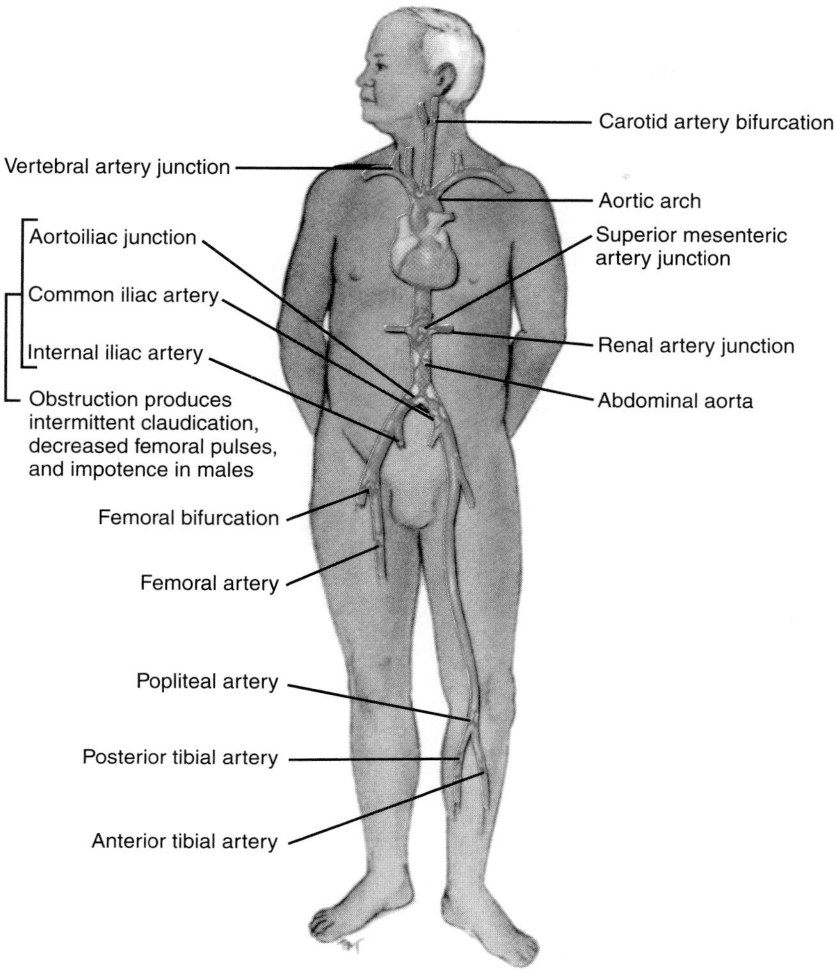

OCCLUSIONS

FIGURE 3-20 ■ Peripheral artery disease: Occlusions. (From Jarvis C. *Physical Examination and Health Assessment.* 2nd ed. Philadelphia, PA: Saunders; 1996:597.)

  iv. Rupture and death are likely when the diameter exceeds 6 cm for the thoracic aorta or 5 cm for the abdominal aorta.

  v. Common sites for aneurysms

   (a) Abdominal aortic aneurysm: Location between the renal and iliac arteries is the most common site

   (b) Thoracic aortic aneurysm

    (1) Ascending, transverse, or descending aorta

    (2) Most common in men aged 60 to 70 years or older

   (c) Aneurysms of the iliac, femoral, and popliteal arteries

b. Aortic dissection

  i. Intima of the ascending and/or descending aorta is weakened by atherosclerosis or congenital disease of the media.

  ii. Hypertension causes or contributes to the injury in 80% of cases.

  iii. Tear develops through the intima and is propagated up and down the aorta by a dissecting column of blood.

  iv. False channel is created.

  v. Some organs may be perfused by the true lumen and some by the false lumen.

      vi. Occasionally, a dissection of the ascending aorta extends to the aortic valve, and aortic insufficiency and even bleeding into the pericardium can result.

      vii. End-organ ischemia and injury can occur.

  c. Peripheral artery disease

      i. Atherosclerotic disease develops from the same risk factors and process as those for CAD.

      ii. Stenosis and hypoperfusion result, culminating in ischemia, occlusion, and infarction (unless supported by collateral circulation).

      iii. Occluded lesions generally occur at bifurcations.

      iv. Occlusions can also result from thrombus or embolus.

      v. Common sites for peripheral artery disease include the carotid, renal, popliteal, aortoiliac, and femoral arteries (but any artery including the mesenteric can be involved).

2. Etiology and risk factors

  a. Atherosclerosis

  b. Congenital abnormalities (cystic medial necrosis, Marfan's syndrome)

  c. Trauma: Blunt trauma can create tears in the intima of the thoracic aorta (causing dissecting aneurysm)

  d. Severe hypertension

  e. Arteritis

  f. Raynaud's disease

  g. Risk factors are the same as for CAD (smoking, hypertension, diabetes, hyperlipidemia, family history)

3. Signs and symptoms: Manifestations usually occur at age 60 years or older

  a. Signs and symptoms vary with the location of the aneurysm or occlusion.

      i. Aneurysm (most common): Often asymptomatic, found on routine examination

         (a) Abdominal aortic aneurysm

           (1) Pulsation in the abdominal area

           (2) Dull abdominal or low back pain or ache (impending rupture)

           (3) Nausea and vomiting (pressure against the duodenum)

           (4) Severe, sharp, sudden abdominal pain: Continuous, radiates to back, hips, scrotum, pelvis (rupture)

           (5) Abdominal tenderness, if an inflammatory process

           (6) Syncope, hypovolemic shock

         (b) Thoracic aortic aneurysm

           (1) Sudden, tearing chest pain radiating to the shoulders, neck, and back

           (2) Cough, hoarseness, weak voice from pressure against the recurrent laryngeal nerve

           (3) Dysphagia due to pressure on the esophagus

      ii. Aortic dissections

         (a) Marked by acute severe and instantaneous chest pain (in 90% of cases), radiating to the back, neck, jaw, or abdomen, associated with an absence of the affected pulses and evidence of end-organ injury

         (b) "Ripping," "tearing" sensations described

         (c) Pain may be differentiated from that of acute MI by its instantaneous, severe onset and the absence of pulses.

         (d) Neurologic symptoms present in 15% of cases

      iii. Peripheral arterial disease

         (a) Intermittent claudication

           (1) Cramping, aching pain with exertion

           (2) Pain in the calf (most often) but may also be in the buttocks

           (3) Reproduced after walking a predictable distance

           (4) Relieved with rest, standing still

         (b) Nonhealing ulcers

         (c) Impotence

         (d) Severe pain in the extremities, pallor, absence of pulses, paresthesias, paralysis (seen in acute thrombosis of an abdominal aortic aneurysm)

(e) Carotid arteries: Transient ischemic attacks, monocular visual disturbances, sensory or motor deficits, expressive or receptive aphasia, stroke

(f) 50% of patients with occlusive arterial disease involving the lower extremities are asymptomatic.

b. History

   i. History of atherosclerosis (CAD, CVA) and hypertension

   ii. Risk factors for atherosclerosis

   iii. Trauma: Blunt, deceleration type

   iv. History of impotence (seen in severe aortoiliac disease)

c. Physical examination: Manifestations depend on the organ perfused (i.e., cerebral vascular disease, renal vascular disease, ischemic or infarcted bowel, ischemic extremities)

   i. Aneurysms: Often asymptomatic except for rupture, when the patient is in obvious severe pain

     (a) Hypertensive or hypotensive

     (b) Obvious discomfort with rupture or expansion

     (c) Stridor, hoarseness, dysphagia (pressure on the esophagus, trachea, pharyngeal nerve)

     (d) Bruits: Abdominal aorta; femoral, renal, popliteal artery

     (e) Murmur of aortic insufficiency, if the aneurysm involves the aortic ring

   ii. Aortic dissection

     (a) Hypertension or hypotension

     (b) Dyspnea

     (c) Stridor, hoarseness, dysphagia (pressure on the esophagus, trachea, pharyngeal nerve)

     (d) Palpation: Wide pulse pressure, absence of various peripheral pulses and pressures (50% of cases)

     (e) Auscultation: Murmur of aortic insufficiency (heard in 50% of cases)

   iii. Peripheral arterial disease

     (a) Pain on elevation of the extremities

     (b) Pale, mottled extremities on elevation: Rubor on dependence of the extremities

     (c) Ulcers, gangrene in the extremities

     (d) Skin changes due to impaired circulation (hair loss, thin and shiny skin)

     (e) Retinal arterial emboli (carotid disease)

     (f) Weak or absent peripheral pulses

     (g) Cool skin

     (h) Sluggish capillary refill

     (i) Pulsatile mass in the popliteal fossa (popliteal aneurysm)

     (j) Auscultation: Bruits

4. Diagnostic study findings

a. Laboratory

   i. CBC: Decreased HCT (anemia)

   ii. Elevated BUN and creatinine levels, proteinuria, hematuria (compromised kidneys)

b. Radiologic

   i. Chest radiograph: Increased aortic diameter, right deviation of the trachea, pleural effusions

   ii. Abdominal films (anteroposterior, lateral views): For abdominal aneurysm

   iii. Provides anatomic information

c. Doppler duplex ultrasonography: To assess peripheral, cerebrovascular blood flow and velocity

d. Ankle-brachial index (ABI): Ankle systolic pressure is divided by the systolic pressure at the brachial artery to derive an index. Used to evaluate for the presence and severity of disease.

   i. Normal ABI = 0.9 to 1.3 (pressure normally higher in the ankle)

   ii. ABI less than 0.9 = positive for peripheral artery disease

   iii. ABI less than 0.4 = indicates severe ischemia

    e. CT: Assesses lumen diameter, wall thickness, aneurysm size, mural thrombi, and origin and extent of dissection, including the blood supply to end organs. Three-dimensional CT with angiography gives vivid three-dimensional views of the vascular system.

    f. MRA: Defines the arterial anatomy, shows the presence and severity of the occlusion

    g. TEE: Assesses for the presence of dissection in the aortic root, proximal ascending aorta, or descending thoracic aorta; aortic insufficiency; pericardial effusion. Used intraoperatively to determine the effectiveness of surgery.

    h. Peripheral angiography: Defines the anatomy and severity of lesions and their suitability for intervention

    i. Aortography: Origin and extent of dissection seen

5. Goals of care

    a. Patient has no pain at rest or with activity.

    b. Perfusion to affected extremities is adequate.

    c. No interventional complications are experienced.

    d. Blood pressure is controlled at the systolic goal set for the patient.

    e. Patient understands medications, follow-up requirements, any limitations on activities, proper diet, when to call for medical help, what symptoms to report.

6. Collaborating professionals on health care team: See Chronic Stable Angina; also vascular specialist, primary care physician, stroke team

7. Management of patient care

    a. Anticipated patient trajectory: Aortic aneurysms and dissections are the most frequently missed preventable causes of sudden cardiac death

        i. Pain management: Relieve pain by administering ordered analgesics

        ii. Skin care: Meticulous attention to the skin because of poor circulation and tissue perfusion. Assess for pressure points, reddened or inflamed areas.

            (a) Frequent repositioning. Turn at least every 2 hours

            (b) Heel protection: Off bed on pillows or foam pads, or in protective boots; elevated

            (c) Ointments, skin barriers as needed

        iii. Nutrition: Dietary consult—Assess nutritional status

        iv. Discharge planning: Teach the patient and significant others about the disease process (aneurysm, peripheral arterial occlusive disease), including the following:

            (a) Risk factor modification (e.g., smoking cessation, blood pressure control, diabetes control)

            (b) Discussion of a walking program, identification of resources to help with follow-up

            (c) Good foot care: Daily washing, nail trimming, use of well-fitting shoes, prompt professional attention to corns, calluses, ulcers

            (d) Weight reduction, if overweight

        v. Pharmacology

            (a) β-Blockers (e.g., propranolol, labetalol) to lower blood pressure

            (b) Simultaneous use of nitroprusside to further lower blood pressure and to decrease contractility and sheer force

            (c) Antiplatelet agents: Aspirin daily (to lower the risk of CVA, MI). May also prevent reocclusions.

            (d) Lipid-lowering agents (statins)

        vi. Treatments

            (a) Dissections: Distal dissections (distal to the left subclavian artery) are usually managed medically. Ascending dissections are treated with medications but require surgery.

            (b) Acute aortic dissections: Surgical emergency

                (1) Goals: Stabilize emergently, prevent complications from rupture. Control systemic blood pressure (100 to 120 mm Hg systolic is the goal)

                (2) Prepare the patient for surgery: Resection, replacement, and/or reconstruction of involved arteries

                    a) Monitor blood pressure continuously.

                    b) Intubation may be necessary, if the patient's condition is unstable.

          c) Assess peripheral pulses and blood pressure, comparing both sides. Pressure differences exceeding 20 mm Hg in the upper extremities indicate possible dissection or occluded subclavian, innominate, brachial, or axillary arteries. Pulses may be impossible to assess by palpating and difficult or impossible to assess with Doppler ultrasonographic studies.

          d) Observe for symptoms of shock.

       (3) Proximal dissections carry a high (80%) mortality rate, but survival rate with surgery is also high.

       (4) Postoperative nursing care for dissection

          a) Monitor hemodynamics.

          b) Watch urinary output, mentation.

   (c) Surgery for descending dissections is performed only if the patient's condition continues to be unstable after medical therapy, with aortic rupture or Marfan's syndrome.

   (d) Endovascular stent grafts are being deployed successfully to cover the descending dissections as a less invasive alternative.

   (e) Endovascular revascularization interventions are widely used before surgery in peripheral arterial disease.

       (1) Percutaneous transluminal angioplasty is used to open occluded arteries, particularly in proximal lesions (iliac, renal).

       (2) Excimer laser technology has also been used to debulk atherosclerotic material.

       (3) Stents are used to reduce restenosis in both native arteries and grafts.

       (4) Patients with acute arterial occlusions may be eligible for low-dose catheter-directed thrombolytic therapy (e.g., t-PA).

       (5) Mechanical thrombolysis or catheter-directed thrombectomy may also be performed for rapid thrombus removal.

       (6) Watch for signs of bleeding, especially if the patient has received thrombolytic therapy.

  b. Potential complications

    i. Aortic aneurysm: Dissection, embolization of thrombus, end-organ compromise

    ii. Large abdominal aneurysms: Disseminated intravascular coagulation is an associated problem

    iii. Ascending aortic dissections: MI, hemorrhagic cerebral infarct, tamponade, AR, death

    iv. Postoperative complications with ascending dissections: Death, CVA, end-organ compromise

    v. Postoperative complications with descending dissections: Ischemia of the spinal cord, paralysis, end-organ compromise

    vi. Postprocedure complications with endovascular intervention: Small bowel infarcts, gangrene

8. Evaluation of patient care

  a. Palpable pulses are felt in the affected extremities.

  b. Limbs are warm with good color and brisk capillary refill.

  c. No signs of bleeding are noted.

  d. Patient is relaxed and free of pain.

  e. Patient and family verbalize an understanding of the treatment plan for home care, medication administration, and risk factor modification and the importance of a walking program.

Shock

In shock, tissue perfusion to vital body organs is inadequate (see Chapter 9).

1. Pathophysiology (Table 3-13)

  a. Diminished tissue perfusion deprives cells of oxygen, nutrients, and energy. Cellular dysfunction and potential cell necrosis ensue, because of the lack of oxygenation and resulting acidosis.

  b. Cellular dysfunction is reversible at first but leads to organ damage if untreated.

■ **TABLE 3-13**
■ ■ **Pathophysiology and Clinical Presentations of Shock**

Type of Shock	Forward Cardiac	CVP	PCWP	SVR	Clinical Examination	Comments
CARDIOGENIC SHOCK						
PUMP FAILURE						
LV MI	↓↓↓	↑↑	↑↑↑	↑↑	+S_3, +S_4	Extensive infarct (>40% LV)
RV MI	↓↓	↑↑↑	↔ or ↓	↑	Right sided +S_3, +S_4	Concomitant inferior wall MI common, consider if elevated right-sided filling pressures with normal or low PCWP or hypotension with clear lung fields
Non-CAD cardiomyopathy	↓↓↓	↑↑	↑↑↑	↑↑	+S_3, +S_4	Includes myocarditis, idiopathic, inflammatory causes
Allograft failure	↓↓↓	↑↑	↑↑↑	↑↑	+S_3, +S_4	Includes cellular and humoral rejection
Infiltrative disease (late)	↓↓↓	↑↑	↑↑↑	↑ or ↔	+S_4 (early)	Characteristic echocardiographic appearance
Trauma	↓↓	↑ or ↔	↑↑	↑ or ↔	Variable	Site involved: RA-RV > LA-LV. May see combined shock (i.e., hypovolemic vs. obstructive with pump failure)
MECHANICAL CAUSES						
Acute aortic regurgitation Native or prosthetic	↓↓	↔	↑↑ or ↑↑↑	↑↑	EDM	Endocarditis most common cause. IABP contraindicated
Acute mitral regurgitation Native or prosthetic	↓↓	↑ or ↔	↑↑↑↑	↑↑	ESM	Prominent PCWP V wave. IABP very effective
Aortic stenosis	↔	↑ or ↔	↑↑	↑↑		Symptoms may become manifest with increased metabolic demand (e.g., pregnancy, exercise, thyrotoxicosis, sepsis)
Mitral stenosis	↔	↑ or ↔	↑↑↑	↑↑		
VSD (acute post-MI)	↓ or ↓↓	↑ or ↑↑	↑ or ↑↑	↑↑	HSM, thrill	May be 3-5 days s/p MI, uncommon event but high mortality
Free wall rupture (post-MI)	↓ or ↓↓	↑ or ↑↑	↑ or ↑↑	↑↑	Silent	Catastrophic presentation 1-3 days s/p MI, earlier presentation with lytics

From Crawford MH, DiMarco JP, Paulus WJ, eds. *Cardiology*. 2nd ed. St Louis, MO: Mosby; 2004:856.
↔, Unchanged; *CAD*, coronary artery disease; *CVP*, central venous pressure; *EDM*, early diastolic murmur; *EDP*, end-diastolic pressure; *ESM*, early systolic murmur; *GI*, gastrointestinal; *HSM*, holosystolic murmur; *IABP*, intra-aortic balloon pump; *LA*, left atrium; *LV*, left ventricle; *MI*, myocardial infarction; *PA*, pulmonary artery; *PCWP*, pulmonary capillary wedge pressure; *RA*, right atrium; *RV*, right ventricle; *s/p*, status post; *SVR*, systemic vascular resistance; *VSD*, ventricular septal defect.

    c. Compensatory mechanisms: To support blood pressure, vasoconstriction is the homeostatic response of the body to hypotension and shock. This response is appropriate for, and probably evolved from, the need to respond to hemorrhagic shock. It is completely inappropriate and detrimental in the management of cardiogenic shock.

d. Major organs begin to malfunction as they are deprived of oxygen, as a result of hypoxemia and metabolic acidosis (respiratory failure, renal failure, decreased cerebral perfusion, and disseminated intravascular coagulation may be seen).

2. Etiology and risk factors

a. Cardiogenic shock: Impaired tissue perfusion as a result of severe cardiac dysfunction

  i. MI, especially if large and/or anterior

  ii. Myocardial ischemia (left main artery disease, multivessel CAD)

  iii. Papillary muscle rupture, acute valvular dysfunction (acute mitral regurgitation, aortic insufficiency)

  iv. Heart failure, cardiac tamponade

  v. Dysrhythmias

  vi. Cardiomyopathy

  vii. Other severe forms of myocardial injury (trauma)

  viii. Risk factors: peripheral vascular disease, decreased LV EF, diabetes

b. Hypovolemic shock: Impaired tissue perfusion resulting from severely diminished circulating blood volume

  i. Hemorrhage: Loss of blood, plasma, and body fluids due to surgery, trauma, gastrointestinal bleeding

  ii. Hypovolemia from fluid shifts (e.g., burns)

  iii. Severe dehydration (vomiting, diarrhea, diabetic ketoacidosis, diabetes insipidus, heat stroke)

  iv. Internal, extravascular fluid loss: Resulting from third-spacing in interstitial space, ascites, ruptured spleen, pancreatitis, hemothorax

  v. Adrenal insufficiency

c. Obstructive shock: Impaired tissue perfusion resulting from some obstruction to blood flow

  i. Pulmonary embolism (see Chapter 2)

  ii. Aortic dissection

d. Anaphylactic shock: Impaired tissue perfusion resulting from antigen-antibody reaction that releases histamine into the blood stream. Capillary permeability increases, and arteriolar dilatation occurs. SVR falls. Blood return to the heart is decreased dramatically. Hypotension results.

  i. Contrast media

  ii. Drug reactions

  iii. Blood transfusion reactions

  iv. Food allergies

  v. Insect bites or stings

  vi. Snake bites

e. Septic shock (systemic inflammatory response syndrome): Impaired tissue perfusion caused by widespread infection and invasion of microorganisms in the body, causing vasodilatation, decreased SVR, and hypotension (see Chapter 9)

f. Neurogenic shock: Impaired tissue perfusion caused by damage to or dysfunction of the sympathetic nervous system. This type of shock is rare and may be associated with trauma, anesthesia, or spinal shock.

3. Signs and symptoms: History and assessments must be done rapidly so that immediate life-preserving therapy can be initiated; information is often obtained from significant others or previous records (e.g., bleeding, trauma, symptoms, fever, drugs, exposure)

a. Clinical picture of cardiogenic shock

  i. Inspection

    (a) Hypotension: Systolic blood pressure lower than 90 mm Hg by cuff, lower than 80 mm Hg by arterial line

    (b) Patient confused, restless, or obtunded

    (c) Shallow, rapid respirations

    (d) Distended neck veins (RV MI, tamponade, pulmonary embolism)

    (e) Large differences in extremity pressures

    (f) Oliguria

    ii.   Palpation
- (a) Cold, clammy extremities (vasoconstricted)
- (b) Peripheral pulses: Threezy, rapid, or absent
- (c) Low temperature

   iii.   Auscultation
- (a) Crackles (pulmonary edema)
- (b) S_3: Gallop
- (c) Systolic murmur (heard with acute mitral regurgitation, VSD, aortic stenosis)
- (d) Diastolic murmur of aortic insufficiency may be heard (short in acute aortic insufficiency)
- (e) Heart sounds distant in tamponade

   iv.   Hemodynamics
- (a) Elevated CVP with neck vein distention (in RV MI, tamponade, massive pulmonary embolism)
- (b) Decreased CO, CI (<2 L/min)
- (c) Elevated PCWP
- (d) Elevated SVR

b. Clinical picture of hypovolemic shock

    i.   Inspection
- (a) Anxiety, irritability
- (b) Decreased level of consciousness
- (c) Poor capillary refill
- (d) Pale, gray skin
- (e) Increased heart rate
- (f) Hypotension
- (g) Collapsed neck veins
- (h) Tachypnea
- (i) Urinary output decreased or absent

c. Clinical picture of anaphylactic shock

    i.   Inspection
- (a) Altered mental status, headache
- (b) Stridor, tachypnea, wheezing
- (c) Increased heart rate, decreased blood pressure
- (d) Hives; itching; flushed, warm skin
- (e) Abdominal cramping, nausea, vomiting, diarrhea
- (f) Chills

    ii.   Hemodynamics
- (a) Decreased CVP

d. Clinical picture of septic shock

    i.   Inspection
- (a) Confusion, decreased level of consciousness
- (b) Fever, chills
- (c) Tachycardia
- (d) Tachypnea
- (e) Warm skin
- (f) Cyanosis
- (g) Oliguria

    ii.   Hemodynamics
- (a) Decreased CVP

e. Clinical picture of neurogenic shock

    i.   Inspection
- (a) Mentation changes (restlessness, confusion)
- (b) Warm, dry skin
- (c) Bradycardia
- (d) No sweating (temperature-regulating center altered): Risk for overheating, chilling
- (e) Paralysis

(f) Apnea, tachypnea, diaphragmatic breathing

(g) Profound hypotension

(h) Nausea, vomiting

(i) Decreased urinary output

   ii. Hemodynamics

(a) Decreased CVP

4. **Diagnostic study findings**

   a. Laboratory

   i. ABG levels

(a) Cardiogenic shock: Metabolic acidosis on ABG testing (hypocapnia, hypoxemia)

(b) Hypovolemic shock: Respiratory alkalosis, metabolic acidosis

   ii. HCT: Decreased with hemorrhage

   iii. Leukocytosis (bacteremia in septic shock)

   iv. Thrombocytopenia (disseminated intravascular coagulation, septic shock)

   v. Abnormal electrolyte levels: Check potassium, sodium, chloride, magnesium

   vi. Troponin levels elevated in acute MI

   b. Radiologic findings: Chest radiograph for

   i. Cardiomegaly

   ii. Pulmonary congestion

   iii. Dilated aortic arch (see Aortic Dissection and Peripheral Arterial Disease)

   iv. Pleural effusion

   v. Cervical and thoracic spinal evaluation (for neurogenic shock)

   c. ECG

   i. Ischemia, infarction

(a) RV infarction: ST elevation in RV leads (lead V_4R)

(b) Anterior MI commonly associated with cardiogenic shock

(c) Prior MI

   ii. Dysrhythmias, conduction defects

   iii. New right-axis deviation: With tachycardia, pulmonary embolism

   d. Echocardiography

   i. LV and RV dysfunction (abnormal wall motion, chamber sizes)

   ii. Tamponade, pericardial effusions

   iii. Valvular disease

   iv. Hypovolemia (small, hyperdynamic chamber)

   v. VSD

   e. Bedside right-sided heart catheterization: To assess hemodynamics (i.e., CO, CI, SVR, PCWP), monitor volume status; evaluate the effectiveness of vasoactive agents and other therapies

   f. TEE: To look for aortic dissection, valvular disease, VSD

   g. Cardiac catheterization: Assesses

   i. CAD severity

   ii. LV function

   iii. Valvular function

   iv. Hemodynamics

   v. Shunts

   vi. Aortography: Dissection, aortic regurgitation

5. **Goals of care**

   a. Systolic blood pressure is increased to adequately perfuse tissues and vital organs. Blood pressure and pulse are within normal limits for the patient.

   b. Sufficient oxygenation is provided.

   c. Pulmonary congestion is decreased.

   d. Fluid and electrolyte balances are maintained.

   e. Intake and output are balanced.

6. **Collaborating professionals on health care team: See Chronic Stable Angina; also critical care specialist, infectious disease specialist**

7. **Management of patient care**

a. Anticipated patient trajectory: Initial management of all forms of shock starts with the ABC of airway, breathing, and circulation. Rapid identification and treatment of the cause(s) will help to avoid end-organ damage and death.

    i. Positioning: Place the patient in reverse Trendelenburg's position for severe drop in blood pressure while other measures are being initiated. Legs can be quickly elevated while the patient is lying flat to shift blood volume from the lower periphery to the central organs instantly.

    ii. Nutrition: Patient will need to receive parenteral or enteral nourishment if on NPO status for a prolonged period

    iii. Infection control: If septic shock, the causative microorganism must be identified and properly treated

    iv. Pharmacology

        (a) Cardiogenic shock

            (1) Inotropic agents: Dobutamine, dopamine, norepinephrine, milrinone, nesiritide

            (2) Vasopressors

            (3) Anticoagulants and antiplatelet agents: Heparin, aspirin, GPIIb/IIIa inhibitors

            (4) Avoidance of negative inotropic agents

            (5) Diuretics, if pulmonary edema present

        (b) Hypovolemic shock

            (1) Administer emergency infusions of volume replacement fluids, blood products.

            (2) Observe for and identify symptoms associated with volume overload, especially if the patient has received large amounts of replacement fluids.

        (c) Anaphylactic shock: IV epinephrine, steroids

        (d) Septic shock: Appropriate antibiotics, volume replacement fluids, vasopressors

        (e) Neurogenic shock: Volume replacement fluids, vasopressors, steroids, atropine (for bradycardia)

    v. Treatments

        (a) Treat hypoxemia and acidosis.

            (1) Give the patient oxygen to maintain the oxygen saturation at 92% or higher.

            (2) Monitor ABG levels, report abnormalities, correct acidotic states: ensure adequate ventilation.

            (3) Provide aggressive respiratory care when the patient is intubated to avoid the complication of pneumonia (especially with neurogenic shock).

            (4) Arterial line may be required.

        (b) Treat hypovolemia (inadequate LV filling volumes).

            (1) Ensure that the patient has good IV access.

            (2) Record vital signs at least every hour, more often as warranted.

            (3) Monitor heart rate and blood pressure to evaluate the patient's response to therapy.

            (4) Maintain a strict hourly record of all intake and output.

            (5) Analyze laboratory results: BUN level, HCT, electrolyte levels; notify the physician of abnormal findings.

            (6) Watch for changes in level of consciousness.

            (7) Observe skin condition: Color, turgor, temperature.

        (c) Early reperfusion in acute MI is vital: patient will need to be prepared for emergent angiography and coronary revascularization efforts such as primary PCI, thrombolysis, CABG.

        (d) LV or biventricular assist devices can be used as a bridge to potential transplantation.

b. Potential complication: Death. Prevention, rapid identification, and appropriate treatment of shock states are vital. Vigilance is the best management for the prevention of death.

8. Evaluation of patient care

    a. Tissue perfusion and oxygenation are adequate.

    b. Vital signs and hemodynamic parameters within normal limits.

    c. Fluid volume and electrolyte balance are maintained.

    d. Coronary blood flow is restored with revascularization, as needed.

REFERENCES AND BIBLIOGRAPHY

Physiologic Anatomy

Crawford MH, DiMarco JP, Paulus WJ, eds. *Cardiology*. 2nd ed. Philadelphia, PA: Mosby; 2004.

Darovic GO. *Hemodynamic Monitoring: Invasive and Noninvasive Clinical Application*. 3rd ed. Philadelphia, PA: Saunders; 2002.

Goldman L, Ausiello D. *Cecil Textbook of Medicine*. 22nd ed. Philadelphia, PA: Saunders; 2004.

Jacobson C, Marzlin K, Webner C. *Cardiovascular Nursing Practice: A Comprehensive Resource Manual and Study Guide for Clinical Nurses*. Burien, WA: Cardiovascular Nursing Education Associates; 2007.

Woods SL, Froelicher ES, Motzer SU, Bridges EJ, eds. *Cardiac Nursing*. 5th ed. Philadelphia, PA: Lippincott Williams & Wilkins; 2005.

Patient Assessment

★ Bates B, Bickley LS, Hoeklman RA. *A Guide to Physical Examination and History-taking*. 6th ed. Philadelphia, PA: Lippincott; 1995.

Braunwald E, ed. *Essential Atlas of Heart Diseases*. New York, NY: McGraw-Hill; 2001.

Braunwald E, Zipes DP, Libby P, eds. *Heart Disease: A Textbook of Cardiovascular Medicine*. 6th ed. Philadelphia, PA: Saunders; 2001.

Crawford MH, DiMarco JP, Paulus WJ, eds. *Cardiology*. 2nd ed. Philadelphia, PA: Mosby; 2004.

Darovic GO. *Hemodynamic Monitoring: Invasive and Noninvasive Clinical Application*. 3rd ed. Philadelphia, PA: Saunders; 2002.

Jacobson C, Marzlin K, Webner C. *Cardiovascular Nursing Practice: A Comprehensive Resource Manual and Study Guide for Clinical Nurses*. Burien, WA: Cardiovascular Nursing Education Associates; 2007.

Diagnostic Studies

Can atherosclerosis imaging techniques improve the detection of patients at risk for ischemic heart disease? In: Proceedings of the 34th Bethesda Conference; October 7, 2002; Bethesda, MD. *J Am Coll Cardiol*. 2003;41(11):1855-1917.

Crawford MH, DiMarco JP, Paulus WJ, eds. *Cardiology*. 2nd ed. Philadelphia, PA: Mosby; 2004.

Goldman L, Ausiello D. *Cecil Textbook of Medicine*. 22nd ed. Philadelphia, PA: Saunders; 2004.

Jacobson C, Marzlin K, Webner C. *Cardiovascular Nursing Practice: A Comprehensive Resource Manual and Study Guide for Clinical Nurses*. Burien, WA: Cardiovascular Nursing Education Associates; 2007.

Landesberg G, Shatz V, Akopnik I, et al. Association of cardiac troponin, CK-MB, and postoperative myocardial ischemia with long-term survival after major vascular surgery. *J Am Coll Cardiol*. 2003;42(9):1547-1554.

Coronary Artery Disease

Canto JG, Iskandrian AE. Major risk factors for cardiovascular disease: debunking the "only 50%" myth. *JAMA*. 2003;290:947-949.

Cardenas GA, Lavie CJ, Milani RV. Importance and management of low levels of high-density lipoprotein cholesterol in older adults. Part I: role and mechanism. *Geriatr Aging*. 2004;7(3):40-45.

Cardenas GA, Lavie CJ, Milani RV. Importance and management of low levels of high-density lipoprotein cholesterol in older adults. Part II: screening and treatment. *Geriatr Aging*. 2004;7(4):41-48.

Chobanian AV, Bakris GL, Black HR, et al. The seventh report of the Joint National Committee on Prevention, Detection, Evaluation, and Treatment of High Blood Pressure: the JNC 7 report. *JAMA*. 2003;289:2560-2572.

Coffey M, Crowder GK, Cheek DJ. Reducing coronary artery disease by decreasing homocysteine levels. *Crit Care Nurse*. 2003;23(1):25-29.

Crawford MH, DiMarco JP, Paulus WJ, eds. *Cardiology*. 2nd ed. Philadelphia, PA: Mosby; 2004.

Greenland P, Knoll MD, Stamler J, et al. Major risk factors as antecedents of fatal and nonfatal coronary heart disease events. *JAMA*. 2003;290:891-897.

Grundy SM, Cleeman JI, Merz CN, et al. Implications of recent clinical trials for the National Cholesterol Education Program Adult Treatment Panel III guidelines. *Circulation*. 2004;110:227-239.

Haskell WL. Cardiovascular disease prevention and lifestyle interventions: effectiveness and efficacy. *J Cardiovasc Nurs*. 2003;18(4):245-255.

Jacobson C, Marzlin K, Webner C. *Cardiovascular Nursing Practice: A Comprehensive Resource Manual and Study Guide for Clinical Nurses*. Burien, WA: Cardiovascular Nursing Education Associates; 2007.

Knot UN, Khot MB, Bajzer CT, et al. Prevalence of conventional risk factors with coronary heart disease. *JAMA*. 2003;290:898-904.

Mosca L, Appel LJ, Benjamin EJ, et al. Evidence-based guidelines for cardiovascular disease prevention in women. *J Am Coll Cardiol*. 2004;43(5):898-921.

Sharis PJ, Cannon CP. *Evidence-based Cardiology*. 2nd ed. Philadelphia, PA: Lippincott Williams & Wilkins; 2003.

Stuart-Shor EM, Buselli EF, Carroll DL. Are psychosocial factors associated with pathogenesis and consequences of cardiovascular disease in the elderly? *J Cardiovasc Nurs*. 2003;18(3):169-183.

Websites

American Diabetes Association. http://www.diabetes.org.

National Heart, Lung, and Blood Institute. http://www.nhlbi.nih.gov/. Practice guidelines, excellent patient resources on weight management, blood pressure guidelines, stroke prevention, cholesterol guidelines, Framingham coronary heart disease risk scoring system.

Office of the Surgeon General, US Department of Human Services. http://www.surgeongeneral.gov/tobacco. Smoking information.

Acute Coronary Syndromes: Unstable Angina Pectoris and Non–ST-Segment Elevation Myocardial Infarction

Blake GJ, Ridker PM. C-reactive protein and other inflammatory risk markers in acute coronary syndromes. *J Am Coll Cardiol.* 2003;41(4 suppl S): 37S-42S.

Cannon CP. Small molecule glycoprotein IIb/IIIa receptor inhibitors as upstream therapy in acute coronary syndromes. *J Am Coll Cardiol.* 2003;41(4 suppl S):43S-48S.

Cohen M. The role of low-molecular-weight heparin in the management of acute coronary syndromes. *J Am Coll Cardiol.* 2003;41(4 suppl S):55S-61S.

Conti R, Fuster V, Badimon JJ. Pathogenetic concepts of acute coronary syndromes. *J Am Coll Cardiol.* 2003;41(4 suppl S):7S-14S.

Crawford PA, ed. *The Washington Manual Cardiology Subspecialty Consult*. Philadelphia, PA: Lippincott Williams & Wilkins; 2004.

Jaffe AS, Davidenko J, Clements I. Diagnosis of acute coronary syndromes including myocardial infarction. In: Crawford MH, DiMarco JP, Paulus WJ, eds. *Cardiology*. 2nd ed. Philadelphia, PA: Mosby; 2004:311-348.

McKay RG. "Ischemia-guided" versus "early invasive" strategies in the management of acute coronary syndrome/non-ST-segment elevation myocardial infarction. *J Am Coll Cardiol.* 2003;41(4 suppl S):96S-102S.

Mehta LSR, Yusuf S. Short- and long-term oral antiplatelet therapy in acute coronary syndromes. *J Am Coll Cardiol.* 2003;41(4 suppl S):79S-88S.

Moliterno DJ, Chan AW. Glycoprotein IIb/IIIa inhibition in early intent-to-stent treatment of acute coronary syndromes: EPISTENT, ADMIRAL, CADILLAC, and TARGET. *J Am Coll Cardiol.* 2003;41(4 suppl S):49S-54S.

Monroe VS, Kerensky RA, Rivera E, Smith KM, Pepine CJ. Pharmacologic plaque passivation for the reduction of recurrent cardiac events in acute coronary syndromes. *J Am Coll Cardiol.* 2003;41(4 suppl S):23S-30S.

Newby LK, Goldmann BU, Ohman EM. Troponin: An important prognostic marker and risk-stratification tool in non-ST-segment elevation acute coronary syndromes. *J Am Coll Cardiol.* 2003;41(4 suppl S):31S-36S.

Sabatine MS, Antman EM. The thrombolysis in myocardial infarction risk score in unstable angina/non-ST-segment elevation myocardial infarction. *J Am Coll Cardiol.* 2003;41(4 suppl S):89S-95S.

Sharis PJ, Cannon CP. *Evidence-based Cardiology*. 2nd ed. Philadelphia, PA: Lippincott Williams & Wilkins; 2003.

Skah PK. Mechanisms of plaque vulnerability and rupture. *J Am Coll Cardiol.* 2003;41(4 suppl S): 15S-22S.

Topol EJ. A guide to therapeutic decision-making in patients with non-ST-segment elevation acute coronary syndromes. *J Am Coll Cardiol.* 2003;41 (4 suppl S):123S-129S.

Topol EJ, ed. *Textbook of Interventional Cardiology*. 4th ed. Philadelphia, PA: Saunders; 2004.

ST-Segment Elevation Myocardial Infarction

Alpert JS. Defining myocardial infarction: "Will the real myocardial infarction please stand up?" *Am Heart J.* 2003;146(3):377-379.

Antman EM, Anbe DT, Armstrong PW, et al. ACC/AHA guidelines for the management of patients with ST-segment elevation myocardial infarction: a report of the American College of Cardiology/American Heart Association Task Force on Practice Guidelines (Committee to Revise the 1999 Guidelines for the Management of Patients with Acute Myocardial Infarction). *J Am Coll Cardiol.* 2004;44(3):E1-E211. Full text and pocket guide available at http://www.acc.org/qualityandscience/clinical/topic/topic.htm.

Archbold RA, Schilling RJ. Atrial pacing for the prevention of atrial fibrillation after coronary bypass graft surgery: a review of the literature. *Heart.* 2004;90:129-133.

Crawford MH, DiMarco JP, Paulus WJ, eds. *Cardiology*. 2nd ed. Philadelphia, PA: Mosby; 2004.

Crawford PA, ed. *The Washington Manual Cardiology Subspecialty Consult*. Philadelphia, PA: Lippincott Williams & Wilkins; 2004.

Schwertz DW, Vaitkus P. Drug-eluding stents to prevent re-blockage of coronary arteries. *J Cardiovasc Nurs.* 2003;18(1):11-16.

Sharis PJ, Cannon CP. *Evidence-based Cardiology*. 2nd ed. Philadelphia, PA: Lippincott Williams & Wilkins; 2003.

Spertus JA, Radford MJ, Every NR, et al. Challenges and opportunities in quantifying the quality of care for acute myocardial infarction: summary from the Acute Myocardial Infarction Working Group of the American Heart Association/American College of Cardiology First Scientific Forum on Quality of Care and Outcomes Research in Cardiovascular Disease and Stroke. *J Am Coll Cardiol.* 2003;41(9):1653-1663.

Topol EJ. *Textbook of Interventional Cardiology*. 4th ed. Philadelphia, PA: Saunders; 2004.

Websites

American College of Cardiology. http://www.acc.org. Cardiology practice guideline updates.

American Heart Association. http://www.americanheart.org.

Cardiology home page of Veterans Health Administration. http://www1.va.gov/cardiology/.

Ischemic heart disease, quality enhancement, research initiative.

Ischemic Heart Disease Quality Enhancement Research Initiative. http://www.hsrd.research.va.gov/queri/

Joint Commission. Acute myocardial infarction, version 1.02. http://www.jointcommission.org/PerformanceMeasurement/PerformanceMeasurement/default.htm

Heart Failure

Albert NM. Cardiac resynchronization therapy through biventricular pacing in patients with heart failure and ventricular dyssynchrony. *Crit Care Nurse.* 2003;23(3 suppl): 2-16.

★ Braunwald E, Zipes DP, Libby P, eds. *Heart Disease: A Textbook of Cardiovascular Medicine.* 6th ed. Philadelphia, PA: Saunders; 2001:503-658.

Cianci P, Lonergan-Thomas H, Slaughter M, et al. Current and potential applications of left ventricular assist devices. *J Cardiovasc Nurs.* 2003;18(1):17-22.

Darovic GO. *Hemodynamic Monitoring: Invasive and Noninvasive Clinical Application.* 3rd ed. Philadelphia, PA: Saunders; 2002.

Eckardt L, Milberg P, Bocker D, et al. Arrhythmias in heart failure. In: Crawford MH, DiMarco JP, Paulus WJ, eds. *Cardiology.* 2nd ed. Philadelphia, PA: Mosby; 2004:905-915.

Frishman WH, Sonnenblick EH, Sica DA, eds. *Cardiovascular Pharmacotherapeutics.* 2nd ed. New York, NY: McGraw-Hill; 2004.

Fuster V, Alexander RW, O'Rourke RA, eds. *Hurst's The Heart.* 10th ed. New York, NY: McGraw-Hill; 2001:655-724.

Givertz MM, Stevenson LW, Colucci WS. Hospital management of heart failure. In: Antman EM, ed. *Cardiovascular Therapeutics: A Companion to Braunwald's Heart Disease.* Philadelphia, PA: Saunders; 2002:357-373.

★ Goldman L, Ausiello D. *Cecil Textbook of Medicine.* 22nd ed. Philadelphia, PA: Saunders; 2004.

Hunt SA, Abraham WT, Chin MH, et al. ACC/AHA 2005 guideline update for the diagnosis and management of chronic heart failure in the adult: a report of the American College of Cardiology/American Heart Association Task Force on Practice Guidelines. *Circulation.* 2005;112:e154-e235. http://www.acc.org/clinical/topic/topic.htm#H.

Joint Commission. Overview of the heart failure (HF) core measure set. http://www.jointcommission.org/PerformanceMeasurement/PerformanceMeasurement/default.htm Published March 22, 2002. Accessed October 14, 2008.

Kirklin J, Young J, McGiffin D. *Heart Transplantation.* New York, NY: Churchill Livingstone; 2002.

MacKlin M. Managing heart failure: a case study approach. *Crit Care Nurse.* 2001;21(2):40-46, 50-51.

Mehra MR, Uber PA, Potluri S, et al. Is heart failure with reserved systolic function an overlooked enigma? *Curr Cardiol Rep.* 2002;4(3):187-193.

Patel AR, Konstam MA. Assessment of the patient with heart failure. In: Crawford MH, DiMarco JP, Paulus WJ, eds. *Cardiology.* 2nd ed. Philadelphia, PA: Mosby; 2004:845-854.

Prahash A, Lynch T. B-type natriuretic peptide: a diagnostic, prognostic, and therapeutic tool in heart failure. *Am J Crit Care.* 2004;13(1):46-55.

Redfield MM, Rodeheffer RJ. Medical therapy of systolic ventricular dysfunction and heart failure. In: Murphy JG, ed. *Mayo Clinic Cardiology Review.* 2nd ed. Philadelphia, PA: Lippincott Williams & Wilkins; 2000:75-92.

Rodeheffer RJ, Redfield MM. Congestive heart failure: diagnosis, evaluation, and surgical therapy. In: Murphy JG, ed. *Mayo Clinic Cardiology Review.* 2nd ed. Philadelphia, PA: Lippincott Williams & Wilkins; 2000:55-74.

Schwarz KA, Elman CS. Identification of factors predictive of hospital readmissions for patients with heart failure. *Heart Lung.* 2003;32(2):88-99.

Websites

Datascope Corp. http://www.datascope.com. Intra-aortic balloon counterpulsation.

Heart Failure Society of America. http://www.hfsa.org/. Practice guidelines, patient education.

Pericardial Disease

Bonnefoy E, Godon P, Kirkorian G, et al. Serum cardiac troponin I and S-T segment elevation in patients with acute pericarditis. *Eur Heart J.* 2000;21:832-836.

Cheitlein MD, Armstrong WF, Aurigemma GP, et al. ACC/AHA/ASE 2003 guideline update for the clinical application of echocardiography: summary article: a report of the American College of Cardiology/American Heart Association Task Force on Practice Guidelines (ACC/AHA/ASE Committee to Update the 1997 Guidelines for the Clinical Application of Echocardiography). *Circulation.* 2003;108:1146-1162.

Hoit BD. Diseases of the pericardium. In: Fuster V, Alexander RW, O'Rourke RA, eds. *Hurst's the Heart.* 10th ed. New York, NY: McGraw-Hill; 2001:2061-2085.

Kabbani SS, LeWinter MM. Pericardial disease. In: Murphy JG, ed. *Mayo Clinic Cardiology Review.* 2nd ed. Philadelphia, PA: Lippincott Williams & Wilkins; 2000:993-1007.

Oh JK. Pericardial diseases. In: Murphy JG, ed. *Mayo Clinic Cardiology Review.* 2nd ed. Philadelphia, PA: Lippincott Williams & Wilkins; 2000:509-532.

Spodick DH. Pericardial diseases. In: Braunwald E, Zipes DP, Libby P, eds. *Heart Disease: A Textbook of Cardiovascular Medicine.* 6th ed. Philadelphia, PA: Saunders; 2001:1823-1876.

Myocarditis

Felker GM, Boehmer JP, Hruban RH, et al. Echocardiographic findings in fulminant and acute myocarditis. *J Am Coll Cardiol.* 2000;36(1):227-232.

Goldman ME. Infectious myocarditis. In: Alpert JS, ed. *Cardiology for the Primary Care Physician.* Philadelphia, PA: Current Medicine; 2001:250-269.

Kirklin J, Young J, McGiffin D. *Heart Transplantation.* New York, NY: Churchill Livingstone; 2002: 221-222.

Sarda L, Colin P, Boccara F, et al. Myocarditis in patients with clinical presentation of myocardial infarction and normal coronary angiograms. *J Am Coll Cardiol.* 2001;37(3):786-792.

Schultheiss H-P, Kuhl U. Myocarditis and inflammatory cardiomyopathy. In: Crawford MH, DiMarco JP, Paulus WJ, eds. *Cardiology.* 2nd ed. Philadelphia, PA: Mosby; 2004:937-949.

Infective Endocarditis

Acar J, Michel P-L. Infective endocarditis. In: Murphy JG, ed. *Mayo Clinic Cardiology Review.* 2nd ed. Philadelphia, PA: Lippincott Williams & Wilkins; 2000:1161-1177.

Cheitlein MD, Armstrong WF, Aurigemma GP, et al. ACC/AHA/ASE 2003 guideline update for the clinical application of echocardiography: summary article: a report of the American College of Cardiology/American Heart Association Task Force on Practice Guidelines (ACC/AHA/ASE Committee to Update the 1997 Guidelines for the Clinical Application of Echocardiography). *Circulation.* 2003;108:1146-1162.

Ewy GA. Infectious endocarditis. In: Alpert JS, ed. *Cardiology for the Primary Physician.* 3rd ed. Philadelphia, PA: Current Medicine; 2001: 271-278.

Karchmer AW. Infective endocarditis. In: Braunwald E, Zipes DP, Libby P, eds. *Heart Disease: A Textbook of Cardiovascular Medicine.* 6th ed. Philadelphia, PA: Saunders; 2001:1723-1750.

Mylonakis E, Callderwood SB. Infective endocarditis in adults. *N Engl J Med.* 2001;345:1318-1330.

Patel R, Steckelberg JM. Infections of the heart. In: Murphy JG, ed. *Mayo Clinic Cardiology Review.* 2nd ed. Philadelphia, PA: Lippincott Williams & Wilkins; 2000:407-444.

Sande MA, Kartalija M, Anderson J. Infective endocarditis. In: Fuster V, Alexander RW, O'Rourke RA, eds. *Hurst's the Heart.* 10th ed. New York, NY: McGraw-Hill; 2001:2087-2125.

Cardiomyopathy

Akkad MZ, O'Connell JB. Dilated and toxic cardiomyopathy. In: Crawford MH, DiMarco JP, Paulus WJ, eds. *Cardiology.* 2nd ed. Philadelphia, PA: Mosby; 2004:951-973.

Bristow MR, Mestroni L, Bohlmeyer TJ, et al. Dilated cardiomyopathies. In: Fuster V, Alexander RW, O'Rourke RA, eds. *Hurst's the Heart.* 10th ed. New York, NY: McGraw-Hill; 2001:1947-1966.

Elliott PM, Reith S, McKenna WJ. Hypertrophic cardiomyopathy. In: Crawford MH, DiMarco JP, Paulus WJ, eds. *Cardiology.* 2nd ed. Philadelphia, PA: Mosby; 2004:961-973.

Hoekstra JW, ed. *Handbook of Cardiovascular Emergencies.* 2nd ed. Philadelphia, PA: Lippincott Williams & Wilkins; 2001.

Kirklin J, Young J, McGiffin D. *Heart Transplantation.* New York, NY: Churchill Livingstone; 2002.

Maron BJ. Hypertrophic cardiomyopathy. In: Fuster V, Alexander RW, O'Rourke RA, eds. *Hurst's the Heart.* 10th ed. New York, NY: McGraw-Hill; 2001:1967-1987.

Maron BJ. Hypertrophic cardiomyopathy. *Circulation.* 2002;106:2419-2421.

Maron BJ, McKenna WJ, et al. ACC/ESC clinical expert consensus document on cardiomyopathy: a report of the American College of Cardiology Task Force on Clinical Expert Consensus Documents and the European Society of Cardiology Committee for Practice Guidelines (Committee to Develop an Expert Consensus Document on Hypertrophic Cardiomyopathy). *J Am Coll Cardiol.* 2003;42(9):1687-1713.

Nishimura RA, Ommen SR, Tajik AJ. Hypertrophic cardiomyopathy: a patient perspective. *Circulation.* 2003;108:e133-e135.

Pereira NL, Dec GW. Restrictive and infiltrative cardiomyopathy. In: Crawford MH, DiMarco JP, Paulus WJ, eds. *Cardiology.* 2nd ed. Philadelphia, PA: Mosby; 2004:983-992.

Sweeney MO, Ellenbogen KA. Implantable devices for the electrical management of heart disease: overview of indications for therapy and selected advances. In: Antman EM, ed. *Cardiovascular Therapeutics: A Companion to Braunwald's Heart Disease.* Philadelphia, PA: Saunders; 2002:516-528.

End-Stage Heart Disease

Albert NM. Cardiac resynchronization therapy through biventricular pacing in patients with heart failure and ventricular dyssynchrony. *Crit Care Nurse.* 2003;23(3 suppl):2-16.

Bolno PB, Kresh JY. Physiologic and hemodynamic basis of ventricular assist devices. *Cardiol Clin.* 2003;21(1):15-27.

Holmes EC. Outpatient management of long-term assist devices. *Cardiol Clin.* 2003;21:91-99.

Hunt SA, Abraham WT, Chin MH, et al. ACC/AHA 2005 guideline update for the diagnosis and management of chronic heart failure in the adult: a report of the American College of Cardiology/American Heart Association Task Force on Practice Guidelines. *Circulation.* 2005;112:e154-e235. http://www.acc.org/clinical/topic/topic.htm#H.

Hunt SA, Schroeder JS, Berry GJ. Cardiac transplantation, mechanical ventricular support, and endomyocardial biopsy. In: Fuster V, Alexander RW, O'Rourke RA, eds. *Hurst's the Heart.* 10th ed. New York, NY: McGraw-Hill; 2001:725-744.

Jessup M, Brozena SC. Epilogue: support devices for end stage heart failure. *Cardiol Clin.* 2003;21: E135-139.

Kirklin J, Young J, McGiffin D. *Heart Transplantation.* New York, NY: Churchill Livingstone; 2002.

Mehra MR, Uber PA. The dilemma of late-stage heart failure. *Cardiol Clin.* 2001;19(4):627-635.

Mehra MR, Uber PA. Emergence of Laplace therapeutics: declaring an end to "end-stage" heart failure. *Congest Heart Fail.* 2002;8:228-231.

Mehra MR, Uber PA, Vivekananthan K, et al. Comparative beneficial effects of simvastatin and pravastatin on cardiac allograft rejection and survival. *J Am Coll Cardiol.* 2002;40(9):1609-1614.

Miniati DN, Robbins RC, Reitz B. Heart and heart-lung transplantation. In: Braunwald E, Zipes DP, Libby P, eds. *Heart Disease: A Textbook of Cardiovascular Medicine.* 6th ed. Philadelphia, PA: Saunders; 2001:615-634.

Park MH, Scott RL, Uber PA, et al. Treatment of pulmonary hypertension. *Catheter Cardiovasc Interv.* 2002;57:395-403.

Patel H, Pagani FD. Extracorporeal mechanical circulatory assist. *Cardiol Clin.* 2003;21(1):29-41.

Remme WJ, Swedberg K. Comprehensive guidelines for the diagnosis and treatment of chronic heart failure, Task Force for the diagnosis and treatment of chronic heart failure of the European Society of Cardiology. *Eur J Heart Fail.* 2002;4:11-22.

Young JB. Surgery, assist devices and cardiac transplantation for heart failure. In: Crawford MH, DiMarco JP, Paulus WJ, eds. *Cardiology.* 2nd ed. Philadelphia, PA: Mosby; 2004:917-930.

Cardiac Trauma

Cummins RO, ed. *ACLS for Experienced Providers.* Dallas, TX: American Heart Association; 2003.

Mattox KL, Estera AL, Wall MJ. Traumatic heart disease. In: Braunwald E, Zipes DP, Libby P, eds. *Heart Disease: A Textbook of Cardiovascular Medicine.* 6th ed. Philadelphia, PA: Saunders; 2001:1877-1907.

Murphy JG, Nobrega TP. Cardiac trauma. In: Murphy JG, ed. *Mayo Clinic Cardiology Review.* 2nd ed. Philadelphia, PA: Lippincott Williams & Wilkins; 2000:1129-1138.

Myers ML, Cheung A, Sibbald WJ. Trauma. In: Crawford MH, DiMarco JP, Paulus WJ, eds. *Cardiology.* 2nd ed. Philadelphia, PA: Mosby; 2004:1577-1582.

Poh KK, Tan HC, Chia BL, et al. A case of broken heart from blunt trauma. *Singapore Med J.* 2002;43(8):423-425.

Symbas PN. Traumatic heart disease. In: Foster V, Alexander RW, O'Rourke RA, eds. *Hurst's the Heart.* 10th ed. New York, NY: McGraw-Hill; 2001:2219-2226.

Website

http://www.surgical-tutor.org.uk/core/trauma/chest_trauma.htm.

Basic Dysrhythmias for Progressive Care
Symptomatic Bradycardia

Crawford MH, DiMarco JP, Paulus WJ, eds. *Cardiology.* 2nd ed. Philadelphia, PA: Mosby; 2004.

Cummins RO. *ACLS—The Reference Book. ACLS: Principles and Practice.* Dallas, TX: American Heart Association; 2003.

Gregoratos G, Epstein AE, Hayes DL, et al. ACC/AHA/NASPE 2002 guidelines update for implantation of cardiac pacemakers and antiarrhythmia devices: summary article: a report of the American College of Cardiology/American Heart Association Task Force on Practice Guidelines (ACC/AHA/NASPE Committee to Update the 1998 Pacemaker Guidelines). *Circulation.* 2002;106:2145-2161.

Hayes DL, Zipes DP. Cardiac pacemakers and cardioverter-defibrillators. In: Braunwald E, Zipes DP, Libby P, eds. *Heart Disease: A Textbook of Cardiovascular Medicine.* 6th ed. Philadelphia, PA: Saunders; 2001:775-814.

Huszar RJ. Basic dysrhythmias: interpretation and management. 3rd ed. Philadelphia, PA: Mosby; 2001.

Lynn-McHale DJ, Carlson KK, eds. *AACN Procedure Manual for Critical Care.* 4th ed. Philadelphia, PA: Saunders; 2001.

★ Moss AJ, Cannom DS, Daubert JP, et al. Multicenter Automatic Defibrillator Implantation Trial II (MADIT II): design and clinical protocol. *Ann Noninvasive Electrocardiol.* 1999;4:83-91.

Murphy JG, ed. *Mayo Clinic Cardiology Review.* 2nd ed. Philadelphia, PA: Lippincott Williams & Wilkins; 2000.

Symptomatic Tachycardia

Blomstrom-Lundqvist C, Aliot EA, Calkins H. ACC/AHA/ESC guidelines for the management of patients with supraventricular arrhythmias: executive summary: a report of the American College of Cardiology/American Heart Association Task Force on Practice Guidelines and the European Society of Cardiology Committee for Practice Guidelines (Writing Committee to Develop Guidelines for the Management of Patients with Supraventricular Arrhythmias). *J Am Coll Cardiol.* 2002;42(8):1493-1531.

★ Braunwald E, Zipes DP, Libby P, eds. *Heart Disease: A Textbook of Cardiovascular Medicine.* 6th ed. Philadelphia, PA: Saunders; 2001.

Crawford MH, DiMarco JP, Paulus WJ, eds. *Cardiology.* 2nd ed. Philadelphia, PA: Mosby; 2004.

Cummins RO. *ACLS—The Reference Book. ACLS: Principles and Practice.* Dallas, TX: American Heart Association; 2003.

Deaton C, Dunbar SB, Moloney M, et al. Patient experiences with atrial fibrillation and treatment with implantable atrial defibrillation therapy. *Heart Lung.* 2003;32(5):291-299.

Fuster V, Rydén LE, Asinger RW, et al. ACC/AHA/ESC guidelines for the management of patients with atrial fibrillation: executive summary: a report of the American College of Cardiology/American Heart Association Task Force on Practice Guidelines and the European

Society of Cardiology Committee for Practice Guidelines and Policy Conferences (Committee to Develop Guidelines for the Management of Patients with Atrial Fibrillation). *J Am Coll Cardiol.* 2001;38(4):1231-1266.

Epstein AE, DiMarco JP, Ellenbogen KA et al. ACC/AHA/HRS 2008 guidelines for device-based therapy of cardiac rhythm abnormalities: a report of the American College of Cardiology/American Heart Association Task Force on Practice Guidelines (Writing Committee to revise the ACC/AHA/NASPE 2002 Guideline update for implantation of cardiac pacemakers and antiarrhythmia devices) Developed in collaboration with the American Association for Thoracic Surgery and Society of Thoracic Surgeons. *J Am Coll Cariol.* 2008;51:e1-e62. Full text available at http://content.online-jacc.org/cgi/content/full/j.jacc.2008.02.032

Hayes DL, Zipes DP. Cardiac pacemakers and cardioverter-defibrillators. In: Braunwald E, Zipes DP, Libby P, eds. *Heart Disease: A Textbook of Cardiovascular Medicine.* 6th ed. Philadelphia, PA: Saunders; 2001:775-814.

Lynn-McHale DJ, Carlson KK, eds. *AACN Procedure Manual for Critical Care.* 5th ed. Philadelphia, PA: Saunders; 2005.

Murphy JG, ed. *Mayo Clinic Cardiology Review.* 2nd ed. Philadelphia, PA: Lippincott Williams & Wilkins; 2000.

Singer DE, Go AS. Antithrombotic therapy in atrial fibrillation. *Clin Geriatr Med.* 2001;17(1):131-147.

Absent or Ineffective Pulse

Crawford MH, DiMarco JP, Paulus WJ, eds. *Cardiology.* 2nd ed. Philadelphia, PA: Mosby; 2004.

Cummins RO. *ACLS—The Reference Book. ACLS: Principles and Practice.* Dallas, TX: American Heart Association; 2003.

Gregoratos G, Epstein AE, Hayes DL, et al. ACC/AHA/NASPE 2002 guidelines update for implantation of cardiac pacemakers and antiarrhythmia devices: summary article: a report of the American College of Cardiology/American Heart Association Task Force on Practice Guidelines (ACC/AHA/NASPE Committee to Update the 1998 Pacemaker Guidelines). *Circulation.* 2002;106:2145-2161.

Murphy JG, ed. *Mayo Clinic Cardiology Review.* 2nd ed. Philadelphia, PA: Lippincott Williams & Wilkins; 2000.

Myerburg RJ, Castellanos A. Cardiac arrest and sudden cardiac death. In: Braunwald E, Zipes DP, Libby P, eds. *Heart Disease: A Textbook of Cardiovascular Medicine.* 6th ed. Philadelphia, PA: Saunders. 2001:890-931.

Hypertensive Crisis

Alper AB, Calhoun DA. Hypertensive emergencies. In: Antman EM, ed. *Cardiovascular Therapeutics: A Companion to Braunwald's Heart Disease.* Philadelphia, PA: Saunders; 2002:817-831.

Beevers DG, Lip GY. Hypertensive crises. In: Crawford MH, DiMarco JP, Paulus WJ, eds. *Cardiology.* 2nd ed. Philadelphia, PA: Mosby; 2004:545-552.

Black HR, Bakris GL, Elliott WJ. Hypertension: epidemiology, pathophysiology, diagnosis, and treatment. In: Fuster V, Alexander RW, O'Rourke RA, eds. *Hurst's the Heart.* 10th ed. New York, NY: McGraw-Hill; 2001:1553-1604.

Chobanian AV, Bakris GL, Black HR, et al. Seventh report of the Joint National Committee on Prevention, Detection, Evaluation, and Treatment of High Blood Pressure. *Hypertension.* 2003;42:1206-1252.

Goldman L, Ausiello D. *Cecil Textbook of Medicine.* 22nd ed. Philadelphia, PA: Saunders; 2004.

Hogan MJ. Hypertension. In: Murphy JG, ed. *Mayo Clinic Cardiology Review.* 2nd ed. Philadelphia, PA: Lippincott Williams & Wilkins; 2000:1067-1082.

Vaughan CJ, Delanty N. Hypertensive emergencies. *Lancet.* 2000;356:411-417.

Weber MA. *Hypertension Medicine.* Totowa, NJ: Humana Press; 2001:429-435.

Websites

American Heart Association Council for High Blood Pressure Research. http://www.americanheart.org/presenter.jhtml?identifier=1115.

American Society of Hypertension. http://www.ash-us.org/.

Aortic and Peripheral Arterial Disease

★ Braunwald E, Zipes DP, Libby P, eds. *Heart Disease: A Textbook of Cardiovascular Medicine.* 6th ed. Philadelphia, PA: Saunders; 2001.

Crawford PA, ed. *The Washington Manual Cardiology Subspecialty Consult.* Philadelphia, PA: Lippincott Williams & Wilkins; 2004.

Erbel R, Alfonso F, Boileau C, et al. Diagnosis and management of aortic dissection. *Eur Heart J.* 2001;22:1642-1681.

Fagrell B. Arterial disease of the limbs. In: Crawford MH, DiMarco JP, Paulus WJ, eds. *Cardiology.* 2nd ed. Philadelphia, PA: Mosby; 2004:109-122.

Fahey VA. *Vascular Nursing.* 3rd ed. Philadelphia, PA: Saunders; 1999.

Garmany R. Diseases of the aorta. In: Crawford PA, ed. *The Washington Manual Cardiology Subspecialty Consult.* Philadelphia, PA: Lippincott Williams & Wilkins; 2004:235-242.

Goldman L, Ausiello D. *Cecil Textbook of Medicine.* 22nd ed. Philadelphia, PA: Saunders; 2004.

Halperin JL, Fuster V. Meeting the challenge of peripheral arterial disease. *Arch Intern Med.* 2003;28:877-878.

Hirsch AT, Criqui MH, Treat-Jacobson D, et al. Peripheral arterial disease detection, awareness, and treatment in primary care. *JAMA.* 2001;281(11):1317-1324.

McPhail IR, Spittel PC, Weston SA, et al. Intermittent claudication: an objective office-based assessment. *J Am Coll Cardiol.* 2001;37:1381-1385.

Mehta R, O'Gara P, Bossone E, et al. Acute type A aortic dissection in the elderly: clinical characteristics, management, and outcomes in the current era. *J Am Coll Cardiol.* 2002;40:685-692.

Wernly JA. Thoracic aorta disease. In: Crawford MH, DiMarco JP, Paulus WJ, eds. *Cardiology.* 2nd ed. Philadelphia, PA: Mosby; 2004:141-152.

Shock

Alexander RW, Pratt CM, Ryan TJ, et al. Diagnosis and management of patients with acute myocardial infarction. In: Fuster V, Alexander RW, O'Rourke RA, eds. *Hurst's the Heart.* 10th ed. New York, NY: McGraw-Hill; 2001:1275-1359.

★ Braunwald E, Zipes DP, Libby P, eds. *Heart Disease: A Textbook of Cardiovascular Medicine.* 6th ed. Philadelphia, PA: Saunders; 2001.

Crawford MH, DiMarco JP, Paulus WJ, eds. *Cardiology.* 2nd ed. Philadelphia, PA: Mosby; 2004.

Darovic GO. *Hemodynamic Monitoring: Invasive and Noninvasive Clinical Application.* 3rd ed. Philadelphia, PA: Saunders; 2002.

★ Goldman L, Ausiello D. *Cecil Textbook of Medicine.* 22nd ed. Philadelphia, PA: Saunders; 2004.

Hochman JS, Califf RM. Acute myocardial infarction. In: Antman EM, ed. *Cardiovascular Therapeutics: A Companion to Braunwald's Heart Disease.* Philadelphia, PA: Saunders; 2002:233-291.

Hoekstra JW, ed. *Handbook of Cardiovascular Emergencies.* 2nd ed. Philadelphia, PA: Lippincott Williams & Wilkins; 2001.

Murphy JG, ed. *Mayo Clinic Cardiology Review.* 2nd ed. Philadelphia, PA: Lippincott Williams & Wilkins; 2000.

The Neurologic System

Physiologic Anatomy

1. **Brain**
   a. Coverings
      i. Scalp
         (a) Dermal layer: Skin
         (b) Subcutaneous fascia: Fibrous fatty layer between the skin and galea that contains blood vessels
         (c) Galea aponeurotica: Freely movable, tendinous tissue; covers the vertex of the skull; absorbs the force of external trauma
         (d) Subaponeurotic or subgaleal space: Contains the diploic and emissary veins
         (e) Periosteum: Thin layer of tissue that covers the skull
      ii. Cranium
         (a) Part of the skull that houses and protects the brain (Figure 4-1)
         (b) Bones: Frontal, sphenoid, ethmoid, occipital, two temporal, and two parietal bones
         (c) Basilar skull: Base of the skull has three depressions—the anterior, middle, and posterior fossae (Figure 4-2)
      iii. Meninges (Figure 4-3)
         (a) Dura mater
            (1) Outermost covering of the brain; consists of two layers of tough fibrous tissue
            (2) Outer layer forms the periosteum of the bone.
            (3) Inner layer folds to form the falx cerebri, tentorium cerebelli, falx cerebelli, and diaphragma sella.
            (4) Meningeal arteries and venous sinuses lie in clefts formed by the inner and outer layers of the dura mater.
            (5) Subdural space lies between the inner dura mater and the arachnoid mater.
         (b) Arachnoid mater
            (1) Fine, fibrous, elastic layer between the dura mater and pia mater
            (2) Subarachnoid space
               a) Lies between the arachnoid mater and pia mater; expanded areas of this space form cisterns at the base of the brain
               b) Contains blood vessels, including the circle of Willis
               c) Contains cerebrospinal fluid (CSF), which completely surrounds the brain and spinal cord; acts as a shock absorber
               d) Contains the arachnoid villi: Projections of the arachnoid mater that absorb CSF into the venous system

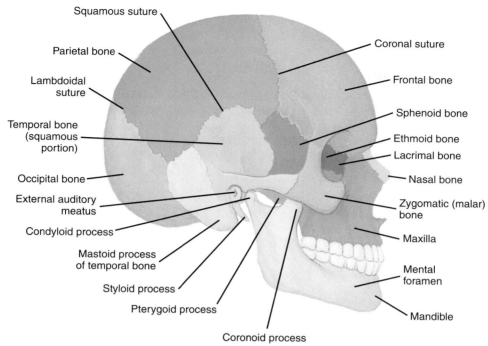

FIGURE 4-1 ■ The skull as seen from the side. (From Slazinski T, Littlejohns LR. Anatomy of the nervous system. In: Bader MK, Littlejohns LR, eds. *AANN Core Curriculum for Neuroscience Nursing*. 4th ed. St Louis, MO: Saunders; 2004:31; modified from Thibodeau GA, Patton K. *Anatomy and Physiology*. 5th ed. St Louis, MO: Mosby; 2003.)

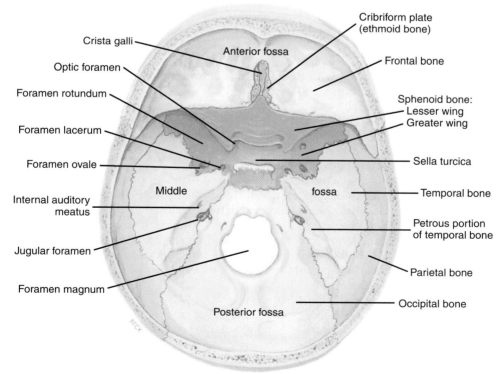

FIGURE 4-2 ■ Base of the skull showing the cranial fossae. (From Slazinski T, Littlejohns LR. *Anatomy of the Nervous System*. In: Bader MK, Littlejohns LR, eds. *AANN Core Curriculum for Neuroscience Nursing*. 4th ed. St Louis, MO: Saunders; 2004:32; modified from Thibodeau GA, Patton K. *Anatomy and Physiology*. 5th ed. St Louis, MO: Mosby; 2003.)

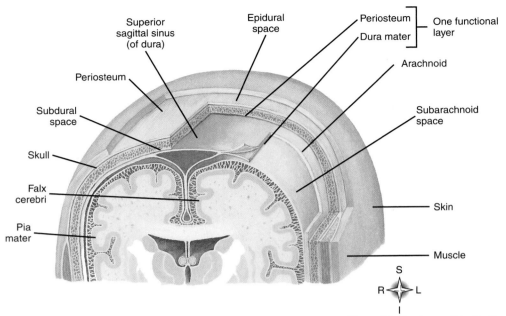

FIGURE 4-3 ■ Coverings of the brain. *I*, Inferior; *L*, left; *R*, right; *S*, superior. (From Thibodeau GA, Patton K. *Anatomy and Physiology*. 5th ed. St Louis, MO: Mosby; 2003:376.)

        (c) Pia mater
            (1) Delicate vascular layer that covers the brain surface, following the sulci and gyri
            (2) Surrounds surface blood vessels and emerging nerves
            (3) Blood vessels of the pia mater form the choroid plexus.
  b. Divisions of the brain
     i. Cerebrum
        (a) Telencephalon: Two cerebral hemispheres separated by a longitudinal fissure; joined by the corpus callosum
            (1) Functional localization in the cerebral cortex, including *cerebral dominance* (Table 4-1)
            (2) Corpus callosum: Commissural fibers that transfer learned discriminations, sensory experiences, and memory from one cerebral hemisphere to corresponding parts of the other
            (3) Basal ganglia (basal nuclei) (Figure 4-4)
                a) Masses of gray matter; includes the caudate, putamen, globus pallidus, claustrum, amygdaloid, and, functionally, the subthalamic and substantia nigra nuclei
                b) Functions: Exert regulating and controlling influences on the coordination of voluntary motion, motor integration, movement initiation, muscle tone, and postural reflexes. A major center of the extrapyramidal motor system.
        (b) Diencephalon (Figure 4-5)
            (1) Thalamus: Two egg-shaped masses of gray matter that abut the lateral walls of the third ventricle; subdivided into several nuclei
                a) Certain nuclei receive, integrate, and process sensory input for relay to the cerebral cortex.
                b) Other nuclei participate in affective aspects of brain function; are functionally related to the association areas of the cortex; or have a role in conscious pain, temperature, and touch awareness, motor function, and the ascending reticular activating system.

▨ TABLE 4-1
▨ ▨ Functional Localization in the Cerebral Cortex

Lobe	Functions
Frontal	Higher mental functions
	Concentration
	Abstract thinking
	Foresight and judgment
	Behavior and tactfulness
	Inhibition
	Memory
	Personality
	Affect
	Conjugate eye movements
	Voluntary motor function
	Motor control of speech (dominant hemisphere*)
Temporal	Hearing
	Comprehension of spoken language (dominant hemisphere*)
	Visual, olfactory, and auditory perception
	Memory
	Learning and intellect
	Emotion
Parietal	Sensory perception of touch, pain, temperature, position, pressure, and vibration
	Body awareness
	Sensory interpretation
Occipital	Visual perception and interpretation
	Control of some visual and ocular movement reflexes

*Cerebral dominance: In right-handed and most left-handed people, the left cerebral hemisphere is dominant for language, mathematical, and analytic functions. The opposite nondominant hemisphere is thought to be concerned with nonverbal, geometric, spatial, visual, and musical functions.

      (2) Hypothalamus: Below the thalamus; regulates
        a) Body temperature
        b) Food and water intake
        c) Behavior: Part of the limbic system; concerned with aggressive and sexual behavior; elicits physical expressions associated with emotions; may be involved with sleep-wake cycles and circadian rhythm control
        d) Autonomic responses: Control center for the autonomic nervous system (ANS); controls numerous visceral and somatic activities (e.g., heart rate, pupil constriction and dilation)
        e) Hormonal secretion of the pituitary gland (see Chapter 6)
          1) Posterior pituitary gland (neurohypophysis): Stores and releases antidiuretic hormone (ADH) and oxytocin, produced by the hypothalamus. ADH causes vasoconstriction and increases renal water reabsorption. Oxytocin stimulates uterine contraction and milk ejection.
          2) Anterior pituitary gland (adenohypophysis): Secretes prolactin and growth-stimulating, thyroid-stimulating, adrenal-stimulating, follicle-stimulating, and luteinizing hormones; hormonal secretion is under the control of pituitary releasing and inhibiting factors produced in the hypothalamus and transported to the anterior pituitary via a pituitary portal system (see Chapter 6)
      (3) Subthalamus: Functionally related to the basal ganglia
      (4) Epithalamus: Dorsal part of the diencephalon
        a) Contains the pineal gland
        b) Thought to regulate circadian rhythms and the food-getting reflex; probable role in growth and development

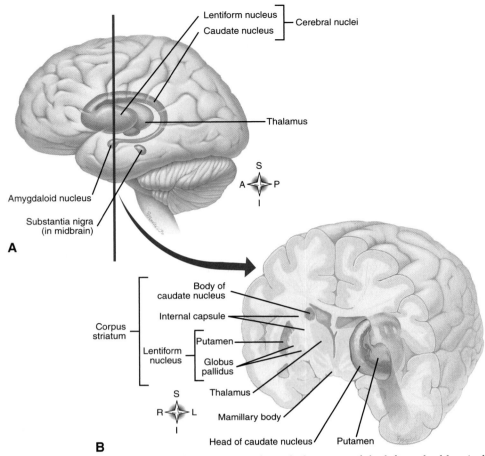

FIGURE 4-4 ■ Basal ganglia or basal nuclei. **A,** As seen through the cortex of the left cerebral hemisphere. **B,** As seen in a frontal (coronal) section of the brain. *A,* Anterior; *I,* inferior; *L,* left; *P,* posterior; *R,* right; *S,* superior. (From Thibodeau GA, Patton K. *Anatomy and Physiology.* 5th ed. St Louis, MO: Mosby; 2003:392.)

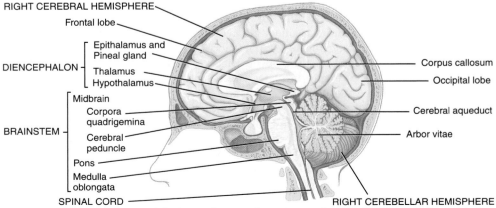

FIGURE 4-5 ■ Midsagittal section of the brain showing the major portions of the diencephalon, brainstem, and cerebellum. (From Applegate EJ. *The Anatomy and Physiology Learning Systems Textbook.* 2nd ed. Philadelphia, PA: Saunders; 2000:167.)

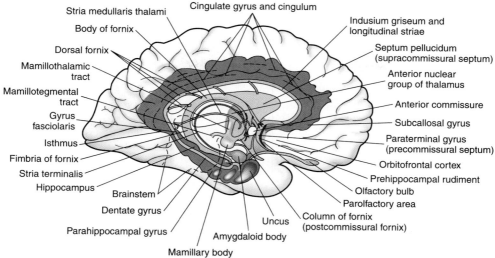

Stria medullaris thalami
Cingulate gyrus and cingulum
Body of fornix
Dorsal fornix
Mamillothalamic tract
Mamillotegmental tract
Gyrus fasciolaris
Isthmus
Fimbria of fornix
Stria terminalis
Hippocampus
Brainstem
Dentate gyrus
Parahippocampal gyrus
Uncus
Amygdaloid body
Mamillary body
Column of fornix (postcommissural fornix)
Parolfactory area
Olfactory bulb
Prehippocampal rudiment
Orbitofrontal cortex
Paraterminal gyrus (precommissural septum)
Subcallosal gyrus
Anterior commissure
Anterior nuclear group of thalamus
Septum pellucidum (supracommissural septum)
Indusium griseum and longitudinal striae

FIGURE 4-6 ■ Anatomy of the limbic system illustrated by the shaded areas of the figure. (From Slazinski T, Littlejohns LR. Anatomy of the nervous system. In: Bader MK, Littlejohns LR, eds. *AANN Core Curriculum for Neuroscience Nursing*. 4th ed. St Louis, MO: Saunders; 2004:41.)

    (c) Limbic system (Figure 4-6)
        (1) Composed of the limbic lobe (cingulate and parahippocampal gyri) plus structures to which it is anatomically and functionally connected such as the amygdala, hippocampus, fornix, hypothalamus, olfactory tract, and thalamus
        (2) Responsible for emotional behavioral responses and accompanying visceral, endocrine, and somatic responses; has a role in basic instinctual drives (e.g., mating, hunger, motivation) and in some aspects of memory and learning
  ii. Brainstem (Figure 4-7; also see Figure 4-5)
    (a) Midbrain (mesencephalon): Located between the diencephalon and pons
        (1) Contains nuclei of cranial nerve (CN) III (oculomotor) and CN IV (trochlear) and some CN V (trigeminal) nuclei
        (2) Contains motor and sensory pathways
        (3) Holds respiratory control centers
        (4) Tectal region (inferior and superior colliculi): Concerned with the auditory and visual systems
        (5) Connects to the cerebellum via the superior cerebellar peduncles
    (b) Pons (metencephalon): Between the midbrain and medulla
        (1) Contains nuclei of CN V, VI (abducens), and VII (facial) and some CN VIII (acoustic) nuclei
        (2) Middle cerebellar peduncles on its basal surface provide extensive connections between the cerebral cortex and cerebellum, ensuring maximal motor efficiency.
        (3) Contains motor and sensory pathways
        (4) Holds respiratory control centers that help coordinate breathing patterns
    (c) Medulla (myelencephalon): Between the pons and spinal cord
        (1) Contains nuclei of CN IX (glossopharyngeal), X (vagus), XI (spinal accessory), and XII (hypoglossal) and some nuclei from CN V, VII, and VIII.
        (2) Motor and sensory tracts of spinal cord continue into the medulla.
        (3) Attaches to the cerebellum via the inferior cerebellar peduncles
        (4) Holds respiratory, cardiac, and vasomotor control centers

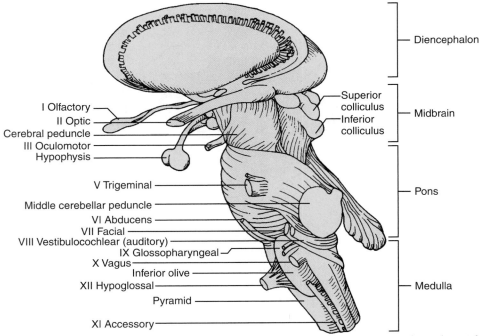

Diencephalon

Midbrain
- Superior colliculus
- Inferior colliculus

Pons

Medulla

I Olfactory
II Optic
Cerebral peduncle
III Oculomotor
Hypophysis

V Trigeminal

Middle cerebellar peduncle
VI Abducens
VII Facial
VIII Vestibulocochlear (auditory)
IX Glossopharyngeal
X Vagus
Inferior olive
XII Hypoglossal
Pyramid

XI Accessory

FIGURE 4-7 ■ Lateral view of the brainstem showing the main subdivisions, surface landmarks, and cranial nerves. (From Barker E. *Neuroscience Nursing: A Spectrum of Care*. 2nd ed. St Louis, MO: Mosby; 2002:23.)

       (d) Reticular formation (RF) (Figure 4-8): Diffuse cellular network in the brainstem, with axons projecting to the thalamus and into the cortex; receives input from the cerebrum, spinal cord, other brainstem nuclei, and the cerebellum; has a role in the control of autonomic and endocrine functions, skeletal muscle activity, and visceral and somatic sensation. The reticular activating system is part of the RF.

          (1) Ascending reticular activating system is essential for arousal from sleep, alert wakefulness, focusing of attention, and perceptual association.

          (2) Descending reticular activating system may inhibit or facilitate motor neurons controlling the skeletal musculature.

    iii. Cerebellum: Lies in the posterior fossa behind the brainstem; separated from the cerebrum by the tentorium cerebelli

       (a) Influences muscle tone in relation to equilibrium, locomotion, posture, and nonstereotyped movements

       (b) Important in the synchronization of muscle action to enable coordinated movement

       (c) Input is from the spinal cord, brainstem, vestibular system, and cerebral centers; output to the brainstem and thalamus influences spinal and cerebral activities.

  c. Cerebral circulation (Figure 4-9)

    i. Arterial system: Supplied by the internal carotid and vertebral arteries

       (a) Circle of Willis: Anastomosis of arteries at the base of the brain formed by a short segment of the internal carotid and anterior and posterior cerebral arteries, which are connected by an anterior communicating artery and two posterior communicating arteries. This anastomosis may permit collateral circulation if a carotid or vertebral artery becomes occluded.

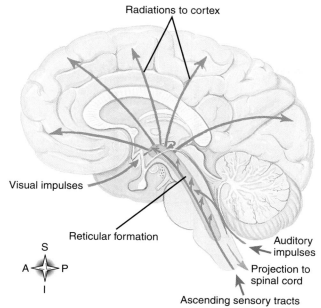

Radiations to cortex

Visual impulses

Reticular formation

S

A ✦ P

I

Auditory impulses

Projection to spinal cord

Ascending sensory tracts

FIGURE 4-8 ■ Reticular activating system. Consists of centers in the brainstem reticular formation plus fibers that conduct to the centers from below and fibers that conduct from the centers to widespread areas of the cerebral cortex. Functioning of the reticular activating system is essential for consciousness. *A,* Anterior; *I,* inferior; *P,* posterior; *S,* superior. (From Thibodeau GA, Patton K. *Anatomy and Physiology.* 5th ed. St Louis, MO: Mosby; 2003:395.)

(b) Internal carotid system: Internal carotid arteries arise from the common carotid arteries. Table 4-2 shows the branches of this system and the areas they supply.

(c) Vertebral system: Vertebral arteries arise from the subclavian arteries and join at the lower pontine border to form the basilar artery. Branches of this system and the areas they supply are summarized in Table 4-2.

(d) Branches of the internal carotid, external carotid, and vertebral arteries (e.g., anterior, middle, posterior meningeal arteries) provide blood supply to the meninges.

ii.   Cerebral blood flow (CBF)

(a) Normal CBF averages 50 ml/100 g of brain tissue per minute.

(b) Cerebral perfusion pressure (CPP) and intrinsic regulatory mechanisms affect CBF.

(1) CPP: Pressure gradient that drives blood into the brain; calculated as the difference between the mean arterial pressure (MAP) and the intracranial pressure (ICP): CPP = MAP − ICP

(2) Regulatory mechanisms influence the diameter of the cerebrovasculature.

a) Pressure or myogenic autoregulation: Alteration in the diameter of the brain's resistance vessels (arterioles) that maintains a constant CBF over a range of pressures between 50 and 150 mm Hg. Chronic hypertension can increase the upper and lower pressure ranges for the range of autoregulation.

b) Elevated arterial partial pressure of carbon dioxide ($Paco_2$) and hypoxemia (arterial partial pressure of oxygen [Pao_2] of <50 mm Hg) cause vasodilatation and increased CBF; decreased $Paco_2$ causes vasoconstriction and reduced CBF.

c) Metabolic autoregulation: CBF varies with metabolic activity. Factors that increase the metabolic rate (e.g., seizures, fever) increase CBF; reduced metabolic requirements (e.g., hypothermia) decrease CBF.

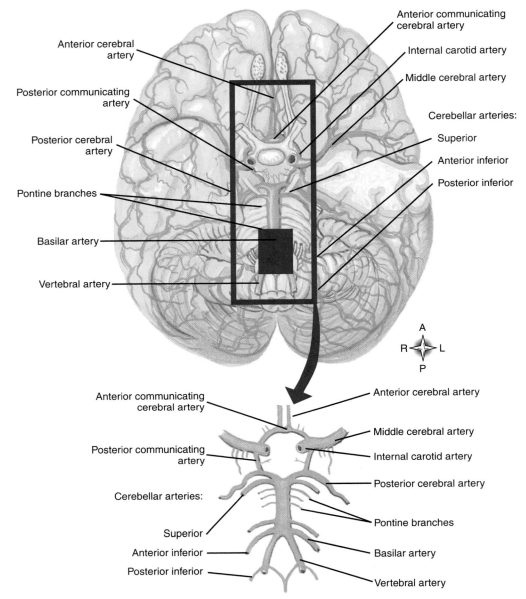

FIGURE 4-9 ■ Arteries at the base of the brain. The arteries that compose the circle of Willis are the two anterior cerebral arteries joined to each other by the anterior communicating cerebral artery and to the posterior cerebral arteries by the posterior communicating arteries. *A,* Anterior; *L,* left, *R,* right, *P,* posterior. (From Thibodeau GA, Patton K. *Anatomy and Physiology.* 5th ed. St Louis, MO: Mosby; 2003:573.)

          (3) Inadequate CBF results in brain tissue ischemia (CBF <18 to 20 ml/100 g/min) and death (CBF <8 to 10 ml/100 g/min).

          (4) CBF higher than metabolic demand is called hyperemia.

    iii. Venous system: Brain surface drains into the superficial veins; the central interior cerebrum drains into the internal veins beneath the corpus callosum (Figure 4-10). Veins have no valves.

        (a) Veins empty into venous sinuses between dural layers (Table 4-3).

        (b) Internal jugular veins collect blood from the large dural venous sinuses and return blood to the heart.

TABLE 4-2
Major Cerebral Arteries and Areas they Supply

Artery	Area of the Brain Supplied
INTERNAL CAROTID ARTERY BRANCHES	
Anterior cerebral artery	Medial aspect of the frontal and parietal lobes; part of the cingulate gyrus and corpus callosum; via the recurrent artery of Heubner supplies part of the basal ganglia and a portion of the internal capsule
Anterior communicating artery	Connects the right and left anterior cerebral arteries
Middle cerebral artery (largest branch of the internal carotid artery)	Most of the lateral surfaces of the frontal, temporal, and parietal lobes; via the lenticulostriate artery, supplies the majority of the basal ganglia and internal capsule
Posterior communicating artery	Connects the posterior cerebral artery with the internal carotid artery; connects the carotid with the vertebrobasilar circulation
VERTEBRAL ARTERY BRANCHES	
Anterior spinal artery	Anterior one half to three quarters of the spinal cord
Posterior inferior cerebellar artery	Undersurface of the cerebellum; choroid plexus of the fourth ventricle; medulla
BASILAR ARTERY BRANCHES	
Posterior cerebral artery	Occipital lobes and the inferior and medial portion of the temporal lobes; thalamus and part of the hypothalamus; choroid plexuses of the lateral and third ventricles; midbrain
Superior cerebellar artery	Upper surface of the cerebellum; midbrain
Anterior inferior cerebellar artery	Inferior surface of the cerebellum; portion of the pons

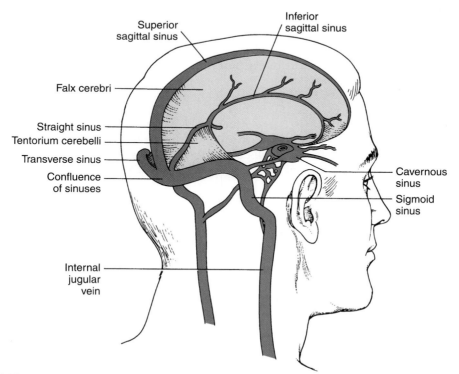

FIGURE 4-10 ■ Diagram showing the pattern of distribution of the major dural venous sinuses and their connection to the internal jugular veins. (From Barker E. *Neuroscience Nursing: A Spectrum of Care*. 2nd ed. St Louis, MO: Mosby; 2002:36.)

▨ **TABLE 4-3**
▨ ▨ **Major Venous Drainage Structures, Their Locations, and Areas Drained**

Venous Structure	Location and Area Drained
Superior sagittal sinus	Courses along the midline at the superior border of the falx cerebri; superior cerebral veins empty into it
Straight sinus	Lies in the midline attachment of the falx cerebri and the tentorium; drains the system of internal cerebral veins (including the inferior sagittal sinus and great cerebral vein of Galen)
Transverse sinuses	Lie in the bony groove along the fixed edge of the tentorium cerebelli; drain the straight sinus and the superior sagittal sinus
Sigmoid sinuses	Lie on the mastoid process of the temporal bone and jugular process of the occipital bone; receive blood from the transverse sinuses and empty into the internal jugular veins
Inferior sagittal sinus	Lies along the free inferior border of the falx cerebri just above the corpus callosum; receives blood from the medial aspects of the hemispheres
Emissary veins	Connect the dural sinuses with veins outside the cranial cavity

    iv. Blood-brain barrier: Specialized permeability of the brain capillaries that limits transfer of certain substances from blood into brain tissue. Barrier formed by tight junctions between brain capillary endothelial cells, reduced transport mechanisms of these cells, and footlike projections from the astrocytes that encase the capillaries.

        (a) Water, carbon dioxide, oxygen, glucose, and lipid-soluble substances cross the cerebral capillaries with ease. Uptake of other substances, such as dyes and ions (e.g., Na^+, K^+), is much slower.

        (b) Regulates the entry or removal of various substances to maintain a homeostatic environment for the central nervous system (CNS)

        (c) Clinically significant in treating and diagnosing CNS disease. Blood-brain barrier disruption and increased permeability occur with brain injury, tumors, infections, and stroke.

  d. Ventricular system and CSF (Figure 4-11)

    i. Ventricles: Four cavities containing CSF

        (a) Lateral ventricles: Largest ventricles, one in each cerebral hemisphere. The anterior (frontal) horns lie in the frontal lobes; the bodies extend back through the parietal lobes to the posterior (occipital) horns, which project into the occipital lobes; the inferior (temporal) horns lie in the temporal lobes.

        (b) Third ventricle: Midline between the two lateral ventricles, surrounded by the diencephalon

        (c) Fourth ventricle: In the posterior fossa bordered by the pons, medulla, and superior cerebellar peduncles; continuous with the cerebral aqueduct (aqueduct of Sylvius) superiorly and the central spinal canal inferiorly

    ii. CSF functions

        (a) Cushions the brain and spinal cord from injury

        (b) Provides support and buoyancy for the brain, decreasing its effective weight on the skull

        (c) Its displacement out of the cranial cavity (and, to an extent, its increased reabsorption) compensates for increases in intracranial volume and pressure.

        (d) Regulates the nervous system chemical environment to preserve homeostasis

        (e) Enables water-soluble metabolites to diffuse from the brain

        (f) Serves as a channel for neurochemical communication within brain

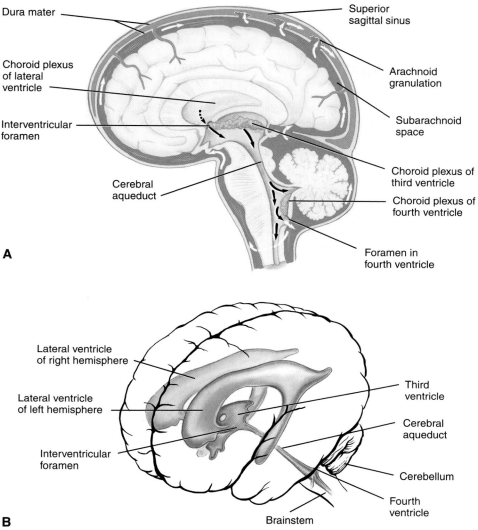

FIGURE 4-11 ■ Ventricular system. **A,** Circulation of cerebrospinal fluid. **B,** Ventricles of the brain. (From Applegate EJ. *The Anatomy and Physiology Learning Systems Textbook.* 2nd ed. Philadelphia, PA: Saunders: 2000:169.)

   iii. CSF properties: See Table 4-4
   iv. CSF formation
      (a) Rate of synthesis estimated as 500 ml/day or 22 to 25 ml/hr
      (b) Choroid plexus: Tuft of capillaries covered by epithelial cells found in all ventricles; principal source of CSF; lateral ventricles produce most
      (c) Small amounts of CSF are produced by the blood vessels of the brain and meningeal linings.
   v. Circulation and absorption of CSF (see Figure 4-11)
      (a) CSF circulates from the lateral ventricles through the interventricular foramina (foramina of Monro) to the third ventricle and to the fourth ventricle via the aqueduct of Sylvius; CSF then circulates to the subarachnoid space via the foramina of Luschka and Magendie.
      (b) Most CSF is absorbed via the arachnoid villi into the dural sinuses.
      (c) When CSF pressure exceeds venous pressure, CSF is absorbed through the unidirectional valves of the arachnoid villi.

■ **TABLE 4-4**
■ ■ **Normal Properties of Cerebrospinal Fluid**

Characteristic	Normal Finding
Appearance	Clear, colorless
Specific gravity	1.007
Glucose level	50-75 mg/dl or approximately 60% of serum glucose level
Protein level	Lumbar: 15-45 mg/dl (*Note:* Increases when blood is present in CSF)
Cells	White blood cells: 0-5/mm³
	Red blood cells: 0/mm³
Lactate level	10-20 mg/dl
pH	7.35
Pressure	70-180 mm water, measured at the lumbar level, with the patient in the lateral decubitus position
Volume	Ventricular system and subarachnoid space contain approximately 125 to 150 ml of CSF

CSF, Cerebrospinal fluid.

vi. Blood-CSF barrier: Choroid plexus epithelium imposes a barrier analogous to the blood-brain barrier; permits selective transport of substances from the blood into the CSF
e. Brain metabolism
   i. Brain has high metabolic energy requirements; energy primarily used for neuronal conductive and metabolic activities.
   ii. At rest, the brain consumes 25% of body glucose and 20% of body oxygen; cerebral oxygen consumption averages 49 ml/min.
   iii. Brain utilizes glucose as its principal energy source.
   iv. Minimal storage of oxygen and glucose in the brain necessitates a constant supply for normal neuronal function.
   v. Anaerobic glucose metabolism (glycolysis) yields insufficient adenosine triphosphate (ATP) to meet cerebral energy demands. Rate of glycolysis increases markedly during hypoxia in an attempt to maintain functional neuronal activity.
   vi. Within seconds to minutes of anoxia, the energy-dependent sodium-potassium pump fails; cytotoxic cerebral edema results.
   vii. Hypoglycemia causes neuronal dysfunction and may lead to convulsions, coma, and death.
f. Cells of the nervous system
   i. Neuron: Basic functional unit of the nervous system; transmits nerve impulses
      (a) Components of each cell (Figure 4-12)
         (1) Cell body: Carries out the metabolic functions of the cell; contains a nucleus, cytoplasm, and organelles surrounded by a lipoprotein cell membrane
         (2) Dendrites: Short branching extensions of the cell body; conduct impulses toward the cell body
         (3) Axon hillock: Thickened area of the cell body from which the axon originates
         (4) Axon: Long extension of the cell body; conducts impulses away from the cell body; usually myelinated. Outside the brain, axons are also covered with neurilemma. Branch into several processes at the terminal end.
         (5) Myelin sheath: White protein-lipid complex that surrounds some axons; laid down by oligodendrocytes in the CNS and by Schwann cells in the peripheral nervous system (PNS)
         (6) Nodes of Ranvier: Periodic interruptions in the myelin covering along the axon. Impulses are conducted from node to node (saltatory conduction), which makes conduction more rapid and efficient.
         (7) Synaptic knobs: At the terminal ends of the axon; contain vesicles that store neurotransmitter substances

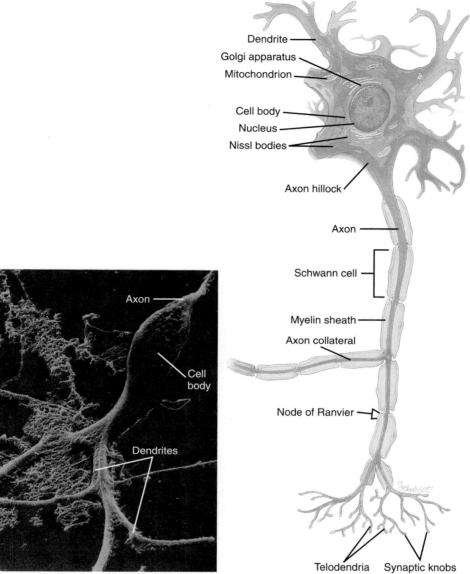

FIGURE 4-12 ■ Structure of a typical neuron. (From Thibodeau GA, Patton K. *Anatomy and Physiology*. 5th ed. St Louis, MO: Mosby; 2003:348.)

    (b) Functions
        (1) Receive input from other neurons, primarily via the dendrites and cell body
        (2) Conduct action potentials or impulses along the axon
        (3) Transfer information by synaptic transmission to other neurons, muscle cells, or gland cells
  ii. Neuroglial cells: Support, nourish, and protect the neurons; about 5 to 10 times as numerous as neurons. Four types:
    (a) Microglia: Phagocytize tissue debris when nervous tissue is damaged
    (b) Oligodendroglia: Responsible for myelin formation on axons in the CNS
    (c) Astrocytes: Contribute to the structure of the blood-brain barrier. Provide nutrients for neurons. Constitute the structural and supporting framework for nerve cells and capillaries. Remove excess potassium and neurotransmitters. Contribute to scar formation in response to neuronal cell injury or death.

(d) Ependyma: Line the ventricles of the brain and the central canal of the spinal cord. Regulate the flow of substances from these cavities into the brain. Aid in CSF production.

g. Synaptic transmission of impulses: Unidirectional conduction of an impulse from a presynaptic neuron across a junction or synapse to a postsynaptic neuron

    i. *Resting membrane potential* (RMP): Voltage difference across the cell membrane when the neuron is resting. Determined by the difference in ion concentrations on either side of the membrane. At rest, cells are positively charged outside and negatively charged inside.

    ii. *Depolarization*: Stimulus causes sodium channels to open, which results in an intracellular influx of sodium ions (Na^+)

        (a) These ionic fluxes decrease RMP.

        (b) This depolarization is called the *excitatory postsynaptic potential* (EPSP).

    iii. *Action potential*: If a transient voltage change that occurs with depolarization is of sufficient magnitude (threshold level), an action potential is produced and transmitted (conducted as an impulse) along the nerve fibers in an active, self-propagating process

    iv. *Summation*: Simultaneous excitation of numerous excitatory presynaptic terminals (or rapidly successive discharges from the same presynaptic terminal) can add together to cause a progressive increase in the postsynaptic potential that may eventually reach threshold to generate an action potential

    v. Neurotransmitters (Table 4-5): Chemicals secreted by presynaptic knobs or vesicles (usually located at the axon terminal) that excite, inhibit, or modify the response of a postsynaptic neuron. When an action potential reaches the synaptic knob, calcium channels are opened, allowing Ca^{++} influx into the knob, which triggers neurotransmitter release.

        (a) Transmitter diffuses across the synapse and binds with postsynaptic membrane receptors, which causes certain ion channels to open.

        (b) Excitatory neurotransmitters open sodium and potassium channels, which results in postsynaptic membrane depolarization.

    vi. Refractory period

        (a) *Absolute refractory period*: Membrane is unresponsive to any stimulus, so that the neuron is incapable of producing an action potential. Occurs for a fraction of a second after the membrane surpasses the threshold potential. Limits the frequency of the impulses that a cell can generate.

        (b) *Relative refractory period*: Neuron can be excited again but only by a very strong stimulus (i.e., summation above threshold); occurs during membrane repolarization

    vii. Repolarization

        (a) At the peak of an action potential, the cell membrane again becomes impermeable to Na^+; potassium channels open and allow rapid efflux of K^+ from the cell, which thereby reestablishes the RMP.

        (b) RMP returns with the aid of the sodium–potassium–adenosine triphosphatase (ATPase) pump, which pumps Na^+ out of the cell and K^+ into the cell.

    viii. Inhibition

        (a) *Inhibitory postsynaptic potential* (IPSP)

            (1) Inhibitory neurotransmitters open potassium and/or chloride channels; this causes increased negativity of the membrane potential, which results in hyperpolarization of the cell membrane.

            (2) Decreases excitability and inhibits impulse transmission

        (b) Presynaptic inhibition: Reduced amount of neurotransmitter is released; this reduces the magnitude of the EPSP to subthreshold levels

2. Spine and spinal cord

    a. Vertebral column (Figure 4-13)

        i. Composed of 33 vertebrae

TABLE 4-5

Major Neurotransmitters: Type, Location, and Action

Neurotransmitter	Location	Action*
Acetylcholine	Distributed throughout the body, including concentrations in the following locations: • Many areas of the brain (e.g., motor cortex, some basal ganglia cells, hypothalamus) • Motor neurons innervating muscles or glands • Cholinergic fibers of the ANS	Usually excitation Inhibitory effect on some of the PNS (e.g., vagus nerve on the heart) Primary neurotransmitter of the PNS
AMINES		
Norepinephrine	Distributed throughout the CNS In the brain, produced by neurons with cell bodies in the pons (in the locus ceruleus nuclei) and medulla, which send axons to all areas of the CNS, including the brainstem, spinal cord, cerebellum, cortex, hypothalamus, and thalamus Found in the adrenergic fibers of the ANS	Excitation and inhibition Primary neurotransmitter of the SNS; regulates SNS effectors Implicated in numerous functions, including motor control, emotional responses, mood, feeding behavior, temperature regulation, and sleep
Dopamine	Produced by neurons of the substantia nigra and distributed throughout the CNS, particularly the basal ganglia Found in the ANS	Mostly inhibition Regulates motor control Also involved in other functions, including emotions, mood, behavior control, and mental functions
Serotonin (5-HT)	Produced in the raphe nuclei of the brainstem that project to several regions in the CNS, including the hypothalamus, brainstem, spinal cord, cortex, basal ganglia, and cerebellum	Mostly inhibition Implicated in a number of functions, including sensory processing, control of body heat, behavior, hunger, emotions, and sleep
AMINO ACIDS		
γ-Aminobutyric acid	Distributed over much of the CNS including neuron terminals in the spinal cord, cerebellum, basal ganglia, and some areas of the cortex	Inhibition
Glutamate	Found in many areas of the CNS High concentrations in the cortex, particularly the hippocampus and basal ganglia Released in large amounts when brain cells are injured by trauma or hypoxia-ischemia; hypoxic-ischemic changes are attributed in part to glutamate, which affects the hippocampus in particular	Excitation Excessive glutamate receptor stimulation opens ionic channels, causing neuronal disintegration from calcium influx through N-methyl-D-aspartate receptors and cellular swelling from influx of sodium and water

ANS, Autonomic nervous system; *CNS*, central nervous system; *PNS*, parasympathetic nervous system; *SNS*, sympathetic nervous system.
*Action is determined by the postsynaptic receptor rather than the neurotransmitter.

(a) Cervical: Seven vertebrae
  (1) Support the head and neck; smallest vertebrae
  (2) Atlas (first cervical vertebra): Supports the head; articulates with the occipital bone superiorly and the axis inferiorly
  (3) Axis (second cervical vertebra)
    a) Odontoid process (dens): Projection of the axis that protrudes upward through the anterior arch of atlas
    b) Allows for rotation of the head
(b) Thoracic: Twelve vertebrae; articulate with the ribs; support the chest muscles

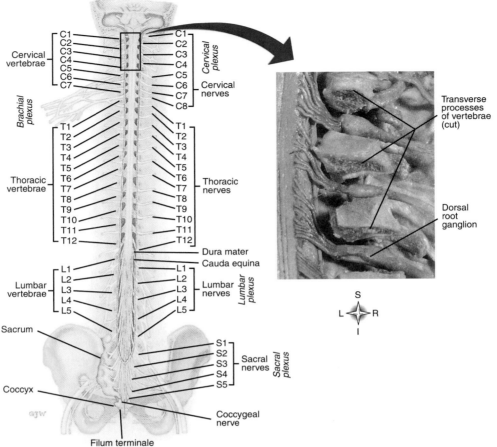

FIGURE 4-13 ■ Spinal nerves. Each of the 31 pairs of spinal nerves exits the spinal cavity from the intervertebral foramina. The names of the vertebrae are given on the left and the names of the corresponding spinal nerves on the right. Note that after leaving the spinal cavity, many of the spinal nerves interconnect to form plexuses. *I*, Inferior; *L*, left; *R*, right; *S*, superior. (From Thibodeau GA, Patton K. *Anatomy and Physiology*. 5th ed. St Louis, MO: Mosby; 2003:414.)

      (c) Lumbar: Five vertebrae; support the lower back muscles; the largest and strongest vertebrae

      (d) Sacral: Five fused vertebrae; form a large triangular bone, the sacrum

      (e) Coccygeal: Four fused rudimentary vertebrae

  ii. Anatomic features of a typical vertebra

      (a) Body: Flat round, solid portion; lies anteriorly

      (b) Arch: Posterior part of the vertebra. Consists of the following:

        (1) Pedicles: Two short bony projections that extend posterior from the body

        (2) Lamina: Joins each pedicle and fuses posteriorly at the midline to complete the arch; processes project from the laminae

        (3) Spinous process: Midline projection protruding posteriorly from the laminae

        (4) Transverse processes: Projections from the laminae on each side of the vertebrae

        (5) Articular processes (facets): Projections from the laminae that protrude upward or downward (superior or inferior articulating processes); inferior processes articulate with the superior processes of the vertebra directly below

(c) Intervertebral foramina: Openings between the vertebrae through which spinal nerves pass

(d) Spinal foramina: Opening between the arch and the body through which the spinal cord passes

   iii. Intervertebral disks

(a) Fibrocartilage layer between the bodies of adjoining vertebrae

(b) Act as shock absorbers

(c) Composed of the annulus fibrosus (tough outer layer) and nucleus pulposus (gelatinous inner layer)

   iv. Spinal ligaments: Hold the vertebrae and disks in alignment; prevent excessive spinal flexion or extension

b. Spinal cord

   i. Location: Extends from the superior border of the atlas to the first or second lumbar vertebra

(a) Continuous with the medulla oblongata

(b) Conus medullaris: Caudal end of the spinal cord

(c) Central canal: In the center of the spinal cord; contains CSF and is continuous with the fourth ventricle

(d) Filum terminale: Nonneural filament that extends downward from the conus medullaris and attaches to the coccyx; helps maintain the position of spinal cord during trunk movement

   ii. Meninges: Continuous with the layers covering the brain

   iii. Gray matter (Figure 4-14)

(a) An H-shaped, internal mass of gray substance surrounded by white matter; consists of cell bodies and their dendrites and axons

(b) Anterior gray column (anterior horn): Contains cell bodies of efferent motor fibers

(c) Lateral column: Contains preganglionic fibers of the ANS

(d) Posterior gray column (posterior horn): Contains cell bodies of afferent sensory fibers

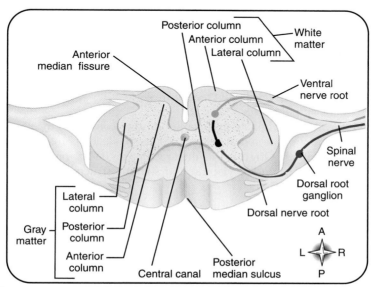

FIGURE 4-14 ■ Transverse section of the spinal cord. *A*, Anterior; *L*, left, *R*, right, *P*, posterior. (From Ozuna JM. Nursing assessment neurologic system. In: Lewis SM, Heitkemper MM, Dirksen SR. *Medical Surgical Nursing: Assessment and Management of Clinical Problems.* 5th ed. St Louis, MO: Mosby; 2000:1584.)

    iv.   White matter (see Figure 4-14)
       (a)   Composed of three longitudinal columns (funiculi): Anterior, lateral, and posterior
       (b)   Contains mostly myelinated axons
       (c)   Funiculi contain tracts (fasciculi): Composed of axons with similar origin, course, and termination that perform specific functions; clinically significant tracts are summarized in Table 4-6; classified as follows (Figure 4-15):
          (1)   Ascending or sensory tracts: Pathways to the brain for impulses that enter the cord via the dorsal roots of the spinal nerves
          (2)   Descending or motor tracts: Transmit impulses from the brain to the motor neurons of the spinal cord that exit via the ventral root of the spinal nerves
       (d)   Most tracts are named to indicate the column in which the tract travels, the location of its cells of origin, and the location of axon termination.
    v.   Upper and lower motor neurons
       (a)   Lower motor neurons (LMNs): Spinal and cranial motor neurons that directly innervate muscles. LMN lesions cause flaccid paralysis, muscular atrophy, absent reflexes.
       (b)   Upper motor neurons (UMNs): Located completely in the CNS; regulate LMN activity. UMN lesions are associated with spastic paralysis, clonus, increased tone, hyperactive reflexes, Babinski's sign.
  c.   Reflexes
    i.   Reflex arc: Requires a receptor, sensory neuron, motor neuron, and effector (e.g., muscle or gland) (Figure 4-16)
    ii.   Monosynaptic reflex arc: Direct synapse between the afferent and efferent neurons
       (a)   Stimulation of afferent nerve fibers sends impulses to the spinal cord through the dorsal roots of spinal nerves.
       (b)   Impulse synapses with anterior motor neurons, sending out an efferent discharge confined to the axons supplying the muscle from which the afferent impulse originated.
    iii.   Polysynaptic reflex arc
       (a)   More than one synapse is required to complete the reflex arc.
       (b)   Most reflexes are polysynaptic; may involve interneurons (neurons in the CNS that transmit impulses from a sensory neuron to or toward a motor neuron) and multiple spinal segments and/or areas of brain.
    iv.   Reciprocal innervation: Impulses that excite motor neurons supplying a particular muscle also inhibit motor neurons of antagonistic muscles

3. PNS
  a.   Spinal nerves
    i.   Thirty-one symmetrically arranged pairs of nerves, each possessing a sensory (dorsal) root and a motor (ventral) root: 8 cervical pairs, 12 thoracic pairs, 5 lumbar pairs, 5 sacral pairs, 1 coccygeal pair (see Figure 4-13)
    ii.   Fibers of the spinal nerves
       (a)   Motor fibers: Originate in the anterior gray column of the spinal cord, form the ventral root of the spinal nerve, and pass to skeletal muscles
       (b)   Sensory fibers: Originate in the spinal ganglia of the dorsal roots; peripheral branches distribute to visceral and somatic structures as mediators of sensory impulses to the CNS
       (c)   Autonomic fibers
          (1)   Sympathetic
             a)   Originate from cells between the posterior and anterior gray columns from the first thoracic to second lumbar cord segment
             b)   Innervate the viscera, blood vessels, glands, and smooth muscle
          (2)   Parasympathetic
             a)   Arise from sacral cord segments S2 to S4
             b)   Pass to the pelvic and abdominal viscera
       (d)   Cauda equina: Spinal nerves that arise from the lumbosacral portion of the spinal cord contained within the lumbar cistern

TABLE 4-6
Major Spinal Cord Tracts

Name	Origin	Termination	Cross	Function
ASCENDING TRACTS				
Posterior dorsal columns: Fasciculus gracilis and fasciculus cuneatus	Fasciculus gracilis: Spinal cord at the lumbar and sacral levels Fasciculus cuneatus: Spinal cord at the cervical and thoracic levels	Medulla → thalamus → sensory strip of the cerebral cortex	Ascend in the posterior funiculus and cross over in the lower medulla	Convey position and vibratory sense, joint and two-point discrimination, tactile localization, pressure and discriminating touch Fasciculus gracilis: Carries impulses from the lower body Fasciculus cuneatus: Carries impulses from the upper body
Lateral spinothalamic tract	Posterior horn	Thalamus → cerebral cortex	Crosses over in the spinal cord to the contralateral anterolateral funiculus before ascending	Conveys pain and temperature sensation
Anterior spinothalamic tract	Posterior horn	Thalamus → cerebral cortex	Crosses over in the spinal cord to the contralateral anterolateral funiculus before ascending	Conveys light touch and pressure sensation
Posterior spinocerebellar tract	Posterior horn	Cerebellum	Ascends uncrossed in the lateral funiculus	Conveys proprioceptive data that influence muscle tone and synergy necessary for coordinated muscle movements
Anterior spinocerebellar tract	Posterior horn	Cerebellum	Mostly crosses in the spinal cord before ascending in the lateral funiculus	Conveys proprioceptive data that influence muscle tone and synergy necessary for coordinated muscle movements
Spinotectal tract	Posterior horn	Tectum (roof) of the midbrain	Ascends crossed in the lateral funiculus	Conveys general sensory information that influences pupil reaction and head and eye movement in response to stimuli
DESCENDING TRACTS				
Rubrospinal tract	Red nucleus of the midbrain	Anterior horn	Crosses in the midbrain and descends in the lateral funiculus	Conveys impulses to control muscle tone and synergy and to maintain posture
Lateral corticospinal tract	Cerebral cortical motor areas	Anterior horn	Up to 90% crosses in the medulla and descends in the lateral funiculus	Carries impulses for voluntary movement
Anterior corticospinal tract	Cerebral cortical motor areas	Anterior horn	Descends in the anterior funiculus and crosses in the cord at the level at which it terminates	Carries impulses for voluntary movement
Tectospinal tract	Superior colliculus of the midbrain	Anterior horn in the cervical spinal cord	Crosses in the midbrain and descends in the anterior funiculus	Mediates optic and auditory reflexes (e.g., reflexive head turning in response to visual or auditory stimuli)

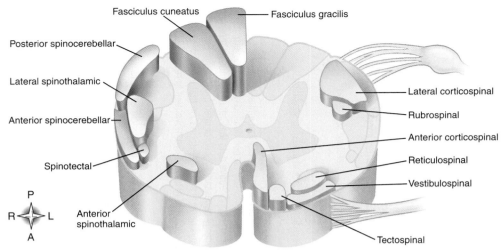

FIGURE 4-15 ■ Major ascending (sensory) and descending (motor) tracts of the spinal cord. *A*, Anterior; *L*, left; *R*, right; *P*, posterior. (From Thibodeau GA, Patton K. *Anatomy and Physiology*. 5th ed. St Louis, MO: Mosby; 2003:382.)

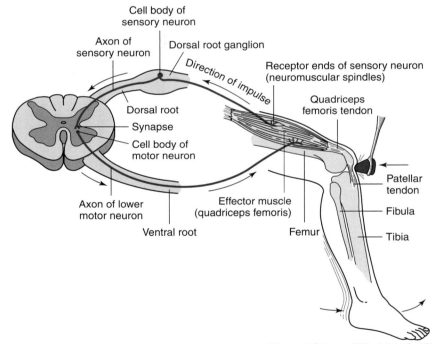

FIGURE 4-16 ■ The two-neuron patellar reflex or "knee jerk." (From Phipps WJ, Marek JF, Monahan FD, et al. *Medical-Surgical Nursing: Health and Illness Perspectives*. 7th ed. St Louis, MO: Mosby; 2003:1311.)

    iii. Dermatomes (Figure 4-17): Skin areas supplied by the dorsal root (sensory fibers) of a given spinal nerve; adjacent dermatomes overlap
    iv. Plexuses: Network of spinal nerve roots (Table 4-7)
  b. Neuromuscular transmission (Figure 4-18)
    i. Physiologic anatomy at the neuromuscular junction
      (a) Motor end plate: Distal end of motor axon loses its myelin sheath and flattens out at the end lying close to the muscle fiber membrane (sarcolemma)

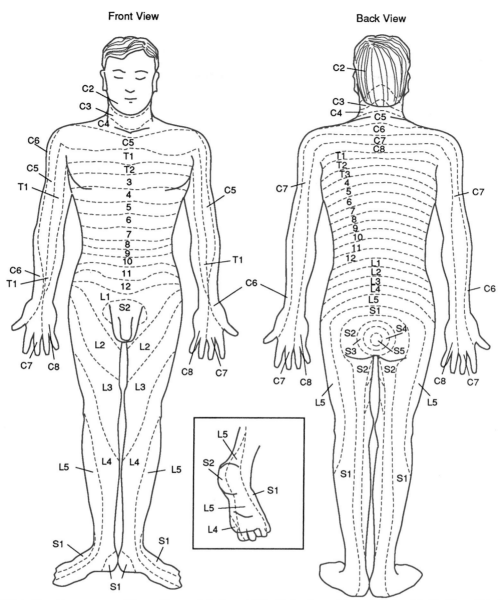

FIGURE 4-17 ■ Dermatomes. (From Russo-McCourt TA. Spinal cord injuries. In: McQuillan KA, Von Rueden KT, Hartsock RL, et al, eds. *Trauma Nursing From Resuscitation Through Rehabilitation*. 3rd ed. St Louis, MO: Saunders; 2002:522.)

  (b) Synaptic cleft: Space between the motor end plate and the muscle fiber membrane
  (c) Synaptic gutter: Invagination of the muscle fiber membrane where numerous folds increase the surface area available for neurotransmitter to act
  (d) Vesicles: Nerve terminal structures that store and release the neurotransmitter acetylcholine (ACh)
  ii. When an action potential reaches the neuromuscular junction, vesicles release ACh into the synaptic cleft. Amount released depends on the magnitude of the action potential and the presence of calcium. ACh attaches to receptor sites on the postjunctional muscle membrane and increases its permeability to Na^+, K^+, and other ions.

■ **TABLE 4-7**
■ ■ **Plexuses and Their Locations and Areas of Innervation**

Name	Spinal Nerve Anterior Branches That Comprise Plexus	Location of Plexus	Important Nerves That Emerge	Areas of Innervation
Cervical	C1-C4	Deep within the neck	Portion of the phrenic nerve	Muscles and skin of a portion of the head, neck, and upper shoulders; diaphragm
Brachial	C5-C8 and T1	Deep within the shoulder	Phrenic, circumflex, musculocutaneous, ulnar, median, and radial nerves	Shoulder, arm, and hand; diaphragm
Lumbar	L1-L4	Lumbar region of the back	Femoral cutaneous, femoral and genitofemoral branches	Anterior abdominal wall and genitalia; thigh and leg
Sacral	L4 and L5 and S1-S4	Inner surface of the posterior pelvic wall	Tibial, common peroneal, sciatic, and pudendal nerves	Skin of the leg; muscles of the posterior thigh, leg, and foot

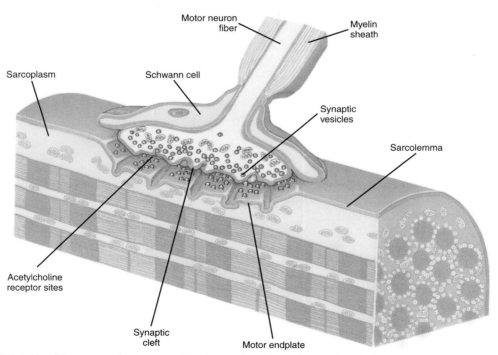

FIGURE 4-18 ■ Neuromuscular junction. This figure shows how the distal end of a motor neuron fiber forms a synapse, or "chemical junction," with an adjacent muscle fiber. Neurotransmitters (specifically, acetylcholine) are released from the neuron's synaptic vesicles and diffuse across the synaptic cleft. There they stimulate receptors in the motor endplate region of the sarcolemma. (From Thibodeau GA, Patton K. *Anatomy and Physiology.* 5th ed. St Louis, MO: Mosby; 2003:316.)

      iii. End-plate potential: Motor nerve action potential that is local (e.g., nonpropagated) and graded, rather than all or nothing

      iv. Muscle contraction: Action potentials subsequently form on either side of the end plate and conduct in both directions along the muscle fiber, initiating a series of events that result in muscle contraction

      v. Acetylcholinesterase: Catalyzes the hydrolysis of ACh to choline and acetic acid and thus limits the duration of ACh action on the end plate, which ensures production of only one action potential

  c. Cranial nerves: 12 pairs of nerves considered part of the PNS (Figure 4-19 and Table 4-8)

  d. ANS (Figure 4-20)

    i. Structure

      (a) Composed of two neuron chains

      (b) Preganglionic cell bodies are located within the lateral gray column of the spinal cord or brainstem nuclei.

      (c) Most preganglionic axons are myelinated and synapse on the cell bodies of postganglionic neurons outside the CNS.

      (d) Axons of postganglionic neurons terminate on visceral effectors (i.e., smooth and cardiac muscle, glandular epithelium).

    ii. Divisions

      (a) Sympathetic (thoracolumbar)

        (1) Preganglionic axons emerge from cell bodies within the lateral horn of the spinal cord gray matter at the thoracic and upper two lumbar levels. Axons leave the spinal cord via the ventral roots and pass to

          a) Paravertebral sympathetic ganglion chain via white rami communicantes, ending on cell bodies of postganglionic neurons

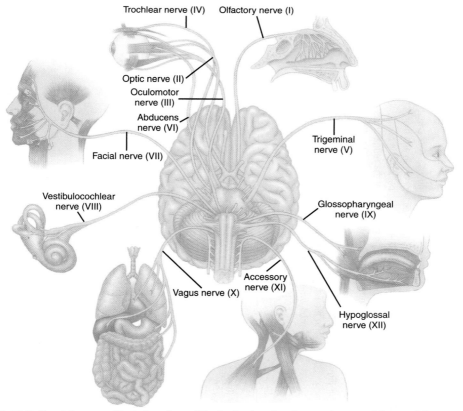

FIGURE 4-19 ■ Cranial nerves. Ventral surface of the brain showing the attachment of the cranial nerves. (From Thibodeau GA, Patton K. *Anatomy and Physiology*. 5th ed. St Louis, MO: Mosby; 2003:421.)

■ TABLE 4-8
■ ■ Cranial Nerves: Origin, Course, and Function

Cranial Nerve	Origin and Course	Function
Olfactory (I)	Receptor cells located in the nasal mucosa. Axons from these cells form the olfactory nerve, which passes to the olfactory bulb and then forms the olfactory tract.	Smell
Optic (II)	Fibers originate from the ganglion cells of the retina. At the optic chiasm, optic nerve fibers from the nasal half of the retina cross; those from the temporal half do not. Fibers continue as optic tracts to the lateral geniculate bodies of the thalamus and then as geniculocalcarine tracts to the occipital cortex.	Vision
Oculomotor (III)	Nuclei are located in the midbrain. Preganglionic parasympathetic fibers originate in the Edinger-Westphal nucleus and accompany other oculomotor fibers into the orbit, where they terminate in the ciliary ganglion. Postganglionic fibers pass to the constrictor papillae and ciliary muscles of the eye.	Pupil constriction Levator palpebrae innervation raises the upper eyelid. Innervates extraocular muscles to move the eye as follows: • Inferior rectus: moves eye downward and outward • Medial rectus: Moves eye medially • Superior rectus: Moves eye upward and outward • Inferior oblique: Moves eye upward and inward
Trochlear (IV)	Originates in the midbrain	Supplies the superior oblique muscle, which moves the eye downward and inward
Trigeminal (V)	Sensory fibers arise from cells in the semilunar (trigeminal) ganglion. Axons from the ganglion attach to the lateral aspect of the pons. Motor fibers leave the pons ventromedial to the sensory roots. Components of this nerve are also located in the midbrain and medulla.	Three sensory divisions 1. Ophthalmic branch provides sensation to the forehead, upper eyelid, cornea, conjunctiva, nose, and part of the nasal mucosa. 2. Maxillary branch provides sensation to the lower eyelid, upper jaw, teeth, gums and lip, upper cheek, hard and soft palates, some of the nasal mucosa, and the lower side of the nose. 3. Mandibular branch provides sensation to the lower jaw, teeth, gums and lip, buccal mucosa, tongue, part of the external ear, and auditory meatus. All three divisions contribute sensory fibers to the meninges. Motor fibers innervate the muscles of mastication.
Abducens (VI)	Arises from nuclei in the pons. Emerges anteriorly at the border of the pons and medulla. Enters the orbit through the superior orbital fissure with cranial nerves III, IV, and the ophthalmic branch of V.	Supplies the lateral rectus muscle, which abducts the eye horizontally
Facial (VII)	Fibers originate in the pons and emerge at the junction of the pons and medulla. The smaller nerve root containing the sensory and parasympathetic fibers is called the *nervus intermedius*. Sensory fibers originate in the geniculate ganglion located within the facial canal of the temporal bone, and parasympathetic fibers originate in the superior salivary nucleus located within the medulla.	Motor portions of the nerve innervate all muscles of facial expression. Sensory portion conveys taste from the anterior two thirds of the tongue and skin sensation from the external auditory meatus and the auricle. Parasympathetic fibers innervate the salivary and lacrimal glands.

Nerve	Description	Function
Acoustic (VIII) (also known as vestibulocochlear)	Nerve enters the brainstem at the pontomedullary junction. Two divisions: • Cochlear nerve: Cell bodies of these bipolar neurons are located in the spiral ganglion of the cochlea. Peripheral fibers of these neurons innervate hair cells located in the organ of Corti of the cochlea, which transduce sounds into neural signals. Central fibers of the neurons project to the ventral and dorsal cochlear nuclei in the medulla. Fibers from these nuclei synapse in the medial geniculate nuclei of the thalamus and then on the auditory cortex of the temporal lobe. • Vestibular nerve: Cell bodies of these bipolar neurons are located in the vestibular ganglion. Peripheral fibers of the vestibular ganglion receive input from receptors in the semicircular canals, the utricle, and the saccule of the inner ear. Central fibers project from the vestibular ganglion to the vestibular nuclei located in the pons and medulla. These nuclei send out projections to the spinal cord, cerebellum, reticular formation, and nuclei of cranial nerves III, IV, and VI.	Cochlear nerve: Hearing Vestibular nerve: Aids in maintaining equilibrium or balance and coordinating head and eye movements
Glossopharyngeal (IX)	Sensory fibers arise from cells at the back of the tongue, the pharynx, and the palate and enter the medulla. Motor fibers originate from the ambiguus nucleus in the medulla to innervate the stylopharyngeus muscle of the pharynx. Preganglionic fibers terminate in the otic ganglion, which is the parasympathetic ganglion that innervates the parotid gland.	Sensory fibers provide sensation to the pharynx, soft palate, and posterior third of the tongue. They also supply special receptors in the carotid body and carotid sinus, which are concerned with reflex control of respiration, blood pressure, and heart rate. Motor fibers participate with the vagus nerve in swallowing.
Vagus (X)	Sensory fibers originate in the cells of ganglia just below the jugular foramen and enter the medulla. Motor fibers leave the medulla and join the sensory part of the nerve. Preganglionic parasympathetic fibers are distributed to the abdominal and thoracic viscera.	Sensory fibers convey sensation from the palate and pharynx (along with IX) and from the larynx, external auditory meatus, and thoracic and abdominal viscera. Motor fibers innervate muscles of the palate, pharynx (along with IX), and larynx. Provides parasympathetic functions to the abdominal and thoracic organs
Spinal accessory (XI)	Motor fibers arise from the medulla and upper cervical spinal cord.	Supplies the trapezius muscle to enable shoulder elevation, and the sternocleidomastoid muscle, which allows the head to tilt, turn, and be thrust forward
Hypoglossal (XII)	Motor fibers originate in the hypoglossal nucleus of the medulla.	Innervates muscles of the tongue

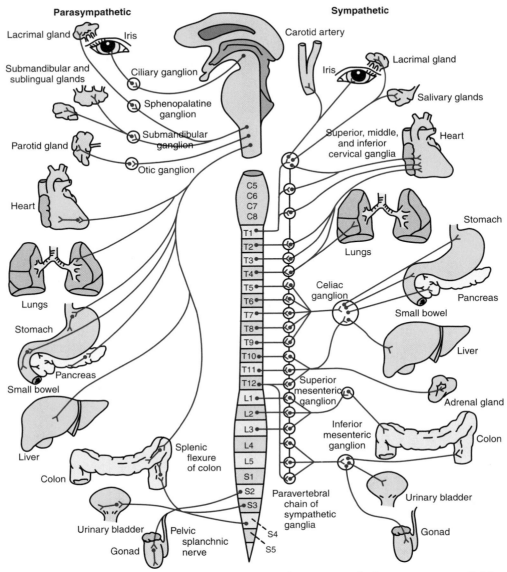

FIGURE 4-20 ■ Diagram of the autonomic nervous system. The parasympathetic nervous system division *(left)* arises from cranial nerves III, VII, IX, and X and from spinal cord segments S2 to S4. The sympathetic division *(right)* arises from spinal cord segments T1 to T12. (From DeMyer W. *Neuroanatomy.* 2nd ed. Baltimore, MD: Williams & Wilkins; 1998:99.)

          b) Collateral ganglia, ending on postganglionic neurons closer to the viscera

          c) Adrenal medulla, ending on modified postganglionic neurons that are secretory endocrine cells

     (2) Postganglionic axons pass to

          a) Viscera via the sympathetic nerves

          b) Gray rami communicantes, which return to the spinal nerve and are distributed to autonomic effectors in areas supplied by these nerves

     (3) Functions (Table 4-9)

          a) Come into widespread activity under emergency conditions ("fight or flight")

          b) Generally antagonistic to parasympathetic activity

          c) Synapse with many postganglionic fibers

TABLE 4-9
Autonomic Nervous System Effects on Various Effector Sites

Effector Organ		Sympathetic Influence	Parasympathetic Influence
Eyes	Pupils	Dilation (mydriasis)	Constriction (miosis)
Glands	Lacrimal	Decreased	Increased
	Nasal	Decreased	Increased
	Salivary	Decreased	Increased
	Sweat	Increased	None
Heart		Increased rate	Decreased rate
		Increased conduction velocity	
		Increased contractility	Decreased contractility
Blood vessels	Coronary	Vasodilation	Minimal dilation
	Skeletal	Vasodilation	None
	Abdominal viscera	Vasoconstriction	None
	Cutaneous	Vasoconstriction	None
Blood pressure		Increased	Decreased
Lungs		Bronchodilation	Bronchoconstriction
Gastrointestinal system	Motility	Decreased peristalsis	Increased peristalsis
	Sphincter	Increased tone	Relaxation
	Secretions	Inhibition	Stimulation
Bladder		Decreased detrusor tone	Increased detrusor tone
Sex organs		Ejaculation	Erection
Skin	Pilomotor muscles	Excited (contraction)	None

From Russo-McCourt T. Spinal cord injuries. In: McQuillan KA, Von Rueden KT, Hartsock RL, et al, eds. *Trauma Nursing: From Resuscitation Through Rehabilitation.* 3rd ed. Philadelphia, PA: Saunders; 2002:512.

 (b) Parasympathetic (craniosacral) (see Table 4-9)
  (1) Preganglionic cell bodies are located in brainstem nuclei and the lateral gray columns of the middle three sacral spinal cord segments (S2 to S4).
  (2) Preganglionic fibers end on short postganglionic neurons located on or near visceral structures.
  (3) Supplies visceral structures in the head via the oculomotor (III), facial (VII), and glossopharyngeal (IX) cranial nerves and those in the thorax and upper abdomen via the vagus (X) nerve
  (4) Sacral outflow supplies the pelvic viscera via the pelvic branches of S2 to S4.
  (5) Produces localized reactions rather than the mass action of sympathetic stimulation
 iii. Chemical mediation: ANS is divided into cholinergic and adrenergic divisions based on the neurotransmitter released
  (a) Cholinergic neurons release ACh and include
   (1) All preganglionic neurons
   (2) Parasympathetic postganglionic neurons
   (3) Sympathetic postganglionic neurons to the sweat glands and skeletal muscle blood vessels (vasodilation)
  (b) Adrenergic neurons release norepinephrine and include
   (1) Sympathetic postganglionic endings, except as noted earlier
   (2) Constrictor fibers of the skeletal muscle blood vessels
4. Physiology of pain
 a. *Core Curriculum* focuses primarily on acute (nociceptive or physiologic) pain. Chronic pain is discussed briefly because unrelieved acute pain can result in the development of chronic (pathologic) pain.
 b. Acute pain results when mechanisms such as surgery, trauma, or disease cause inflammation and cellular damage.

    i.   Warns of potential for, or extent of, tissue damage; initiates protective behaviors to minimize damage and promote tissue repair

    ii.   Usual characteristics include the following:

       (a) Activates sympathetic nervous system (autonomic, involuntary) responses, such as increased heart rate, blood pressure (BP), respiratory rate

       (b) Proportional to intensity and extent of stimuli; however, wide variations exist among patients

       (c) Has a beginning and end, with resolution or healing of the underlying pathologic condition. Research indicates that

          (1) Long-term alterations in neural tissue are initiated within the first few hours after injury

          (2) Inadequately managed acute pain can persist after injured tissue is repaired

    iii.   Classifications of acute pain

       (a) *Somatic*: Arising from tissues (e.g., skin, muscle, bone). Descriptors include *sharp, dull, aching, cramping*. Is localized or diffuse; may radiate.

       (b) *Visceral*: Arising from organs (e.g., liver, pancreas, bowel). Descriptors include *sharp, stabbing, deep ache*. Is well or poorly localized; may be referred.

    iv.   Key physiologic concepts

       (a) *Nociception*: Neurochemical process of transmitting the pain response to a peripheral noxious (thermal, mechanical, or chemical) stimulus to an intact spinal cord and brain

          (1) Pain perception requires cortical integration of many factors (e.g., physiologic factors, psychosocial factors, past experiences); often results in emotional responses (e.g., anger, anxiety).

          (2) Nociception does not always result in pain (e.g., pain perception can be blunted by endogenous endorphin release); pain can occur without nociception (e.g., phantom limb pain).

       (b) *Nociceptors*: Peripheral neurons (primary afferent peripheral fibers) that sense unpleasant or potentially damaging noxious stimuli. Examples are

          (1) *A delta*: Large, thinly myelinated fibers that rapidly conduct impulses generated in response to mechanical or thermal stimuli; usually results in sharp, well-localized pain

          (2) *C*: Smaller, unmyelinated fibers that slowly conduct impulses generated in response to all noxious stimuli; usually poorly localized, dull, aching pain; 75% of nociceptors are C fibers

       (c) *Peripheral sensitization*: Lowering of nociceptor activation threshold following exposure to chemical mediators or repeated noxious stimuli

       (d) Four basic stages of nociception described in Table 4-10 and illustrated in Figure 4-21

  c. Chronic pain: Pain state persisting beyond the period of healing

    i.   Serves no useful purpose

    ii.   Usual characteristics

       (a) Neither tissue pathology nor sympathetic nervous system activation is identifiable.

       (b) Represents a disproportionate response to the stimulus and/or physical findings

       (c) Possibly indicates interpersonal or psychologic problems

    iii.   Often involves *neuropathic pain*: Abnormal processing of sensory input in PNS or CNS due to injury or impairment

       (a) Described as either continuous or intermittent sensations (e.g., burning, shooting, shocklike, tingling, jabbing)

       (b) Examples include pain caused by nerve root compression, diabetic neuropathy, Guillain-Barré syndrome; phantom limb pain, complex regional pain syndrome

    iv.   Key physiologic concepts

       (a) *Neuroplasticity*: Ability of neurons to change their subsequent response to stimuli following long-term or sustained exposure to noxious stimuli

       (b) *Central sensitization*: State of heightened excitability resulting in an exaggerated response to stimuli and an expanded distribution of pain

          (1) *Hyperalgesia*: Lowered threshold for noxious stimuli

          (2) *Allodynia*: Perception of normally benign stimuli as painful

■ **TABLE 4-10**
■ ■ **Basic Stages of Nociception**

Stage	Steps	Mechanisms of Action for Interventions
Transduction	1. Cells damaged by noxious stimuli release nociceptor-activating substances (e.g., prostaglandins, serotonin, substance P, histamine), which cause inflammation, peripheral sensitization, and primary hyperalgesia (increased sensitivity around the area of tissue damage). 2. An action potential leads to generation of an electrical impulse in response to the stimulus.	1. Nonsteroidal antiinflammatory drugs target the inflammatory response. 2. Anticonvulsants and local anesthetics can block various ion exchanges involved in the generation of an action potential.
Transmission	1. Sensitized fibers release neurotransmitters (e.g., glutamate, substance P), which facilitate impulse travel to dorsal horn neurons in the spinal cord. Glutamate binds NMDA receptors and facilitates transmission. 2. Impulses travel on to the brainstem, thalamus (relay station between the brain and spinal f), and cortex via different ascending tracts.	1. Opioids reduce release of substance P. 2. NMDA receptor antagonists (e.g., ketamine, dextromethorphan, possibly methadone) inhibit glutamate binding.
Perception	Once impulses reach the brain, pain processing is thought to include the following: • Reticular activating system: Autonomic response and alerting of the individual to respond to pain • Somatosensory cortex: Localization, characterization, and preservation of information about pain • Limbic system: Site of emotional-behavioral response to pain	1. Opioids binding to their receptors in the brain can alter the perception of pain. 2. Strategies such as distraction or relaxation may modify pain perception by limiting the number of signals the brain has to process.
Modulation	1. Neurons descending from the brainstem synapse on dorsal horn neurons and release inhibitory neurotransmitters: inhibitory amino acids (e.g., GABA, glycine) and neuropeptides (e.g., endogenous opioids), serotonin, and norepinephrine. • These substances bind with receptors to raise the threshold for nociceptor activation and prevent the release of other neurotransmitters (e.g., substance P). • Neurotransmitters are then recycled and stored for future use. 2. Emotions (e.g., fear, anxiety, anticipation, stress) can increase pain.	1. Baclofen binds to GABA receptors and mimics its inhibitory effects. 2. Opioids activate descending inhibitory pathways. 3. Tricyclic antidepressants prevent the reuptake and storage of serotonin and norepinephrine, which makes them more available.

Compiled from Ballantyne J, Fishman SM, Abdi S, eds. *The Massachusetts General Hospital Handbook of Pain Management.* Philadelphia, PA: Lippincott Williams & Wilkins; 2002; Blakely WP, Page GG. Pathophysiology of pain in critically ill patients. *Crit Care Nurs Clin North Am.* 2001;12(2):167-179; McCaffery M, Pasero C. *Pain: Clinical Manual.* 2nd ed. St Louis, MO: Mosby; 1999; Melzack R, Wall PD, eds. *Handbook of Pain Management.* Edinburgh, Scotland: Churchill Livingstone; 2003; and National Pharmaceutical Council. *Pain: Current Understanding of Assessment, Management, and Treatment.* Reston, VA: National Pharmaceutical Council; 2001.
GABA, γ-Aminobutyric acid; *NMDA*, *N*-methyl-D-aspartate.

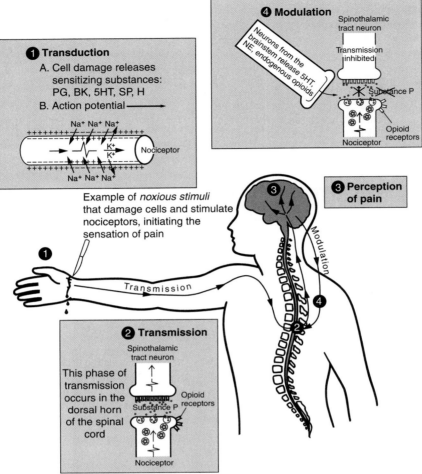

FIGURE 4-21 ■ Four basic processes involved in nociception. *BK*, Bradykinin; *5HT*, 5-hydroxytryptamine (serotonin); *H*, histamine; *NE*, norepinephrine; *PG*, prostaglandin; *SP*, substance P. (From McCaffery M, Pasero C. *Pain: Clinical Manual*. St Louis, MO: Mosby; 1999:21.)

Patient Assessment

1. **Nursing history**
   a. Current health issues
      i. Current symptoms, including chronologic sequence of onset, duration, location, and frequency
      ii. Factors that relieve or exacerbate symptoms
      iii. Difficulties performing activities of daily living (ADLs)
   b. Patient health history: Significant medical and surgical history, including traumatic injury and childhood diseases
   c. Medication history: Use of over-the-counter and prescription drugs, nutritional and herbal supplements, including amount, frequency, duration, last dose, effectiveness, adverse response. Especially note use of analgesics, anticonvulsants, tranquilizers, sedatives, anticoagulants, platelet aggregation inhibitors, stimulants, antihypertensives, cardiac medications.
   d. Allergies
   e. Family history: Note history of disease that may impact current illness (e.g., cardiac disease, stroke [especially early onset], aneurysms, arteriovenous malformations, seizures, migraines, dementia, autoimmune disorders)

  f. Social history and habits
  i. Significant others affected by the patient's illness
  ii. Support systems available to assist the patient and family
  iii. Alcohol and tobacco use: Past and present, amount, duration
  iv. Illicit drug use or abuse: Particularly cocaine, amphetamines
  v. Type of work; impact of symptoms on work
  vi. Hobbies, recreational activities
  vii. Current dwelling, including layout and number of stairs
2. Nursing examination of patient
  a. Physical examination data
  i. First ABC: Evaluate *a*irway patency, sufficiency of *b*reathing, and *c*irculation
  ii. Inspection then palpation of the head, face, and spine: Shape, symmetry, bony contour, coloration and skin integrity; irregularities may indicate injury, ventricular shunt, previous surgery, or congenital abnormality. Note nares or ear drainage.
  iii. Auscultation: Heart for murmurs and clicks; carotid arteries and over eyes for bruits
  iv. Assessment of neurologic function
    (a) Level of consciousness (LOC) (Box 4-1)
    (b) Glasgow Coma Scale (GCS) (Table 4-11): Used to assess LOC; total score also used to classify severity of brain injury. Limitations include inability to assess eye opening in patients with periorbital swelling or verbal response in intubated patients. Hypoxia, hypotension, hypothermia, drug intoxication, postictal state, and administration of sedatives, analgesics, or paralytic agents can interfere with GCS responses. Presence of any confounding variable should be noted when reporting score. Neurologic deterioration that affects only one side of the body is not reflected in GCS score.

■ **BOX 4-1**
■ **ASSESSMENT OF LEVEL OF CONSCIOUSNESS**

Consciousness is an awareness of self and the environment. A disturbance in consciousness is a sensitive indicator of neurologic dysfunction. Unconsciousness (coma) can result from extensive bilateral cerebral lesions, injury to the diencephalon or pontomesencephalic (pons-midbrain) reticular formation, or metabolic abnormalities. Unilateral lesions of the cerebrum (without prior contralateral injury) and lesions of the medulla or spinal cord do not cause coma.

   Arousal: Evaluate what stimulus is necessary to elicit a response. Determine if the patient responds spontaneously; if not, apply the following stimuli in progressive order until a response is obtained: Address the patient by name, shake the patient, apply a peripheral pain stimulus (i.e., nail bed pressure), apply a deep central pain stimulus (i.e., sternal rub, supraorbital pressure).

   Awareness or the content of consciousness reflects higher cortical functions; can be assessed via the following:
   ■ General behavior and appearance; appropriateness to the situation
   ■ Attention span, long- and short-term memory, insight, orientation, and calculation
   ■ Intellectual capacity appropriate for educational level, judgment
   ■ Emotional state, affect
   ■ Thought content: Illusions, hallucinations, delusions
   ■ Execution of intentional motor activity: *Apraxia* is the inability to perform these movements
   ■ Recognition and interpretation of sensations
   ■ Language: Fluency, clarity, content, comprehension of written and spoken word, ability to name objects and repeat phrases, patient's awareness of a language disorder
Aphasia: Difficulty in the expression of language (expressive aphasia) or understanding of language (receptive aphasia) indicates dominant hemisphere dysfunction
Motor speech apraxia: Inability to perform the mouth movements to produce the sounds for the intended words; a motor speech programming disorder indicates a lesion in Broca's speech area
Dysarthria: Difficulty with articulation due to impaired movement of the speech musculature may result from dysfunction of cranial nerves V, VII, IX, X, or XII or cerebellar dysfunction that interferes with the coordination of the muscles innervated by these nerves; represents speech impairment without a language deficit

■ **TABLE 4-11**
■ ■ **Glasgow Coma Scale**

Response	Score
EYE OPENING	
Assesses arousal state	
"Spontaneously": Patient opens eyes without stimulation	4
"To voice": Patient opens eyes when spoken to	3
"To pain": Patient opens eyes when a noxious stimulus is applied	2
"None": Patient does not open eyes to any stimulus	1
BEST VERBAL RESPONSE	
Assesses the content of consciousness in terms of the ability to produce speech and quality of speech. It is controversial whether points should be added to the score when patients nod or gesture indicating they would speak appropriately if able.	
"Oriented": Patient can state his or her name, where he or she is, and the date	5
"Confused": Patient speaks words but cannot state either who he or she is, where he or she is, or the date	4
"Inappropriate words": Patient speaks words with no specific intent at communicating	3
"Incomprehensible sounds": Patient grunts, groans, or makes other sounds	2
"None": Patient makes no attempt to vocalize. (*Note*: A "T" may be written after the score to indicate the presence of a tracheal tube.)	1
BEST MOTOR RESPONSE	
Assesses both arousal and the content of consciousness. Ensure consistent stimuli and limb position with each assessment to avoid influencing the patient's response.	
"Obeys": Follows commands	6
"Localizes": Attempts to remove noxious stimulus	5
"Withdraws": Pulls away from noxious stimulus	4
"Abnormal flexion": Decorticate posturing*	3
"Abnormal extension": Decerebrate posturing†	2
"No response": No motor movement of any kind to any stimulus	1
SCORING	
The patient's responses are graded and the best scores achieved for the eye opening, verbal, and motor categories are summed.	
Total score ranges from 3 to 15, with 15 being normal.	

*Rigid flexion, internal rotation, and adduction of the upper extremity; extension, internal rotation, and plantar flexion of the lower extremity.
†Rigid extension, adduction, and internal rotation of the upper extremity; extension, internal rotation, and plantar flexion of the lower extremity.

(c) Motor function
   (1) Assess size and contour of muscles: Note atrophy, hypertrophy, asymmetry, and joint malalignments.
   (2) Observe for involuntary movements, such as fasciculations, tics, tremors, abnormal positioning.
   (3) Determine motor response to stimuli.
      a) Ability to follow simple commands such as "Hold up two fingers." Do not ask the patient to squeeze your hand because this may be a reflex response to palmar stimulation.
      b) Localization: Able to locate a noxious stimulus (e.g., deep pain stimulus) and attempt to remove it; indicates cortical dysfunction
      c) Withdrawal: Pulls limb(s) away from painful stimuli with normal flexor movement; indicates extensive cortical damage

d) Abnormal flexion (decorticate posturing; see Table 4-11): Associated with lesions to the corticospinal tract just above the brainstem near or in the cerebral hemispheres, in the area of the diencephalon

e) Extensor (decerebrate) posturing (see Table 4-11): Indicates damage to the midbrain or upper pons

f) No response: Associated with lower brainstem or high spinal cord dysfunction

(4) Perform strength testing (if the patient is able to follow commands).

a) Evaluate the integrity and function of UMNs and LMNs that innervate a specific muscle or muscle group (Table 4-12).

b) Grade strength on a 0 to 5 scale (Table 4-13).

c) Note whether weakness follows a distributional pattern (proximal-distal, right-left, or upper-lower extremity).

(5) Perform strength testing for a patient unable to follow commands.

a) Observe which extremities move spontaneously or to noxious stimuli.

b) Hemiparesis or hemiplegia may be detected by lifting both arms off the bed and releasing them simultaneously. The limb on the hemiparetic side will fall more quickly and more limply than that on the normal side.

(6) Assess muscle tone: state of muscle tension is assessed by palpating muscles at rest and during passive range-of-motion (ROM) movement; possible abnormalities include the following:

TABLE 4-12
Muscle Groups, Associated Level of Spinal Cord Innervation, and Method of Testing

Muscle(s) Tested	Primary Level(s) of Spinal Nerve Innervation	Method of Testing
Deltoids	C5	Raising of arms
Biceps	C5	Flexion of elbow
Wrist extensors	C6	Extension of wrist
Triceps	C7	Extension of elbow
Hand intrinsics	C8-T1	Hand squeezing, finger flexion, finger abduction
Iliopsoas	L1, L2	Hip flexion
Hip adductors	L2-L4	Adduction of hips (squeezing legs together)
Hip abductors	L4, L5, S1	Abduction of hips (separating hips)
Quadriceps	L3, L4	Knee extension
Hamstrings	L5, S1, S2	Knee flexion
Tibialis anterior	L4, L5	Dorsiflexion of foot
Extensor hallucis longus	L5	Extension of great toe
Gastrocnemius	S1	Plantar flexion of foot

Adapted from McIlvoy L, Meyer K, McQuillan KA. Traumatic spine injuries. In: Bader MK, Littlejohns LR, eds. *AANN Core Curriculum for Neuroscience Nursing*. 4th ed. St Louis, MO: Saunders; 2004:345.

TABLE 4-13
Muscle Strength Grading Scale

Score	Muscle Function
0	Absent, no muscle contraction
1	Contraction of muscle felt or seen
2	Movement through full range of motion with gravity removed
3	Movement through full range of motion against gravity
4	Movement against resistance but can be overcome
5	Full strength against resistance

a) *Rigidity*: Increased muscular resistance throughout passive ROM movement; seen with a basal ganglia lesion

b) *Spasticity*: Increased muscular resistance to joint movement often followed by release of resistance; increased tone indicates corticospinal tract lesion

c) *Hypotonia* (flaccidity): Decreased muscle tone associated with LMN lesions, cerebellar dysfunction, or spinal shock related to acute spinal cord injury

(7) Assess deep tendon or muscle stretch reflexes: elicited by percussing the tendon with a reflex hammer, which causes stretching of the muscle spindles and subsequent contraction of muscle fibers when the monosynaptic reflex arc is intact. Compare responses side to side.

a) Hyperreflexia usually indicates UMN lesion.

b) May be diminished initially after an acute intracranial injury because of cerebral shock·or at and below the level of spinal cord injury because of spinal shock

c) Areflexia most often due to LMN lesions

d) Deep tendon reflexes commonly tested: See Table 4-14

e) Grade deep tendon reflexes on a 0 to 4 scale: See Table 4-15

(8) Assess superficial reflexes: tested by stroking the skin with a moderately sharp object (Table 4-16). These reflexes are lost or abnormal with UMN or LMN lesions.

(9) Assess pathologic reflexes: See Box 4-2.

(10) Assess abnormal movements: See Box 4-2.

(11) Assess balance and coordination: See Box 4-2.

(d) Sensory function

(1) In an unresponsive or uncooperative patient, a cursory sensory examination is performed by noting the patient's response to painful stimuli applied while performing various interventions (e.g., venipuncture).

■ **TABLE 4-14**
■ ■ **Deep Tendon or Muscle Stretch Reflexes and Level of Spinal Cord Innervation**

Reflex	Level of Spinal Cord Innervation
Biceps	C5, C6
Brachioradialis	C5, C6
Triceps	C7, C8
Quadriceps (patellar)	L2-L4
Achilles (ankle jerk)	S1, S2

■ **TABLE 4-15**
■ ■ **Grading Scale for Strength of Deep Tendon Reflexes**

Score	Reflex Response
4+	Hyperreactive, clonus
3+	Very brisk
2+	Normal, average
1+	Diminished
0	No response, flaccid

From McIlvoy L, Meyer K, McQuillan KA. Traumatic spine injuries. In: Bader MK, Littlejohns LR, eds. *AANN Core Curriculum for Neuroscience Nursing.* 4th ed. St Louis, MO: Saunders; 2004:346.

TABLE 4-16

Superficial Reflexes, Level of Spinal Nerve Innervation, and Method for Assessment

Reflex	Spinal Nerve Innervation	Stimulus	Response
Upper abdominal	T8-T10	Stroke upper abdomen.	Abdominal wall contraction that causes umbilicus to move toward the stimulus
Lower abdominal	T10-T12	Stroke lower abdomen.	Abdominal wall contraction that causes umbilicus to move toward the stimulus
Cremasteric	L1, L2	Stroke medial thigh.	Testicular elevation
Bulbocavernous	S3, S4	Apply pressure to glans penis.	Contraction of the anus
Perianal	S3-S5	Stroke perianal area.	Contraction of the external anal sphincter

Adapted from McIlvoy L, Meyer K, McQuillan KA. Traumatic spine injuries. In: Bader MK, Littlejohns LR, eds. *AANN Core Curriculum for Neuroscience Nursing.* 4th ed. St Louis, MO: Saunders; 2004:347.

BOX 4-2

ASSESSMENT OF PATHOLOGIC REFLEXES, ABNORMAL MOVEMENTS, BALANCE, AND COORDINATION

Pathologic reflexes
- Primitive reflexes present in infants but normally absent in adults may reappear in association with frontal lobe impairment. Examples include the following:
  1. Grasp reflex: In response to palmar stimulation
  2. Sucking reflex: In response to lip stimulation
  3. Rooting reflex: Mouth opens, head deviates toward a stimulus applied to the lower lip or cheek
- Babinski's sign
  1. Stroking the lateral aspect of the sole of the foot from the heel upward and across the ball causes abnormal dorsiflexion of the great toe and extensor fanning of the other toes.
  2. In an adult, indicates a lesion of the corticospinal tract anywhere from the motor cortex to the anterior horn of the spinal cord

Abnormal movements: Note the distribution, rate, duration, and relationship to activity of any involuntary movements, such as the following:
- Seizures (refer to Seizures under Specific Patient Health Problems)
- Tremors: Rhythmic trembling movement of muscles
- Clonus: Abrupt onset of brief jerking movements of a muscle or muscle group (e.g., oscillation of the foot between flexion and extension with sudden passive extension of the foot)

Balance and coordination: Primarily evaluate cerebellar function; tested in patients able to perform voluntary movements
- Romberg's test: Patient stands erect with the feet together, first with the eyes open and then with the eyes closed. Positive test result indicating posterior column or cerebellar dysfunction occurs when the patient loses balance and sways or falls when the eyes are closed.
- Observe the patient while he or she is sitting; swaying indicates cerebellar dysfunction.
- Evaluate for *dystaxia* or *ataxia* (muscle incoordination with volitional movements) and *dysmetria* (inability to halt a movement at a desired point), which indicate cerebellar dysfunction.
  1. Have the patient first touch the examiner's finger, positioned at the length of patient's arm from the face, and then touch his or her nose.
  2. Have the patient slap the thigh first with the palm and then with the back of the hand in quick, alternating movements.
  3. Have the patient run the heel from the opposite knee down the shin.
  4. Rebound test: Have the patient extend the arms forward while the examiner taps the patient's wrist; in cerebellar disease, the arm moves markedly out of place and overshooting occurs as the patient attempts to move the arm back into position
- Gait
  1. Observe the gait and have the patient perform tandem (heel-to-toe) walking.
  2. A wide-based, staggering gait and the inability to perform tandem walking indicate cerebellar dysfunction.
  3. Gait disturbances with different clinical characteristics can be correlated with other specific neurologic or muscular dysfunction (e.g., spastic hemiparesis following an upper motor neuron lesion causes the patient to walk with the arm flexed close to the body and the spastic leg to move outward and forward in a semicircle, often with the toe dragged).

(2) In an awake, cooperative patient able to understand and follow commands, a complete sensory assessment can be performed. Test with the patient's eyes closed and compare one side of the body with the other.

(3) Sensory function is scored by using a 0 to 2 scale: See Table 4-17.

(4) When possible, delineate sensory impairments on the basis of dermatome distribution (see Figure 4-17).

(5) Assess spinothalamic tracts: See Box 4-3.

(6) Assess posterior columns: See Box 4-3.

(7) Assess cortical discriminatory sensation: See Box 4-3.

■ **TABLE 4-17**
■ ■ **Sensory Function Scoring**

Score	Sensory Function
0	Absent
1	Impaired or hyperesthetic
2	Normal or intact

Adapted from McIlvoy L, Meyer K, McQuillan KA. Traumatic spine injuries. In: Bader MK, Littlejohns LR, eds. *AANN Core Curriculum for Neuroscience Nursing*. 4th ed. St Louis, MO: Saunders; 2004:344.

■ **BOX 4-3**
■ **ASSESSMENT OF SPINOTHALAMIC TRACTS, POSTERIOR COLUMNS, AND CORTICAL DISCRIMINATORY SENSATION**

Lesions or dysfunction of the peripheral nerves, ascending nerve tracts, or sensory perceptive areas of the cerebral cortex (i.e., parietal lobe) may impair sensory function.

SPINOTHALAMIC TRACTS (ANTERIOR AND LATERAL)
■ Test either pain or temperature sensation, because both functions are carried in the same lateral spinothalamic tracts.
■ Pain: Have the patient distinguish sharp from dull stimuli randomly applied; gently touch the skin using a clean pin for sharp sensation and using a blunt edge (head of a pin) for dull sensation
■ Temperature: Ask the patient to distinguish between hot and cold stimuli when randomly touched with test tubes filled with hot or cold water
■ Light touch: Lightly touch the patient with a wisp of cotton

POSTERIOR COLUMNS (FASCICULUS GRACILIS AND FASCICULUS CUNEATUS)
■ Test either proprioception or vibration sense, because both are carried in the same tracts.
■ Vibration: Apply a vibrating tuning fork to bony prominences; ask the patient to report when vibration is felt; apply first to the distal aspect of each extremity and move proximally
■ Proprioception (position sense): Ask the patient to close the eyes and report whether a finger or toe is being moved up or down; assess in all four extremities

CORTICAL DISCRIMINATORY SENSATION
In addition to the sensory pathways, assesses the association portions of the cortex (i.e., the parietal lobe). Deficits are called *agnosias* (not knowing). Examples include the following:
■ *Stereognosis*: Ask the patient, without the aid of vision, to identify familiar objects placed in his or her hand. The inability to identify objects is *astereognosis*.
■ *Graphesthesia*: Ask the patient to identify numbers or letters traced on the palm. Inability to discern what is written is *agraphesthesia*.
■ *Simultaneous double stimulation*: With the patient's eyes closed, touch the patient's limb and then touch both sides of the body in corresponding locations. Determine if the patient can detect the number and location of stimuli. Inability to identify that he or she is being touched on both sides of body simultaneously is *tactile inattention*. Inability to locate a single touch sensation is *atopognosia*.

(e) Cranial nerves: See Table 4-18 and Figure 4-22
(f) Eye and pupil signs: In addition to cranial nerve assessment, other findings may include the following:
  (1) Pupil abnormalities (Table 4-19)
  (2) Gaze deviation or gaze preference: Horizontal or vertical gaze deviations indicate a cortical or brainstem lesion
    a) Eyes deviate toward the side of a destructive hemispheric lesion affecting the frontal gaze centers.
    b) Gaze deviates away from irritative foci (seizures) affecting the frontal gaze centers.
    c) Inability to gaze upward is associated with dorsal midbrain lesions.
    d) Eyes deviate away from the side of a unilateral pons lesion.
  (3) Nystagmus (rhythmic, oscillatory eye movements)
    a) Detected by having the patient follow your finger through the fields of gaze
    b) Due to lesions of the cerebellum, vestibular system, or brainstem pathways, or toxic-metabolic disorders; clinical features vary with the part of the pathway affected
(g) Vital signs
  (1) Temperature
    a) Hyperthermia increases cerebral oxygen consumption by 10% for every 1.8° F (1° C) elevation. Higher metabolic demand increases the risk for CNS ischemia. Neurogenic fever can be caused by damage to the hypothalamus, where the thermoregulation center is located.
    b) Hypothermia, if extreme, can lead to cardiac dysrhythmias, coagulopathies, other complications. Seen with hypothalamic lesions, spinal cord injury with autonomic dysfunction, and metabolic or toxic encephalopathy.
  (2) Respirations: Respiratory dysrhythmias often correlate with lesions at specific locations in the brain, although effects may vary and may be influenced by other factors (Table 4-20)
  (3) Pulse and BP
    a) Both are notoriously unreliable parameters in detecting CNS disease or neurologic deterioration. May change late in the course of increased ICP and thus are of limited clinical use.
    b) Cardiac dysrhythmias may be seen with neurologic disorders, particularly with blood in the CSF, after posterior fossa surgery, with increased ICP, or with stroke in certain locations.
    c) Tachycardia and hypertension may be seen with injury or compression of the hypothalamus that results in sympathetic nervous system stimulation.
    d) Cushing's response occurs when intracranial hypertension causes compression of the medullary vasomotor center. Systolic pressure rises, widens pulse pressure, and may slow pulse.
  (4) Pain—the fifth vital sign
    a) Pain that is assessed at regular intervals and treated with the same zeal as abnormalities in other vital signs has a much better chance of being treated effectively
    b) Key concepts in pain assessment: See Box 4-4
    c) Components of pain assessment: See Table 4-21
    d) Adequate pain assessment poses a special challenge in the critically ill patient.
    e) Acute pain assessment tools
      1) Pain tools should estimate the severity of pain and accurately reflect changes in pain intensity after interventions.
      2) General guidelines for successful use include the following:
        a) Tool should be valid, reliable, and appropriate for the patient's age and cognitive, cultural, developmental, and physical status.

TABLE 4-18

Cranial Nerve Assessment and Anticipated Deficits

Cranial Nerve	Assessment in Conscious Patient	Assessment in Unconscious or Uncooperative Patient	Anticipated Deficit
Olfactory (I)	Test each nostril separately. Ask the patient to identify familiar nonirritating odors, such as coffee or perfume.	Unable to assess	Loss of sense of smell (anosmia)
Optic (II)	1. Inspect the optic disc (fundus), macula, and blood vessels with an ophthalmoscope. 2. Test visual acuity with a Snellen chart or printed material; test each eye individually. 3. Determine visual field using the confrontation test. Have the patient cover one eye and fixate on you with the other. Position yourself about 24 inches directly in front of the patient and close your eye that is opposite the patient's covered eye. With your finger halfway between yourself and the patient, bring your finger from the periphery into the patient's field of vision, evaluating the upward, downward, nasal, and temporal fields. Compare your visual field with the patient's. Repeat the test with the other eye.	Evaluate the pupillary light reflex (provides the sensory limb for this reflex) as part of the assessment with CN III described later.	1. Papilledema (optic disc swollen and distorted with a reddish hue), which is indicative of increased intracranial pressure 2. Decrease or loss of central vision; blindness 3. Visual field defect (see Figure 4-22)
Oculomotor (III)	1. Evaluate the width and symmetry of the palpebral fissures and eyelid position. 2. Assess pupil shape, size, and equality. Describe size in millimeters. 3. Test the direct light reflex (constriction of the pupil when stimulated by light). This tests the afferent limb of CN II and the efferent limb of CN III. Describe the reflex as brisk, sluggish, or nonreactive. 4. Test the consensual light reflex (constriction of the opposite pupil when light stimulates one eye). Differentiates CN II and CN III lesions. Reflex is "present" or "absent." 5. Test the accommodation reflex: Have the patient look at an object (e.g., finger, pen) positioned 2 to 3 ft in front of the patient; as the object is moved toward the patient, the patient's eyes converge toward the midline, pupils constrict, and the lenses thicken. 6. Assess extraocular movement as part of the assessment for CN IV and VI described later.	1. Assess pupil shape, size, equality, and reactivity to light as was done for a conscious patient. 2. Evaluate extraocular movement as described later.	1. Eyelid droops (ptosis). 2. Irregularly shaped pupils can be caused by direct trauma, cataracts, or other ocular dysfunction; an irregularly shaped or oval pupil may accompany tentorial herniation that compresses CN III. 3. Disruption or compression of parasympathetic fibers from CN III and/or the nucleus (e.g., from a mass lesion or tentorial herniation) causes the ipsilateral pupil to dilate, which results in unequal pupils (anisocoria). 4. The direct light reflex is lost with oculomotor (parasympathetic) or optic nerve injury but retained with sympathetic disruption. 5. A blind eye (CN II lesion) does not have a direct light reflex; it has a consensual light reflex if CN III and midbrain connections are intact; cortical blindness does not affect either direct or consensual reflexes. 6. The accommodation reflex is lost.

Cranial Nerve	Assessment		Findings
Oculomotor (III), trochlear (IV), and abducens (VI)	1. Check the range of EOMs by having the patient's eyes follow your finger through all fields of gaze. Observe for nystagmus at rest and during ocular movements. 2. Ask the patient whether double vision is experienced in any visual field	In patients who open their eyes, determine whether they can move both their eyes medially (CN III), laterally outward (CN VI), or up and down (more difficult to elicit) in response to a verbal or noxious stimulus. Evaluate whether the eyes move together (conjugate movement).	1. Impairment of EOM • Inability to move eye(s) downward and outward, medially, upward and inward, or upward and outward indicates CN III involvement. • Impaired downward and inward movement indicates CN IV involvement. • Inability to move the eye(s) horizontally outward indicates CN VI involvement. 2. Diplopia
Trigeminal (V)	Sensory examination 1. Test the forehead, cheeks, and jaw on each side of the face. To evaluate light touch sensation, use a wisp of cotton; to evaluate temperature sensation, use test tubes of warm and cold water. 2. Corneal reflex: Touch the cornea of each eye with a wisp of cotton. Observe for reflex blinking. This tests the afferent limb of CN V and the efferent limb of CN VII. Motor examination 1. Ask the patient to clench his or her teeth and palpate the masseter and temporal muscles. Assess the symmetry and strength of muscle contraction. Assess the strength of the masseter muscles by pushing down on the mandible (chin) against the patient's resistance. 2. Assess the patient's ability to chew.	Test the corneal reflex.	1. Absent, unequal, or uncomfortable sensation when the face is stimulated 2. Absence or weakness of blink response to corneal stimuli 3. Weakness of masseter and/or temporal muscles
Facial (VII)	1. Ask the patient to raise his or her eyebrows, frown, smile, and open the eyes against resistance. Note the strength and symmetry of facial movement. 2. Test taste on the anterior two thirds of the tongue by applying salt and then sugar to both sides of the tongue. Ask the patient to identify the taste before closing the mouth. 3. Assess the corneal reflex.	Test the corneal reflex.	1. Weakness on one or both sides of the upper and/or lower face; if only the lower portion of the face is weak the cause is an upper motor neuron lesion (e.g., stroke) on the contralateral side of the facial weakness; weakness of the entire side of the face is due to an ipsilateral lower motor neuron lesion of the facial nerve 2. Loss of taste sensation 3. Absence or weakness of the corneal reflex

Continued

■ **TABLE 4-18**
■ ■ Cranial Nerve Assessment and Anticipated Deficits—Cont'd

Cranial Nerve	Assessment in Conscious Patient	Assessment in Unconscious or Uncooperative Patient	Anticipated Deficit
Acoustic (vestibulocochlear) (VIII)	Cochlear (hearing) 1. Hearing acuity: Cover one ear, and test the other with a watch or a whisper. 2. Weber's test: Place the stem of a vibrating tuning fork on the midline vertex of the skull. Ask the patient if the sound is heard equally in both ears or more on one side. Normally, there is no lateralization of sound. 3. Rinne's test: Place the stem of a vibrating tuning fork on the mastoid bone. When sound is no longer heard, invert the tuning fork and place it in front of the ear. Ask the patient to tell you when sound is no longer heard. Vestibular (balance) 1. Assess the patient for complaints of vertigo, nausea, anxiety, nystagmus, postural deviation, and vomiting. All may indicate vestibular nerve dysfunction. 2. Observe gait. 3. Evaluate balance. 4. Perform the caloric irrigation test (to test the oculovestibular reflex): Position the patient with the head of the bed elevated 30 degrees. After checking to ensure an unoccluded ear canal and intact tympanic membrane, irrigate the canal with cold water. In the awake patient, when the pathway from the vestibular portion of CN VIII through the brainstem to CN III and CN VI is intact, the response will consist of slow conjugate eye deviation toward the irrigated ear and then rapid eye movement away from the irrigated ear. The cerebral cortex controls the fast phase. Awake patients may also experience vertigo, nausea, and vomiting.	The vestibular portion of CN VIII and its connections via the medial longitudinal fasciculus with CN III, IV, and VI provide information regarding the integrity of the brainstem; can be tested by the oculocephalic or oculovestibular reflex: 1. Oculocephalic reflex (doll's eye test): In a comatose patient who has had a cervical spine injury ruled out, turn the patient's head quickly from side to side while holding open the patient's eyes and noting the direction of eye movement. With intact connections between CN VIII and CN III and VI, the eyes move bilaterally in the opposite direction of the head movement. This is described as "doll's eyes present." 2. Oculovestibular reflex (caloric irrigation test): Tested the same as described for a conscious patient. Conjugate eye deviation toward the irrigated ear indicates that the pathway from the vestibular portion of CN VIII to CN III and VI is intact. (When the cerebral cortex is depressed, the fast eye deviation is lost.)	1. Impaired hearing 2. Negative result on Weber's test: When sound is referred to the better-hearing ear, decreased hearing is due to impaired function of the cochlear nerve 3. Negative result on Rinne's test: Because air conduction is normally greater than bone conduction, middle ear disease is suspected in a patient who can hear the tuning fork when it is placed on the mastoid bone as well as or better than near the ear 4. Presence of complaints seen with vestibular dysfunction 5. Imbalance 6. Abnormal oculocephalic reflex: There is no eye movement or the eyes move asymmetrically in response to head rotation 7. Abnormal oculovestibular reflex (showing the brainstem pathways to be impaired): The eyes stay in midposition when the ear is irrigated

Glosso-pharyngeal (IX) and vagus (X)	1. Ask the patient to open his or her mouth and say, "Ahh." Observe for symmetric elevation of the palatal arch and midline uvula. 2. Test for the gag reflex: Stroke the palatal arch with a tongue blade. The palate should elevate, and the patient should have a gag response. This tests the afferent limb of CN IX and the efferent limb of CN X. 3. Appraise articulation and voice quality. 4. Assess the ability to swallow. 5. Evaluate the ability to taste salt and sugar placed on the posterior third of the tongue.	1. Test by evaluating the gag and cough reflexes, usually accomplished by observing the patient's response to suctioning or movement of the endotracheal tube or to direct stimulation of the palatal arch. 2. Evaluate the patient's ability to handle oral secretions by swallowing.	1. Deviation of the uvula to the unaffected side 2. Palate does not rise on the affected side. 3. Absent gag reflex 4. Difficulty with vocalization (dysphonia): • No voice • Hoarseness related to vocal cord paralysis; laryngoscopic examination may be indicated • Whisper, nasal-sounding voice indicates soft palate paralysis. 5. Difficulty swallowing (dysphagia) 6. Loss of taste sensation on the posterior third of the tongue
Spinal accessory (XI)	1. Assess the SCM and trapezius muscles for size, symmetry, and spasticity. 2. Ask the patient to turn his or her head to one side. Place one hand on the patient's cheek and the other on the patient's shoulder for stability. Instruct the patient to resist your attempt to forcibly turn the head back to midline. Repeat on other side. 3. Ask the patient to push the head forward against your hand. Assess the strength of both SCM muscles. 4. Ask the patient to shrug his or her shoulders upward against the resistance of your downward pressure on the shoulders. Note the strength of the trapezius muscles.	Not typically assessed in the unconscious patient	1. Atrophy or spasticity of the SCM or trapezius muscles 2. Weakness or inability to turn or lift the head or shrug the shoulder
Hypoglossal (XII)	1. Inspect the tongue for atrophy or fasciculation with the patient at rest. 2. Have the patient protrude the tongue and assess for alignment and symmetry. 3. Ask the patient to move the tongue to the right and left and then press the tongue against the inside of the cheek while you assess its strength. 4. Note articulation.	Not typically assessed in the unconscious patient	1. Tongue deviation to the paralyzed side 2. Tongue movement weakness or paralysis 3. Dysarthria

CN, Cranial nerve; *EOM*, extraocular movements; *SCM*, sternocleidomastoid.

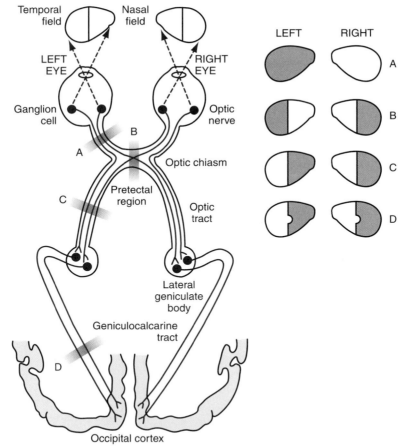

FIGURE 4-22 ■ Visual pathways. Transection of the pathways at the locations indicated by the letters causes the visual field defects shown in the diagrams on the right. Occipital lesions may spare fibers from the macula (as in *D*) because of the separation in the brain of these fibers from the others subserving vision. (From Ganong WF. *Review of Medical Physiology.* 21st ed. New York, NY: Lange Medical Books/McGraw-Hill; 2003:153.)

■ **TABLE 4-19**
■ ■ **Pupil Abnormalities Associated with Specific Areas of Brain Dysfunction**

Pupil Finding	Related Brain Dysfunction
Small, equal, reactive	Bilateral diencephalic damage that affects the sympathetic innervation originating from the hypothalamus; metabolic dysfunction
Nonreactive, midpositioned	Midbrain damage
Fixed and dilated	Ipsilateral oculomotor (cranial nerve III) compression or injury
Bilateral fixed and dilated	Brain anoxia and ischemia; bilateral cranial nerve III compression
Pinpoint, nonreactive	Pons damage, often from hemorrhage or ischemia that interrupts the sympathetic nervous system pathways
One pupil smaller that the other, but both reactive to light; associated with ptosis and an inability to sweat on the same side as the smaller pupil (Horner's syndrome)	Interruption of ipsilateral sympathetic innervation that can be caused by a lesion of the anterolateral cervical spinal cord or lateral medulla, damage to the hypothalamus, or occlusion or dissection of the internal carotid artery

▓ TABLE 4-20
▓ ▓ Respiratory Patterns Associated with Specific Areas of Brain Dysfunction

Breathing Pattern	Description	Location of Brain Lesion or Type of Dysfunction
Cheyne-Stokes	Regular cycles of respirations that gradually increase in depth to hyperpnea and then decrease in depth to periods of apnea	Usually bilateral lesions deep within the cerebral hemispheres, basal ganglia, or diencephalon; metabolic disorders
Central neurogenic hyperventilation	Deep, rapid respirations	Midbrain, upper pons
Apneustic	Prolonged inspiration followed by a 2- to 3-second pause; occasionally may alternate with an expiratory pause	Pons
Cluster	Cluster of irregular breaths followed by an apneic period lasting a variable amount of time	Lower pons or upper medulla
Ataxic or irregular	Irregular, unpredictable pattern of shallow and deep respirations and pauses	Medulla

Adapted from McQuillan KA, Mitchell PH. Traumatic brain injuries. In: McQuillan KA, Von Rueden KT, Hartsock RL, et al, eds. *Trauma Nursing From Resuscitation Through Rehabilitation*. 3rd ed. St Louis, MO: Saunders; 2002:420.

▓ BOX 4-4
▓ BASIC PAIN ASSESSMENT "PEARLS"

- All patients have the right to appropriate assessment and management of pain and should be educated and encouraged to report unrelieved pain.
- Pain is an individual, subjective sensation. It cannot be proved or disproved.
- Your attitudes and beliefs about pain can affect the way you treat pain.
- Pain assessment is conducted and documented as appropriate to the patient's condition.
    1. Include pain intensity, quality, location, pain-related complications, and adverse effects of treatment whenever possible.
    2. Increase assessment frequency during times of inadequately controlled pain.
    3. Obtain a detailed pain assessment, history, and focused physical examination as the patient improves to ensure an accurate diagnosis of pain.
- Make every effort to obtain the patient's self-report of pain, because this is the most reliable indicator of pain. (Do not assume that a patient cannot provide a self-report without asking.)
    1. Ask simple questions, allow time for response, and repeat or rephrase as needed.
    2. Documenting a simple "yes" or "no" (or nod or shake of head) is acceptable.
- Assess pain in a patient unable to provide a self-report of pain.
    1. Never assume that a sedated and/or chemically paralyzed patient does not feel pain—medications such as propofol and midazolam do not provide analgesia.
    2. The absence of observable signs does not mean that pain does not exist.
    3. When conditions exist that are known to be painful, assume that pain is present.
- Reassessment after intervention has taken effect is essential and should include these questions:
    1. How much relief was obtained and how long did it last?
    2. Were there any adverse effects?

    b) Patient and caregivers should be educated on tool use and purpose.
    c) Whenever possible, the same tool should be used consistently with a given patient.
    d) Whenever possible, a pain tool in the patient's language should be used.
   3) Unidimensional tools measure a single element of pain (e.g., intensity). Figure 4-23 shows examples of reliable and valid self-reporting tools for measuring intensity.

■ **TABLE 4-21**
■ ■ **Components of Pain Assessment**

Component	Sample Questions/Comments
Location and radiation	Where is the pain? Can you point to where you hurt? Does the pain go anywhere else? Consider that there may be more than one location of pain to be assessed.
Intensity or severity	Assessed via pain scales, words, gestures See the section on pain assessment in patients who cannot communicate under Patient Assessment.
Character or quality	What does the pain "feel" like? Give words to choose from (e.g., sharp, dull, aching, shooting, burning, pins and needles). Description of pain quality helps determine treatment (e.g., neuropathic pain may respond better to adjuvant medications than to opioids).
Timing	When did the pain start? How long did it last? Is it there all the time? Does it come and go?
Alleviating and aggravating factors	What lessens the pain? What makes it worse? Considerations include medications or other remedies, activities, position, foods.
Associated factors and symptoms	What else occurs with the pain? Considerations include nausea, vomiting, constipation, confusion, depression.
Impact on life and functionality	What can't you do that you'd like to do? What is your expectation of pain relief? Consider the pain's effect on, for example, appetite, sleep, mood, work, home life, hobbies.
Relevant medical history	Past surgeries, trauma, coexisting medical conditions, psychiatric illness (e.g., depression) Prior pain experiences Past or current tobacco, drug, or alcohol use Past or present pain management strategies and outcomes (e.g., how much pain relief was obtained, how long did it last) Other medication history

    a) Numeric rating scale (NRS)
       i) 0 to 10 range
       ii) Use horizontally or vertically.
       iii) Present verbally or visually.
    b) Faces rating scales
       i) Patient selects face.
       ii) Often used with other scales
    c) Verbal descriptor scales
       i) Present verbally or visually.
       ii) Use words the patient understands.
    d) Visual analogue scale (0 to 100): May be difficult for critically ill patients to use
   f) Pain assessment when the patient cannot communicate
    1) Lack of self-report can lead to undertreatment.
    2) When self-report is not possible, assume pain is present on the basis of the presence of a painful condition or procedure
    3) Behavioral and physiologic signs are not always reliable indicators of pain but may be useful to confirm suspicion of pain or evaluate the response to intervention when no alternative exists.
      a) Behaviors are often more reliable indicators than physiologic signs.
      b) Physiologic signs are temporary, may resolve before pain resolves, and may reflect other phenomena (e.g., anxiety).
    4) Hierarchy of importance of basic measures of pain intensity is as follows (criteria are listed in order of reliability):

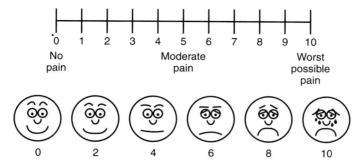

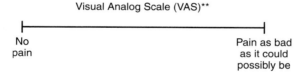

Numerical rating scale (NRS) and Wong-Baker faces scale: Patient indicates number or face that best describes their pain intensity either verbally or by gestures

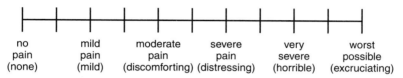

| no pain (none) | mild pain (mild) | moderate pain (discomforting) | severe pain (distressing) | very severe (horrible) | worst possible (excruciating) |

Verbal Descriptor Scale: Patient selects words/phase that best represents their pain intensity

Visual Analog Scale (VAS)**

No pain   Pain as bad
                                                        as it could
                                                        possibly be

Visual Analog Scale (VAS): **A 10-cm baseline is recommended
Patient places a mark on the line to represent pain intensity. Measure in millimeters
from "no pain" to patient's mark. Score ranges from "0" to "100."

FIGURE 4-23 ■ Pain assessment tools. (Numeric rating scale, Wong-Baker faces scale, and Visual Analog Scale from McCaffery M, Pasero C. *Pain: Clinical Manual.* 2nd ed. St Louis, MO: Mosby; 1999:62, 67; faces pain scale modified by McCaffery and Pasero from Whaley LF, Wong DL. *Essentials of Pediatric Nursing.* St Louis, MO: Mosby; 1997:1215-1216; Verbal Descriptor Scale from Acute Pain Management Guideline Panel. *Acute Pain Management in Adults: Operative Procedures, Quick Reference Guide for Clinicians No 1.* Rockville, MD: Agency for Health Care Policy and Research; 1992:116. AHCPR Pub No 92-0019.)

    a) patient's self-report of pain
    b) Pathology (e.g., fractures, incisions)
    c) Behaviors (e.g., grimacing, frowning, wincing) (Table 4-22)
    d) Report of a parent, family member, or other person close to the patient ("proxy pain rating")
    e) Physiologic indices (e.g., increased heart rate, BP) (Table 4-23)
  5) Behavioral pain tools designed for use in critically ill patients require further testing before general use can be recommended.
    a) If used, evaluate each time a low score is obtained with potentially painful conditions because patients may not be able to demonstrate specific behaviors required for scoring.
    b) Examples include Behavioral Pain Scale, Nonverbal Pain Scale, Checklist of Nonverbal Pain Indicators.

3. Appraisal of patient characteristics: Patients with acute neurologic problems enter progressive care units with a wide range of clinical characteristics. During their stay, their clinical status may slowly or abruptly improve or deteriorate. Changes in the patient's condition may involve one or all life-sustaining functions, and functions can be easy or nearly

■ **TABLE 4-22**
■ ■ **Behaviors Often Associated with Pain in Nonverbal Patients**

Category	Behavioral Examples	Comments
Facial expressions	Grimacing, frowning, wincing, wrinkled forehead, eyes either closed or wide open with eyebrows raised, mouth wide open with exposed teeth and tongue, clenched teeth	Grimacing, frowning, and wincing may represent involuntary responses to acute pain and are felt to be valid indicators of acute pain, even in sedated patients Some medical conditions (e.g., Parkinson's disease, stroke, chemical paralysis) may result in distorted or absent facial expressions apart from pain. Eye signals may be used to communicate pain by patients unable to otherwise communicate.
Movement	Restlessness, splinting, guarding, shaking, flailing, fidgeting, rigidity or tenseness, arching, clenching of fists, holding or rubbing of affected area, resistance to movement or care procedures, slow or cautious or no movement, repositioning, rocking, withdrawing	Some patients who are unable to verbally communicate may seek attention to their pain through gestures or other arm and leg movements, or by hitting the bed.
Vocalizations	Verbal complaints of pain, whimpering, crying, groaning, moaning, yelling, screaming, verbal outbursts, protest words (e.g., "Stop," "Don't")	For patients with nonspecific vocalizations (e.g., screaming or yelling) a trial of analgesics should be made rather than relying solely on sedatives and/or anxiolytics.
Other	Agitation, aggression, change in usual activity or behavior, confusion, altered sleep, fatigue	Other conditions besides pain can lead to agitation (e.g., hypoxia, hypercarbia, sepsis).

Summary	All behaviors
	• Although self-report of pain is optimal, behaviors may be the only way pain can be communicated in the patient unable to verbalize.
	• The degree of behavioral response factors into the degree of pain intensity and distress patients experience (Puntillo et al, 2004).
	• The absence of "pain" behaviors does not mean that the patient is not experiencing pain.
		• Pain behaviors are influenced by many factors (e.g., culture, duration of pain, coping skills).
		• Some patients, such as the following, cannot exhibit pain behaviors of any kind:
		  • Sedated or chemically paralyzed patients
		  • Nonresponsive trauma patients
		  • Comatose patients
		  • Patients sedated for painful procedures
		• Behaviors should be used as only one assessment technique.

impossible to monitor with precision. Examples of clinical attributes that the nurse should assess when caring for a patient with an acute neurologic disorder are the following:

a. Resiliency
  i. Level 1—*Minimally resilient*: A frail, 84-year-old woman admitted with a left-sided ischemic stroke who is experiencing severe dysphagia and in whom aspiration pneumonia has developed
  ii. Level 3—*Moderately resilient*: A 63-year-old woman admitted with a left-sided hemorrhagic stroke resulting from hypertension who is experiencing some right-sided weakness
  iii. Level 5—*Highly resilient*: A 42-year-old man admitted after a bowel resection complaining of pain 7/10
b. Vulnerability
  i. Level 1—*Highly vulnerable*: A 78-year-old man transferred from the intensive care unit (ICU) who is comatose after a massive intracranial hemorrhage several days earlier
  ii. Level 3—*Moderately vulnerable*: A 37-year-old woman admitted after a grand mal seizure preceded by complaints of severe headache and confusion

■ **TABLE 4-23**
■ ■ **Harmful Effects and Clinical Manifestations of Acute Pain**

Body System	Harmful Effects of Unrelieved Pain	Clinical Manifestations
Endocrine	↑Catabolic hormones (e.g., adrenocorticotropic hormone, cortisol, catecholamines, antidiuretic and growth hormones, glucagon, renin, angiotensin II, aldosterone); ↓insulin, testosterone	Alterations in water and electrolyte handling (e.g., decreased urine output, fluid overload, sodium retention, hypokalemia); ↑demands on various body systems
Metabolic	Gluconeogenesis; glycogenolysis; glucose intolerance; insulin resistance; carbohydrate, fat, and protein catabolism	Hyperglycemia, weight loss, alterations in wound healing, impaired immune function, fever, enhanced tumor development and metastasis
Cardiovascular	Activation of the sympathetic nervous system leading to ↑cardiac demands; ↓fibrinolysis. Activation of the autonomic nervous system	↑Heart rate, blood pressure, peripheral vascular resistance, cardiac output, cardiac workload, myocardial oxygen consumption (with possible ischemia, angina and infarction); ↓blood flow to extremities, hypercoagulability (e.g., ↑risk for deep venous thrombosis, pulmonary embolism)
	Parasympathetic nervous system activation	↓Heart rate and blood pressure, atrioventricular block
Respiratory	Alteration in respiratory mechanics: Involuntary spinal reflex response and voluntary reduction of muscle movement in thorax and diaphragm	↑Respiration rate, ↓tidal volume, vital capacity, and alveolar ventilation; shunting, hypoxemia, hypercarbia, muscle spasm, grunting noncompliance with ventilator, poor cough, atelectasis, retained secretions, infection
Musculoskeletal	Involuntary reflex motor activity	↑Muscle tone, spasm, splinting, limitation of movement, rigidity, impaired muscle function (e.g., atrophy, weakness)
Gastrointestinal	↑Intestinal secretions and smooth muscle sphincter tone; ↓gastric motility and contractility. Activation of the autonomic nervous system	Nausea and vomiting, gastric distention, stasis, ileus, constipation, appetite changes (delayed gastric emptying can also be related to opioids)
Genitourinary	↑Sphincter activity. Activation of the autonomic nervous system	Urinary retention with associated discomfort
Neurologic and skin	Activation of the autonomic nervous system	Dilated pupils, tearing, diaphoresis, pallor, flushing
Cognitive	Negative psychologic and emotional impact	Sleep disturbances, anxiety, depression, confusion

Compiled from Graf C, Puntillo K. Pain in the older adult in the intensive care unit. *Crit Care Clin.* 2003;19(4):749-770; Hamill-Ruth RJ, Marohn ML. Evaluation of pain in the critically ill patient. *Crit Care Clin.* 1999;15(1):35-54; McCaffery M, Pasero C. *Pain: Clinical Manual.* 2nd ed. St Louis, MO: Mosby; 1999; Melzack R, Wall PD, eds. *Handbook of Pain Management.* Edinburgh, Scotland: Churchill Livingstone; 2003; Pasero C. Pain in the critically ill patient. *J Perianesth Nurs.* 2003;18(6):422-425; and Payen JR, Bru O, Bosson JL, et al. Assessing pain in critically ill sedated patients by using a behavioral pain scale. *Crit Care Med.* 2001;29(12):2258-2263.

    iii. Level 5—*Minimally vulnerable*: A 63-year-old woman admitted after a carotid endarterectomy

  c. Stability

    i. Level 1—*Minimally stable*: A 56-year-old man admitted with a right-sided stroke who has become increasingly disoriented and is having progressive weakness with vomiting

    ii. Level 3—*Moderately stable*: A 50-year-old woman transferred from the ICU 1 week after a subarachnoid hemorrhage with aneurysm clipping in whom diabetes insipidus has developed with fluctuations in blood pressure

    iii. Level 5—*Highly stable*: A 72-year-old woman admitted after falling at home and hitting her forehead. She is taking warfarin (Coumadin) because of chronic atrial fibrillation. She is awake and neurologically intact.

  d. Complexity

    i. Level 1—*Highly complex*: A 57-year-old man admitted for left-sided ischemic stoke who is completely aphasic and experiencing dysphagia. He is in atrial fibrillation and has uncontrolled diabetes.

       ii. Level 3—*Moderately complex*: A 60-year-old woman transferred from the ICU in whom hydrocephalus has developed requiring a shunt after an intraventricular hemorrhage

       iii. Level 5—*Minimally complex*: A 40-year-old woman admitted for a transient ischemic attack (TIA) who is anxious to go home

  e. Resource availability

       i. Level 1—*Few resources*: A 59-year-old man admitted for a decreased LOC due to a chronic subdural hematoma. He is homeless and an alcoholic.

       ii. Level 3—*Moderate resources*: A 30-year-old woman admitted 1 week earlier with a small right parietal arteriovenous malformation (AVM) that hemorrhaged. She is neurologically intact. She is not married and has no family in the area, but a close friend has been visiting. She is insured and is a candidate for outpatient focused-beam radiation therapy.

       iii. Level 5—*Many resources*: A 67-year-old woman admitted 5 days ago with a left-sided stroke. She has a right hemiparesis that will require inpatient rehabilitation. She is married, has insurance, and has two sisters and parents who live near her.

  f. Participation in care

       i. Level 1—*No participation*: An 82-year-old man admitted several days ago from a skilled nursing facility after having a massive stroke. He has been transferred from the ICU. He is comatose and areflexic and has no known family.

       ii. Level 3—*Moderate level of participation*: A 76-year-old man admitted with a left-sided stroke several days ago. He does not speak English and is being discharged home tomorrow with a moderate expressive dysphasia The patient's primary support person at home is a daughter who works as a nursing assistant and speaks English.

       iii. Level 5—*Full participation*: A 56-year-old man admitted after having a grand mal seizure at work 2 days ago. He is awake and neurologically intact. He is being discharged home with his wife.

  g. Participation in decision making

       i. Level 1—*No participation*: A 55-year-old man admitted with a left-sided stroke. He is having expressive and receptive aphasia.

       ii. Level 3—*Moderate level of participation*: A 46-year-old woman transferred from the ICU after being admitted 19 days ago with an anterior communicating artery aneurysm rupture. She is lethargic with periods of disorientation.

       iii. Level 5—*Full participation*: A 45-year-old woman admitted after having a seizure in the grocery store. She provided a history of having switched medications several days earlier because of changing her health insurance. She is requesting additional information on her medication options under her current health plan.

  h. Predictability

       i. Level 1—*Not predictable*: A 79-year-old woman admitted after a right-sided stroke who is having left-sided neglect and spatial perceptual deficits. She needs continual reorientation and refuses to remain in bed. She becomes more confused at night.

       ii. Level 3—*Moderately predictable*: An 18-year-old man admitted after a grand mal seizure. He is being transitioned from intravenous (IV) to oral anticonvulsants.

       iii. Level 5—*Highly predictable*: A 25-year-old woman admitted with a severe headache. Results of her computed tomographic (CT) scan are negative, and she is neurologically intact.

4. Diagnostic studies

  a. Laboratory

       i. Complete blood cell count (CBC) and differential

       ii. Blood glucose level

       iii. Blood chemistry tests, including osmolality, electrolyte levels

       iv. Clotting profile, including prothrombin time (PT), international normalized ratio (INR), partial thromboplastin time (PTT), D-dimer levels, fibrinogen levels

       v. Arterial blood gas (ABG) levels

   vi. Toxicology screen
   vii. Urinalysis
   viii. CSF analysis: Compare with normal values and request a culture and sensitivity test
  b. Radiologic
   i. Skull series: In the absence of CT scans, skull radiographs may be useful in diagnosing skull abnormalities (e.g., fractures, erosion), noting shift of the pineal gland, and detecting intracranial air or abnormal calcifications
   ii. Spine series: Assesses vertebral integrity and alignment to diagnose fractures, dislocations, bony defects, or degenerative processes; CT (Box 4-5) or magnetic resonance imaging (MRI) (Box 4-6 and Table 4-24) often used to further delineate abnormalities
   iii. CT scan (see Box 4-5)
   iv. Perfusion CT (see Box 4-5)
   v. Myelography

■ **BOX 4-5**
■ **COMPUTED TOMOGRAPHIC STUDIES**

COMPUTED TOMOGRAPHY (CT)
TECHNIQUE
■ X-ray beam is projected through narrow section of brain or spine; detectors at opposite side measure attenuation of radiation after it passes through tissues. Readings are fed into a computer that derives absorption of x-rays by tissues in path of beam. Computer-generated images are printed as serial thin slices of adjacent anatomy.
■ Hyperdense tissue (e.g., bone) absorbs more x-rays and appears whiter on final image. Hypodense features (e.g., air, fluid) absorb fewer x-rays and appear darker.
■ Scan may be repeated after patient has received intravenous (IV) contrast agent to delineate vasculature and enhance tissues where there is disruption of blood-brain barrier.

CLINICAL USES
■ Brain: Valuable in detection of intracranial hemorrhage, especially subarachnoid hemorrhage, cerebral edema, contusions, hydrocephalus, larger mass lesions, and evidence of probable increased intracranial pressure. Bone windows provide exquisite detail of skull architecture. Limitations include poor visibility of posterior fossa, base of brain, and brainstem.
■ Spine: Provides clear look at bony structures to better visualize vertebral fractures, dislocations, degenerative changes, canal stenosis, congenital abnormalities, and surgical fixation; may identify mass lesions
■ CT angiogram: Postcontrast CT scan reconstructed to outline cerebral vasculature. Useful in screening for vascular lesions (e.g., aneurysm, arteriovenous malformation). Sometimes helpful in delineating architecture of aneurysm before surgical clipping or endovascular intervention.

PREPROCEDURE AND POSTPROCEDURE CARE
■ Agitated patients may require sedation to optimize image quality.
■ If contrast enhancement used, assess for allergy to contrast medium, secure informed consent. Patients with renal insufficiency are at risk for contrast-induced nephropathy (see Chapter 5 for interventions to reduce risk of contrast-induced nephropathy).

PERFUSION CT
TECHNIQUE
■ CT scan performed during IV bolus administration of iodinated contrast material
■ Computer calculations provide measures of regional cerebral blood volume, mean transit time, and regional cerebral blood flow.

CLINICAL USES
■ Used in acute stroke and other cerebrovascular diseases to identify infarcted and marginally perfused areas

PREPROCEDURE AND POSTPROCEDURE CARE
■ Same as for CT

■ **BOX 4-6**
■ **MAGNETIC RESONANCE IMAGING**

TECHNIQUE
■ Magnetic fields and radiofrequency waves create signals that generate an image.
■ Factors that contribute to image can be manipulated to emphasize different characteristics of normal and abnormal tissue.
■ Gadolinium, a contrast agent, may be used to enhance some lesions.

CLINICAL USES
■ Brain: Tissue contrast resolution is superior to that of computed tomography (CT); magnetic resonance imaging (MRI) generally better detects contusions, tumors, infection, edema, subacute and chronic hemorrhage, ischemia or infarction, vascular abnormalities, and degenerative diseases. Better visualizes tissues in posterior fossa, basilar skull, and brainstem; better differentiates gray and white matter. Gadolinium enhances areas of increased vascularity or blood-brain barrier disruption.
■ Spine: MRI is far superior to CT in visualizing soft tissues and defining lesions such as cysts, vascular abnormalities, contusions, tumors, edema, hemorrhage, ischemia or infarction of spinal cord, and degenerative processes (e.g., disk disease, stenosis).

PREPROCEDURE AND POSTPROCEDURE CARE
■ All metal objects must be removed from patient before scanning.
■ MRI is contraindicated in patients with metallic implants such as cardiac pacemakers or ferromagnetic aneurysm clips. MRI safety guidelines recommended for other implanted devices must be followed.
■ Patient must be able to tolerate removal from metallic life-support devices (i.e., ventilator, intravenous infusion pump), or nonmetallic alternatives may be used during the study.
■ Inform patient that he or she will need to lie very still, will be in a small, confined space, and will hear a loud, clunking noise. Patient may need sedation if claustrophobic or agitated.
■ No specific postprocedure care or complications
■ *See* Table 4-24 *for other MRI technology.*

    (a) Principle: Radiographic examination of the spinal canal after a radiopaque substance is injected into the subarachnoid space (usually in the lumbar area or occasionally at C1-C2)
    (b) Clinical use: To detect spinal cord or nerve root compression; diagnose obstructions to contrast flow (e.g., intervertebral disk herniation, spinal cord tumors or stenosis, vertebral displacement)
    (c) Preprocedure and postprocedure care: Avoid contrast-induced nephropathy. Before study, ensure that coagulation parameters are within normal limits; discontinue medications that lower the seizure threshold (e.g., phenothiazides). After the procedure, keep the head of the bed elevated at least 30 to 45 degrees to prevent upward migration of the contrast agent (causes headache and seizures).
  vi. Cerebral angiography
    (a) Principle: Contrast material is injected into the vertebral and carotid arteries to enable radiographic visualization of the intracranial and extracranial vasculature
    (b) Clinical uses: Diagnosis of vascular abnormalities such as aneurysms, AVMs, vasospasm, thrombosis, or occlusion, as well as cerebral vasculitis and vascular tumors. Aids diagnosis of other intracranial abnormalities that cause stretching, displacement, or altered diameter of vessels. Evaluates collateral circulation.
    (c) Preprocedure and postprocedure care: Obtain consent. Patient may be premedicated and should be well hydrated. Avoid contrast-induced nephropathy. BP should be controlled and coagulation parameters within an acceptable range. After the procedure observe for potential complications: reaction to contrast medium, stroke, vascular damage, thrombosis, seizures, transient or permanent neurologic dysfunction, carotid sinus sensitivity, circulatory insufficiency of

■ **TABLE 4-24**
■ ■ **Some Types of MRI Technology and Their Clinical Uses**

MRI Technology	Clinical Uses
Diffusion-weighted imaging	Detects small movements of water; visualizes acute ischemic lesions and cytotoxic edema Enables immediate assessment of stroke-related vasospasm and neurovascular changes Differentiates acute from chronic lesions and irreversible from reversible infarction
Fluid-attenuated inversion recovery imaging	Suppresses signals from certain fluids, such as cerebrospinal fluid, and provides a high signal for brain tissue lesions Superior capability in detecting hemorrhage, stroke, infections, and white matter lesions that abut the ventricles
Echoplanar imaging	Uses ultrafast imaging technology to assist with diagnosis of quickly evolving disease processes
Functional MRI	Detects changes in the brain's oxygen consumption and blood flow in response to sensory stimuli or performance of a motor activity Provides functional data in addition to anatomic information for brain mapping and identifying disease
Magnetic resonance spectroscopy	Provides neurochemical data related to tissue metabolism, including brain pH, levels of metabolites and some neurotransmitters May aid in determining tumor malignancy, differentiating tumors from other brain lesions, and locating epileptogenic foci
Magnetic resonance angiography/ magnetic resonance venography	Flowing blood affects radiofrequency signals emitted during MRI, and these effects are manipulated to create an image of the cerebral and extracranial vasculature; less risk-prone alternative to cerebral angiography, although not as sensitive. Used for visualizing larger vessels, screening neck vessels for abnormalities (although it typically overemphasizes degree of stenosis), evaluating patency of major veins and venous sinuses, and identifying vascular malformations (e.g., aneurysms)
Diffusion tensor imaging	Measures diffusion of water in the brain tissue to enable visualization of anatomic substructures, particularly white matter fiber tracts Can detect disruption or damage to white matter tracts from injury/disease

MRI, Magnetic resonance imaging.

the catheterized extremity, bleeding or hematoma at the injection site. After the application of direct manual pressure, a pressure dressing or ice may be applied to the catheter insertion site.

vii. Spinal angiography: Used to diagnose the source of bleeding, vessel injuries, and vascular abnormalities (e.g., AVMs) in or around the spinal cord. See the description of cerebral angiography earlier for further information.

viii. Digital subtraction angiography

(a) Principle: Fluoroscopic images are taken before and after the IV (occasionally intra-arterial) administration of radiographic contrast material; computer digitally subtracts the initial (precontrast) image from the later (postcontrast) image to enhance visualization of cerebral vessels.

(b) Clinical uses: Aids diagnosis of occlusive vascular disease, vascular abnormalities (e.g., aneurysm, AVM), vessel injury, and tumors. Evaluates vascular surgical repair (e.g., aneurysm clipping). Potentially safer, less invasive, and cheaper and requires less contrast material than regular angiography.

(c) Preprocedure and postprocedure care: Patient may require sedation to lie still during study. After the procedure, observe for unlikely potential complications: reaction to the contrast medium, stroke, hemorrhage, and thrombosis.

ix. Nuclear medicine studies (Box 4-7)

■ **BOX 4-7**
■ **NUCLEAR MEDICINE AND ELECTROPHYSIOLOGIC STUDIES**

NUCLEAR MEDICINE STUDIES
RADIOISOTOPE BRAIN SCAN
Technique
- Radioactive substance introduced into blood before brain scanning
- In some disorders, radioisotope accumulates in abnormal areas of brain, probably owing to blood-brain barrier breakdown or increased vascularity of lesion.

Clinical uses
- Used to screen for brain tumors and evaluate cerebrovascular disease, some infectious processes

Preprocedure and postprocedure care
- Radioisotope injected at varying time intervals before scanning. Agitated patients may require sedation.

SINGLE PHOTON EMISSION TOMOGRAPHY (SPECT)
Principle
- Rotating gamma camera system detects disintegration of single-photon–emitting radioisotopes, such as technetium-99m, thallium-201, iodine-123, or hexamethylpropyleneamine oxime (HMPAO), administered to patient.
- Delineates regional brain perfusion because tracer distribution depends on blood flow

Clinical uses
- Adjunct measurement or a primary modality if other blood flow techniques not available
- May be used to detect tumors or seizure foci or to determine effects of stroke or brain injury

Preprocedure and postprocedure care
- Radioisotope may be administered at varying times before scanning. Patient must lie still during study.

POSITRON EMISSION TOMOGRAPHY (PET)
Principle
- Positron-emitting radiopharmaceuticals of C, F, N, or O_2 are administered and gamma rays emitted are recorded by pairs of detectors around head.
- Provides high-sensitivity quantitative measurements of regional cerebral blood flow, oxygen metabolism, glucose uptake and metabolism, and blood volume

Clinical uses
- Identifies abnormalities in brain's functional metabolism that precede structural alterations associated with disease
- Provides information about seizures, tumors, neurodegenerative disease, cerebrovascular disease, and brain injury. Limited availability due to expense of equipment.

Preprocedure and postprocedure care
- Patient should take nothing by mouth for prescribed period before testing.
- Study may last over 1 hour and requires patient to lie still.

ELECTROPHYSIOLOGIC STUDIES
ELECTROMYOGRAPHY (EMG)
Principle
- Needle electrodes inserted into skeletal muscle record electrical potentials from resting and contracting muscle fibers and display them on oscilloscope.

Clinical uses
- Aids in diagnosis of lower motor neuron disease, neuromuscular junction, and muscle disorders
- Differentiates lesions of muscles, peripheral nerves, and anterior horn cells

Preprocedure and postprocedure care
- No risk to patient, although needle electrodes are uncomfortable
- Muscle damage from needle electrodes may elevate creatine phosphokinase level after procedure.

NERVE CONDUCTION VELOCITY (NCV)
Principle
- Large motor nerve stimulated at two or more locations; response is measured in muscle innervated by that nerve. Nerve conduction velocity and amplitude of muscle response can be determined.

- Pure sensory fiber may be stimulated and response recorded along course of same nerve.

Clinical use

- Diagnoses peripheral neuropathies and nerve compression or trauma

Preprocedure and postprocedure care

- No risk to patient, although needle electrodes are uncomfortable

ELECTROENCEPHALOGRAPHY (EEG)

Principle

- Electrodes attached to scalp are used to record electrical activity of brain.
- Amplitude, frequency, and characteristics of brain electrical impulses are evaluated.

Clinical uses

- Most helpful in diagnosis of seizures
- May detect changes associated with space-occupying lesions, infectious processes, dementia, drug intoxication, or brain injury
- May be used to verify absence of electrocerebral activity to support diagnosis of brain death

Preprocedure and postprocedure care

- Preprocedure care varies, depending on the institution and type of EEG. Verify whether certain medications should be withheld from patient.
- Postprocedure: Wash conductive paste from hair. No risks.

EVOKED POTENTIALS (EPs)

Principle

- Electrodes are placed on scalp in locations appropriate for type of evoked response (potential) tested: Brainstem auditory evoked response (BAER), visual evoked response (VER), or somatosensory evoked response (SER).
- Stimulus is applied (e.g., clicking noise for BAER, strobe light or pattern shift for VER, and electrical stimulation of a peripheral nerve for SER), and evoked responses are measured and recorded by computer, which calculates an average curve. Evoked potential latencies and amplitudes are compared with normal responses and compared for the two sides of the body.

Clinical uses

- Evaluates functional integrity of sensory pathways
- BAER is useful in determining brainstem function.
- VER is useful index of hemispheric function; helps diagnose optic nerve disorders.
- SER may demonstrate lesions of peripheral pathways, spinal cord, or brainstem.
- May aid in detecting lesions, disease, or injury that affects specific sensory path
- Useful in determining prognosis in severe head injury
- May be used during intracranial or spinal surgery to monitor patient's response to procedure

Preprocedure and postprocedure care

- No specific care needed

    (a) Radioisotope brain scan
    (b) Single-photon emission computed tomography (SPECT)
    (c) Positron emission tomography (PET)
  c. Electrophysiologic (see Box 4-7)
    i. Electromyography
    ii. Nerve conduction velocity
    iii. Electroencephalogram (EEG)
    iv. Evoked potentials
  d. Lumbar puncture
    i. Principle: Needle placed into the subarachnoid space below the conus medullaris, usually at L4-L5 interspace
    ii. Clinical uses

        (a) Obtain CSF for laboratory examination.

        (b) Measure or reduce CSF pressure.

        (c) Administer medication.

        (d) Prepare for other diagnostic studies (e.g., myelography).

    iii. Preprocedure and postprocedure care

        (a) Contraindicated with coagulopathies; extreme caution must be used with increased ICP, because CSF removal may lead to brainstem herniation

        (b) Patients should increase fluid intake and lie flat for a few hours after the procedure.

        (c) Potential complications: Infection, headache, backache, temporary voiding difficulties

        (d) Postprocedure CSF leak may require a "blood patch" (small volume of the patient's blood is slowly injected into the epidural space, where it congeals and seals the leak) or in rare cases surgical repair.

  e. Brain biopsy

    i. Purpose: Tissue is removed from the brain for histologic evaluation. May be guided by CT scan; stereotactic methods frequently used.

    ii. Clinical uses: Can diagnose tumors, certain degenerative diseases, infections, and inflammatory processes

    iii. Preprocedure and postprocedure care: Ensure that consent is obtained. After the procedure observe for neurologic changes, hemorrhage, and infection.

Patient Care

1. **Inability to establish or maintain a patent airway because of decreased LOC or impaired protective airway reflexes (e.g., gag, cough, swallow): See Chapter 2**
2. **Myocardial repolarization abnormalities, cardiac dysrhythmias due to ANS disruption or catecholamine release: See Chapter 3**
3. **Fluid and electrolyte imbalance associated with intracranial pathology resulting from inadequate fluid intake, use of diuretics, or ADH imbalance**

  a. Description of problem: May occur with

    i. Diabetes insipidus: Intracranial pathologic condition affecting hypothalamic or posterior pituitary system can impede or stop the production or secretion of ADH, causing diabetes insipidus (Table 4-25). Also see Chapter 6.

    ii. Syndrome of inappropriate secretion of antidiuretic hormone (SIADH): CNS pathology impairs feedback mechanism responsible for ADH suppression (see Table 4-25 and Chapter 6)

    iii. Cerebral salt wasting: Excessive Na^+ excretion with subsequent diuresis may be associated with acute CNS disease. Thought to be caused, at least in part, by impaired Na^+ reabsorption from the proximal tubules due to an increase in circulating natriuretic peptides (one of which is produced in the brain). Effects of natriuretic factors include vasodilation, natriuresis, diuresis, and suppression of the renin–angiotensin II–aldosterone axis. Brain natriuretic peptide has been found in the hypothalamus; edema or infarction of the hypothalamus may trigger its release. Increased sympathetic nervous system activity related to brain injury may also contribute to renal Na^+ excretion (see Table 4-25).

  b. Goals of care

    i. Vital signs and neurologic status remain stable.

    ii. Electrolyte levels, osmolality, and intravascular volume are maintained within the desired ranges.

  c. Collaborating professionals on health care team

    i. Nurse

    ii. Physician

    iii. Laboratory personnel

  d. Interventions (see also Chapters 5 and 6)

    i. Monitor vital signs, neurologic status, input and output, and hemodynamics at least hourly until condition is stable.

▓ **TABLE 4-25**

▓ ▓ **Manifestations and Treatment of Neurogenic Diabetes Insipidus, SIADH, and Cerebral Salt Wasting**

Parameter	Diabetes Insipidus	SIADH	Cerebral Salt Wasting
Urine specific gravity	Low	Elevated	Elevated
Urine osmolality	Low	Increased	Increased
Urine sodium level	Low in relation to serum	Elevated	Elevated
Serum osmolality	Elevated	Decreased	Decreased
Serum sodium level	Elevated	Decreased	Decreased
Clinical manifestations	Hypovolemia, dehydration Intensive thirst (if mechanism is not impaired) Large volumes of poorly concentrated urine Urine osmolality increase of 9% or more in response to administration of aqueous vasopressin (Pitressin)	Euvolemia or hypervolemia Usually low urine output, low BUN level Muscle cramps, weight gain without edema, lethargy, confusion, personality change, irritability, sluggish deep tendon reflexes, nausea and vomiting, diarrhea, abdominal cramps, fatigue, headache, restlessness Severe signs Coma, seizures, death	Hypovolemia, dehydration Increased BUN levels, high urine output, net sodium loss

Treatment	• Administer fluid to replace urine output and insensible losses.
	• Administer exogenous ADH:
	  • Aqueous Pitressin—often used in critical phase
	  • Pitressin tannate in oil
	  • dDAVP (desmopressin)
	  • Nasal lysine vasopressin
		Restrict fluids. For severe symptoms:
		• Give hypertonic saline solution.
		• Diurese with furosemide.
		• Give demeclocycline hydrochloride to produce renal resistance to ADH.
			Replete salt and fluid volume. Give fludrocortisone acetate to increase renal tubule sodium reabsorption.

Adapted from McQuillan KA, Mitchell PH. Traumatic brain injuries. In: McQuillan KA, Von Rueden KT, Hartsock RL, et al, eds. *Trauma Nursing From Resuscitation Through Rehabilitation.* 3rd ed. St Louis, MO: Saunders; 2002:445.
ADH, Antidiuretic hormone; *BUN,* blood urea nitrogen; *dDAVP,* 1-deamino-8-D-arginine vasopressin; *SIADH,* syndrome of inappropriate secretion of antidiuretic hormone.

     ii. Monitor serum and urine electrolyte levels, osmolality, fluid balance, and daily weight; report abnormal values.

     iii. Provide prescribed fluid and electrolyte replacements and pharmacologic agents to correct imbalances (see Table 4-25).

   e. Evaluation of patient care

     i. Vital signs, neurologic status, and fluid and electrolyte balance are maintained within the desired ranges.

     ii. Urine output is maintained above 30 ml/hr.

5. Infection related to invasive lines, monitoring and therapeutic devices, and traumatic and surgical wounds: See Chapter 9

6. Seizures: See Seizures under Specific Patient Health Problems

7. Potential for gastrointestinal ulceration and bleeding resulting from ANS disruption, stress, lack of enteral nutrition, possible steroid use: See Chapter 8

8. Dysphagia

a. Description of problem: Dysphagia can occur as a result of dysfunction of the muscles used for mastication and swallowing or to deficits in CN V, VII, IX, X, XI, and XII involved in swallowing. May lead to aspiration and inadequate oral food intake.

b. Goals of care
   i. Nutritional and fluid intake are adequate.
   ii. No aspiration occurs.

c. Collaborating professionals on health care team
   i. Nurse
   ii. Physician
   iii. Speech therapist
   iv. Nutritional specialist

d. Interventions
   i. Involve a nutrition specialist to identify the patient's caloric needs and the best diet to achieve nutritional goals.
   ii. Ensure that swallow function is intact before starting oral food intake.
   iii. If dysphagia is present, have a speech therapist evaluate swallowing and recommend food consistency and feeding techniques to minimize aspiration risk.
   iv. Until dysphagia resolves, provide feedings via a nonoral route. In the acute phase, a gastric or postpyloric feeding tube may be used. If dysphagia is likely to persist, a feeding tube may be inserted surgically.
   v. Take precautions to avoid aspiration (also see Chapters 2 and 8).
      (a) Keep suction readily available.
      (b) Elevate the head of the bed at least 30 degrees unless contraindicated; discontinue tube feedings if head-down position needed.
      (c) Secure the feeding tube to prevent dislodgment.
      (d) Regularly assess for proper feeding tube placement.
      (e) Evaluate tube feed residuals. If residuals exceed a predetermined volume, withhold tube feedings.
      (f) During oral feeding: Have the patient sit up with the head forward; place food on the unaffected side of the oral cavity; encourage small mouthfuls and thorough chewing; ensure that the mouth is clear of food after each bite; do not leave the patient unattended while the patient is eating

e. Evaluation of patient care
   i. Patient receives adequate nutrition and hydration.
   ii. Aspiration is prevented.

9. Pain
   a. Description of problem
      i. Overview
         (a) Pain is a subjective perception consisting of complex sensory, emotional, and cognitive elements.
         (b) Many progressive care patients experience continuous pain related to their condition or treatments; pain management should be a priority.
         (c) Despite advances in pain management, the critically ill are at high risk for undertreatment of pain
      ii. Definitions: See Chapter 10
      iii. Clinical manifestations: Table 4-23 outlines various harmful effects and clinical manifestations of pain (see also Chapter 10); adequate analgesia may lessen the harmful effects of pain
      iv. Factors complicating pain assessment and impeding effective pain management: See Table 4-26
      v. Diagnostic studies
         (a) Imaging studies to outline underlying pathology
         (b) Blood work to identify organ dysfunction(s)
         (c) Electrodiagnostic tests to identify myopathies, some neuropathies
         (d) Nerve blocks to distinguish source or types of pain

■ **TABLE 4-26**
■ ■ **Factors Complicating Accurate Pain Assessment and Effective Pain Management**

Factor	Issues	Suggestions for Management
IMPAIRED ABILITY TO COMMUNICATE		
Altered level of consciousness, mental status (e.g., agitation, coma, sedation)	Potential difficulty obtaining pain assessment (e.g., self-report of pain) Failure to recognize pain as a potential cause for agitation	Assume pain is present and treat accordingly. Use behaviors and physiologic signs to confirm suspicion of pain.
Sensory deficits		Obtain and have patient use glasses or hearing aids as needed.
MEDICATION EFFECTS		
Combining of opioids and sedatives	Potential for oversedation	When these agents are given together, less of each medication may achieve desired effect and avoid adverse effects.
PHYSIOLOGIC CONDITIONS		
Hemodynamic instability Respiratory instability Weaning from ventilator Head trauma Renal or hepatic impairment	Withholding of opioids related to fear of • Exacerbating hemodynamic or respiratory instability • Delaying extubation • Impairing neurologic assessment Impaired excretion of opioid metabolites can increase opioid adverse effects (e.g., sedation).	Give intravenous fluids and vasopressors as ordered. Splinting related to pain can also impair gas exchange. Titrate small doses slowly and more often. Perform frequent assessment for opioid adverse effects. Consider fentanyl (short acting, less histamine release), nonopioids, epidural opioids, blocks. Use opioids with no clinically relevant metabolites (e.g., hydromorphone, fentanyl). Avoid meperidine; use morphine cautiously.
PREEXISTING (CHRONIC) PAIN STATES		
Regular use of pain medications (e.g., opioids, adjuvants)	Potential for undertreatment of pain and development of withdrawal syndrome (signs and symptoms similar to those of pain, such as increased heart rate, restlessness, sleeplessness)	Accept patient's report of pain. Higher than "normal" starting dosages of analgesics may be required. Continue other routine medications whenever possible.

   b. Goals of care
      i.   Development of potentially harmful far-reaching physical and psychosocial effects of pain is prevented by aggressive and proactive pain management.
      ii. Patient comfort and rapid functional recovery are promoted by the achievement of optimal analgesia with the fewest adverse effects.
   c. Collaborating professionals on health care team for pain management
      i.   Nurses play a pivotal role in coordinating care and achieving effective pain management for patients.
      ii. Other disciplines represented can include anesthesia, physical medicine and rehabilitation, neurosurgery, interventional radiology, physical therapy, pain management, pharmacy, psychology, and social and chaplain services.
   d. Interventions
      i.   Pharmacologic methods
         (a) Choice of an analgesic depends on many factors (e.g., clinical judgment, patient history, type and severity of pain, patient response to interventions).
         (b) Optimal use requires the understanding of a drug's pharmacokinetics (e.g., time to onset, peak effect, duration of action) and pharmacodynamics (e.g., mechanism of action, metabolism, and excretion).

(c) Three broad categories of analgesics are used in pain management (Tables 4-27, 4-28, and 4-29).

(1) Nonopioids: Include acetaminophen and nonsteroidal anti-inflammatory drugs (NSAIDs) (see Table 4-27)

(2) Opioids: Primarily μ-agonists, such as morphine, hydromorphone (see Table 4-28)

    a) Duration of action

        1) Most parenteral, immediate-release, and short-acting (oral) formulations can last up to 3 to 4 hours.

■ **TABLE 4-27**
■ ■ **Commonly Used Nonopioids to Treat Pain**

Overview: A group of analgesics that includes NSAIDs and acetaminophen (see examples later). Limited use in the critically ill because of adverse effects and limited availability of parenteral formulations. Reduce dosages in the elderly and in those with renal or hepatic insufficiency.

Indications: Acute and chronic pain related to many causes, including surgery, trauma, arthritis, and cancer. May be effective for relief of mild pain when used alone. Both acetaminophen and NSAIDs have analgesic and antipyretic effects; NSAIDs are also effective for inflammatory pain.

Mechanism of action: NSAIDs have both peripheral and central actions. Nonselective NSAIDs inhibit two isoforms of COX (COX-1 and COX-2). Inhibition of COX-1, normally found in tissues (e.g., platelets, GI tract, kidneys), results in well-known adverse effects of NSAIDs (see later). Inhibition of COX-2 decreases inflammation by inhibiting prostaglandin formation. COX-2–selective NSAIDs inhibit COX-2 and do not decrease platelet aggregation. They pose less risk of GI ulceration and bleeding, but no less risk of renal toxicity, compared with nonselective NSAIDs (American Pain Society, 2003). Acetaminophen is believed to cause a central inhibition of prostaglandin, perhaps via a third isoform of COX.

Benefits: Nonopioids provide analgesia without the sedative and respiratory adverse effects of opioids, so their concurrent use allows lower opioid dosages to be given without reducing analgesia (known as "opioid dose–sparing" effect).

AEs: NSAIDs: (1) Inhibition of platelet aggregation; (2) adverse GI effects (e.g., ulcerations, bleeding); (3) renal insufficiency and acute renal failure; (4) central nervous system dysfunction (e.g., decreased attention span, headache); and (5) hypersensitivity. Acetaminophen: Can cause severe hepatotoxicity in patients with chronic alcoholism or liver disease and in fasting patients. COX-2–selective NSAIDs: Risk of renal toxicity similar to that of nonselective NSAIDs.

Examples	Method of Administration	Typical Dosage	Comments
Nonselective NSAIDs (e.g., ibuprofen, ketorolac)	Oral except ketorolac (both oral and parenteral)	Ibuprofen: 200-400 mg q 4-6 hr Ketorolac: 15-30 mg intravenously q 6 hr	Ibuprofen: Limit to 2400 mg/day Ketorolac: Limit to 5 days; may precipitate renal failure in dehydrated patients; do not exceed 60 mg/day in patients >65 yr old or in those with elevated creatinine levels Naproxen: possible increased risk of CV AEs
COX-2–selective NSAIDs (e.g., celecoxib)	Oral	Celecoxib: 200-400 mg q 12-24 hr	Possible increased risk of CV AEs
Salicylates (e.g., aspirin)	Oral, rectal	500-1000 mg q 4-6 hr	Usually avoided in critically ill patients
Acetaminophen	Oral, rectal	500-1000 mg q 4-6 hr	Less risk of GI and renal complications compared with NSAIDs; decrease dosage in patients with chronic alcohol use or liver insufficiency

Data from American Pain Society. *Principles of Analgesic Use in the Treatment of Acute Pain and Cancer Pain.* 5th ed. Glenview, IL: American Pain Society; 2003; Pasero C, McCaffery M. Multimodal balanced analgesia in the critically ill. *Crit Care Nurs Clin North Am.* 2001;13(2):195-206; and McCaffery M, Pasero C. *Pain: Clinical Manual.* 2nd ed. St Louis, MO: Mosby; 1999.

AE, Adverse effect; *COX,* cyclooxygenase; *CV,* cardiovascular; *GI,* gastrointestinal; *NSAID,* non-steroidal anti-inflammatory agent; q, every.

■ **TABLE 4-28**
■ ■ **Commonly Used Opioids to Treat Pain**

Overview: Foundation of effective pain management in critically ill patients, procedural pain

Indications: Moderate to severe acute and cancer pain, some chronic pain syndromes, procedural pain

Mechanism of action: Bind to opioid receptors (μ, κ, and δ) in the brain, spinal cord, and periphery, inhibiting the release of neurotransmitters (e.g., substance P, glutamate), which blocks transmission of pain impulses

Routes of administration: Oral, parenteral, intraspinal, transdermal, transmucosal; avoid intramuscular route

Adverse effects: Sedation, respiratory depression, nausea, vomiting, mental clouding, pruritus, and urinary retention usually occur with initiation of opioid therapy; however, tolerance develops, usually within a matter of days. Tolerance does not develop to constipation, and regular assessment with prophylactic treatment is required.

Achievement of effective analgesia: Titrate frequent, small, increasing doses to achieve therapeutic effect, then initiate continuous infusion or scheduled boluses to provide steady blood levels. No analgesic ceiling with single-entity opioids.

Management of adverse effects: Most adverse effects are dose related. Initial treatment includes (1) appropriate medications as indicated (e.g., antiemetic); (2) addition of nonopioid, if possible; and (3) reduction in opioid dose. May need to change opioid or route of administration.

Opioid	Method of Administration	Starting Dosages	Comments

Morphine sulfate
Oral formulations
Elixirs
Immediate release
Sustained release
Suppository
	IV loading dose
	Continuous infusion
	IV rescue bolus
	Intraspinal
		2.5-5 mg q
		  10 min prn
		1.25-2 mg/hr
		1-2 mg q
		  10 min prn
		Immediate release/short acting: 15-30 mg q 3-4 hr prn
		Controlled release: 30 mg q 8-12 hr ATC
			Active metabolites may cause most adverse effects and accumulate in renal insufficiency.
			Histamine release and vasodilatation can cause hypotension.
			Do NOT crush or break sustained-release tablets. 10 mg IV $\approx$ 30 mg PO

Fentanyl Other formulations Transdermal Transmucosal Intraspinal	IV loading (over 2-5 min) Continuous infusion IV bolus (over 2-5 min)	25-50 mcg q 10 min prn 10-25 mcg/hr 10-25 mcg q 10 min prn Transmucosal: 200-400 mcg sucked (not chewed) over 15 min	No active metabolites and less histamine release than morphine Good choice with hemodynamic instability or renal insufficiency Risk of chest wall rigidity with rapid large IV doses Transdermal form not for acute pain Fentanyl 25 mcg IV $\approx$ morphine 2 mg IV
Hydromorphone Oral, suppository	IV loading dose (over 2-3 min) Continuous infusion IV bolus	0.4-0.8 mg q 10 min prn 0.2-0.4 mg/hr 0.2-0.4 mg q 10 min prn	Metabolites have minimal clinical effect. Good alternative in renal insufficiency Hydromorphone IV 1.5 mg morphine 10 mg IV
Oxycodone Elixirs Immediate release	Oral formulation only	Varies Oxycodone starting dosage: 5-10 mg q 4-6 hr	Metabolites have minimal clinical effect. Good alternative in renal insufficiency
Supplemental analgesia Acetaminophen with oxycodone Sustained release		OxyContin: q 12 hr 10-20 mg	Do not crush or break sustained-release tablets.
Hydrocodone with acetaminophen	Oral formulation only	5-10 mg q 4-6 hr prn	Combinations come in varying strengths of hydrocodone and acetaminophen; watch daily acetaminophen intake.

ATC, Around the clock; *IV*, intravenous; *PO*, by mouth; *prn*, as needed; *q*, every.

TABLE 4-29
Commonly Used Adjuvant Medications to Treat Pain

Category/Example	Mechanism of Action	Indication	Adverse Effects	Comments
Anticonvulsants (e.g., gabapentin, topiramate)	Cell membrane stabilizer, decreases ectopic neuron firing	Shooting or knifelike neuropathic pain (e.g., diabetic or postherpetic neuropathy)	Sedation, mental clouding, dizziness, gastrointestinal upset	Gabapentin usually dosed tid, titrate slowly up to 3600 mg/day until symptoms resolve or adverse effects occur. Reduce dose in renal insufficiency.
Tricyclic antidepressants (e.g., amitriptyline, nortriptyline)	Block reuptake of serotonin and norepinephrine	Continuous burning or hypersensitive neuropathic pain; also migraines, fibromyalgia	Potent anticholinergic effects (e.g., orthostatic hypotension, sedation, constipation, delirium)	Daily dosing (give at night to promote sleep). Analgesic dosages less than antidepressant dosages. Coronary artery disease (conduction abnormalities) is a relative contraindication.
Local anesthetics (e.g., lidocaine 4% spray, 5% patch; EMLA cream; lidocaine via IV, oral, neuraxial route or as nerve block); benzocaine topical lubricant	Block sodium channels to inhibit impulses from damaged neurons	Procedure-related pain (e.g., IV starts, intubation), neuropathic pain (e.g., stump pain, complex regional pain syndrome)	Topical administration: Few adverse effects Systemic administration: Dizziness, tremor, paresthesias, seizures	Bupivacaine and ropivacaine also used as regional anesthetic (e.g., nerve blocks, epidural injections, continuous neuraxial analgesia). "Caine" drugs may cause methemoglobinemia. EMLA: Onset in 1 hr; lasts 1-2 hr after removal
Antihistamines (e.g., diphenhydramine, hydroxyzine)	Mild central nervous system depressant	Itching, nausea, anxiety	Mild sedative activity Anticholinergic effects	Carefully monitor for increased sedation levels when used with opioids; no data to support analgesic effect (American Pain Society, 2003). IV hydroxyzine is contraindicated.
Benzodiazepines (e.g., diazepam), lorazepam	Relieve pain by relaxing spasm	Acute anxiety or muscle spasm	Sedation, respiratory depression, risk of dependence	Are not effective analgesics
Antispasmodics (e.g., baclofen)	Relax spasms and potentiate analgesia by enhancing γ-aminobutyric acid neurotransmitter	Spasm related to muscle injury, fractures Spasticity Neuropathic pain	Sedation, risk of dependence	Opioids alone are not effective for muscle spasms. Baclofen can be given orally or intrathecally.

Other adjuvants (with general indications for use)

Corticosteroids: For bony, inflammatory, cancer, and neuropathic pain; nausea; mood and appetite stimulation

α_2-Adrenergic agonist (e.g., clonidine): For neuropathic pain, chronic headache, withdrawal symptoms

N-Methyl-D-aspartate receptor blockers (e.g., ketamine, dextromethorphan): For neuropathic pain

Propranolol: For migraine prophylaxis

Data from American Pain Society. *Principles of Analgesic Use in the Treatment of Acute Pain and Cancer Pain*. 5th ed. Glenview, IL: American Pain Society; 2003; National Pharmaceutical Council (NPC). Pain: current understanding of assessment, management, and treatment, 2001. http://www.npcnow.org. Accessed 2003; McCaffery M, Pasero C. *Pain: Clinical Manual*. 2nd ed. St Louis, MO: Mosby; 1999.

EMLA, Eutectic mixture of local anesthetics; *IV*, intravenous; *tid*, three times per day.

          2) Controlled-release formulations last 8 to 12 hours; should be given "around the clock," not as needed.

          3) Oral extended-release formulations last 12 to 24 hours.

          4) Transdermal patches last 48 to 96 hours (usually 72 hours).

        b) Use as necessary before procedures and before pain gets out of control.

      (3) Adjuvants or coanalgesics: Drugs that are analgesic under some conditions, with a primary indication other than pain (e.g., tricyclic antidepressants) (see Table 4-29)

    (d) Multimodal balanced analgesia combines analgesic regimens to reduce the likelihood of adverse effects from a single agent.

  ii.   Nonpharmacologic methods (see Chapter 10, Table 10-4)

  e. Evaluation of patient care (see also Chapter 10)

    i.   Pain intensity is maintained at a level that allows the patient the best opportunity to heal with the minimum amount of discomfort (usually at or below a rating of 4 on a scale of 10).

    ii.   Ongoing assessments appropriate to the patient identify ineffective pain management and result in revision of the analgesic plan.

10. Corneal abrasion resulting from impaired corneal reflex

  a. Description of problem: Impaired corneal reflex caused by CN V, CN VII, or brainstem dysfunction makes the cornea vulnerable to injury

  b. Goal of care: Eyes are protected from corneal injury

  c. Collaborating professionals on health care team

    i.   Nurse

    ii.   Physician

  d. Interventions

    i.   Assess corneas for abrasions, irritation, or drainage.

    ii.   Cleanse exudate from eyes at least once a shift.

    iii.   Apply lubricant to the eyes as prescribed.

    iv.   Protect the eyes from injury; in some cases, the eyes may be taped closed or protective shields may be applied.

  e. Evaluation of patient care: No corneal injury occurs

11. Inability of the patient to communicate needs effectively

  a. Description of problem: Barriers to effective communication may include tracheostomy tube, decreased LOC, expressive or receptive dysphasia, motor speech apraxia, or dysarthria

  b. Goals of care: Effective communication is maintained so the patient's needs can be met

  c. Collaborating professionals on health care team

    i.   Nurse

    ii.   Speech therapist

  d. Interventions

    i.   Collaborate with a speech therapist to assess the patient's comprehension and expression of written and spoken language and to identify the best interventions.

    ii.   Explain the nature of and reason for communication deficits to the patient and family; encourage patience with communication difficulties.

    iii.   Speak slowly in a normal tone. Use short phrases. If the patient has a hearing loss, speak to the patient on the unaffected side; repeat or rephrase, as necessary.

    iv.   Stand so the patient can see your lip movements and nonverbal expressions. Allow time for the patient to respond.

    v.   Use alternative strategies for communicating (e.g., gestures, yes or no questions, pointing, pictures, alphabet board).

    vi.   Communicate for short periods to avoid tiring and frustrating the patient; be supportive and understanding of the patient's frustrations.

    vii.   Involve the family in using effective communication techniques.

  e. Evaluation of patient care: Patient effectively communicates needs

12. **Weakness or paralysis of one or more extremities**
    a. Description of problem: Neurologic disorders can decrease muscle strength, control, mass, or endurance. Loss of motor function leaves the patient unable to perform purposeful activities, including repositioning, transfers, and ambulation. Skin breakdown, contractures, and deep venous thrombosis (DVT) may occur as a result. Spasticity, which often occurs in body areas affected by UMN lesions, may also reduce ROM and further impair functional mobility.
    b. Goals of care
        i.   Full joint ROM is maintained.
        ii. If possible, muscle strength is regained.
        iii. Patient demonstrates how to compensate for weakness or paralysis so independence is regained.
        iv. Patient exhibits no evidence of complications, such as contractures, skin breakdown, or DVT.
        v.   Problematic spasticity is controlled.
    c. Collaborating professionals on health care team
        i.   Physical therapist
        ii. Occupational therapist
        iii. Nurse
        iv. Physician
    d. Interventions
        i.   Assess motor strength every shift.
        ii.   Use pressure-relief devices as appropriate.
        iii. Reposition the patient frequently. Assess skin integrity while turning. Maintain functional anatomic alignment; protect bony prominences; keep head and trunk straight to normalize posture and tone and to encourage symmetry.
        iv.   Position hemiplegic patients in opposition to spastic adduction and flexion in the arm and extension in the leg.
        v.   Position proximal joints (pelvis, shoulders) correctly to reduce tone in extremities.
        vi.   Follow the recommendations of an occupational therapist and a physical therapist on how to move and position the patient, and use splints, braces, and elastic gloves; teach ROM and transfer techniques.
        vii. If necessary, administer prescribed antispasmodics (e.g., dantrolene sodium, baclofen, diazepam).
        viii. Perform ROM exercises to joints; progress from passive to active as tolerated. Do not pull on a paretic limb.
        ix.   Encourage progressive independent activity as tolerated; encourage movement toward the paretic side.
        x.   Place items within reach of the unaffected arm.
        xi.   Involve the family in therapy as appropriate.
    e. Evaluation of patient care
        i.   Joint mobility is maintained.
        ii. If possible, muscle strength is regained.
        iii. Patient participates in therapy to strengthen muscles and learns strategies to compensate for motor dysfunction.
        iv. Complications of paresis or paralysis are prevented.

13. **Cognitive deficits**
    a. Description of problem: Brain pathology can cause a number of cognitive deficits, including the following:
        i.   Disorientation to time, place, person, and situation
        ii. Diminished attention span and problem-solving abilities, impulsiveness, poor judgment, belligerence
        iii. Memory loss and lack of sequential thought (i.e., inability to recall events in the order in which they occurred)
        iv. Inability to follow requests or instructions
        v.   Inability to recognize deficits

   b. Goals of care
      i. Patient responds to the environment appropriately.
      ii. Patient organizes thoughts and uses appropriate judgment to carry out ADLs with minimal assistance.
      iii. Patient is able to compensate for cognitive deficits.
      iv. Patient does not injure self.
   c. Collaborating professionals on health care team
      i. Nurse
      ii. Physician
      iii. Physical therapist
      iv. Occupational therapist
      v. Speech therapist
   d. Interventions
      i. In an unresponsive patient, increase environmental awareness by providing familiar stimulation to all five senses. Provide only one stimulus at a time for brief periods to avoid sensory overload.
      ii. Orient to the environment frequently.
         (a) Call the patient by name; tell the patient your name.
         (b) Inform the patient about time and location.
         (c) Provide tools to help maintain orientation (e.g., calendar, clock, newspapers, radio, television).
         (d) Keep the patient's items in the same place.
      iii. Establish and maintain a predictable schedule.
      iv. Provide simple instructions frequently in a calm tone.
      v. With therapists, teach ADLs using cues and drills.
      vi. Protect the patient from injury (e.g., use restraints only if necessary, keep side rails up and call light within reach, locate the patient near the nurses' station).
      vii. Remove unnecessary or aggravating stimuli; provide prescribed pharmacologic agent(s) to control agitation.
      viii. Teach and involve the family in care as appropriate.
   e. Evaluation of patient care
      i. Patient is oriented and responds appropriately to environmental stimuli.
      ii. Patient uses adaptive strategies to make appropriate decisions and carry out ADLs with minimal assistance.
      iii. Injury is prevented.
14. **Situational crisis for the patient resulting from neurologic deficits causing loss of control and independence, and a change in role: See** Chapter 10
15. **Situational crisis for the family resulting from disruption of the usual family roles, burden of care, and concern about the family member's pathologic condition and deficits: See Chapter 10**

SPECIFIC PATIENT HEALTH PROBLEMS

Increased Intracranial Pressure

1. **Pathophysiology**
   a. Nondistensible intracranial cavity is filled to capacity with CSF, intravascular blood, and brain tissue.
   b. *Monro-Kellie hypothesis*: If the volume of one of the intracranial constituents increases, a reciprocal decrease in the volume of one or both of the others must occur or ICP will increase
   c. Principal spatial buffers that resist elevations in ICP with volume increases include displacement of CSF from the cranial vault and compression of the low-pressure venous system. Decreased CSF production and increased CSF absorption may also contribute to spatial compensations.
      i. Volume of fluid that can be displaced for spatial compensation is finite; when intracranial volume exceeds the amount of fluid displaced, ICP rises.

ii.   Relationship between ICP and volume can be plotted as a pressure-volume curve that depicts the effects of increasing intracranial volume on ICP (Figure 4-24). Flat portion of the curve reflects the phase in which spatial buffers compensate for increases in intracranial volume so there is little change in ICP. *Brain compliance*, a measure of the brain's adaptive capacity, is high at this portion of the curve. Once compensatory mechanisms are exceeded, the curve turns sharply upward, which indicates that small increases in volume then cause significant ICP elevations. At this part of the curve, brain compliance is low. Patient response to changes in intracranial volume depends, in part, on where the patient's condition is on this curve.

d. As ICP increases and approaches the MAP, CPP decreases. When perfusion pressure falls below a critical point (usually around 40 mm Hg), autoregulation becomes impaired and CBF gradually falls, which leads to cerebral ischemia.

e. Herniation syndromes: ICP elevations cause displacement of brain structures (Figure 4-25)

   i.   *Cingulate or subfalcine herniation*: Unilateral cerebral lesion shifts brain tissue laterally across the midline, which causes distortion of the cingulate gyrus under the falx cerebri

   ii.   *Uncal or lateral transtentorial herniation*: Expanding lesion forces the uncus of the medial temporal lobe over the edge of the tentorium

   iii.   *Central transtentorial herniation*: Midline, bilateral, or unilateral cerebral lesions displace one or both hemispheres, the diencephalon, and the midbrain downward through the tentorial notch, which causes midbrain compression; can progress to tonsillar herniation

   iv.   *Tonsillar herniation*: Posterior fossa contents, particularly the cerebellar tonsils, are displaced through the foramen magnum, which causes brainstem distortion

2. Etiology and risk factors

   a. Rate and extent of ICP elevation depend on the following:

   i.   Amount of volume increase

   ii.   Rate of volume change (i.e., the faster volume is added, the greater the rise in ICP)

   iii.   Total volume within the intracranial cavity

   iv.   Intracranial compliance (i.e., the capacity for compensation)

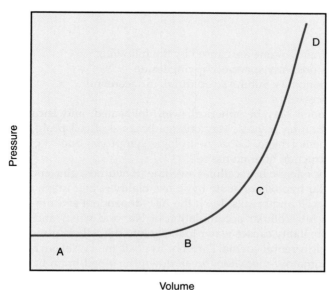

Volume

FIGURE 4-24 ■ Pressure-volume curve. From point *A* to point *B*, intracranial pressure (ICP) remains constant with the addition of volume, and brain compliance is high. At point *B* brain compliance begins to change, and ICP rises slightly. From point *B* to point *C*, compliance is low, and ICP rises with increases in intracranial volume. From point *C* to point *D*, small increases in volume cause significant ICP elevations. (From McQuillan KA, Mitchell PH. Traumatic brain injuries. In: McQuillan KA, Von Rueden KT, Hartsock RL, et al, eds. *Trauma Nursing From Resuscitation Through Rehabilitation*. 3rd ed. St Louis, MO: Saunders; 2002:413.)

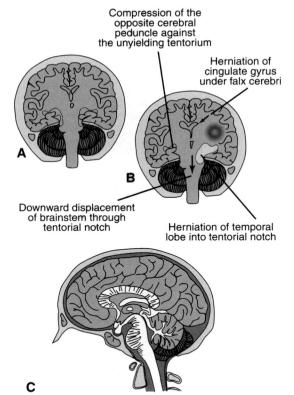

FIGURE 4-25 ■ Brain herniation. **A,** Normal relationship of intracranial structures. **B,** Shift of intracranial struc-tures. **C,** Downward herniation of the cerebellar tonsils into the foramen magnum. (From Kerr ME. Nursing management intracranial problems. In: Lewis SM, Heitkemper MM, Dirksen SR. *Medical Surgical Nursing: Assessment and Management of Clinical Problems.* 5th ed. St Louis, MO: Mosby; 2000:1614.)

    b. Increases in brain volume are caused by the following:
        i. Mass lesions: Any space-occupying lesion
           (a) Hematomas: Subdural, epidural, intracerebral
           (b) Abscesses
           (c) Tumors: May be spherical, well delineated, and encapsulated or diffuse and infiltrating masses. May enlarge because of cell proliferation, necrosis, edema, or hemorrhage. Cause neurologic symptoms due to compression, invasion, or destruction of brain tissue.
        ii. Cytotoxic edema: Intracellular swelling of neurons, glia, and endothelial cells caused by cellular hypoxia or acute hypo-osmolality (water intoxication). Hypoxia depletes cellular ATP and breaks down the ATP-dependent sodium-potassium pump, which leads to intracellular accumulation of Na^+ and water and cellular swelling. Acute hypo-osmolality causes water to move into the cell via osmosis.
        iii. Vasogenic cerebral edema: Direct or hypoxic injury, severe hypertension, endotoxins, or inflammatory mediators break down the blood-brain barrier; this allows osmoti-cally active molecules such as proteins to leak into the interstitium, which draws water from the vascular system and cells into the interstitial space. Seen around contusions, tumors, or abscesses or generalized, as with meningitis or diffuse brain injury.
        iv. Interstitial edema: High intraventricular pressure (e.g., hydrocephalus) causes fluid to extravasate into tissues around the ventricles
    c. Increases in cerebral blood volume (CBV) may be caused by the following:
        i. Venous outflow obstruction

(a) Head rotation, neck hyperextension or hyperflexion, or tight tracheal tube ties can compress the jugular veins, diminish venous return, and cause venous engorgement.

(b) Thrombus or another venous lesion may block the outflow of intracranial blood.

(c) Raised intrathoracic and/or intra-abdominal pressure may impede venous return.

   ii.   Hyperemia: CBF exceeds metabolic demand

(a) Increased ICP can reduce CPP and CBF, causing vasodilation, increasing CBV, and further elevating ICP.

(b) Autoregulation may be impaired, globally or regionally, by cerebral injury or insult. When impaired, arterioles passively dilate with elevated arterial BP, increasing CBF and CBV.

(c) BP that exceeds the limits of autoregulation can increase CBV.

(d) Increased $Paco_2$ and Pao_2 lower than 60 mm Hg cause cerebral vasodilatation, increasing CBF.

(e) Certain anesthetics (e.g., halothane, nitrous oxide) and other drugs (e.g., nitroprusside, nitroglycerin) cause cerebral vasodilatation, which increases CBV. Use these cautiously with neurosurgical patients.

  d. Increases in CSF volume (hydrocephalus) are caused by the following:

   i.   Increased production of CSF (an uncommon cause)

   ii.   Decreased reabsorption of CSF

(a) Obstruction of CSF circulation (see Figure 4-11) due to a mass lesion, edema, hemorrhage, or inflammatory process in or near the ventricular system or on the convexity of the brain blocking the subarachnoid space (*noncommunicating hydrocephalus*)

(b) Impaired reabsorption of CSF from the subarachnoid space into the venous system due to meningeal inflammation or the obstruction of arachnoid villi by debris (e.g., blood cells, infectious matter) (*communicating hydrocephalus*)

3. Signs and symptoms

  a. Clinical presentation may show little or no change if the cause is a slow, progressive pathologic condition (e.g., slow-growing tumor).

  b. Papilledema may be the initial sign if ICP rises gradually but is a late sign with acute ICP elevations.

  c. More commonly, trends in LOC; motor activity; pupillary size, shape, and reactivity; cranial nerve function; and vital signs will indicate possible ICP elevations over time.

   i.   LOC changes may present as restlessness, agitation, disorientation, or lethargy, which may progress to less responsive or comatose states, or coma may be evident at the outset.

   ii.   Increased ICP can exert pressure on the motor and sensory nerve tracts, leading to impairment or loss of function, usually on the side contralateral to the compression. Sometimes ipsilateral hemiparesis or hemiplegia is seen if brain tissue is displaced laterally and the contralateral cerebral peduncle is compressed (*Kernohan's notch phenomenon*). See section on motor function under Patient Assessment for a description of other abnormal motor responses.

   iii.   Pupil abnormalities are described in Table 4-9. Transtentorial herniation typically compresses the ipsilateral CN III, causing the pupil on the same side to enlarge and have a sluggish or absent direct light reflex. Occasionally, the pupil opposite the side of herniation may dilate if uncal herniation causes contralateral midbrain and CN III compression against the opposite tentorial edge.

   iv.   See also section on vital signs under Patient Assessment.

  d. Other findings suggesting ICP elevation must be evaluated in light of the history and clinical presentation.

   i.   Increasing headache, blurred vision, diplopia

   ii.   Seizures

   iii.   Vomiting: May result from lesions that involve the vestibular nuclei, impinge on the floor of the fourth ventricle, or produce medullary compression

4. **Diagnostic study findings**
   a. CT scan: Axial CT without contrast shows indications of mass effect and probable increased ICP
      i. Shift of the ventricles and falx away from the mass
      ii. Effacement of the sulci and ventricles
      iii. Compressed or absent basal cisterns
5. **Goal of care: patient's neurologic status improves**
6. **Collaborating professionals on health care team**
   a. Nurse, physician, pharmacist, nutritionist, laboratory personnel
   b. Respiratory, physical, speech, and occupational therapists
   c. Case manager or discharge coordinator, social worker, chaplain
7. **Management of patient care**
   a. Anticipated patient trajectory: As the volume in the intracranial compartment is reduced, the patient's ICP will decrease to within normal levels and recovery from the precipitating event will run its course
      i. Delivery of care: Depending on the severity of the patient's signs and symptoms or the frequency or type of interventions required, the patient may need to be transferred to the ICU for treatment
      ii. Positioning
         (a) Facilitate venous return.
            (1) Elevate the head of the bed to a level that minimizes ICP and optimizes CPP (and, if monitored, CBF and oxygenation), usually 30 degrees.
            (2) Avoid hyperextension, flexion, or rotation of the head and neck.
            (3) Ensure that tracheal tube ties are not wrapped tightly around the head or neck.
            (4) If a cervical collar is used, ensure proper fit and placement.
         (b) Avoid sharp hip flexion.
         (c) With each patient position change, ensure that the external transducer and intraventricular catheter drainage chamber are appropriately positioned.
      iii. Skin care: Provide meticulous care to prevent breakdown in patients with sensory or motor deficits
      iv. Pain management: Short-acting or easily reversible analgesics (e.g., morphine, fentanyl) may be used to control pain and reduce ICP. Avoid causing hypotension; monitor pain relief.
      v. Discharge planning: Discharge destination (e.g., home, rehabilitation or skilled nursing facility) is determined in large part by the patient's cognitive capabilities and motor or sensory deficits. Educate the family about what the course of the patient's condition is likely to be and what should be expected in the postacute phase of care.
      vi. Pharmacology: See Box 4-8
      vii. Psychosocial issues: Family presence reduces ICP in some patients. Help alleviate the family's fear and anxiety by providing information and encouraging the use of appropriate coping mechanisms and support systems (see Chapter 10).
      viii. Treatments
         (a) Noninvasive
            (1) Eliminate any unnecessary noxious stimuli that may elevate ICP.
            (2) Maintain normothermia. Use antipyretic agents and other cooling methods to reduce hyperthermia, which increases CBF approximately 6% for every $1.8°$ F ($1°$ C) temperature increase and thereby raises ICP.
            (3) Note the effects of various interventions (e.g., suctioning) on ICP, CPP, and other parameters. If the patient evidences poor brain compliance, provide prescribed sedation before performing interventions or space activities to minimize ICP elevations.
            (4) Suction only when clinically indicated to avoid excessive ICP elevations; limit the number of suction catheter passes (one or two times); pass the catheter for 10 seconds or less; hyperoxygenate with 100% fraction of inspired oxygen (F_{IO_2}), and hyperinflate with 135% of the tidal volume for four breaths

■ **BOX 4-8**
■ **PHARMACOLOGIC MANAGEMENT OF INCREASED INTRACRANIAL PRESSURE**

- Supplemental oxygen: To prevent hypoxia and insufficient cerebral oxygen delivery, which can cause or worsen brain ischemia and increased intracranial pressure (ICP)
- Prescribed fluids: To maintain euvolemic state, and normal electrolyte levels. Typically, isotonic crystalloids are administered. Hypotonic and glucose-containing solutions are generally avoided. Colloids, hypertonic saline solutions, and, if indicated, blood products may also be used.
- Sedation: Often effective in reducing ICP, particularly in restless or agitated patients. Short-acting or easily reversible agents preferred (e.g., midazolam). Rule out other physiologic causes of agitation that require different treatment (e.g., hypoxia, electrolyte imbalance). Avoid hypotension.
- Diuretics: Ensure adequate hydration before administration; replace fluids to avoid dehydration and hypotension.
  Mannitol: Osmotic diuretic administered as bolus (0.25 to 1.0 g/kg) to reduce ICP by creating osmotic gradient that pulls fluid from brain tissue into intravascular space; expands plasma volume, which reduces blood viscosity, improves cerebral blood flow (CBF) and oxygen delivery
  Loop diuretics (e.g., furosemide): May lower ICP by reducing sodium and water transport into brain, causing diuresis, and decreasing cerebrospinal fluid production
- Hypertonic saline solutions: Lower ICP by pulling interstitial fluid from brain tissue into intravascular space, expanding intravascular volume, which improves CBF and oxygen delivery, and perhaps by modifying the injury-induced inflammatory response
- Lidocaine: Reduces cerebral metabolic rate and suppresses cough reflex to prevent or lower high ICP. Given intravenously or endotracheally before respiratory maneuvers (e.g., intubation, suctioning) to attenuate ICP elevations. Lowers seizure threshold; frequent dosing can cause toxicosis.

at 20-second intervals before each catheter pass; may administer sedative or lidocaine before procedure.
- (5) Maintain normoglycemia. Hypoglycemia or hyperglycemia can worsen cerebral edema and outcome from brain insult.
- (6) Decompress the gut and bladder to prevent increased intra-abdominal pressure, which can raise ICP.
- (7) Avoid the patient's straining, coughing, or using the Valsalva maneuver, which raises ICP via increased intrathoracic pressure and impeding of cerebrovenous outflow.
- (8) Purposeful touch may help reduce ICP.
  - (b) Invasive
    - (1) Surgical interventions to reduce ICP
      - a) Removal of a mass lesion, débridement of necrotic brain tissue, resection of a portion of the brain
      - b) Unilateral or bilateral decompressive craniectomy (i.e., removal of the cranium and opening of the dura), which allows room for the edematous brain to control refractory ICP elevations
      - c) Placement of a ventricular shunt for long-term CSF removal
  - iv. Ethical issues: May consider with the family halting further treatment or withdrawing therapy when the patient has refractory ICP elevations and concurrent findings that indicate a dismal prognosis
- **b.** Potential complications
  - i. Brain ischemia and death
    - (a) Mechanism: Uncontrolled intracranial hypertension compromises CPP and CBF leading to brain ischemia; irreversible brain death ensues when CBF ceases. Criteria for brain death in an adult include unresponsiveness and lack of movement (spinal reflexes may persist); absence of pupillary, oculocephalic, oculovestibular, corneal, cough, and gag reflexes and spontaneous respirations; presence of a known irreversible cause for coma; body temperature above 90° F (32.2° C); absence of the use of masking neuromuscular or sedative agents;

absence of any metabolic or endocrine abnormality. Tests (EEG, angiography, transcranial Doppler ultrasonography, or somatosensory evoked potentials) may be performed to confirm brain death in patients who have one or more components of the clinical examination that cannot be reliably assessed.

(b) Management: Interventions to minimize ICP and optimize CPP and oxygenation to prevent ischemia. Once brain death occurs, the family should be notified and organ donation considered.

8. **Evaluation of patient care: patient's neurologic status improves**

Ischemic Stroke

1. **Pathophysiology: Cerebral artery becomes narrowed or occluded, interrupting CBF and oxygen delivery and causing brain ischemia in that vascular territory. Lack of oxygen halts ATP energy–dependent cell functions, which renders neurons inactive. Depending on the degree of CBF reduction, nonfunctional, ischemic neurons may remain viable and recover function. If the energy supply remains insufficient or is further reduced, numerous intracellular biochemical and molecular cascades are triggered (e.g., ionic shifts; excessive lactic acid production; accumulation of excitatory neurotransmitters; activation of proteases, endonucleases, and phospholipases; increased free radical formation), which produces cytotoxic edema and neuronal death. Area of brain infarction forms surrounded by a marginally perfused dysfunctional but viable ischemic tissue (called the *penumbra*). Tissue in the penumbra is vulnerable to cell death if CBF and oxygen delivery are not quickly restored or if secondary insults occur (e.g., hypoxia, hypotension, metabolic derangements). Approximately 80% to 85% of all strokes are ischemic. Mechanisms include the following**:

   a. Thrombosis (most common cause of stroke)
      i. Atherosclerosis of large cerebral vessels causes injury and plaque formation along the vessel wall. Platelets aggregate with fibrin, and a thrombus forms. Progressive vessel narrowing occurs, eventually occluding the vessel or precluding adequate perfusion.
      ii. Plaques may embolize and occlude smaller vessels.
   b. Embolus
      i. Emboli may originate from atherosclerotic plaques in the extracranial or large intracranial vessels; a diseased heart; infection; particulate matter, fat, or air that gains access to the vasculature; hypercoagulability; or clots caused by vascular injury.
      ii. Emboli usually lodge at arterial bifurcations, where blood flow is the most turbulent and atherosclerotic narrowing is more common. Tiny emboli or fragments may become lodged in smaller vessels.
   c. Small-vessel disease (lacunar strokes)
      i. Lipohyalinosis (hyaline-lipid material lines small penetrating arteries, causing vessel wall thickening) and microatheroma occlude small penetrating arteries that perfuse deep cerebral white matter. Affected brain tissue softens and sloughs away, forming a small cavity or lacuna.
      ii. Condition is most prevalent in the basal ganglia, thalamus, and white matter of the pons and internal capsule.
      iii. Hypertension is a primary risk factor.
   d. Other less common mechanisms: Hematologic diseases, migraine or vasospasm, arteritis, arterial dissection, infection
   e. Cryptogenic: Diagnostic workup fails to identify the stroke origin
2. **Etiology and risk factors**
   a. Previous stroke or TIA
   b. Family history of stroke
   c. Age: Risk doubles every 10 years after age 55 years
   d. Gender: Males have a 9% higher incidence than females but more than 60% of deaths occur in females
   e. Race: African Americans have a higher incidence of stroke and nearly twice the risk of death compared with white Americans

  f. Hypertension, hypercholesterolemia, diabetes mellitus

  g. Hypercoagulable states such as polycythemia, sickle cell anemia, pregnancy

  h. Vascular inflammatory processes, vasospasm, migraine, cerebral artery atherosclerosis, carotid artery stenosis

  i. Cardiac disease: Atrial fibrillation (most common source of cardioemboli), coronary artery disease, heart failure, valvular disease, myocardial infarction, patent foramen ovale with atrial septal aneurysm, left atrial or ventricular thrombi

  j. Behavioral risk factors: Smoking, heavy alcohol use, illicit drug use, sedentary lifestyle, obesity

  k. Medication history

   i. Oral contraceptive use, especially in women over 30 years of age who smoke

   ii. Nonaspirin NSAIDs: Can interfere with the antiplatelet effects of drugs such as aspirin, clopidogrel, and aspirin with dipyridamole

3. Signs and symptoms

 a. Report of a prior TIA: Ischemic event that results in a reversible, short-lived neurologic deficit (<24 hours but may be only minutes). Deficits are the same as for stroke but are short-lived; the highest risk of stroke is within 24 hours of a TIA, so emergent patient evaluation and treatment for secondary prevention are important to avoid a disabling stroke.

 b. Onset of focal neurologic deficits that correlate with a known vascular territory and persist for more than 24 hours

 c. Varying clinical presentation, depending on the area of the brain involved and the extent of injury (Tables 4-30 and 4-31).

 d. Headache present in about 25% of patients

 e. Spontaneous BP elevations: Common after acute stroke, although low-normal BP may be seen with stroke affecting the entire anterior circulation or if coronary artery events occur simultaneously

 f. National Institutes of Health Stroke Scale: Routinely used to measure neurologic function after acute ischemic stroke. Scores range from 0 to 42, with higher scores indicating greater neurologic impairment. Used to determine stroke severity and to guide decisions about thrombolytic use. (Scale available at http://www.ninds.nih.gov/doctors/NIH_Stroke_Scale.pdf.)

4. Diagnostic study findings

 a. Laboratory

  i. Serum glucose level, electrolyte levels, CBC, liver and renal function studies, lipid panel, tests for prothrombic states (e.g., levels of protein S, lupus anticoagulant): To assess stroke risk factors, identify imbalances that warrant treatment, and rule out conditions that mimic stroke

▥ **TABLE 4-30**

▥ ▥ **Signs and Symptoms of Stroke Syndromes Associated with Specific Vessel Involvement**

Occluded Vessel	Signs and Symptoms*
Internal carotid artery	Contralateral face, arm, and leg paralysis and sensory deficits
	Homonymous hemianopsia (loss of half of field of vision)
	Transient monocular blindness (amaurosis fugax) due to retinal artery emboli
	Ipsilateral Horner's syndrome (see Table 4-19)
	Headache behind ipsilateral eye
	Dominant hemisphere: Aphasia
	Nondominant hemisphere: Neglect and/or agnosia
ACA	Motor and sensory deficits in contralateral lower extremity with distal weakness (i.e., foot) worse; impaired gait
	Possible mild contralateral upper extremity weakness
	Abulia (slowness to react)
	Cognitive impairment: Perseveration, amnesia
	Apraxia
	Personality changes, flat affect, easy distractibility, lack of initiative
	Urinary incontinence

Continued

■ **TABLE 4-30**
■ ■ **Signs and Symptoms of Stroke Syndromes Associated with Specific Vessel Involvement—Cont'd**

Occluded Vessel	Signs and Symptoms*
MCA	Contralateral paralysis and sensory loss in arm with leg spared or with less deficit
	Contralateral lower face paralysis
	Homonymous hemianopsia
	Dominant hemisphere: Aphasia, dyslexia, agraphia (inability to express thoughts in writing), acalculia (inability to do simple math)
	Nondominant hemisphere: Constructional apraxia (inability to reproduce or complete a drawing, drawing left half incomplete), dressing apraxia (inability to dress self), loss of sense of spatial relationships, autotopagnosia (inability to recognize parts of body)
Vertebral artery	Wallenberg's syndrome (see posterior inferior cerebellar artery, discussed later)
	Ipsilateral facial weakness and numbness, facial and eye pain Clumsiness, ataxia, dizziness or vertigo
	Nystagmus
	Dysphagia, dysarthria
Basilar artery	Nausea and vomiting
	Progressive decline in level of consciousness
	Impaired ocular movement, conjugate gaze paralysis, diplopia
	Pupillary changes: Pupils miotic (pontine) or large and less light responsive (midbrain)
	Facial sensory loss; facial, pharyngeal, and lingual muscle weakness Dysarthria, dysphagia
	Alternating hemiparesis
	Possible "locked-in syndrome" (no movement except eyelids; consciousness and cortical function, including sensation, are preserved)
	Dysmetria
	Ataxia, vertigo
	Acute deafness
PCA	Manifestations can vary widely:
	• Homonymous hemianopsia; visual deficits—loss of depth perception, blindness, visual hallucinations
	• Memory loss
	• Thalamus involvement: Contralateral sensory loss (all modalities), hemiparesis, intention tremors, spontaneous pain
	• Cerebral peduncle involvement: Weber's syndrome (contralateral hemiplegia with cranial nerve III palsy)
Posterior inferior cerebellar artery (Wallenberg's syndrome)	Nausea and vomiting
	Dysphagia, impaired gag reflex and swallowing
	Dysarthria
	Nystagmus, diplopia
	Hiccups
	Vertigo, ataxia
	Ipsilateral facial numbness and Horner's syndrome
	Loss of pain and temperature sensation over contralateral trunk and extremities
Small penetrating arteries (e.g., lenticulostriate branches of ACA and MCA, paramedian branches of basilar artery, thalamoperforate branches of PCA)	Contralateral hemiplegia equally affecting leg, arm, and face without aphasia, visual impairment, or sensory loss
	Sensory loss in leg, trunk, arm, and face; may be associated with pain without motor loss
	Dysarthria
	Clumsiness, ipsilateral ataxia

*Some or all of the deficits may be evident when a particular vessel is occluded; syndromes frequently overlap.
ACA, Anterior cerebral artery; *MCA,* middle cerebral artery; *PCA,* posterior cerebral artery.

■ **TABLE 4-31**
■ ■ **Signs and Symptoms of Stroke Syndromes Associated with Specific Stroke Location**

Location	Signs and Symptoms
Right (nondominant) hemisphere	Left hemiparesis and sensory loss
	Left visual field deficit
	Right gaze preference
	Dysarthria
	Flat affect
	Spatial perception deficits
	Constructional and dressing apraxia
	Neglect of left side (inattention to objects in the left visual field and to left auditory stimuli)
	Anosognosia (unawareness or denial of deficits on affected side)
Left (dominant) hemisphere	Right hemiparesis and sensory loss
	Right visual field deficit
	Left gaze preference
	Acalculia, agraphia
	Aphasia (expressive, receptive, or global)
	Apraxia of left limbs
	Finger agnosia (inability to identify the finger touched)
	Right-left disorientation
Brainstem, cerebellum	Diplopia
	Dysmetria
	Hemiparesis or quadriparesis
	Hemisensory loss or sensory loss in all four limbs and face
	Ocular movement abnormalities
	Acute hearing loss
	Nausea and vomiting, oropharyngeal weakness, dysarthria
	Vertigo, tinnitus, ataxia
	Dysmetria

Adapted from Hinkle JL, Guanci MM, Bowman L, et al. Cerebrovascular events of the nervous system. In: Bader MK, Littlejohns LR, eds. *AANN Core Curriculum for Neuroscience Nursing.* 4th ed. St Louis, MO: Saunders; 2004:544.

    ii.   Platelet count, PT, PTT, INR: To check adequacy of coagulation
    iii.   Toxicology screen: May identify drug (e.g., cocaine) that precipitated stroke
  b. Radiologic
    i.   CT scan without contrast: To exclude hemorrhage or mass lesions as the cause of deficits. Ischemia and infarctions often are not seen for 24 hours or more after the occlusive event, whereas hemorrhage is seen immediately. Ideally the CT scan is done within 25 minutes of the physician's writing the order and is interpreted within 20 minutes of scan completion.
    ii.   CT scan with contrast: To rule out lesions mimicking a TIA or stroke
    iii.   CT angiography: Helpful to identify acute vascular occlusion and vascular lesions
    iv.   Perfusion CT scan: Identifies ischemic stroke, shows area of infarct and penumbra
    v.   Cerebral angiography: Reveals vessel abnormalities, occlusion, stenosis, spasm, or displacement
    vi.   MRI: May reveal acute infarction, hemorrhage
    vii.   Diffusion-weighted MRI: Detects ischemia from within the first few minutes to 2 weeks
    viii. Magnetic resonance angiography (MRA): Reveals abnormal (occluded, stenosed, atherosclerotic) blood vessels
    ix.   PET scan: Provides quantitative values for CBF, CBV, and brain cell metabolism to define infarction size and location; generally not performed in the acute phase after a stroke

      x.   SPECT scan: May be used to determine regional and global CBF; generally not used in the acute phase after a stroke

  c. Twelve-lead ECG, continuous ECG monitoring: To detect dysrhythmias or cardiac disease contributing to stroke

  d. Lumbar puncture: Done if a subarachnoid hemorrhage (SAH) is suspected but not seen on CT scan; not used if the patient is a candidate for thrombolytics

  e. Once the patient is stable, additional diagnostic tests to identify the underlying disease that contributed to stroke may be performed.

5. Goals of care

  a. Adequate brain perfusion is maintained to minimize ischemia.

  b. Optimal recovery of neurologic function occurs.

  c. Potential complications are prevented or are recognized and appropriately managed.

  d. Patient and family are prepared for interventions, possible complications, and outcomes.

6. Collaborating professionals on health care team

  a. Nurse, physician, pharmacist, nutritionist, laboratory personnel

  b. Respiratory, physical, speech, and occupational therapists

  c. Case manager or discharge coordinator, social worker, chaplain

7. Management of patient care

  a. Anticipated patient trajectory: patient's clinical course and outcome are influenced by the location and extent of brain ischemia and infarction; the neurologic deficits that result; the occurrence and severity of complications; age; and preexisting health problems. Specific needs for patients with ischemic stroke in the acute care setting include the following:

      i. Delivery of care: Depending on the severity of the patient's signs and symptoms or the frequency or type of interventions required, the patient may need to be transferred to the ICU for treatment

      ii. Positioning

        (a) Keep the head of the bed flat for 24 hours after stroke; then the head can be raised. Get the patient out of bed as early as possible.

        (b) Protect the patient's neglected, paralyzed, or insensate side during positioning.

        (c) Position patient items in the unaffected visual field initially; gradually move objects to the affected side and encourage the patient to attend to that side.

      iii. Skin care: Provide meticulous care to prevent breakdown in patients with sensory or motor deficits

      iv. Pain management: Short-acting or easily reversible analgesics (e.g., morphine, fentanyl) may be used to control pain. Avoid causing hypotension; monitor pain relief.

      v. Nutrition: Maintain normoglycemia. If LOC or dysphagia precludes oral intake, employ alternative methods of feeding early (see Dysphagia under Patient Care).

      vi. Transport: When possible, the stroke victim should be rapidly transported to the emergency department for quick assessment and diagnostic studies. If CT scanning is unavailable, the patient's condition should be stabilized and the patient should be transferred to an appropriate facility.

      vii. Discharge planning: Discharge destination (e.g., home, rehabilitation or skilled nursing facility) is determined in large part by the patient's cognitive capabilities and motor or sensory deficits. Educate the family about what the course of the patient's condition is likely to be and what should be expected in the postacute phase of care.

      viii. Pharmacology: See Box 4-9

      ix. Psychosocial issues: Depression is common after stroke and if present should be treated with appropriate pharmacotherapy and supportive care. Ensure that the possibility of developing depression is discussed with the patient and family before discharge.

      x. Treatments

        (a) Noninvasive

          (1) Monitor neurologic status closely and report changes to the physician.

          (2) Maintain normothermia.

          (3) Initiate occupational, speech, and physical therapy early.

■ **BOX 4-9**
■ **PHARMACOLOGIC THERAPY FOR ISCHEMIC STROKE**

- Supplemental oxygen to maintain adequate systemic and brain tissue oxygenation
- Tissue plasminogen activator (t-PA)
  1. Thrombolytic agent that breaks up clot causing vessel occlusion, thereby restoring cerebral blood flow to ischemic tissues and improving neurologic outcome
  2. Intravenous (IV) administration considered if within 3 hours of stroke symptom onset and patient meets recommended criteria; dose is 0.9 mg/kg to a maximum dose of 90 mg; 10% of dose given over 1 minute and remaining 90% over 1 hour via infusion pump
  3. Intra-arterial administration may be considered for anterior circulation stroke if within 6 hours of symptom onset; for posterior circulation stroke, typically given up to 8 to 12 hours after symptoms begin but under some circumstances may be given when symptoms have been present even longer; catheter is threaded through the vasculature to the site of the cerebral occlusion, where a small amount of t-PA is delivered; intra-arterial administration not yet approved by the US Food and Drug Administration
- Antihypertensives to maintain the blood pressure (BP) within desired range; sublingual calcium channel blockers should not be used; hypotension must be avoided to prevent worsening ischemia!
  1. When no thrombolytic agent is used, treatment of hypertension is deferred unless acute myocardial infarction, aortic dissection, hypertensive encephalopathy, or severe left ventricular failure is present or BP exceeds 220 mm Hg systolic, 120 mm Hg diastolic, or mean arterial pressure of 130 mm Hg; use IV labetalol or nitroprusside to achieve BP control.
  2. For patients who are candidates for thrombolytic administration, systolic BP must be maintained below 185 mm Hg and diastolic below 110 mm Hg to reduce risk of hemorrhage; IV labetalol, nitroprusside, nicardipine, or hydralazine may be used to control BP.
- Prescribed IV fluids, isotonic crystalloids without glucose (e.g., normal saline), to maintain hypervolemia or normovolemia
- Vasoactive or inotropic agents if necessary to maintain desired BP
- Insulin as necessary to maintain blood glucose level below 110 mg/dl; hyperglycemia can increase infarct size and cerebral edema
- Antiplatelet agents such as aspirin, clopidogrel (Plavix), and extended-release dipyridamole and aspirin (Aggrenox) to inhibit platelet aggregation and prevent recurrent stroke; initiate once hemorrhage is ruled out in patient not receiving thrombolytics; in patients receiving t-PA, start antiplatelet agent 24 hours after t-PA administration

    (b) Invasive
        (1) Avoid any invasive procedures in patients who are candidates for therapy with tissue plasminogen activator (t-PA). Place a gastric tube or Foley catheter before t-PA is administered.
        (2) Interventional radiology
            a) May be used to deliver thrombolytics to the occlusion site (Box 4-10)
            b) Angioplasty via balloon inflation at the site of stenosis of a cerebral vessel
            c) Intravascular stenting used with angioplasty to maintain vessel patency
        (3) Surgical interventions to prevent stroke
            a) Carotid endarterectomy: Removes atherosclerotic plaque and clot from the intra-arterial lumen
            b) Extracranial-intracranial bypass: Used selectively to provide collateral circulation for patients with severe major vessel stenosis
    xi. Ethical issues: May consider with the family halting further treatment or withdrawing therapy when the patient has findings that indicate a dismal prognosis
  b. Potential complications: See Box 4-11; also see health problems described under Patient Care
8. Evaluation of patient care
  a. Brain infarct is minimized, and ischemia resolves.
  b. Optimal neurologic outcome is achieved.

■ **BOX 4-10**
■ **CRITERIA FOR ADMINISTRATION OF THROMBOLYTIC THERAPY**

PATIENT CHARACTERISTICS
■ Head computed tomography scan negative for hemorrhage
■ Age older than 18 years
■ Time of symptom onset less than 3 hours earlier
■ No history of intracranial surgery, head trauma, or stroke within past 3 months
■ Neurologic signs that are not clearing rapidly and spontaneously
■ Neurologic signs that are not minor and isolated
■ No myocardial infarction within the past 3 months
■ No gastrointestinal or urinary tract hemorrhage in the previous 21 days
■ No major surgery in the previous 14 days
■ No arterial puncture at a noncompressible site in the previous 7 days
■ No evidence of acute bleeding or acute trauma (fracture) on examination
■ No seizure with postictal residual neurologic impairments
■ Systolic blood pressure less than 185 mm Hg and diastolic blood pressure less than 110 mm Hg

LABORATORY DATA
■ Prothrombin time longer than 15 seconds
■ No prolongation of partial thromboplastin time or international normalized ratio less than 1.5
■ Platelet count higher than 100,000/mm³
■ Blood glucose level above 50 mg/dl (2.7 mmol/L) and below 400 mg/dl
■ Patient cannot be lactating or have a positive pregnancy test result.

From Hinkle JL, Guanci MM, Bowman L, et al. Cerebrovascular events of the nervous system. In: Bader MK, Littlejohns LR, eds. *AANN Core Curriculum for Neuroscience Nurses.* St Louis, MO: Saunders; 2004:545.

c. Complications are prevented or minimized.
d. Patient and family are prepared for interventions, necessary lifestyle changes, possible complications, and outcomes.

Hemorrhagic Stroke

1. **Pathophysiology**
   a. Rupture of a blood vessel within the cranium. Includes intracerebral hemorrhage (ICH), epidural hematoma (EDH), subdural hematoma (SDH), intraventricular hemorrhage (IVH), and SAH.
      i. ICH: Hemorrhage into brain parenchyma produced by shearing and tensile stresses within brain tissue that result in rupture of intracerebral vessels. Frequently occurs in white matter of frontal and temporal regions, less commonly deep in hemispheres or cerebellum. May be single or multiple, often associated with other intracranial lesions, penetrating injuries, aneurysm rupture, AVM rupture, or hypertension.
      ii. EDH: Blood accumulation beneath skull and above dura; most often from arterial source. Most commonly associated with temporal bone fracture that lacerates middle meningeal artery. EDH compresses brain yet is associated with little underlying primary brain injury.
      iii. SDH: Blood accumulation beneath dura, usually due to venous bleeding from torn bridging veins. As SDH expands it compresses brain and increases ICP. Categorized into three groups according to timing of presentation:
         (a) Acute: Often associated with more underlying primary brain injury than EDH; poor prognosis
         (b) Subacute: Prognosis better than that of acute SDH because of less severe underlying brain injury and lower likelihood of progressing to brainstem compression.
         (c) Chronic: SDH accumulates slowly, likely because of small rebleeds; over 2 to 4 days blood congeals and thickens. After about 2 weeks, clot breaks down and

▓ **BOX 4-11**
▓ **POTENTIAL COMPLICATIONS OF ISCHEMIC STROKE**

HEMORRHAGE
MECHANISM
- Energy depletion and acidosis in tissue surrounding infarction can allow red blood cell extravasation, creating hemorrhagic infarction.
- Risk is increased if thrombolytics, anticoagulants, or antiplatelet agents given or if severe hypertension occurs.

MANAGEMENT
- Hold anticoagulants and antiplatelet agents for 24 hours after administration of tissue plasminogen activator.
- Monitor vital signs and neurologic status frequently.
  1. With thrombolytic therapy: Every 15 minutes for 2 hours, every 30 minutes for 6 hours, hourly for 16 hours, then every 2 to 4 hours
  2. Without thrombolytic therapy, hourly for 8 hours, then every 2 hours
- Hold infusion of thrombolytic agent if neurologic condition changes. Report changes to physician and prepare patient for computed tomographic (CT) scan. If CT excludes hemorrhage, may resume thrombolytics per order.
- Monitor for bleeding at puncture sites, sclera, oropharynx, nares, gastrointestinal and genitourinary tracts.
- Maintain blood pressure and coagulation parameters within the desired ranges.
- Monitor coagulation parameters (platelet count, prothrombin time, partial thromboplastin time, international normalized ratio, fibrinogen) and complete blood cell count.

REPERFUSION INJURY
MECHANISM
- Restoration of perfusion to ischemic tissue causes activation of oxygen free radicals that further injure compromised cells. May occur hours to weeks after initial stroke; new or same stroke symptoms may appear.

MANAGEMENT
- Monitor neurologic status closely after reperfusion is established (e.g., after thrombolytic therapy).

RECURRENT STROKE
MECHANISM
- Most recurrences occur within hours to days of first stroke; highest risk is within first 30 days.

MANAGEMENT
- Identify and treat modifiable risk factors that contribute to stroke.
- Administer antiplatelet and antithrombotic therapy as prescribed.
- Provide patient and family education about lifestyle changes needed.

INCREASED INTRACRANIAL PRESSURE
MECHANISM
- Cerebral edema (usually peaks 2 to 5 days after stroke) and intracranial hemorrhage can increase intracranial volume and pressure.

MANAGEMENT
- Refer to Increased Intracranial Pressure under Specific Patient Health Problems.

SEIZURES
- Refer to Seizures under Specific Patient Health Problems.

eventually becomes xanthochromic fluid encased by membranes. SDH eventually reabsorbs or becomes calcified.
- iv. IVH: Bleeding into ventricles; may be associated with extension of SAH or ICH
- v. SAH: Bleeding into subarachnoid space due to rupture of an aneurysm or AVM or traumatic brain injury

The following section focuses on stroke associated with spontaneous ICH

    b. ICH compresses and irritates cerebral tissues, causing ischemic cellular responses, cerebral edema, intracranial hypertension, and CPP compromise. Functional loss and death of neurons result.

    c. ICH associated with hypertension and cerebral amyloid angiopathy usually involves small, deep cortical arteries; most commonly occurs in the basal ganglia, thalamus, cerebellum, or brainstem but may affect more superficial areas of cerebrum.

    d. Hemorrhagic strokes account for approximately 15% to 20% of strokes.

2. Etiology and risk factors

    a. Hypertensive vascular disease (most common cause)

    b. Cerebral amyloid angiopathy: β-amyloid protein deposits in small meningeal and cortical blood vessel walls make them more friable

    c. Ischemic stroke with a hemorrhagic conversion; traumatic ICH

    d. Vasculitis, vascular brain tumor, venous infarction (e.g., thrombosis in the sagittal sinus)

    e. Use of anticoagulants or platelet aggregation inhibitors; systemic hemorrhagic disorders and diathesis

    f. Use of illicit drugs, particularly cocaine, amphetamines

    g. Increased age; race—young and middle-aged African Americans have a higher incidence than whites of the same age

3. Signs and symptoms

    a. Sudden, spontaneous onset; may progress in minutes to hours

    b. Specific clinical presentation varies, depending on the location, extent, and rate of bleeding. Symptoms may include severe headache, decreased LOC, nausea and vomiting, ataxia, seizures, hemiplegia or hemiparesis (arm, leg, or both), aphasia, cranial nerve dysfunction, impaired swallowing, and gaze deviations.

    c. Table 4-32 shows distinguishing signs and symptoms of hemorrhagic stroke into deep cortical structures.

4. Diagnostic study findings (also see Ischemic Stroke for studies used in generic stroke evaluation)

    a. Laboratory

        i. Clotting profile (platelet count, PT, PTT, INR): To check the adequacy of clotting

        ii. CBC, sedimentation rate: May indicate cause related to infection, inflammation, or malignancy

        iii. Serum glucose and electrolyte levels

        iv. Toxicology screen: To identify drugs that may have precipitated stroke

▪ **TABLE 4-32**

▪ ▪ **Distinguishing Signs and Symptoms Associated with Hemorrhagic Stroke**

Deep Cortical Structure	Distinguishing Signs and Symptoms*
Cerebellum	Dizziness
	Vertigo
	Ataxia
	Occipital headache
	Nystagmus, ipsilateral gaze deficit
	Dysarthria
Pons	Contralateral hemiparesis and, with more extensive hemorrhage, quadriparesis and "locked-in" syndrome
	Impaired lateral eye movement
	Small, poorly reactive pupils
	Possible abnormal respiratory patterns (see Table 4-20)
Thalamus	Contralateral hemiparesis and sensory loss, equal in the face, arm, and leg; or hemisensory loss alone
Putamen (often involving the internal capsule)	Contralateral hemiparesis and sensory loss
	Dysarthria

*In addition to these distinguishing features, signs and symptoms of increased intracranial pressure will likely be present.

b. Radiologic
   i. CT scan: Reveals acute hemorrhage size, location, possibly cause (e.g., tumor), complications (e.g., herniation, hydrocephalus)
   ii. MRI: Reveals hemorrhage and areas of edema; may reveal cause
   iii. Studies to rule out vascular lesions, such as CT angiography, MRA, cerebral angiography
c. Lumbar puncture: For suspected SAH with no evidence of blood on CT scan and no signs of increased ICP. If hemorrhagic stroke extends into the ventricle or SAH exists, the CSF contains red blood cells and appears xanthochromic. CSF protein and white blood cell levels are elevated. CSF pressure may be elevated.

5. Goals of care
a. Recovery of neurologic functions is optimal.
b. Potential systemic and neurologic complications are prevented or recognized and appropriately managed.
c. Patient and family are prepared for interventions, possible complications, and outcomes.

6. Collaborating professionals on health care team
a. Nurse, physician, pharmacist, nutritionist, laboratory personnel
b. Respiratory, physical, speech, and occupational therapists
c. Case manager or discharge coordinator, social worker, chaplain

7. Management of patient care
a. Anticipated patient trajectory: Numerous factors influence the clinical course and outcome, including the location and extent of the hemorrhage, the occurrence and severity of complications; age; and preexisting health problems. Hemorrhagic stroke carries much higher mortality and morbidity than ischemic stroke. Anticipated patient trajectory for increased ICP is relevant for these patients (see Increased Intracranial Pressure). Other needs specific to patients with hemorrhagic stroke include the following:
   i. Delivery of care: Depending on the severity of the patient's signs and symptoms or the frequency or type of interventions required, the patient may need to be transferred to the ICU for treatment
   ii. Positioning: Maintain the head of the bed at 30 degrees to promote cerebrovenous outflow
   iii. Skin care: Provide meticulous care to prevent breakdown in patients with sensory or motor deficits
   iv. Pain management: Short-acting or easily reversible analgesics (e.g., morphine, fentanyl) may be used to control pain. Avoid causing hypotension; monitor pain relief.
   v. Nutrition: Maintain normoglycemia. If LOC or dysphagia precludes oral intake, employ alternative methods of feeding early (see Dysphagia under Patient Care).
   vi. Transport: When possible, the stroke victim should be rapidly transported to the emergency department for quick assessment and diagnostic studies. If CT scanning is unavailable, the patient's condition should be stabilized and the patient should be transferred to an appropriate facility.
   vii. Discharge planning: Discharge destination (e.g., home, rehabilitation or skilled nursing facility) is determined in large part by the patient's cognitive capabilities and motor or sensory deficits. Educate the family about what the course of the patient's condition is likely to be and what should be expected in the postacute phase of care.
   viii. Pharmacology
      (a) Provide supplemental oxygen.
      (b) Administer prescribed IV fluids, typically isotonic non–glucose-containing solutions.
      (c) Administer prescribed antihypertensives; generally IV labetalol is used initially. Typically a systolic BP of 150 to 170 mm Hg and an MAP of less than 130 mm Hg is desired. Avoid hypotension or reduction of MAP by 15% or more of baseline over 24 hours.
      (d) Fresh frozen plasma, platelets, and/or vitamin K may be used to correct coagulopathy.
      (e) Sedation may be prescribed for agitation, which can elevate BP and ICP.

      ix. Psychosocial issues: Depression is common after stroke and if present should be treated with appropriate pharmacotherapy and supportive care. Ensure that the possibility of developing depression is discussed with the patient and family before discharge.

      x. Treatments
        (a) Noninvasive
          (1) Monitor neurologic status closely and report changes to the physician.
          (2) Maintain normothermia.
          (3) Initiate occupational, speech, and physical therapy early.

      xi. Ethical issues: May consider with the family halting further treatment or withdrawing therapy when the patient has findings that indicate a dismal prognosis

  b. Potential complications (see also health problems described under Patient Care)
      i. Increased ICP (see Increased Intracranial Pressure section)
      ii. Hydrocephalus
        (a) Mechanism: Ventricular extension of the bleed can impair CSF flow or reabsorption. Cerebral edema and clot formation can obstruct CSF flow.
        (b) Management: Temporary or permanent placement of a shunt

8. Evaluation of patient care
  a. Brain infarct is minimized, and ischemia resolves.
  b. Optimal recovery of neurologic function is achieved.
  c. Complications are prevented or minimized.
  d. Patient and family are prepared for interventions, possible complications, and outcomes.

Intracranial Aneurysms

1. Pathophysiology
  a. Localized dilatation of an artery resulting from weakness of the vessel wall
  b. In adults, 85% occur in the anterior circulation, usually at bifurcations in the anterior circle of Willis. Common sites in the posterior circulation include the basilar artery apex, basilar artery junctions with the adjoining vertebral, anterior inferior cerebellar, and superior cerebellar arteries, and the vertebral and posterior inferior cerebellar artery junction.
  c. Some 10% to 20% of patients have multiple aneurysms.
  d. Aneurysm growth is not thoroughly understood but is affected by hemodynamic factors and arterial wall integrity. As the aneurysm enlarges it can compress surrounding nerves and brain tissue, causing neurologic deficits.
  e. Enlargement further weakens the vessel wall, so rupture can occur. Each year, there is a 1% to 2% risk of rupture. Rupture most often causes SAH and less frequently intracerebral, intraventricular (common with anterior communicating artery aneurysms), or subdural hemorrhage.

2. Etiology and risk factors
  a. Etiology of most aneurysms is unclear. Although they were once thought due to congenital defects, research indicates that the likely cause is hemodynamically induced degenerative changes.
  b. Familial association in some patients, but causes are not known. Risk of aneurysm-related SAH (aSAH) increases if a first-degree family member has had an aSAH. Risk of aSAH increases with age (highest incidence in 40- to 60-year age group), hypertension, heavy alcohol consumption, amphetamine abuse, use of oral contraceptives, atherosclerosis, and hypercholesterolemia.
  c. Higher risk of aneurysm formation and rupture in association with female gender, ischemic heart disease in women, cigarette smoking, and diseases such as adult polycystic kidney disease and Ehlers-Danlos syndrome
  d. Traumatic aneurysm: Trauma injures the vessel wall
  e. Mycotic aneurysm: Bacterial or fungal infections send septic emboli that attach to the cerebral vessel wall and destroy it
  f. Atherosclerotic aneurysm: Deposition of atheromatous material damages vessel walls, which causes formation of fusiform aneurysms (arterial wall outpouching with no defined aneurysm stem or neck)

3. **Signs and symptoms**
   a. Before rupture, most patients are asymptomatic.
   b. Large aneurysms may compress nearby brain tissue causing focal neurologic symptoms. Examples of focal symptoms include the following:
      i. Cranial nerve deficits, especially CN III, IV, or VI dysfunction
      ii. Pain behind or above the eye
      iii. Localized headache
   c. Patient usually comes for treatment with signs of intracranial hemorrhage (usually SAH) from aneurysm rupture. Specific signs and symptoms vary with the severity and location of the hemorrhage. Aneurysmal SAH is graded most commonly using the Hunt and Hess scale: good outcomes are correlated with Hunt and Hess scores of I to III and worse outcomes with scores of IV and V.
      i. Grade I: Asymptomatic, or mild headache and slight nuchal rigidity
      ii. Grade II: Cranial nerve palsy (e.g., III and VI), moderate to severe headache, nuchal rigidity
      iii. Grade III: Mild focal deficit, lethargy, or confusion
      iv. Grade VI: Stupor, moderate to severe hemiparesis, early decerebrate rigidity
      v. Grade V: Deep coma, decerebrate rigidity, moribund appearance
   d. Other signs and symptoms of aSAH
      i. Presenting complaint: "Worst headache of my life"
      ii. Nausea, vomiting, dizziness
      iii. Usually brief loss of consciousness but may be prolonged if the hemorrhage is large or causes hydrocephalus or brain edema
      iv. Symptoms of meningeal irritation
         (a) *Nuchal rigidity*: Resistance to flexion of the neck
         (b) *Brudzinski's sign*: Adduction and flexion of the legs as the examiner flexes the patient's neck
         (c) *Kernig's sign*: When the patient's hip is flexed and the knee is at a right angle, the examiner's attempts to extend the leg elicit resistance or hamstring pain and spasm
         (d) *Headache, photophobia*
      v. Cranial nerve deficits (pupillary and eye movement dysfunction)
      vi. Motor deficits (e.g., hemiparesis, decerebrate posturing)
      vii. Alterations in vital signs may be seen
   e. Evidence of ICH due to rupture
   f. Evidence of increased ICP (see Increased Intracranial Pressure)
4. **Diagnostic study findings**
   a. CT scan (initial study of choice) reveals ICH, SDH, intraventricular blood, amount and distribution of SAH, and hydrocephalus.
   b. CT angiogram affords rapid visualization of arterial anatomy, a three-dimensional image that assists in determining the shape of the aneurysm before therapeutic intervention.
   c. Cerebral angiogram illustrates the size, shape, and location of aneurysms and the presence of vasospasm.
   d. MRI reveals evidence of hemorrhage and hydrocephalus but is not the study of choice.
   e. MRA may diagnose aneurysms larger than 3 mm.
   f. Transcranial Doppler ultrasonography may reveal vasospasm, altered blood flow states, increased ICP, impaired autoregulation, or brain death after aSAH.
   g. Lumbar puncture: Performed in patients with suspected SAH for whom there are no evidence of blood on CT scan and no signs of increased ICP. After SAH, the CSF contains red blood cells and appears xanthochromic (yellowish) after centrifuging, which indicates that hemorrhage occurred several hours earlier. CSF protein and white blood cell counts are elevated. CSF pressure may be elevated.
5. **Goals of care**
   a. Brain ischemia is minimized to optimize neurologic outcomes.
   b. Rebleeding, vasospasm, hydrocephalus, increased ICP, seizures, hyponatremia, and cardiac dysrhythmias are prevented or, if they occur, are recognized and appropriately managed.
   c. Patient and family are prepared for interventions, possible complications, and outcomes.

6. Collaborating professionals on health care team
   a. Nurse, physician, pharmacist, nutritionist, laboratory personnel
   b. Respiratory, physical, speech, and occupational therapists
   c. Case manager or discharge coordinator, social worker, chaplain
   d. Interventional radiologist
7. Management of patient care
   a. Anticipated patient trajectory: Numerous factors influence the clinical course and outcome, including the location and extent of hemorrhage; the occurrence and severity of complications; age; and preexisting disorders. Anticipated patient trajectory for ICP is also relevant if aneurysm rupture precipitates intracranial hypertension (see Increased Intracranial Pressure).
      i. Delivery of care: Depending on the severity of the patient's signs and symptoms or the frequency or type of interventions required, the patient may need to be transferred to the ICU for treatment
      ii. Positioning: Elevate the head of the bed 30 degrees to promote cerebrovenous outflow
      iii. Skin care: Provide meticulous care to prevent breakdown in patients with sensory or motor deficits
      iv. Pain management: Administer prescribed analgesics for headache and surgical incision pain. Short-acting or easily reversible agents preferred; avoid hypotension; monitor pain relief.
      v. Nutrition: Maintain normoglycemia. If LOC or dysphagia precludes oral intake, employ alternative methods of feeding early (see Dysphagia under Patient Care).
      vi. Discharge planning: Discharge destination (e.g., home, rehabilitation or skilled nursing facility) is determined in large part by the patient's cognitive capabilities and motor or sensory deficits. Educate the family about what the course of the patient's condition is likely to be and what should be expected in the postacute phase of care.
      vii. Pharmacology
         (a) Administer supplemental oxygen to prevent hypoxia and insufficient cerebral oxygen delivery.
         (b) Administer prescribed fluids and antihypertensives (e.g., labetalol) or vasopressors to maintain BP at the desired level; carefully avoid even transient incidents of hypotension. Generally, before aneurysm repair the desired systolic BP is 120 to 150 mm Hg; after repair the desired systolic BP is more than 160 to 200 mm Hg.
         (c) Calcium channel blocker (i.e., nimodipine) may be prescribed for vasospasm.
         (d) Sedation may be prescribed to control agitation, which can elevate BP and ICP.
         (e) Stool softeners may be prescribed to prevent straining, which can elevate BP and ICP.
         (f) Prophylactic anticonvulsants may be prescribed, at least in the acute phase.
         (g) Antibiotics may be prescribed for mycotic aneurysm.
      viii. Psychosocial issue: Intervene to help alleviate the patient's and family's fear and anxiety by providing information and encouraging the use of appropriate coping mechanisms and support systems (see Chapter 10).
      ix. Treatments
         (a) Noninvasive
            (1) SAH patients in poor neurologic and medical condition may be managed medically until status improves.
            (2) Before aneurysm repair, avoid BP elevations, which increase the risk of rupture: manage pain; have the patient avoid straining and performing the Valsalva maneuver; provide a private room and quiet environment; limit visitors.
            (3) Monitor neurologic status closely and report changes to the physician.
         (b) Invasive

(1) Surgical or endovascular interventions may be performed to seal off the aneurysm and prevent bleeding or rebleeding. Research demonstrates that performing intervention within the first 24 to 48 hours after rupture improves outcome. Once the aneurysm is obliterated, vasospasm and other complications can be treated more aggressively.

(2) Surgical repair may include the following:

    a) Clipping of the aneurysm neck to obliterate

    b) Resecting or wrapping of aneurysms not amenable to clipping to reinforce the vessel wall

(3) Interventional neuroradiologists may insert devices such as coils, detachable balloons, and/or stents to occlude the aneurysm.

    x. Ethical issues: Halting further treatment or withdrawing current therapy may be considered with the family when diagnostic study findings and neurologic examination indicate a dismal prognosis

b. Potential complications: See Box 4-12; also see health problems under Patient Care

8. Evaluation of patient care

    a. Patient achieves optimal neurologic outcomes.

    b. Complications are prevented or are recognized and treated.

    c. Patient and family are prepared for interventions, possible complications, and outcomes.

Arteriovenous Malformations

1. Pathophysiology: Abnormal vascular network consisting of one or more direct connections between arteries and veins without an intervening capillary network. May be localized or extensive; most often located in the supratentorial structures; commonly involve the cortex. Affected vessels develop thin walls and become passively enlarged. Seven percent to 17% of patients with AVMs have aneurysms, usually in major feeding arteries. Brain parenchyma between AVM vessels consists of nonfunctional neuroglia. Brain tissue around an AVM may receive insufficient perfusion because of the diversion of blood to the AVM (vascular steal phenomenon). High flow volume and increased venous pressure predispose the fragile vessels of the AVM to rupture, most often causing ICH and, less frequently, IVH, SAH, or SDH. Smaller AVMs are more likely to bleed than larger lesions.

2. Etiology and risk factors: Congenital lesions caused by an embryonic vascular malformation

3. Signs and symptoms: May be caused by mass effect of malformation, inadequate perfusion to adjacent brain tissue, venous hypertension, or hemorrhage from the lesion

    a. AVM may be found incidentally during diagnostic tests.

    b. Most are not symptomatic until the third decade of life.

    c. Clinical signs and symptoms associated with hemorrhage into the parenchyma (see Hemorrhagic Stroke), subdural space, ventricles, or subarachnoid space (see Intracranial Aneurysms) are the most common presentation; other signs and symptoms depend on the extent and location of bleeding.

    d. Seizures: Second most common presenting sign; more common initial symptom in patients with large AVMs

    e. Headache: Recurrent, unresponsive to traditional therapy

    f. Pulsatile tinnitus

    g. Progressive neurologic deficits; depend on the area of the brain affected

4. Diagnostic study findings

    a. CT: Noncontrast scan may show areas of calcification in and around the AVM and may detect hemorrhage. Contrast-enhanced scan often shows large tortuous feeding arteries or draining veins.

    b. CT angiography: Reveals composition of the AVM

    c. Cerebral angiography: Most definitive, revealing the anatomy of feeding and draining vessels; the size and location of the AVM; intracranial hemorrhage; and vasospasm

    d. MRI: Identifies AVM location and size; may reveal cerebral edema, as well as an old hemorrhage indicated by the presence of hemosiderin

    e. MRA: Reveals the composition of the vessels in the lesion

■ **BOX 4-12**
■ **POTENTIAL COMPLICATIONS OF INTRACRANIAL ANEURYSMS**

REBLEEDING
MECHANISM
- Most common during first 2 weeks after rupture when aneurysm not repaired
- Peak incidence in first 24 to 28 hours and at 7 to 10 days after initial subarachnoid hemorrhage (SAH)
- Typically causes sudden severe headache, nausea, vomiting, and neurologic deterioration
- Associated with significant mortality and morbidity

MANAGEMENT
- Early surgical or endovascular repair is most effective intervention to prevent rebleed.
- Correct any coagulopathy that may be present.

VASOSPASM
MECHANISM
- Sustained arterial contraction reduces distal cerebral blood flow (CBF) and may cause brain ischemia and infarct.
- Commonly occurs 3 to 14 days after rupture, but may be delayed up to 3 weeks after SAH
- Incidence and degree are directly related to amount of blood in subarachnoid space.
- Neurologic symptoms may not occur or there may be subtle or dramatic deterioration in neurologic function.
- Signs and symptoms may include the following:
  1. Headache, altered level of consciousness, focal neurologic signs (e.g., speech impairment, hemiparesis), seizures; hypotension can worsen ischemia and exacerbate neurologic deficits
  2. Transcranial Doppler ultrasonography, usually done daily for 14 days after SAH, may detect vasospasm (blood flow velocity >120 cm/s indicates vasospasm, flow velocities >200 cm/s are diagnostic of severe spasm; ratio of middle cerebral artery velocity to internal carotid artery velocity >3 indicates cerebral vasospasm rather than hyperemia; ratio >6 indicates severe vasospasm).
  3. Cerebral angiography used to diagnose or confirm vasospasm
  4. Brain tissue partial pressure of oxygen ($Pbto_2$) or CBF decreases if sensor located in region fed by the spastic vessel.

MANAGEMENT
- Immediately after SAH diagnosis, calcium channel blocker (i.e., nimodipine) is given prophylactically to reduce vasospasm and improve long-term outcomes. Dosage is 60 mg every 4 hours or, if hypotension occurs, 30 mg every 2 hours for 21 days.
- After aneurysm repair, hypervolemia, hemodilution, and hypertension (so-called triple-H therapy) are used to enhance cerebral perfusion. Before aneurysm repair a modified version of this intervention may be used. Fluids, vasopressors (e.g., phenylephrine), and inotropic agents (e.g., dobutamine) are used to maintain systolic blood pressure above 160 to about 200 mm Hg but not higher than 240 mm Hg. (Desired systolic blood pressure before aneurysm repair is 120 to 150 mm Hg.) Hemodilution and hypervolemia are accomplished by administration of colloid (e.g., albumin, hetastarch) and isotonic crystalloid solutions.
- Goals are to maintain cerebral perfusion pressure above 60 to 70 mm Hg; pulmonary artery wedge pressure of 10 to 20 mm Hg; central venous pressure of 8 to 12 mm Hg; cardiac index higher than 2.2; and hematocrit below 40% (usual target level is 32% to 38%). Therapeutic goals vary depending on neurologic, pulmonary, and cardiac status. Neurologic, hemodynamic, pulmonary, and fluid and electrolyte status require close monitoring during triple-H therapy so that complications (pulmonary edema, heart failure, myocardial ischemia, stroke, electrolyte imbalance) can be prevented or minimized.
- Endovascular intervention may be used to treat confirmed vasospasm unresponsive to nimodipine or triple-H therapy.
  1. Balloon angioplasty may be done to enlarge a stenotic vessel.
  2. A vascular smooth muscle relaxant (e.g., papaverine, verapamil) may be injected into a spastic artery during angiography to relax and dilate the vessel. Effects may be temporary and may cause intracranial pressure (ICP) elevation.

HYDROCEPHALUS
MECHANISM
- Clot formed at rupture site may obstruct flow of cerebrospinal fluid (CSF), and blood in subarachnoid space may obstruct arachnoid villi, impeding reabsorption of CSF.

- Onset may be delayed days or weeks after SAH.
- Symptoms may include diminished level of consciousness, ataxia, headache, blurred vision, diplopia, nausea, vomiting, incontinence, and signs of increased ICP.

MANAGEMENT
- Initially ventriculostomy tube is placed to drain CSF until ICP is normal and ventricular and subarachnoid spaces are clear of blood. With less-acute onset, lumbar drain may be placed to remove CSF.
- Ventricular size is monitored with serial computed tomographic (CT) scans.
- If frequent CSF drainage is required to keep ICP below 20 mm Hg and the ventricular system remains enlarged on CT scan, a ventriculoperitoneal shunt is usually placed.

INCREASED ICP AND RELATED COMPLICATIONS
- Refer to Increased Intracranial Pressure under Specific Patient Health Problems.

SEIZURES
- Refer to Seizures under Specific Patient Health Problems.

HYPONATREMIA
MECHANISM
- Usually secondary to syndrome of inappropriate secretion of antidiuretic hormone or cerebral salt wasting
- May precede or occur during vasospasm

MANAGEMENT
- Refer to Fluid and Electrolyte Imbalance under Patient Care; Chapter 5.

CARDIAC DYSRHYTHMIAS AND REPOLARIZATION ABNORMALITIES
MECHANISM
- Associated with SAH; may relate to systemic release of catecholamines

MANAGEMENT
- Refer to Chapter 3.

5. **Goals of care**
   a. AVM is obliterated without hemorrhage or brain tissue injury.
   b. patient's neurologic status remains normal or improves.
   c. Complications such as hemorrhage, cerebral edema, hydrocephalus, increased ICP, and seizures are prevented or minimized.
   d. Patient and family are prepared for interventions, possible complications, and outcomes.
6. **Collaborating professionals on health care team**
   a. Nurse, physician, pharmacist, nutritionist, laboratory personnel
   b. Respiratory, physical, speech, and occupational therapists
   c. Case manager or discharge coordinator, social worker, chaplain
   d. Interventional radiologist or neuroradiologist
7. **Management of patient care**
   a. Anticipated patient trajectory: Numerous factors influence the clinical course and outcome, including the location, size, and characteristics of the AVM; the occurrence and severity of complications; the effectiveness of interventions to obliterate the lesion; the patient's age; and the presence of comorbidities. If the AVM ruptures, the patient is managed similarly to other patients with intracranial hemorrhage, intracranial aneurysms, and hemorrhagic stroke. Morbidity, mortality, and risk of vasospasm are lower from AVM hemorrhage than from aneurysmal hemorrhage.

    i.   Delivery of care: Depending on the severity of the patient's signs and symptoms or the frequency or type of interventions required, the patient may need to be transferred to the ICU for treatment

    ii.   Positioning: Elevate the head of the bed 30 degrees to promote cerebrovenous outflow

    iii.   Skin care: Provide meticulous care to prevent breakdown in patients with sensory or motor deficits

    iv.   Pain management: Administer prescribed analgesics for headache and surgical incision pain. Short-acting or easily reversible agents preferred; avoid hypotension; monitor pain relief.

    v.   Discharge planning: Discharge destination (e.g., home, rehabilitation or skilled nursing facility) is determined in large part by the patient's cognitive capabilities and motor or sensory deficits. Educate the family about what the course of the patient's condition is likely to be and what should be expected in the postacute phase of care.

    vi.   Pharmacology
        (a) IV fluids to maintain normovolemia
        (b) Antihypertensives to maintain BP in the desired range
        (c) Anticonvulsants to prevent or treat seizures

    vii.   Psychosocial issues: Intervene to help alleviate the patient's and family's fear and anxiety by providing information and encouraging the use of appropriate coping mechanisms and support systems (see Chapter 10)

    viii.   Treatments: May include conservative management, a single treatment, or a combination of interventions. Choice of treatment depends on AVM size, location, and characteristics; the patient's clinical condition, preexisting comorbidities, and age; and the capabilities of health care providers.
        (a) Noninvasive: Radiosurgery (e.g., gamma knife, proton beam): Uses stereotactically directed radiation to initiate vessel wall inflammation, which causes thickening and eventually thrombosis and obliteration of the AVM vessels. Obliterates or shrinks AVMs up to 3 cm in diameter with little collateral damage to normal brain tissue. AVM is vulnerable to hemorrhage until vessels thrombose (takes 1 to 3 years).
        (b) Invasive
            (1) Craniotomy and microsurgery to resect the AVM
            (2) Embolization: Flow-directed and flow-assisted microcatheters are navigated through the vasculature to the pathologic area, where a solid or liquid embolic agent is delivered to obliterate some or all of the AVM. May be curative, palliative, or an adjunct to surgery or radiosurgery.

    ix.   Ethical issues: Halting further treatment or withdrawing current therapy may be considered with the family when diagnostic study findings and neurologic examination indicate a dismal prognosis

b. Potential complications

    i.   Rebleeding
        (a) Mechanism: Slightly increased risk for a year after initial hemorrhage; causes sudden neurologic deterioration
        (b) Management
            (1) Obliterate the AVM; treatment is generally elective unless an ICH or SDH requires urgent intervention.
            (2) Maintain BP within the ordered range.
            (3) Monitor neurologic status often in the first 24 to 48 hours.

    ii.   Seizures (see Seizures section): AVM obliteration may reduce the incidence of seizures

    iii.   Hydrocephalus
        (a) Mechanism: May occur from SAH, IVH, or compression of the ventricle or aqueduct of Sylvius by the AVM
        (b) Management: See Potential Complications under Intracranial Aneurysms

    iv.   Postoperative cerebral edema and hemorrhage

(a) Mechanism: May result from normal CPP breakthrough as a result of the shunting of high-pressure arterial blood into low-pressure veins. Usually occurs early in the postoperative period; may be complicated by hypertension. Neurologic deterioration, especially a change in LOC, typically signals onset.

(b) Management: Monitor BP and neurologic status closely for the first 24 to 48 hours; keep BP within the ordered range

    v. Hemorrhage or ischemia with endovascular therapy

(a) Mechanism: Vessel rupture or a thromboembolic event may occur during or after an endovascular procedure

(b) Management   .

    (1) Administer prescribed heparin therapy to prevent thromboembolism and maintain coagulation within the desired range. If hemorrhage occurs, heparin reversal indicated.

    (2) Monitor BP and neurologic status closely for the first 24 to 48 hours; keep BP within the ordered range.

    vi. Increased ICP

(a) Mechanism: Cerebral edema, intracranial hemorrhage, venous outflow obstruction, and hydrocephalus can all increase ICP

(b) Management: See Increased Intracranial Pressure

8. Evaluation of patient care

    a. AVM is successfully obliterated.

    b. patient's neurologic status remains normal or improves.

    c. Complications are prevented or are recognized and minimized.

    d. Patient and family are prepared for interventions, possible complications, and outcomes.

Seizures

1. Pathophysiology

    a. *Seizures* are paroxysmal episodes of desynchronized and excessive electrical discharges from neurons that result in a sudden transient alteration in brain function.

    b. In *status epilepticus*, the brain's excitatory and inhibitory circuits become reconfigured, which allows prolonged or frequently recurring seizures. The longer status epilepticus lasts, the more difficult it is to control.

    c. Seizures increase cerebral metabolic demand and can deplete high-energy phosphates (e.g., ATP), causing failure of energy-dependent functions (e.g., sodium-potassium-ATPase pump).

    d. CBF can increase to three to five times the normal level.

    e. Aspiration and trauma may occur during a seizure. Prolonged seizures can cause cerebral edema, neuronal dysfunction and injury, hyperthermia, metabolic derangements, dysrhythmias, rhabdomyolysis, and death.

    f. Seizures that occur in the acute phase of a neurologic insult can worsen neurologic outcome.

2. Etiology and risk factors (for seizures in critical care)

    a. Inadequate levels of or withdrawal from anticonvulsant therapy

    b. Acute withdrawal from the chronic use of sedatives or depressants (e.g., alcohol, benzodiazepines, barbiturates)

    c. Drug toxicity or adverse drug reaction

    d. Metabolic disorders (e.g., uremia, hypoglycemia, electrolyte disorders, fever)

    e. Neurologic pathologic conditions such as traumatic brain injury, CNS infections, brain tumors, cerebral edema, stroke, cerebral anoxia, AVM, increased ICP

3. Signs and symptoms (of seizures commonly seen in critical care)

    a. *Tonic-clonic seizure* (grand mal seizure): Involves the whole body without a focal onset. Loss of consciousness is followed by brief period of muscle rigidity (tonic phase) and then rhythmic muscle jerking (clonic phase). In the tonic phase, apnea may occur momentarily and cyanosis may develop. Hyperventilation may accompany the clonic phase or occur as the seizure terminates. Incontinence, profuse salivation, and diaphoresis are common during the seizure, which usually lasts 1 to 5 minutes. Headache, amnesia for the seizure, confusion, myalgia, and fatigue are common in the postictal phase.

b. *Myoclonic seizure*: Sudden, brief muscular contractions that may occur singly or repetitively; usually involve the extremities or face, but can be generalized

c. *Partial seizure*: If the patient remains conscious, the seizure is referred to as a *simple partial seizure*; if loss of consciousness occurs, it is referred to as a *complex partial seizure*. May progress and become generalized. Signs and symptoms relate to the area of the brain affected:

    i. Motor events, such as face twitching or limb jerking

    ii. Automatisms (e.g., lip smacking, fidgeting, blinking): Common with complex partial seizures

    iii. Sensory events: Numbness or tingling; visual, auditory, gustatory, or vertiginous symptoms

    iv. Psychic events (e.g., hallucinations, illusions)

    v. Autonomic events (e.g., diaphoresis, vomiting)

d. *Status epilepticus*: Seizures occur for a prolonged period (>5 to 10 minutes) or repetitively without full recovery between ictal episodes. May be generalized convulsive, nonconvulsive (without visible movement), or, less commonly, focal motor seizures.

4. Diagnostic study findings

  a. Laboratory

    i. Electrolyte or metabolic abnormalities (e.g., sodium imbalance, hypomagnesemia, hypoglycemia, hypoxemia) may precipitate or result from seizures.

    ii. Serum enzyme levels, particularly creatine phosphokinase levels, are elevated after seizures.

    iii. Myoglobinuria is common after prolonged seizures.

    iv. Other tests (e.g., toxicology screen) may reveal disorders that precipitated the seizure.

  b. Radiologic: To determine precipitating or complicating cause

  c. EEG: Identifies seizure activity and localizes the foci

5. Goals of care

  a. Oxygenation and ventilation are maintained.

  b. Seizure activity is controlled.

  c. No injuries or other complications result from the seizures.

  d. No toxic effects are experienced from anticonvulsants.

6. Collaborating professionals on health care team

  a. Nurse

  b. Physician, may include neurologist and infectious disease specialist

  c. EEG technician, respiratory therapist

  d. Pharmacist

7. Management of patient care

  a. Anticipated patient trajectory: Seizures are controlled and, if identified, the precipitating factor is effectively treated. Specific needs of patients with seizures may include the following:

    i. Positioning: After seizures, turn the patient on the side to prevent aspiration

    ii. Discharge planning: After seizures and precipitating factors are controlled and metabolic responses to seizure are resolved, the patient can typically be discharged to home. Unresolved neurologic impairment from seizures may require discharge to a rehabilitation center or skilled nursing care facility.

    iii. Pharmacology

      (a) Supplemental oxygen

      (b) Prescribed IV fluids to maintain euvolemia

      (c) Anticonvulsant(s) to control seizures. Monotherapy preferred, but if one anticonvulsant is not effective, another may be added. Monitor and maintain therapeutic plasma levels, observe for toxic effects.

        (1) Benzodiazepines (e.g., lorazepam, midazolam, diazepam) are generally used to control acute seizures. Another anticonvulsant drug (usually phenytoin or fosphenytoin) is given simultaneously to prevent recurrent seizures (Table 4-33).

■ **TABLE 4-33**
■ ■ **Anticonvulsants Commonly Used to Treat Status Epilepticus**

Drug	Typical Dosage	Onset	Desired Drug Level	Major Adverse Effects
Lorazepam (Ativan)	4 mg (0.1 mg/kg) IV at 2 mg/min; repeat after 10-15 min if seizures persist	Usually around 5 min	Not typically assessed	Sedation; respiratory depression (more common with use of diazepam); may cause hypotension
Diazepam (Valium)	10-20 mg IV at 5 mg/min; can repeat after 10 min if seizures persist	Almost immediate	Not typically assessed	Sedation; respiratory depression, hypotension may occur
Midazolam (Versed)	2-5 mg IV; for refractory seizures, 0.1-0.4 mg/kg/hr IV	1-5 min	Not typically assessed	Sedation, neuromuscular block, respiratory depression and arrest, hypotension
Phenytoin (Dilantin)	15-20 mg/kg IV no faster than 50 mg/min in saline solution; then 300-400 mg/day in divided doses; do not give intramuscularly	30-60 min	10-20 mcg/ml; free level 1-2 mcg/ml	Dysrhythmias (e.g., bradycardia); cardiovascular collapse; use cautiously in patients with heart block or Stokes-Adams syndrome; hypotension may occur
Fosphenytoin (Cerebyx)	Dosed as PE, 20 mg/kg PE IV at 150 mg PE/min; can be given faster than phenytoin IV; may be given intramuscularly; converted to phenytoin; compatible in standard IV solutions, including those with glucose	Conversion to phenytoin half-life is 15 min.	Same as for phenytoin (actually assess phenytoin levels)	Same as for phenytoin
Valproic acid (Depakote)	15-60 mg/kg/day IV or PO; infuse IV over 60 min (≤20 mg/min)	Peaks in 1-4 hr	50-100 mcg/ml	Sedation, tremors, hepatic toxicity, thrombocytopenia, gastrointestinal disturbance, alopecia
Levetiracetam (Keppra)	1000-3000 mg/day PO	Peaks in 1 hr	Not assessed	Sedation, weakness, incoordination, behavioral abnormalities, leukopenia
Phenobarbital (Luminal)	10-20 mg/kg IV at 50-75 mg/min	5-20 min	20-40 mcg/ml	Sedation, hypotension, respiratory depression may occur.
Pentobarbital (Nembutal)	Loading dose 10 mg/kg IV over 30 min, followed by 5-10 mg/kg/hr for 3 hr, then 1-3 mg/kg/hr infusion	About 1 min	10-50 mcg/ml	Hypotension, myocardial and respiratory depression, immune suppression, and CNS depression, which obscures the neurologic examination
Propofol (Diprivan)	10 mcg/kg/min IV, then titrated to desired effect	Less than 1 min	Not typically assessed	Hypotension, respiratory depression and arrest; propofol infusion syndrome—metabolic acidosis, cardiac failure, rhabdomyolysis, renal failure

CNS, Central nervous system; *IV*, intravenously; *PE*, phenytoin equivalents; *PO*, by mouth

           (2) Valproic acid or levetiracetam may be added for repeated seizures refractory to phenytoin.

           (3) If seizure activity is not halted with these medications in the usual dosages, high-dose pentobarbital, propofol, or midazolam may be used (see Table 4-33).

    iv. Psychosocial issues: Depression and social isolation may occur; ensure provision of counseling and support for dealing with seizures and potentially necessary life changes

    v. Treatments

      (a) Noninvasive

           (1) If the patient has a neurologic disease or injury that puts the person at high risk for seizures, implement seizure precautions: maintain the bed in a low position with side rails up and padded; ensure that harmful objects are out of reach; keep suction and airway equipment readily available.

           (2) Facilitate repeat EEG or provide continuous EEG monitoring to detect subclinical seizures and evaluate the effectiveness of anticonvulsant therapy.

           (3) Observe, record, and report seizures, including the body parts involved, the order of involvement, and the nature of movements; eye deviation, nystagmus, and pupil size change; respiratory pattern and function; neurologic status throughout the seizure and postictal phase; the duration of each phase.

           (4) Maintain a patent airway; ensure adequate ventilation and circulation during and after a seizure; suction airway as necessary.

           (5) Prevent injury during seizures: Stay with the patient; never force anything into the patient's mouth; do not restrain the patient; remove harmful objects from the vicinity; loosen tight clothes; if the patient is out of bed, lower the patient to the floor.

           (6) Reorient the patient after the seizure.

           (7) Investigate and treat the underlying cause.

           (8) Educate the patient and family about seizures, actions to take for another seizure, planned diagnostic tests and interventions, prescribed anticonvulsants.

      (b) Invasive: Intubation and ventilator support if necessary

b. Potential complications

    i. Metabolic complications: May include acidosis, hypoxemia, hypoglycemia, electrolyte imbalances

      (a) Mechanism: Seizures cause increased metabolic demands and imbalances

      (b) Management: Identify and correct imbalances

    ii. Cerebral edema, ischemia, and brain dysfunction

      (a) Mechanism: Seizures increase the cerebral metabolic rate; if cerebral oxygen delivery does not keep up with metabolic demand, brain ischemia, edema, neuronal dysfunction, and death can occur. Hyperemia from increased cerebral metabolic rate encourages vasogenic edema.

      (b) Management: Control seizures. Monitor neurologic status. Avoid hypoxia. Optimize cerebral oxygen delivery.

    iii. Increased ICP

      (a) Mechanism: Cerebral edema and hyperemia

      (b) Management: See Increased Intracranial Pressure

    iv. Renal failure

      (a) Mechanism: Myoglobinuria from muscle breakdown during prolonged seizure activity can lead to acute renal failure

      (b) Management: See Chapter 5

v. Hyperthermia
  (a) Mechanism: Seizures increase the metabolic rate and muscle activity, which elevates body temperature
  (b) Management: Antipyretics, cooling measures as warranted

8. **Evaluation of patient care**
   a. No evidence of seizure activity is present.
   b. There is no injury or neurologic deterioration from seizures.
   c. Adverse effects of anticonvulsant therapy are absent or controlled.
   d. If possible, the underlying cause of the seizures is effectively treated.
   e. Metabolic responses to seizures are resolved.

REFERENCES AND BIBLIOGRAPHY

Physiologic Anatomy

Bader MK, Littlejohns LR, eds. *AANN Core Curriculum for Neuroscience Nursing*. 4th ed. St Louis, MO: Saunders; 2004.

Barker E. *Neuroscience Nursing: A Spectrum of Care*. 3rd ed. St Louis, MO: Mosby; 2008.

DuPen A, Shen D, Ersek M. Mechanisms of opioid-induced tolerance and hyperalgesia. *Pain Manage Nurs*. 2007;8(3):113-121.

Geotz CG. *Textbook of Clinical Neurology*. 3rd ed. Philadelphia, PA: Saunders; 2007.

Guyton AC, Hall JT. *Textbook of Medical Physiology*. 11th ed. Philadelphia, PA: Saunders; 2006.

Han CY, Backous DD. Basic principles of cerebrospinal fluid metabolism and intracranial pressure homeostasis. *Otolaryngol Clin North Am*. 2005;38(4):569-576.

McCance KL, Huether SE, eds. *Pathophysiology: The Biologic Basis for Disease in Adults and Children*. 5th ed. St Louis, MO: Mosby; 2006.

Winn HR, ed. *Youmans Neurological Surgery*. Vols 1–4. 5th ed. Philadelphia, PA: Saunders; 2004.

Patient Assessment

Armon C, Evans RW. Addendum to assessment: Prevention of post-lumbar puncture headaches: report of the Therapeutics and Technology Assessment Subcommittee of the American Academy of Neurology. *Neurology*. 2005;65(4):510-512.

Bader MK, Littlejohns LR, eds. *AANN Core Curriculum for Neuroscience Nursing*. 4th ed. St Louis, MO: Saunders; 2004.

Barker E. *Neuroscience Nursing: A Spectrum of Care*. 3rd ed. St Louis, MO: Mosby; 2008.

Devereaux MW. Anatomy and examination of the spine. *Neurol Clin*. 2007;25(2):331-351.

Feldman HH, Jacova C, Robillard A, et al. Diagnosis and treatment of dementia: 2. Diagnosis. *CMAJ*. 2008;178(7):825-836.

Kidwell CS, Wintermark M. Imaging of intracranial haemorrhage. *Lancet Neurol*. 2008;7(3):256-267.

Mark DG, Pines JM. The detection of nontraumatic subarachnoid hemorrhage: still a diagnostic challenge. *Am J Emerg Med*. 2006;24(7):859-863.

Pasero C. Pathophysiology of neuropathic pain. *Pain Manage Nurs*. 2004;5:3-8.

Sessler CN, Varney K. Patient-focused sedation and analgesia in the ICU. *Chest*. 2008;133(2):552-565.

Stevens RD, Bhardwaj A. Approach to the comatose patient. *Crit Care Med*. 2006;34(1):31-41.

Thompson HJ. *Neurologic Assessment of the Older Adult*. Glenview, IL: American Association of Neuroscience Nurses; 2007.

Urden LD, Stacy KM, Lough ME. *Thelan's Critical Care Nursing: Diagnosis and Management*. 5th ed. St Louis, MO: Mosby; 2006.

Vanderah TW. Pathophysiology of pain. *Med Clin North Am*. 2007;91(1):1-12.

Winn HR, ed. *Youmans Neurological Surgery*. Vols 1–4. 5th ed. Philadelphia, PA: Saunders; 2004.

Patient Care

Adler SM, Verbalis JG. Disorders of body water homeostasis in critical illness. *Endocrinol Metab Clin North Am*. 2006;35(4):873-894.

American Pain Society. *Principles of Analgesic Use in the Treatment of Acute Pain and Cancer Pain*. 5th ed. Glenview, IL: American Pain Society; 2003.

Ashley J, Duggan M, Sutcliffe N. Speech, language, and swallowing disorders in the older adult. *Clin Geriatr Med*. 2006;22(2):291-310.

Dahlin C, Lynch M, Szmuilowicz E, Jackson V. Management of symptoms other than pain. *Anesthesiol Clin*. 2006;24(1):39-60.

Dunwoody CJ, Krenzischek DA, Pasero C, Rathmell JP, Polomano RC. Assessment, physiological monitoring, and consequences of inadequately treated acute pain. *J Perianesth Nurs*. 2008;23(1 Suppl):S15-S27.

Gordon DB, Dahl J, Phillips P, et al. The use of "as-needed" range orders for opioid analgesics in the management of acute pain: a consensus statement of the American Society for Pain

Management Nursing and the American Pain Society. *Pain Manage Nurs.* 2004;5(2): 53-58.

Loh JA, Verbalis JG. Disorders of water and salt metabolism associated with pituitary disease. *Endocrinol Metab Clin North Am.* 2008;37(1):213-234.

Polomano RC, Rathmell JP, Krenzischek DA, Dunwoody CJ. Emerging trends and new approaches to acute pain management. *J Perianesth Nurs.* 2008;23(1 Suppl):S43-S53.

Ranger M, Campbell-Yeo M. Temperament and pain response: a review of the literature. *Pain Manag Nurs.* 2008;9(1):2-9.

Increased Intracranial Pressure

Bader MK, Littlejohns LR, eds. AANN *Core Curriculum for Neuroscience Nursing.* 4th ed. St Louis, MO: Saunders; 2004.

Ball AK, Clarke CE. Idiopathic intracranial hypertension. *Lancet Neurol.* 2006;5(5):433-442.

Barker E. *Neuroscience Nursing: A Spectrum of Care.* 3rd ed. St Louis, MO: Mosby; 2008.

Blissitt PA. Hemodynamic monitoring in the care of the critically ill neuroscience patient. *AACN Adv Crit Care* 2006;17(3):327-340.

Josephson L. Management of increased intracranial pressure: a primer for the non-neurocritical care nurse. *Dimens Crit Care Nurs.* 2004;23(5):194-207.

Lee EL, Armstrong TS. Increased intracranial pressure. *Clin J Oncol Nurs.* 2008;12(1):37-41.

Littlejohns L, Bader MK. Prevention of secondary brain injury: targeting technology. *AACN Clin Issues.* 2005;16(4):501-514.

Rangel-Castillo L, Robertson CS. Management of intracranial hypertension. *Crit Care Clin.* 2006;22(4):713-732.

Vincent JL, Berré J. Primer on medical management of severe brain injury. *Crit Care Med.* 2005;33(6):1392-1399.

Stroke

Adams HP Jr, del Zoppo G, Alberts MJ, et al. Guidelines for the early management of adults with ischemic stroke: a guideline from the American Heart Association/American Stroke Association Stroke Council, Clinical Cardiology Council, Cardiovascular Radiology and Intervention Council, and the Atherosclerotic Peripheral Vascular Disease and Quality of Care Outcomes in Research Interdisciplinary Working Groups. *Stroke.* 2007;38:1655-1711.

Alexander S, Gallek M, Presciutti, Zrelak P. *Care of the Patient With a Subarachnoid Hemorrhage.* Glenview, IL: American Association of Neuroscience Nurses; 2007.

Bader MK, Littlejohns LR, eds. *AANN Core Curriculum for Neuroscience Nursing.* 4th ed. St Louis, MO: Saunders; 2004.

Baker WF Jr. Thrombolytic therapy: Current clinical practice. *Hematol Oncol Clin North Am.* 2005;19(1):147-181.

Barker E. *Neuroscience Nursing: A Spectrum of Care.* 3rd ed. St Louis, MO: Mosby; 2008.

Broderick J, Connolly S, Feldmann E, et al. Guidelines for the management of spontaneous intracerebral hemorrhage in adults: 2007 update: a guideline from the American Heart Association/American Stroke Association Stroke Council, High Blood Pressure Research Council, and the Quality of Care and Outcomes in Research Interdisciplinary Working Group. *Stroke.* 2007;38:2001-2023.

Chaturvedi S, Bruno A, Feasby T, et al. Carotid endarterectomy—an evidence-based review: report of the Therapeutics and Technology Assessment Subcommittee of the American Academy of Neurology. *Neurology.* 2005;65:794-801.

Finley Caulfield A, Wijman CA. Critical care of acute ischemic stroke. *Crit Care Clin.* 2006; 22(4):581-606.

Giles MF, Rothwell PM. Risk of stroke early after transient ischaemic attack: a systematic review and meta-analysis. *Lancet Neurol.* 2007;6(12):1063-1072.

Jamieson DG. Secondary prevention of ischemic stroke: evolution from a stepwise to a risk stratification approach to care. *Dis Manage.* 2007;10(5):273-284.

Janjua N, Brisman JL. Endovascular treatment of acute ischaemic stroke. *Lancet Neurol.* 2007;6(12):1086-1093.

Pugh S, Mathiesen C, Meighan M, Summers D. *Guide to the Care of the Patient With Ischemic Stroke.* Glenview, IL: American Association of Neuroscience Nurses; 2004.

Semplicini A, Benetton V, Macchini L, et al. Intravenous thrombolysis in the emergency department for the treatment of acute ischaemic stroke. *Emerg Med J.* 2008;25(7):403-406.

Somes J, Bergman DL. ABCDs of acute stroke intervention. *J Emerg Nurs.* 2007;33(3):228-234.

Urrutia VC, Wityk RJ. Blood pressure management in acute stroke. *Crit Care Clin.* 2006;22(4): 695-711.

Intracranial Aneurysms and Arteriovenous Malformations

Bader MK, Littlejohns LR, eds. *AANN Core Curriculum for Neuroscience Nursing.* 4th ed. St Louis, MO: Saunders; 2004.

Barker E. *Neuroscience Nursing: A Spectrum of Care.* 3rd ed. St Louis, MO: Mosby; 2008.

Dhar R, Diringer MN. The burden of the systemic inflammatory response predicts vasospasm and outcome after subarachnoid hemorrhage. *Neurocrit Care.* 2008;8(3):404-412.

Gross BA, Hage ZA, Daou M, et al. Surgical and endovascular treatments for intracranial aneurysms. *Curr Treat Options Cardiovasc Med.* 2008; 10(3):241-252.

Hedlund M, Ronne-Engstrom E, Ekselius L, Carlsson M. From monitoring physiological functions to using psychological strategies. Nurses' view of caring for the aneurysmal subarachnoid haemorrhage patient. *J Clin Nurs*. 2008;17(3): 403-411.

Keedy A. An overview of intracranial aneurysms. *McGill J Med* 2006;9(2):141-146.

Koebbe CJ, Veznedaroglu E, Jabbour P, Rosenwasser RH. Endovascular management of intracranial aneurysms: current experience and future advances. *Neurosurgery*. 2006;59(5 Suppl 3):S93-S102.

Lantz ER, Meyers PM. Neuropsychological effects of brain arteriovenous malformations. *Neuropsychol Rev*. 2008;18(2):167-177.

Pritz MB. Thrombosis, growth, recanalization, and rupture of a saccular, non-giant cerebral aneurysm. *J Stroke Cerebrovasc Dis*. 2008;17(3):158-160.

Schatlo B, Pluta RM. Clinical applications of transcranial Doppler sonography. *Rev Recent Clin Trials*. 2007;2(1):49-57.

Stone SD. Patient concerns posthaemorrhagic stroke: a study of the Internet narratives of patients with ruptured arteriovenous malformation. *J Clin Nurs*. 2007;16(2):289-297.

Wagner M, Stenger K. Unruptured intracranial aneurysms: using evidence and outcomes to guide patient teaching. *Crit Care Nurs Q*. 2005;28(4):341-354.

Wermer MJ, van der Schaaf IC, Algra A, Rinkel GJ. Risk of rupture of unruptured intracranial aneurysms in relation to patient and aneurysm characteristics: an updated meta-analysis. *Stroke*. 2007;38(4):1404-1410.

Young WL. Anesthesia for endovascular neurosurgery and interventional neuroradiology. *Anesthesiol Clin*. 2007;25(3):391-412.

Seizures

Adams SM, Knowles PD. Evaluation of a first seizure. *Am Fam Physician*. 2007;75(9):1342-1347.

Bader MK, Littlejohns LR, eds. *AANN Core Curriculum for Neuroscience Nursing*. 4th ed. St Louis, MO: Saunders; 2004.

Fisher RE, Long L. *Care of the Patient With Seizures*. 2nd ed. Glenview, IL: American Association of Neuroscience Nurses; 2007.

Krumholz A, Wiebe S, Gronseth G, et al. Practice parameter: evaluating an apparent unprovoked first seizure in adults (an evidence-based review): report of the Quality Standards Subcommittee of the American Academy of Neurology and the American Epilepsy Society. *Neurology*. 2007;69:1996-2007.

Mirski MA, Varelas PN. Seizures and status epilepticus in the critically ill. *Crit Care Clin*. 2008;24(1):115-147.

The Renal System

Physiologic Anatomy

1. **Process of urine formation: Urine formation occurs in the renal nephron and involves four processes—filtration, reabsorption, secretion, and excretion**
   a. Anatomic structures of the kidney: Most humans are born with two kidneys; a small number are born with one. The kidneys are located in the retroperitoneal space above the waist (Figure 5-1).
      i.   Cortical (outermost) layer
           (a) Metabolically active portion of the kidney, where aerobic metabolism occurs and where ammonia and glucose are formed
           (b) Metabolic needs more than satisfactorily met by an abundant oxygen supply
           (c) Contains all glomeruli and portions of the proximal and distal tubules
      ii. Medullary (middle) layer
           (a) Region of active glycolytic metabolism; supplies energy for active transport
           (b) Metabolism demands high oxygen consumption, yet oxygen supply is limited.
           (c) Plays role in concentration of urine
           (d) Composed of 6 to 10 renal pyramids, formed by collecting ducts and extending into the renal pelvis
           (e) Site of the deepest part of the long loops of Henle and the collecting ducts of the nephron
      iii. Renal sinus, pelvis, and collecting system
           (a) Papillae: Rounded projections of renal tissue located at the apical ends of the renal pyramids positioned with the base facing the cortex and the apices facing the renal pelvis; the apical portion opens into the minor calices
           (b) Corticomedullary junction: Point of division between the cortex and the medulla formed by the base of the pyramids
           (c) Renal lobe: Composed of a pyramid plus the surrounding cortical tissue
           (d) Calix
               (1) Minor calix wraps around the papilla; receives urine from the collecting duct.
               (2) Major calix channels urine from the renal sinus to the renal pelvis.
               (3) Urine flows from the renal pelvis to the ureter.
      iv. Nephron: Anatomic microscopic structure (Figure 5-2)
           (a) Structural and functional unit of the kidney
           (b) Approximately 1 million in each kidney
           (c) Compensates for a significant degree of nephron destruction by

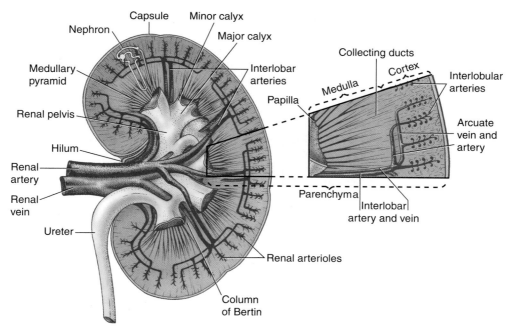

FIGURE 5-1 ■ Major structures of the kidney shown in a diagram of the cut surface of a bisected kidney. (From Brenner BM. *Brenner and Rector's the Kidney.* 6th ed. Philadelphia, PA: Saunders; 2000.)

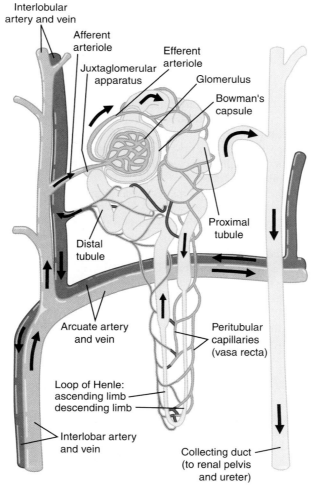

FIGURE 5-2 ■ The functional nephron. (From Guyton AC. *Textbook of Medical Physiology.* 8th ed. Philadelphia, PA: Saunders; 1996.)

(1) Filtering a greater solute load
(2) Hypertrophy of the remaining functional nephrons
(d) Types of nephrons, based on location and function
  (1) Cortical nephrons located in the outer region of the cortex; contain short loops of Henle with a low capacity for sodium reabsorption
  (2) Juxtamedullary nephrons located in the inner cortex adjacent to the medulla; have long loops of Henle that penetrate deep into the medulla and have a greater capacity for concentration of urine because they are sodium-retaining nephrons
(e) Functional segments of the nephron
  (1) Renal corpuscle
    a) Bowman's capsule: Specialized portion of the proximal tubule that supports the glomerulus
    b) Glomerulus: Capillary bed with semipermeable membrane
      1) Normally permeable to water, electrolytes, nutrients, wastes; relatively impermeable to large protein molecules, albumin, erythrocytes
      2) Composed of three cellular layers: Fenestrated endothelial layer, basement membrane, and epithelium podocyte cells that contribute to characteristic semipermeability of this membrane
      3) Characteristics of cellular layers: Endothelial cells contain fenestrations 50 to 100 nm wide, favoring the movement of water and solute; remaining layers are less porous, with openings 1500 nm thick, which may explain the impedance of macromolecules
      4) Major factor influencing filtration is molecular size.
      5) Ionic charge also affects filtration.
        a) Electrical potential of the glomerular membrane possesses a negative charge, which favors the passage of positively charged molecules and impedes negatively charged molecules, such as albumin.
        b) Loss of membrane electrical potential in glomerular disease is reason for proteinuria.
  (2) Renal tubules
    a) Segmentally divided into the proximal convoluted tubule, descending loop of Henle, ascending loop of Henle, distal convoluted tubule, and collecting duct
    b) Each segment has a specific cellular structure and function.

b. Physiologic processes
  i. Glomerular ultrafiltration is the first step in the formation of urine.
    (a) Characteristics of glomerular filtrate
      (1) Normal: Protein-free and red blood cell (RBC)–free, plasmalike substance with a specific gravity (SG) of 1.010. Filtrate contains water, electrolytes, glucose, amino acids, acid-base components, wastes, and other solutes. Pharmaceutical agents can also be included in filtrate.
      (2) Small and middle-sized molecules (up to 60 to 75 kDa): Pass freely through the glomerular membrane (i.e., inulin 5 kDa, albumin >60 kDa)
      (3) Abnormal: Increased permeability of the glomerular membrane allows erythrocytes and protein to be filtered into urine. SG of urine may artificially increase because of the presence of protein or glucose.
      (4) Increased osmotically active substances (glucose, urea): Can cause diuresis
    (b) Filtration is determined by the glomerular pressure and presence of a normal semipermeable glomerular membrane.
      (1) Glomerular hydrostatic pressure is 50 mm Hg and favors filtration; this capillary hydrostatic pressure reflects cardiac output.
      (2) Colloid osmotic pressure of 25 mm Hg and Bowman's capsule hydrostatic pressure of 10 mm Hg oppose hydrostatic pressure and thus oppose filtration.

a) Colloid osmotic pressure results from oncotic pressure of plasma proteins in the glomerular blood supply.

b) Bowman's capsule pressure reflects renal interstitial pressure.

(3) Net filtration pressure is derived by using the following formula:

Glomerular hydrostatic pressure(facilitates):	+50 mm Hg
Colloid osmotic pressure(opposes):	−25 mm Hg
Bowman's capsule pressure(opposes):	−10 mm Hg
Net pressure favoring filtration:	+15 mm Hg

(c) Glomerular filtration rate (GFR)

(1) Clinical assessment tool to determine renal function

(2) Definition: Volume of plasma cleared of a given substance per minute (may be determined by using endogenous creatinine)

(3) GFR equation:

$$GFR = \frac{(Ux \times V)}{Px}$$

where

x = A substance freely filtered through the glomerulus and not secreted or reabsorbed by tubules (e.g., creatinine)

P = Plasma concentration of x

V = Urine flow rate (ml/min)

U = Urine concentration of x

(4) Normal adult GFR: 125 ml/min or 180 L/day

(5) Normal adult urine volume: 1 to 2 L/day, reflecting greater than 99% reabsorption of filtrate

(6) Factors affecting GFR

a) Changes in glomerular hydrostatic pressure

1) Secondary to changes in systemic blood pressure (BP)

2) Caused by variation in afferent or efferent arteriolar tone; increased afferent arteriole resistance decreases GFR; increased efferent arteriole tone increases GFR

b) Alterations in oncotic pressure due to dehydration, hypoproteinemia, or hyperproteinemia

c) Alterations in Bowman's capsule pressure due to urinary tract or nephron destruction, or interstitial edema of kidney

ii. Tubular functions of reabsorption, secretion, and excretion comprise the following steps in urine formation (Figure 5-3):

(a) Conversion of 180 L of plasma filtered per day to 1 to 2 L of excreted urine

(b) Absorption and secretion by two processes:

(1) Passive mechanisms: Solute moves without the expenditure of metabolic energy

a) Diffusion: Solute following either a concentration or an electrical gradient

1) A solute moves from a solution of higher concentration through a semipermeable membrane to a solution of lower concentration.

2) Selectivity of the membrane's permeability and electrical gradient determine diffusion of the solute.

3) The electrical gradient causes a solute to passively migrate to the oppositely charged compartment (e.g., Na^+, a positive ion, migrates to a negatively charged compartment, whereas Cl^-, a negative ion, moves toward a positively charged compartment).

b) Osmosis: Water following an osmotic gradient

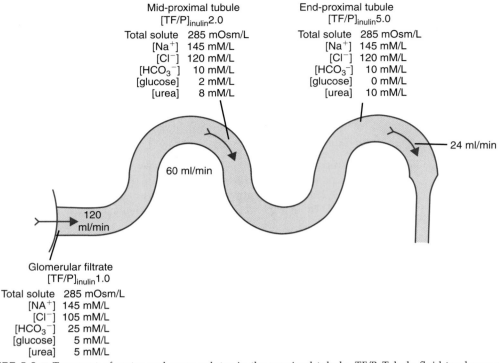

Mid-proximal tubule
$[TF/P]_{inulin}2.0$

Total solute	285 mOsm/L
$[Na^+]$	145 mM/L
$[Cl^-]$	120 mM/L
$[HCO_3^-]$	10 mM/L
[glucose]	2 mM/L
[urea]	8 mM/L

End-proximal tubule
$[TF/P]_{inulin}5.0$

Total solute	285 mOsm/L
$[Na^+]$	145 mM/L
$[Cl^-]$	120 mM/L
$[HCO_3^-]$	10 mM/L
[glucose]	0 mM/L
[urea]	10 mM/L

24 ml/min

60 ml/min

120 ml/min

Glomerular filtrate
$[TF/P]_{inulin}1.0$

Total solute	285 mOsm/L
$[NA^+]$	145 mM/L
$[Cl^-]$	105 mM/L
$[HCO_3^-]$	25 mM/L
[glucose]	5 mM/L
[urea]	5 mM/L

FIGURE 5-3 ■ Transport of water and some solutes in the proximal tubule. *TF/P*, Tubule fluid-to-plasma ratio. (From Maude DL. *Kidney Physiology and Kidney Disease*. Philadelphia, PA: Lippincott; 1977.)

1) Water normally moves from an area of low concentration to an area of higher concentration.
2) An osmotic agent, such as sodium or mannitol, normally remains within a single compartment.
(2) Active mechanisms:
   a) Ion transport requires energy; adenosine triphosphate (ATP) permits ions to move against the concentration gradient.
   b) Maximal tubular transport capacity: Active reabsorption mechanisms in the tubule have limited capacity for reabsorption of certain substances such as glucose. Plasma glucose level of 375 mg/min (transport maximum [Tm]), results in no excretion in urine; plasma glucose level above 375 mg/min results in glucose excretion in urine. Tm for glucose can vary from one nephron to another; as a result, glucose can sometimes spill into the urine at lower serum levels.
   c) Proximal convoluted tubule
(1) Reabsorbs 60% to 80% of filtrate, which remains isotonic to plasma
(2) Major function is active reabsorption of sodium chloride (NaCl) with passive reabsorption of water.
(3) Also reabsorbs glucose, amino acids, phosphates (PO_4^{3-}), uric acid, potassium ion (K^+)
(4) Regulates acid-base balance through reabsorption of carbonic acid (H_2CO_3) and bicarbonate (HCO_3^-) and secretion of hydrogen ions (H^+)
(5) Secretes K^+, ammonium ion (NH_4^+), organic acids, bases, foreign substances (e.g., drugs)
(d) Loop of Henle
(1) Variations in length depend on the type of nephron (i.e., juxtamedullary with long loops or cortical with short loops).

(2) Has two distinct segments
    a) Descending segment, the thin limb, is permeable to water and impermeable to Na^+.
    b) Ascending segment, the thick limb, has active NaCl pump and is impermeable to water; target site for loop diuretics.
(3) Major function is concentration or dilution of urine, accomplished by a countercurrent mechanism that maintains hyperosmolar concentration in the interstitium of the renal medulla.

  (e) Distal convoluted tubule
    (1) Receives hypo-osmotic (or hypotonic) urine from the ascending loop of Henle
    (2) Major functions
      a) Reabsorption of water, NaCl, and sodium bicarbonate
      b) Secretion of K^+, NH_4^+, and H^+ ions
      c) Regulation of composition, tonicity, and volume
    (3) Water permeability here is controlled by antidiuretic hormone (ADH); Na^+ reabsorption is determined by aldosterone.

  (f) Collecting duct
    (1) Receives urine, which is isotonic to plasma, from the distal convoluted and collecting tubules
    (2) Functions with the distal convoluted tubule; affected by ADH and aldosterone
    (3) Final urinary adjustments for composition, tonicity, and volume made here before urine enters the renal pelvis and progresses to the ureter and bladder

2. Renal hemodynamics: Normal blood flow patterns
  a. Renal vasculature
    i. Specialized arrangement of renal blood vessels reflects interdependence of blood supply with kidney function.
    ii. Pathway of blood supply
      (a) Kidney: Aorta → segmented renal arteries → interlobar artery → arcuate artery → interlobular artery → (nephron) → interlobular vein → arcuate vein → interlobar vein → renal vein → inferior vena cava
      (b) Nephron: Afferent arteriole → glomerular capillary → efferent arteriole → peritubular capillary → vasa recta adjacent to tubules → interlobular vein → renal vein → inferior vena cava
    iii. Juxtaglomerular apparatus: Site of renin synthesis
      (a) Specialized cells composed of juxtaglomerular cells and macula densa
        (1) Juxtaglomerular granular cells: Smooth muscle cells containing granules of inactive renin
        (2) Macula densa: Portion of the distal tubule making contact with afferent arterioles of its respective glomerulus
      (b) Responds to arterial BP in afferent and efferent arterioles and to sodium in distal tubule
  b. Renal blood flow (RBF) parameters
    i. Kidney receives 20% to 25% of cardiac output or 1200 ml/min, which translates to flow rate of 4 ml/g/min to the kidney.
    ii. Oxygen extraction from renal cells is high, but the amount is not significant enough to account for flow rate; rather, the flow is required to support normal renal function.
    iii. RBF is
      (a) Higher in males than in females
      (b) Increased with increasing age (until maturity), in the supine position, and in the afternoon
      (c) Decreased in the elderly, at night, and with exercise
  c. Distribution of RBF
    i. Renal tissue

       (a) Cortex: Metabolically active region, receives most (80%) of the blood supply

       (b) Medulla: Site of anaerobic metabolism, receives 20% of blood supply

    ii. Nephrons: Receive 600 to 650 ml/min of renal plasma flow

  d. Intrarenal autoregulation: General principles

    i. Mean arterial pressure (MAP) is maintained in a range of 80 to 180 mm Hg to prevent large changes in GFR.

    ii. Major site of autoregulation is the afferent arteriole.

    iii. Increase in the renal arterial pressure causes afferent vasoconstriction; decrease causes efferent vasoconstriction, producing an increased GFR/RBF ratio.

    iv. Changes in vascular tone of the efferent arteriole (primarily vasoconstriction) complement efforts to maintain GFR by compensating for reduced blood flow.

    v. Autoregulation is essentially absent at an MAP of 70 mm Hg or below.

  e. Neural control

    i. Route of nerve supply is along renal blood vessels; renal neurologic intervention is vasoconstrictive.

    ii. Hypotension decreases systemic arterial pressure, stimulating the carotid sinus and aortic arch baroreceptors to trigger the sympathetic response (release of epinephrine), which decreases RBF and GFR by vasoconstricting both afferent and efferent arterioles.

    iii. Other factors that stimulate increased sympathetic tone are stress, fear, and exercise.

    iv. This neuronal effect is not the primary factor in autoregulation; a denervated kidney can be transplanted and still be able to compensate for changes in BP.

  f. Hormonal modulation of RBF (see Renal Regulation of Blood Pressure)

    i. Renin-angiotensin system: A mechanism to sustain systemic BP and plasma volume

       (a) Responds to a decreased afferent arteriolar pressure by increasing angiotensin II levels

       (b) Angiotensin II vasoconstricts renal blood vessels, particularly the efferent artery, which reduces RBF but increases GFR.

    ii. Renal prostaglandins: Modulate the effects of vasoactive substances, such as angiotensin II, on the kidney by causing vasodilatation

  g. Pharmacologic effects

    i. Epinephrine and norepinephrine: Cause efferent arterioles to vasoconstrict, which leads to a rise in the filtration fraction and a dose-related decrease in RBF

    ii. Furosemide and mannitol: Increase GFR initially by increasing blood flow to the kidney and later by decreasing intratubular pressure

    iii. Calcium channel blockers: Relax renal arteriole and ameliorate renal failure related to renal transplantation and nephrotoxicity due to radiocontrast dyes or cyclosporine

    iv. Atrial natriuretic factor (atrial natriuretic peptide, or ANP): Improves function in oliguric acute renal failure (ARF), but not preventive

3. Body water regulation

  a. Thirst: Regulator of water intake

    i. Thirst center is located in the anterior hypothalamus.

    ii. Neuronal cells are stimulated by intracellular dehydration, which causes sensation of thirst.

    iii. Role is maintenance of satiety state (i.e., drinking exact amount of fluid to return body to normal hydration state).

  b. ADH: Sodium osmoreceptor mechanism for control of extracellular fluid (ECF) osmolality and sodium concentration

    i. ADH is synthesized in the paraventricular and supraoptic nuclei of the hypothalamus and travels along the axons of the supraopticohypophysial tract for storage or release from the posterior pituitary. The supraoptic area of the hypothalamus may overlap with the thirst center, providing integration of the thirst mechanism, osmolality detection, and ADH release.

      ii. Release of ADH occurs with the following:

         (a) Increased serum osmolality stimulates osmoreceptor cells in the hypothalamus that transmit along the neurohypophysial tracts, leading to ADH release from the posterior pituitary; normal serum osmolality is 285 to 295 mOsm/L.

         (b) Volume contraction states reverse the inhibitory effect on ADH release; controlled by stretch receptors in the left atrium that activate the ADH mechanism.

      iii. In the presence of ADH, water reabsorption occurs in the distal tubule and collecting ducts, which results in a hypertonic urine, hypotonic medullary interstitium, and eventual correction of contracted ECF.

      iv. ADH secretion is inhibited when serum osmolality decreases (water intoxication). When this occurs, the distal tubule and collecting duct become relatively impermeable to water, so that large volumes of hypotonic filtrate are delivered to the collecting duct; this results in dilute urine and excess water loss (compared with extracellular solute concentration), which returns serum osmolality to normal limits.

  c. Countercurrent mechanism of the kidney: Mechanism for the concentration and dilution of urine; adjusts urine osmolality from 50 to 1200 mOsm/L

      i. Isotonic glomerular filtrate leaves the proximal tubule and enters the loop of Henle at 300 mOsm/L.

      ii. Descending limb of the loop of Henle is permeable to water only. Water is gradually drawn into the hypertonic medullary interstitium, which gradually increases the osmolality of the filtrate as it becomes dehydrated. At the hairpin turn of the loop, osmolality is dramatically increased by the removal of water and NaCl pump action; osmolality can reach 1000 to 1200 mOsm/L. Concurrently, the medullary interstitium becomes hypotonic.

      iii. Thick ascending limb of the loop of Henle is permeable to NaCl but impermeable to water. The medullary interstitium becomes more hypertonic as its sodium concentration is increased by pumping action at the ascending limb.

      iv. A dilute filtrate reaches the distal tubule. If ADH is absent, dilute filtrate is excreted unchanged, which results in dilute urine with water excretion in excess of solute. If ADH is present, the collecting duct reabsorbs water, and concentrated urine is excreted.

4. Electrolyte regulation

  a. Sodium regulation: Normal serum concentration is 136 to 145 mEq/L solute

      i. Na^+ is the major extracellular cation and osmotically active solute. Because variation in body sodium can be associated with an exchange of water between intracellular and extracellular compartments, sodium affects ECF volume.

      ii. Renal reabsorption sites: Normal percentages of reabsorbed filtered sodium

         (a) Proximal tubule: 65% of filtered Na^+

         (b) Loop of Henle: 25%

         (c) Distal tubule: 6%

         (d) Collecting duct: 2% to 4%

      iii. Major factors that influence Na^+ excretion include GFR, the sympathetic nervous system, aldosterone, the renin-angiotensin-aldosterone system, vasopressin (ADH), and ANP (a peptide hormone that plays a role in regulating and monitoring fluid, electrolyte, and cardiovascular balance).

      iv. Sodium reabsorption increases at the renal tubules under the following conditions:

         (a) Decreased GFR resulting from renal hypoperfusion (e.g., shock): Less sodium is delivered to the renal tubules, and less is excreted

         (b) Secretion of aldosterone (a mineralocorticoid secreted by the adrenal cortex)

            (1) Major effects are to increase renal tubular reabsorption of Na^+ and to control selective renal excretion of K^+.

            (2) Increases Na^+ in ECF, which promotes water reabsorption; at the same time, K^+ is secreted into the distal tubule and collecting duct to be excreted

            (3) Regulated by K^+ concentration in the ECF, the renin-angiotensin-aldosterone mechanism, total body sodium, and adrenocorticotropic hormone (ACTH)

  (c) ANP action: Causes natriuretic, diuretic, and hypotensive effects secondary to its potent vasodilatory properties; the increased urinary excretion of Na^+ is matched by an accompanying loss of K^+ and PO_4^{3-}

  v. Sodium reabsorption decreases at the renal tubules under the following conditions:
  (a) Increased GFR (excess ECF volume): Increases renal perfusion and GFR; more sodium is delivered to the renal tubules and more is excreted in urine
  (b) Inhibition of aldosterone secretion, which results in renal Na^+ excretion
  (c) Secretion of ANP and ADH, administration of diuretics, especially loop-affecting diuretics

b. Potassium regulation: Normal serum concentration is 3.5 to 5.5 mEq/L
  i. Potassium is a major intracellular cation (K^+) necessary for the maintenance of osmolality and electroneutrality of cells.
  ii. Renal transport sites: K^+ is actively reabsorbed in the proximal tubule (60% to 70%) and thick ascending loop (10%); active and passive secretion in the distal tubule and collecting duct maintain the electroneutrality of urine. This electrical gradient is determined primarily by reabsorption of Na^+ from urine.
  iii. Factors enhancing K^+ excretion
  (a) Increase in cellular potassium via increased exchange with Na^+ (K^+ excreted in urine whereas Na^+ is reabsorbed) or via acute metabolic or respiratory alkalosis (causes movement of K^+ ions into cells)
  (b) High-volume tubular flow rates in the distal portion of the nephron: Increase the number of available K^+ ions and thus increase the excretion of potassium
  (c) Aldosterone (provides feedback mechanism for maintenance of K^+ in ECF)
  (1) Elevation of serum potassium stimulates the secretion of aldosterone.
  (2) Aldosterone acts on the distal nephrons and collecting ducts, enhancing the retention of Na^+ and excretion of K^+.
  (3) Excretion of excess K^+ eventually returns levels to normal.
  (d) Hydrogen ions: Alkalemia (associated decrease in H^+) stimulates K^+ secretion
  (e) Diuretics: Loop and thiazide diuretics block NaCl and waste reabsorption, increasing tubular flow and secretion of K^+

c. Calcium regulation: Normal serum concentration is 8.5 to 10.5 mg/dl or 2.20 to 2.60 mmol/L
  i. Major functions of calcium ions (Ca^{2+}): Generation of cardiac action potential and pacemaker function, contraction of cardiac and vascular smooth muscle, transmission of nerve impulses, blood coagulation, formation of bones and teeth, and maintenance of cellular permeability
  ii. Total serum Ca^{2+}: 40% bound to protein, 50% ionized, and 10% combined with carbonate, phosphate, citrate, and various ions
  iii. Renal transport sites: 98% of filtered Ca^{2+} is reabsorbed. Reabsorptive pathways are similar to those for sodium transport. Most active reabsorption occurs in the proximal tubule. Other sites include the loop (20% to 25%) and the distal tubule (10%).
  iv. Factors influencing Ca^{2+} reabsorption:
  (a) Parathyroid hormone (PTH)
  (1) Decrease in serum calcium stimulates secretion of PTH.
  (2) PTH stimulates tubular reabsorption of Ca^{2+} at the distal portion of the nephron, stimulates increased phosphate excretion, and mobilizes calcium and phosphate from bone.
  (b) Vitamin D: Calcium absorption from the small intestine depends on the presence of activated vitamin D (1,25-dihydroxycholecalciferol)
  (1) Activation process: Absorption of ultraviolet light converts 7-dehydrocholesterol in skin to cholecalciferol. The liver hydroxylates vitamin D to form 25-hydroxycholecalciferol. The kidney further hydroxylates to the final activated form of vitamin D (1,25-dihydroxycholecalciferol) in the proximal tubule. PTH stimulates this activation process.
  (2) Decreased serum calcium level reduces urinary Ca^{2+} excretion, so activated vitamin D must be available to absorb Ca^{2+} from the small intestine to maintain adequate serum calcium levels.

(c) Corticosteroid effect: Large doses decrease Ca^{2+} absorption in the intestines; may influence the activation of vitamin D in the liver

(d) Diuretic effect: Diuretics can cause Na^+ and Ca^{2+} excretion. Ultimate effect of reduced serum calcium is decreased excretion. A decrease in total body fluid volume leads to diminished GFR and reduced calcium excretion.

d. Phosphate regulation: Normal serum concentration is 3.0 to 4.5 mg/dl

    i. About 90% of phosphate is found in bone, 10% in intracellular and extracellular fluid spaces. Phosphates (PO_4^{3-}) play significant role in intracellular energy production and may also influence DNA, RNA, and genetic code information. Phosphates are used by the kidneys to buffer H^+.

    ii. Renal transport sites: Reabsorption of phosphate is an active process that occurs in the proximal tubule and requires Na^+. Factors influencing phosphate excretion include the following:

        (a) PTH secretion: Inhibits phosphate reabsorption (and thus promotes its excretion)

        (b) Alterations in GFR: Increased GFR decreases reabsorption of plasma phosphates and vice versa

e. Magnesium regulation: Normal serum concentration is 1.5 to 2.2 mEq/L

    i. The magnesium ion (Mg^{2+}) is the second major intracellular cation and is a significant factor in cellular enzyme systems and biochemical reactions.

    ii. Mg^{2+} may have a role in the management of acute myocardial infarction (MI), because magnesium administration decreases the mortality rate in MI by 24% and improves ventricular function by 25%. Benefits may be attributed to magnesium's ability to enhance coronary blood flow, conserve potassium, improve cellular function, and diminish dysrhythmias.

    iii. Renal transport site: The reabsorptive process is similar to that of Ca^{2+} and is linked to Na^+ reabsorption along the renal tubules

    iv. Factors influencing reabsorption include the availability of sodium (Na^+ is necessary for reabsorption) and the availability of PTH (has minimal effect on Mg^{2+} reabsorption).

f. Chloride regulation: Normal serum concentration is 96 to 106 mEq/L

    i. Renal transport sites: Reabsorbed with Na^+ at all Na^+ absorptive sites in the nephron

    ii. Factors influencing excretion include acidosis (HCO_3^- reabsorbed whereas Cl^- excreted to maintain electrochemical balance) and alkalosis (HCO_3^- excreted as Cl^- reabsorbed)

5. Excretion of metabolic waste products: Excretion is a primary renal function. The kidney excretes more than 200 metabolic waste products. The products measured for interpretation of renal function are blood urea nitrogen (BUN) and serum creatinine.

a. Urea: Nitrogen waste product of protein metabolism filtered and reabsorbed along the entire nephron

    i. Is an unreliable indicator of GFR, because urea excretion is influenced by

        (a) Urine flow (decrease in urine flow rate may allow for reabsorption of urea)

        (b) Extrarenal factors (e.g., hypoperfusion states or drugs such as corticosteroids)

        (c) Gastrointestinal (GI) bleeding or catabolic states such as fever or infection

        (d) Changes in protein intake or metabolism

    ii. Elevation in BUN level without an associated rise in creatinine level (>25:1 ratio) suggests

        (a) Volume depletion, low renal perfusion pressure

        (b) Severe catabolic process or trauma with massive muscle injury (e.g., burns)

        (c) GI bleeding with blood collection in intestines

    iii. Elevated levels of both BUN and creatinine (at a 10:1 ratio) indicate renal disease.

b. Creatinine: A waste product of muscle metabolism

    i. Amount produced daily is proportional to muscle mass, and production occurs at a constant rate.

    ii. Normal kidney excretes creatinine at a rate equal to RBF or GFR.

    iii. Creatinine is freely filtered, so its production normally equals its excretion, which makes it a reliable indicator of kidney function.

    iv. Elevated serum creatinine level is directly correlated with deterioration in renal function.

6. **Renal regulation of acid-base balance: The kidneys regulate acid-base balance by minimizing wide variations in body fluid balance in conjunction with retaining or excreting hydrogen ions. Acid-base balance is also regulated by the lungs and the body buffers (serum bicarbonate, blood, and plasma proteins).**

  a. Bicarbonate (HCO_3^-) reabsorption

    i. Primarily occurs in the proximal tubule with less in the distal tubule; occurs with reabsorption of Na^+

    ii. Occurs if the filtrate contains more than 28 mEq/L (Tm) as in acidemia, volume contraction

  b. Hydrogen ion secretion

    i. Passive secretion occurs in the proximal tubule; active secretion occurs distally in exchange for Na^+.

    ii. Acid is buffered by ammonia (NH_3^+) or phosphate (HPO_4^{2-}) before excretion, which provides for hydrogen (H^+) excretion without lowering pH.

    iii. H secretion is increased during acidemia and decreased during alkalemia.

  c. Renal buffers of hydrogen ions

    i. Buffers that are filtered by the glomerulus

      (a) HCO_3^- is completely reabsorbed (up to 28 mEq/L).

      (b) Phosphate (PO_4^{3-}) is secreted and then reacts with hydrogen.

      (c) $H^+ + HPO_4^{2-} = H_2PO_4^-$

    ii. Buffers produced by the kidney tubule

      (a) HCO_3^- can be synthesized in the distal tubule when H^+, excreted into urine as HCO_3^-, is delivered by ECF with Na^+. H^+ and HCO_3^- both come from the distal tubule cell as a result of ionization of carbonic acid (H_2CO_3); thus

$$H_2CO_3 \underset{}{\overset{CA}{\rightleftharpoons}} H^+ + HCO_3^-$$

      where CA is carbonic anhydrase.

      (b) Carbonic acid comes from hydration of carbon dioxide (CO_2) via CA:

$$H_2O + CO_2 \underset{}{\overset{CA}{\rightleftharpoons}} H_2CO_3$$

      (c) CO_2 is derived from either cellular metabolism or dissolved CO_2 in venous blood; thus new HCO_3^- can be made in the distal tubule from extraurinary sources.

      (d) Complete equation

$$H_2O + CO_2 \overset{CA}{\rightleftharpoons} H_2CO_3 \overset{CA}{\rightleftharpoons} H^+ + HCO_3^-$$

  d. Summary of renal responses to acidemia

    i. H^+ secretion is increased at the distal tubule with increased excretion of titratable acids (HPO_4^{2-}).

    ii. All HCO_3^- is reabsorbed in the proximal tubule.

    iii. Ammonium is produced to accommodate H^+ excretion: $NH_3^+ + H^+ \rightleftharpoons NH_4^+$.

    iv. Urinary pH can be as low as 4.5 for excretion of a more acid urine in the presence of acidemia.

  e. Summary of renal responses to alkalemia

    i. H^+ secretion in the distal tubule is decreased.

    ii. Excess HCO_3^- is excreted.

    iii. Production of NH_4^+ is decreased.

    iv. Urine is alkaline, with a pH over 7.

7. **Renal regulation of blood pressure: Involves five mechanisms:**

  a. Maintenance of volume and composition of ECF

    i. Normal plasma volume is essential for control of BP.

    ii. Alterations in plasma volume eventually affect BP. Reduction of plasma volume lowers arterial BP, leading to compensation by vasoconstriction. Expansion of plasma volume increases cardiac preload and, in accordance with Starling's curve, raises BP.

  b. Aldosterone–body sodium balance, which determines ECF volume: Aldosterone stimulates renal tubular reabsorption of Na^+ in exchange for excretion of primarily K^+ ions

  c. Renin-angiotensin-aldosterone system: Preserves BP and avoids serious volume reduction

    i. Juxtaglomerular apparatus: Granular cells contain inactivated renin. Factors that trigger juxtaglomerular cells to release renin reflect diminished GFR (e.g., reduced arterial BP in afferent and efferent arterioles, reduced Na^+ content or concentration at distal tubule, sympathetic stimulation of kidneys).

    ii. Renin, an enzyme, is released from juxtaglomerular cells into the afferent arteriole.

    iii. On entering the circulation, renin acts on angiotensinogen to split away the vasoactive peptide angiotensin I and convert it to angiotensin II. Requires the presence of angiotensin-converting enzyme (ACE), found primarily in the lung and liver but also in the kidney and all blood vessels. Angiotensin II is a potent systemic vasoconstrictor.

    iv. Circulatory effect of angiotensin II on arterial BP

      (a) Significant peripheral arteriole constriction with moderate venous constriction occurs, which results in the reduction of vascular volume.

      (b) Renal arteriolar constriction results in the renal retention of sodium and water; this expands ECF volume, thus increasing arterial BP.

    v. Fluid volume response to angiotensin II restores effective circulating volume in the following ways:

      (a) Angiotensin II stimulates aldosterone release, which enhances Na^+ reabsorption.

      (b) Vasoconstriction to further decrease GFR leads to Na^+ reabsorption.

      (c) The thirst mechanism is stimulated.

  d. Renal prostaglandins: Modulating effect

    i. Major renal prostaglandins are prostaglandins E_2, D_2, I_2 (vasodilators), and A_2 (vasoconstrictor).

    ii. Physiologic role is modulation, amplification, and inhibition. Vasoactive substances (angiotensin, norepinephrine, bradykinins) stimulate the synthesis and release of prostaglandins. Prostaglandins modulate the action of the vasoactive substances.

    iii. Prostaglandins diminish arterial BP and increase RBF by arterial vasodilation and inhibition of the distal tubules' response to ADH. Suppressed ADH response leads to sodium and water excretion, which ultimately decreases the effective circulatory volume.

    iv. Pharmacologic prostaglandin inhibitors are the nonsteroidal anti-inflammatory drugs (NSAIDs). In cases of compromised renal function avoid the use of NSAIDs (i.e., salicylic acid, ibuprofen [Motrin], indomethacin [Indocin], and naproxen [Naprosyn]).

    v. Loop diuretics stimulate prostaglandin secretion, which leads to vasodilation and decreased preload.

  e. Kallikrein-kinin system: Renal kallikreins are proteases that release kinins and are excreted in the urine. Kinins stimulate both the renin-angiotensin and prostaglandin systems, appearing to link renal hemodynamics and fluid-electrolyte excretion.

8. RBC synthesis and maturation

  a. Erythropoietin secretion: Stimulates the production of erythrocytes in the bone marrow and prolongs the life of erythrocytes

  b. Mechanism of erythropoietin synthesis and secretion

    i. Renal cortical interstitial cells produce erythropoietin, a glycosylated, 165-amino-acid protein.

    ii. Renal erythropoietin production accounts for 90% of RBC production; the remaining 10% is produced by the liver.

    iii. Hypoxia stimulates renal erythropoietin production; the liver is not as responsive to hypoxia and therefore cannot support erythropoiesis in renal failure.

  c. Erythropoietin deficiency: Primary cause of anemia in chronic renal failure (CRF); bleeding is the second most common cause

9. **Aging kidney**
   a. Age-related changes can occur as early as 20 to 40 years of age. Changes include a decrease in tubular length and, at and over age 40 years, a progressive decrease in the percentage of glomeruli. Generally, renal function is diminished by 10% at age 65 years; may diminish further with aging.
   b. Renal response in the elderly
      i. Decreased renal mass associated with a diminished number of nephrons
      ii. Decreased GFR; diminished RBF secondary to age-related changes in vasculature
      iii. Diminished creatinine production ($10 \, mL/min/1.73 \, m^2$ per decade) and diminished ability to excrete creatinine; therefore, change in serum creatinine level may not be evident. Uric acid levels are slightly increased.
      iv. Decreased serum renin and aldosterone levels reduce the ability to conserve sodium, impair urinary water excretion, and limit urinary concentration.

Patient Assessment

1. **Nursing history**
   a. Patient health history
      i. Previous health problems: Indicate the presence of or predisposition to renal disease
         (a) Kidney and/or urinary tract disease
         (b) Cardiovascular disease
            (1) Hypertension: BP control and treatment may prevent or halt renal damage; hypertension develops in 70% to 80% of patients with advanced renal failure
            (2) Heart failure with diminished renal perfusion
            (3) Atherosclerosis
         (c) Diabetes mellitus: Renal disease caused by vascular disease alterations, infection, or neuropathy
         (d) Immunologic disorders, recent infections (streptococcal)
         (e) Pulmonary disease (Goodpasture's syndrome)
         (f) Allergies, recent blood transfusions (history of incompatibility reaction)
         (g) Other: Toxemia of pregnancy, renal transplantation, anemia, recent surgery, dialysis, exposure to drugs and toxins, renal calculi, azotemia, hematuria, exposure to chemicals or poisons
      ii. History of specific signs and symptoms
         (a) Signs and symptoms of urinary tract disorders
            (1) Dysuria
            (2) Abnormal appearance of urine
               a) Hematuria (grossly bloody)
               b) Pyuria (cloudy)
               c) Biliuria or bilirubinuria (orange)
               d) Myoglobinuria (usually clear; red-brown urine; Hematest positive)
            (3) Urine frequency, urgency, incontinence, hesitancy; nocturia
            (4) Polydipsia
            (5) Patterns of urine output
               a) Normal volume: Approximately 1500 ml/24 hr
               b) Oliguria: Less than 400 ml/24 hr
               c) Anuria: Less than 50 ml to no output over 24 hours
               d) Polyuria: Excessive output exceeding 24-hour intake
               e) Nonoliguria: Normal or excess urine volume in the presence of ARF
            (6) Fever
            (7) Pain in costovertebral angle, flank, or groin
            (8) Pattern of weight gain or loss; dry weight is the ideal weight that minimizes symptomatology for a patient with renal failure as achieved by a dialysis treatment
   b. Family health history: Genetic renal disease accounts for about 30% of azotemia. Genetically transmitted diseases that can cause or precipitate renal disease include the following:

          i.   Cardiovascular disease, hypertension
          ii. Diabetes mellitus
          iii. Gout
          iv. Malignancy
          v.   Polycystic kidney disease and medullary cystic disease
          vi. Hereditary nephritis (Alport's syndrome)
          vii. Renal calculi

c. Social history and habits
      i.   Social history: Sexual activity prior to renal disease and sexual dysfunction related to renal disease
      ii. Habits
          (a) Dietary habits
              (1) Dietary and fluid restrictions; compliance or noncompliance with these restrictions
              (2) Dietary intake: Number and nutritional value of meals
          (b) Exercise
          (c) Frequency, type, quantity of caffeine, tobacco, alcohol, or illicit drugs

d. Medication history
      i.   Nephrotoxic agents: Radiocontrast dye and antibiotic therapy (tetracyclines, aminoglycosides, gentamicin, amphotericin B)
      ii. Diuretics, antihypertensives
      iii. Cardiac glycosides (digoxin), antiarrhythmic agents
      iv. Electrolyte replacement therapy
      v.   Immunosuppressives
          (a) Corticosteroids
          (b) Azathioprine, cyclophosphamide, antithymocyte globulin (ATG), cyclosporine, monoclonal antibody (OKT3), tacrolimus (FK-506)
      vi. Analgesics such as meperidine (Demerol)

2. Nursing examination of patient
  a. Physical examination data
      i.   Inspection
          (a) Diminished level of consciousness (lethargy, coma)
          (b) Skin
              (1) Abnormal color: Grayish tinge from anemia, yellowish tinge if retained carotenoids or urochrome pigments in uremia
              (2) Capillary integrity: Easily bruised
              (3) Skin turgor
              (4) Purpura lesions: Present in some forms of renal failure
          (c) Eye: Cataracts, periorbital edema
          (d) Ear: Nerve deafness (Alport's syndrome)
          (e) Edema
              (1) Significance depends on amount of water and Na^+ retained.
              (2) Edema of renal failure is often related to hypoalbuminemia.
          (f) Respiration: May see rate and pattern similar to Kussmaul's respirations
          (g) Muscle tremors, weakness, weight loss with uremic syndrome
          (h) Tetany: Positive Chvostek's and Trousseau's signs; rarely observed; result from severe hypocalcemia or very rapid correction of acidosis
          (i) Asterixis: Indicates progressive uremic state
              (1) Ask the patient to face the examiner and raise the upper extremities in a fixed hyperextension position.
              (2) Palms (fingers separated) must be visible to the examiner.
              (3) Positive sign—irregular movements of the wrists, flapping movements of the fingers—occurs within 30 seconds.
          (j) Fatigue: Occurs with activities of daily living and exercise, and at rest
          (k) Mobility: Extent and strength with ambulation
          (l) Nutritional status

(1) Triceps skinfold thickness (normal is >25 mm for men, >15 mm for women)
(2) Anemia: Pale skin, weakness, shortness of breath
(3) Tolerance of diet: Nausea and vomiting; likes and dislikes
(4) Weight loss
(m) Arteriovenous access: Type, patency, signs of infection
ii. Palpation: To determine size and shape of the kidney and to check for tenderness, cysts, and masses
(a) Right kidney is easier to palpate because it is lower in the abdomen.
(b) Palpate the bladder for urinary distention due to obstruction.
(c) Palpate the flank area to elicit tenderness or pain.
(d) Palpate pulses for a baseline reading and to determine abnormalities.
iii. Percussion
(a) At costovertebral angles to elicit pain or tenderness associated with
(1) Pyelonephritis
(2) Calculi
(3) Renal abscess
(4) Intermittent hydronephrosis
(b) At abdomen for the presence of ascites
iv. Auscultation: Listen for aortic and renal artery bruits (heard in flanks or intercostal regions of anterior abdomen)
b. Monitoring data: Intake and output (I&O), body weight, and central venous pressure (CVP) to determine relationship between cardiac filling pressures and hydration status; correlate findings with daily weight
3. **Appraisal of patient characteristics: Patients with acute, life-threatening renal problems come to progressive care units with a wide range of biochemical, metabolic, and psychosocial clinical characteristics. During their stay, their clinical status may significantly improve or deteriorate, slowly or abruptly change, involve one or all life-sustaining functions, and be readily monitored or nearly impossible to monitor with precision. Some attributes of patients with acute renal disorders that the nurse needs to assess are the following:**
a. Resiliency
i. Level 1—*Minimally resilient:* Any patient with end-stage CRF receiving hemodialysis, whose condition is deteriorating and who is awaiting transfer to a critical care unit
ii. Level 3—*Moderately resilient:* A 58-year-old patient on postoperative day 5 after uncomplicated coronary artery bypass graft surgery who received prophylactic intraoperative IV therapy to prevent renal involvement but still developed and is recovering from nonoliguric ARF
iii. Level 5—*Highly resilient:* Any patient with an isolated episode of a prerenal ARF resulting from dehydration with no significant alteration in hemodynamics, receiving hydration
b. Vulnerability
i. Level 1—*Highly vulnerable:* A 65-year-old male patient with diabetes and cardiovascular complications who has a inaccessible graft and whose condition becomes unstable during insertion of a temporary catheter
ii. Level 3—*Moderately vulnerable:* A 24-year-old woman with acute postrenal failure from infected renal calculi who is scheduled for surgery today
iii. Level 5—*Minimally vulnerable:* A 32-year-old single woman with a urinary tract infection (UTI)
c. Stability
i. Level 1—*Minimally stable:* Any patient whose condition is unstable and who is awaiting transfer to a critical care unit
ii. Level 3—*Moderately stable:* A patient with end-stage CRF and malignant hypertension whose BP is beginning to respond to a new therapeutic regimen of antihypertensive agents including ACE inhibitors
iii. Level 5—*Highly stable:* A 36-year-old patient with lupus nephritis in early stages of CRF who requires a protein-restricted diet and is compliant with the medical regimen

d. Complexity

    i. Level 1—*Highly complex:* A 36-year-old elementary school teacher with chronic diabetic renal disease who decided to terminate dialysis treatment and is now in a uremic coma, and whose family does not agree with her decision

    ii. Level 3—*Moderately complex:* A 21-year-old college student who is approaching end-stage renal failure and feels conflicted because two of his younger siblings are a tissue match and are both eager to donate a kidney

    iii. Level 5—*Minimally complex:* A 46-year-old man with CRF who complies with his medical regimen, is given dialysis at home by his supportive wife, and is now admitted for an acute repair of his arteriovenous fistula

e. Resource availability

    i. Level 1—*Few resources:* A 50-year-old Russian immigrant who has been in the United States 2 weeks when it is determined that he requires hemodialysis; he is not insured and is not eligible for state assistance, and his family cannot offer financial support

    ii. Level 3—*Moderate resources:* A middle-aged patient who needs renal transplantation; he has four siblings who offered to donate but none is a tissue match, so he places himself on the cadaveric organ donor list

    iii. Level 5—*Many resources:* Mrs. Jones, a well-respected elementary school nurse for the past 15 years, who has been effectively managing her own continuous ambulatory peritoneal dialysis for 5 years

f. Participation in care

    i. Level 1—*No participation:* A 26-year-old quadriplegic patient with nephrotoxic acute tubular necrosis (ATN) secondary to carbenicillin administered for an antibiotic-resistant UTI who requires 2 weeks of dialysis after which kidney function should return

    ii. Level 3—*Moderate participation:* A blind man with diabetes who is taught how to perform his own peritoneal dialysis at night with the assistance of his wife

    iii. Level 5—*Full participation:* A patient who has had a successful renal transplant for the past 3 years and makes a practice of visiting local hemodialysis units and teaching the benefits of transplantation as a treatment option

g. Participation in decision making

    i. Level 1—*No participation:* A 70-year-old mentally retarded male patient with advanced chronic kidney disease who is approaching the need for dialysis and lives with his 95-year-old mother, who has periods of senility

    ii. Level 3—*Moderate participation:* A 32-year-old woman in whom renal cancer was recently diagnosed and who has a history of admissions for psychosis and is estranged from most of her family except her 29-year-old sister

    iii. Level 5—*Full participation:* A patient who, after running a marathon, spends a week in the intensive care unit (ICU) recovering from an episode of ARF secondary to rhabdomyolysis; he is surrounded by his family, friends, and representatives from his community, who offer their support during his recovery at home

h. Predictability

    i. Level 1—*Not predictable:* Any patient in whom ATN develops after an extensive period of hypotension and who has repeated episodes of severe dehydration, systemic infection, and exposure to nephrotoxic agents during recovery

    ii. Level 3—*Moderately predictable:* Any patient in whom contrast media–induced ATN develops, when renal involvement is identified early and hydration and loop diuretics are administered

    iii. Level 5—*Highly predictable:* A patient with a relatively uncomplicated condition in whom nonoliguric ATN develops after a short episode of hypotension, which is easily reversed, and who has an uneventful recovery period

4. Diagnostic studies

    a. Laboratory

        i. Blood

            (a) Complete blood cell count: Reduced hematocrit and hemoglobin levels may reflect bleeding or a lack of erythropoietin

            (b) Serum creatinine: To estimate GFR (normal level, 0.6 to 1.2 mg/dl)

■ **TABLE 5-1**
■ ■ **Interpretation of BUN and Serum Creatinine Levels**

Condition	Ratio of BUN to Creatinine	BUN	Serum Creatinine
Normal	20:1	10-20 mg/100 ml	0.6-1.2 mg/100 ml
Prerenal disease	≥25:1	↑	Normal or slight elevation
Renal disease (acute or chronic)	10:1	↑	↑

BUN, Blood urea nitrogen.

(1) Creatinine excretion is proportional to its production.
(2) A significant elevation in creatinine level is associated with renal disease and correlates with percentage of nephrons damaged.
(c) BUN: Normal level, 10 to 20 mg/dl (Table 5-1)
  (1) Prerenal problem: Ratio of BUN to serum creatinine equal to or greater than 25:1 suggests extrarenal problem (dehydration, catabolic state). Elevation in both BUN and creatinine results from decreased GFR.
  (2) Renal failure: Caused by nephron damage
(d) Serum chemistry tests (calcium, phosphate, alkaline phosphatase, bilirubin, uric acid, sodium, potassium, chloride, carbon dioxide, magnesium, glucose, cholesterol)
(e) Baseline arterial blood gas (ABG) levels, clotting profile
(f) Serum osmolality, total protein and albumin
ii. Urine
  (a) Visual examination for color and clarity
    (1) Clear and colorless in hyposthenuria
    (2) Cloudy when infection is present
    (3) Foamy when albumin is present
  (b) Osmolality (50 to 1200 mOsm/kg)
  (c) SG: Wide range of normal values (1.003 to 1.030); provides reasonable estimate of urinary osmolality; actually measures density
    (1) Low normal (<1.010): Suspect diabetes insipidus, overhydration, or heart failure
    (2) Above normal (>1.030): Occurs in proteinuria, glycosuria, severe dehydration, presence of x-ray contrast medium
  (d) Creatinine clearance (C_{cr}): 24-hour urine collection
    (1) Purpose: To determine the presence and progression of renal disease, estimate percentage of functioning nephrons, or determine specific medication dosages
    (2) In 24 hours, the following occurs:

$$\frac{(U_{cr} \times V)}{P_{cr}} = C_{cr}$$

where
U_{cr} = Amount of urinary creatinine excreted
V = Urine volume per minute
P_{cr} = Plasma creatinine level
    (3) In average-sized patients, a satisfactory 24-hour urine collection always has approximately 1 g of creatinine, regardless of the degree of renal function.
  (e) Culture and sensitivity: Check for infection
  (f) pH (normal range, 4.5 to 8; average value, 6); alkaline urine is frequently seen with infection; in absence of infection, possibly indicates renal tubular acidosis if both alkaline urine and systemic acidosis are present

(g) Glucose: In urine when renal threshold for glucose exceeded
(h) Acetone: In urine with starvation or diabetic ketoacidosis; a false-positive result can occur in patients taking salicylates
(i) Protein: Expressed quantitatively as 1+ to 4+; diagnostic for the presence of glomerular membrane disease (nephritic syndrome) and allows the detection of myeloma proteins causing renal failure
(j) Spot urine electrolytes
    (1) Measure urinary concentrations of Na^+, K^+, Cl^-.
    (2) Screening test for tubular function; assess the kidney's ability to conserve sodium and concentrate urine
(k) Urinary sediment
    (1) Casts: Precipitations of protein in the kidney that take the shape of the tubules in which they are formed
        a) Hyaline casts: Entirely protein; small amounts are normal in urine; if large amounts, suspect significant proteinuria such as albumin or myeloma protein in urine
        b) Erythrocyte casts: Diagnostic for active glomerulonephritis or vasculitis
        c) Leukocyte casts: Indicative of an infectious process and intrarenal inflammation
        d) Granular casts: Small number, possibly the result of degenerating erythrocyte or leukocyte casts indicative of an infectious process or an allergic interstitial nephritis
        e) Fatty casts: Abundant in nephrotic syndrome
        f) Renal tubular casts: Seen in ARF
    (2) Bacteria: Presence determined by Gram stain
    (3) Erythrocytes: Small numbers normal; in abundance during active glomerulonephritis, interstitial nephritis, malignancies, and infection
    (4) Leukocytes: Small numbers normal; present in infection and interstitial nephritis
    (5) Renal epithelial cells: Rarely seen; present in abundance during ATN, nephrotoxic injury, and allergic reaction in the kidney
    (6) Crystals: Seen in diseases of stone formation or following certain intoxications
    (7) Eosinophils: Indicate allergic reaction in the kidney
b. Radiologic
    i. Plain abdominal x-ray study: Determines position, shape, and size of the kidney and identifies calcification in the urinary system
    ii. Intravenous pyelography (IVP)
        (a) Visualizes the urinary tract for diagnosing partial obstruction, renovascular hypertension, tumor, cyst, congenital abnormality
        (b) Complications include allergic reaction to dye, dehydration
        (c) Contraindicated in the presence of the following:
            (1) Poor renal function: Dye's dehydrating effect and nephrotoxicity may further compromise function
            (2) Multiple myeloma: IVP dye may precipitate myeloma protein in the kidney
            (3) Pregnancy: Abdominal irradiation should be avoided
            (4) Heart failure: Osmotic effect of dye can compromise cardiac function by expanding vascular volume
            (5) Diabetes mellitus
            (6) Sickle cell anemia: Dye's elevation of renal oncotic pressure can promote renal tissue sickling, infarction
    iii. Renal scan: Determines renal perfusion and function; can provide information about obstructions and renal masses. Radioactive dye is taken up by normal kidney tubule cells. A decrease in uptake indicates hypoperfusion. Often used to assess renal transplants.
    iv. Retrograde pyelography: Used to examine upper region of collecting system

    v. Retrograde urethrography: Used to examine the urethra

    vi. Cystoscopy: Detects bladder or urethral pathology

    vii. Renal arteriography (angiography): Identifies tumors and distinguishes type of renal or renovascular disease. Potential complications can be serious:

        (a) Allergic reaction to dye can cause same complications seen with IVP dye.

        (b) Puncture of a peripheral artery, with consequent hematoma, embolism, or thrombus formation, is the greatest technical risk.

    viii. Voiding cystourethrography: Identifies abnormalities of lower urinary tract, urethra, bladder to detect reflux and residual urine

    ix. Diagnostic ultrasonography: Identifies hydronephrosis, differentiates solid and cystic tumors, localizes cysts or fluid collections

    x. Computed tomography (CT): Identifies tumors and other pathologic conditions that create variations in body density (e.g., abscess or lymphocele); used in renal trauma to determine reason for acute flank pain

    xi. Magnetic resonance imaging (MRI)

        (a) Provides better tissue characterization than CT; provides direct imaging in several planes for detection of renal cystic disease, inflammatory processes, and renal cell carcinoma

        (b) Detects alterations in blood flow (i.e., slow or absent flow)

        (c) Identifies morphologic changes in renal transplant

    xii. Magnetic resonance urography: A form of magnetic imaging that offers results similar to those of an IVP, without the use of dye

    xiii. Chest radiography: Identifies pulmonary edema, cardiomegaly, left ventricular hypertrophy, uremic lung, Goodpasture's disease, and infection

  c. Kidney biopsy: The most common invasive diagnostic tool

    i. For renal disease that cannot be definitively diagnosed by other means

    ii. Determines cause and extent of lesions; helpful in planning treatment

    iii. Types of biopsy

        (a) Open: For severe anatomic deformities or if a "deep specimen" is needed for diagnosis; contraindications to open biopsy include bleeding tendency, hydronephrosis, hypertension, cystic disease, and neoplasms

        (b) Closed: A simple percutaneous procedure; used more frequently than open procedure

Patient Care

1. Overhydration: A state in which an individual experiences fluid retention and edema because kidneys are unable to excrete excess body water

  a. Description of problem

    i. Intake greater than output

    ii. Weight gain with oliguria or anuria, low SG (≤1.015), dilute urine

    iii. Elevated BP, bounding pulses, neck vein distention; elevated CVP, and muffled heart sounds

    iv. Edema: Peripheral, anasarcous, ascitic, periorbital, pulmonary

    v. Dyspnea, orthopnea, crackles on auscultation, pulmonary congestion

    vi. Decreased (diluted) hemoglobin, hematocrit, and electrolyte values

    vii. Anxiety, restlessness, stupor (seen with water intoxication)

  b. Goals of care

    i. Patient maintains dry weight.

    ii. BP and CVP are normal.

    iii. Patient is free of edema.

    iv. Breath sounds are clear bilaterally.

    v. I&O are balanced.

  c. Collaborating professionals on health care team

    i. Progressive care nurse

    ii. Intensivist or physician

    iii. Nurse practitioner, clinical nurse specialist, or physician assistant

      iv. Case manager

      v. Dietitian

      vi. Nephrology consultant

      vii. Hemodialysis nurse (if dialysis indicated)

  d. Interventions

      i. Identify presence of common causes of fluid volume excess.

         (a) Expanded total body water volume secondary to renal failure with oliguria or anuria

         (b) Expanded blood volume due to renal sodium retention

         (c) Lower plasma oncotic pressure due to loss of plasma proteins

         (d) Increased capillary permeability

      ii. Document I&O; compare with daily weight; consider insensible losses—fluid losses via lungs, skin, and bowel (600 to 800 ml/day).

      iii. Assess renal function.

         (a) Urine volume, urinalysis, creatinine clearance, and BUN/creatinine ratio

         (b) Spot electrolytes, urine concentration (SG, osmolality)

         (c) 24-Hour urine collection for protein evaluation

      iv. Restrict fluids in overhydration associated with impaired renal function, impaired cardiac function, or syndrome of inappropriate secretion of antidiuretic hormone (SIADH).

      v. Administer diuretics (preferably loop) if renal response is a GFR of 25 ml/min or higher.

      vi. Consider acute dialysis with ultrafiltration for rapid volume removal.

  e. Evaluation of patient care

      i. 24-Hour I&O balance is negative or zero.

      ii. There is no edema, as evidenced by absence of adventitious breath sounds and hypertension.

2. Dehydration: A state in which an individual experiences vascular, cellular, or intracellular volume depletion due to active fluid loss. Dehydration may occur in the diuretic phase of ARF or as a result of aggressive diuretic therapy.

  a. Description of problem

      i. Output greater than intake

      ii. Weight loss with elevated SG ($\geq$1.020), concentrated urine, variable urinary output

         (a) Polyuric phase: Large volume of dilute urine with low SG

         (b) Dehydration with normal renal function: Oliguria, concentrated urine with an elevated SG

      iii. Hypotension, increased pulse, decreased CVP

      iv. Thirst, dry skin and mucous membranes, poor skin turgor

      v. Increased body temperature

      vi. Weakness, stupor (seen with severe hypovolemia)

  b. Goals of care

      i. Patient's weight is normal and stable.

      ii. Vital signs and hemodynamic parameters are normal.

      iii. Fluid balance and urine output are within normal limits (WNL).

  c. Collaborating professionals on health care team: See Overhydration

  d. Interventions

      i. Identify common causes of fluid deficit.

         (a) Renal water losses

            (1) Diuretic abuse

            (2) Salt-wasting nephropathies

            (3) Diabetes insipidus (nephrogenic, central)

            (4) Osmotic or postobstruction diuresis

         (b) GI losses

            (1) Diarrhea, vomiting, nasogastric suction

            (2) Fistula and wound drainage

            (3) GI bleeding

           (c) Skin: Insensible losses

           (d) Third-spacing (ECF) phenomena

    ii.   Document I&O; compare with daily weight.

    iii. Administer fluid therapy.

           (a) Fluid challenge to increase RBF and urinary excretion

           (b) Caution for fluid challenge: Monitor for pulmonary edema and renal failure unresponsive to volume expansion (i.e., no increase in urinary output)

           (c) Follow with replacement fluid therapy until volume goal achieved, then proceed to maintenance fluid regimen.

    iv. Assess renal function.

           (a) Urine volume, creatinine clearance, BUN/creatinine ratio

           (b) Urinalysis; urine concentration (SG, urine osmolality), spot electrolytes

           (c) 24-Hour urine collection for protein evaluation

e. Evaluation of patient care

    i.   The 24-hour I&O balance is positive or zero.

    ii.   Patient has stable, normal weight.

    iii. Vital signs and hemodynamic parameters are normal.

    iv. Urine volume and SG are normal.

3. Malnutrition

  a. Description of problem: Malnutrition is associated with increased morbidity in CRF, especially in the presence of hypoalbuminemia. Dietary protein intake is restricted to preserve kidney function in early stages of chronic kidney disease. Protein restriction can contribute to malnutrition.

  b. Goals of care

    i.   Patient's intake meets nutritional requirements.

    ii.   Patient maintains stable baseline weight and adequate muscle mass.

    iii. Serum protein and albumin, BUN, and creatinine levels are normal.

  c. Collaborating professionals on health care team: See Overhydration

  d. Interventions

    i.   Identify cause of inadequate nutritional intake; direct care there.

    ii.   Teach appetite-enhancing measures.

           (a) Provide oral hygiene before meals.

           (b) Give small, frequent meals.

           (c) Identify preferred foods, especially those high in complex carbohydrates and essential amino acids.

    iii. Teach the necessary elements of the renal patient's diet.

           (a) Essential amino acids, adequate calories, vitamin and iron supplements (folic acid, multivitamins) as warranted

           (b) Adjusted protein and electrolyte intake (Na^+ and K^+) to avoid uremic symptoms and electrolyte imbalances. Excessively diminished protein intake causes use of protein stored in muscles, which leads to body muscle wasting. Providing increased calories can help avoid this situation.

    iv. Monitor pattern of changes in weight and nutritional intake.

    v.   Assess for noncompliance with dietary instructions.

  e. Evaluation of patient care

    i.   Body weight and muscle mass remain WNL.

    ii.   Serum protein, albumin, BUN, and creatinine levels are at or approach normal limits.

4. Hypertension

  a. Description of problem

    i.   In renal failure, the hypertensive state (diastolic BP >90 mm Hg, systolic BP >140 mm Hg) is usually created by fluid retention and/or stimulation of the renin-angiotensin mechanism; preexisting hypertension is common.

    ii.   Clinical findings: See Chapter 3

  b. Goals of care (see Chapter 3): Goal in CRF is systolic BP 130 mm Hg or lower and diastolic BP 80 to 85 mm Hg or lower

c. Collaborating professionals on health care team: See Chapter 3
d. Interventions (see Chapter 3): Treatment of hypertension in an aggressive manner with a diuretic, ACE inhibitor, β-blocker, and/or possibly calcium channel blocker has the benefit of slowing the progression of CRF

    i. Administer diuretics, as ordered, to treat edema and hypertension.

        (a) General characteristics of diuretics

            (1) Diuretics inhibit the active transport of sodium or chloride, resulting in an increase in urine output.

            (2) The diuretic effect reduces effective plasma circulating volume, thereby lowering BP.

        (b) Complications

            (1) Volume depletion

            (2) Hypokalemia, hyponatremia, hypochloremia

            (3) Hyperkalemia, hyperuricemia, azotemia

            (4) Metabolic alkalosis

        (c) Types of diuretics: Used as single therapy to treat hypertension or with other antihypertensive agents to enhance their therapeutic effect

            (1) Osmotic diuretic: A nonabsorbable solute (mannitol)

                a) Exerts an osmotic effect, causing water diuresis in excess of NaCl

                b) Side effects: Blurred vision, rhinitis, rebound plasma volume expansion, thirst, urinary retention, and fluid and electrolyte imbalance

            (2) Loop diuretics: The most potent diuretics available (furosemide, indapamide, bumetanide, torsemide, and ethacrynic acid). The primary site of action is the thick segment of the medullary ascending loop of Henle.

                a) Block the reabsorption of NaCl, thus contributing to a large diuresis of isotonic urine; potassium excretion also enhanced

                b) Increase RBF by stimulating increased secretion of prostaglandin, which exerts a vasodilatory effect on renal vasculature leading to reduction in preload

                c) Vasodilatory effect of loop diuretics can be minimized, if the cardiovascular effect is negative, by the administration of ACE inhibitors.

                d) Increase GFR even with a decrease in ECF volume, because the tubuloglomerular feedback mechanism is blocked

                e) Side effects: Volume depletion, agranulocytosis, thrombocytopenia, transient deafness, abdominal discomfort, hypokalemia, hypomagnesemia, metabolic alkalosis, and hyperglycemia

                f) Prolonged use without electrolyte replacement results in all other electrolyte imbalances.

            (3) Thiazides (hydrochlorothiazide, chlorthalidone, and metolazone)

                a) Sodium reabsorption inhibited in the ascending loop of Henle and the beginning portion of the distal tubule

                b) Increased potassium excretion occurs with a weak carbonic anhydrase inhibitory effect.

                c) Side effects: Rashes, leukopenia, thrombocytopenia, hypercalcemia, and acute pancreatitis

            (4) Potassium-sparing diuretics (spironolactone, amiloride, triamterene): Aldosterone inhibitors

                a) Promote Na^+ secretion into the distal tubule and K^+ reabsorption; cause mild diuresis and protect K^+ level

                b) Usually selected for patients receiving digoxin and diuretic therapy who cannot tolerate low serum K^+ levels or when a mild diuretic effect is desirable

                c) Side effects: Hyperkalemia, hyponatremia, headache, rash, nausea, diarrhea, urticaria, and gynecomastia or menstrual disturbances

(5) Carbonic anhydrase inhibitors (acetazolamide sodium)
  a) Inhibit the enzyme carbonic anhydrase
  b) Increase the excretion of Na^+ by interfering with HCO_3^- reabsorption. Sodium bicarbonate is lost in the urine, which creates a hyperchloremic metabolic acidosis.
  c) Are beneficial when an alkaline urine is desirable, such as with metabolic alkalosis
  d) Side effects: Hyperchloremic acidosis, renal calculi, rash, nausea, vomiting, anorexia, diminished renal function
(6) Other agents: Pharmacologic agents that increase both cardiac output and GFR contribute to diuresis (e.g., xanthines [theophylline, aminophylline] and digoxin)
(d) General nursing considerations in the administration of diuretics
  (1) Collaborate with the physician to determine the weight and fluid balance desired at the conclusion of diuretic therapy.
  (2) Observe for fluid, electrolyte, and acid-base disorders.
  (3) Maintain I&O records; correlate with daily weights.
  (4) Monitor serum K^+ levels, especially if the patient is taking digoxin (hypokalemia increases risk of digitalis toxicosis).
  (5) Administer potent or high doses of diuretics in the early morning or afternoon unless a Foley catheter is in place.
  (6) Monitor BP during aggressive diuresis because hypotension can indicate dehydration and impending circulatory collapse.
  (7) Advise the patient to report the onset of side effects such as difficulty hearing.
  (8) Be aware that a diminished response to diuretics may be related to electrolyte imbalances, particularly hyponatremia, hypochloremia, and hypokalemia.
ii. Administer antihypertensive agents as ordered (see Chapter 3).
e. Evaluation of patient care: See Chapter 3
5. **Metabolic acidosis: A condition commonly associated with renal failure caused by the inability of the kidney to excrete hydrogen ions (see** Chapter 2)
6. **Anemia: In renal disease, anemia is related primarily to a lack of erythropoietin synthesis and secretion by the kidney but can also be caused by actual blood loss (e.g., stress ulcer)**
   a. Description of problem: See Chapter 7
   b. Goals of care: See Chapter 7
   c. Collaborating professionals on health care team: See Overhydration; include hematology consult if the patient is unresponsive to therapies
   d. Interventions
     i. Identify common causes of anemia associated with renal failure.
       (a) Suppression of erythropoietin synthesis and secretion
       (b) Actual blood losses
       (c) Uremic syndrome
     ii. Treat chronic anemia associated with renal failure.
       (a) Oral or IV iron unless the patient has excess body iron stores
       (b) Folic acid and pyridoxine (vitamin B_6): Important, especially in patients undergoing dialysis, because these are dialyzable vitamins
       (c) Epogen (recombinant human erythropoietin): Stimulates erythrocyte production and prevents the anemia of CRF; effect does not begin until 2 to 6 weeks, with peak results in 3 months after administration; as a result, it is not used in ARF
   e. Evaluation of patient care
     i. Patient maintains acceptable hematocrit level (usually 20% to 24% with traditional therapy and 33% to 36% with epoetin alfa therapy).
     ii. Patient complies with pharmacologic and nutritional supplement therapy regimen.
7. **Uremic syndrome**
   a. Description of problem: Uremic state results from the kidney's inability to excrete toxic waste products; uremic symptoms usually occur at BUN levels above 100 mg/dl or at a GFR below 10 to 15 ml/min (Table 5-2)

■ **TABLE 5-2**
■ ■ **Clinical Findings in Uremic Syndrome**

Uremic syndrome affects every organ, producing a constellation of symptoms that can occur in any combination.

System	Findings
Neurologic	Sensorium changes (loss of attention span, lethargy, fatigue, coma)
	Headache
	Peripheral neuropathy
	Tremors
	Uremic seizures
Skin	Pale yellow tinge
	Pruritus
	Dryness
	Ecchymoses
	Edema
	Uremic frost (rare)
Hematologic and immunologic	Bleeding secondary to platelet dysfunction
	Diminished immune response
	Anemia secondary to erythropoietin loss or bleeding
Gastrointestinal	Nausea and/or vomiting
	Anorexia, weight loss
	Stomatitis
	Uremic fetor
	Dysgeusia (metallic, unpleasant taste)
	Gastritis, colitis (rare)
	Constipation
	Carbohydrate intolerance
Metabolic	Carbohydrate intolerance
	Hyperkalemia
	Hyponatremia or hypernatremia
	Hypocalcemia
	Hyperphosphatemia
	Hypermagnesemia
Musculoskeletal	Renal osteodystrophy—soft tissue calcification
	Bone pain
	Diminished mobility with decreased strength and change in gait
	Muscle atrophy and weakness to paralysis
Genitourinary	Flank pain
	Hematuria
	Proteinuria
	Dysuria, urinary frequency, polyuria
	Normal urine volume to oliguria or anuria
	Urinary tract infections
	Sexual dysfunction
Cardiac	Pericarditis
	Heart murmurs
	Increased rate of atherosclerosis
	Hypertension
	Pulse: Normal, bradycardia, or tachycardia secondary to uremia or electrolyte imbalance
	12-Lead electrocardiogram changes consistent with uremic pericarditis, hyperkalemia, or hypocalcemia
	Chest pain—pleuritic, pericardial, or caused by ischemic heart disease
Endocrine	Hyperparathyroidism (secondary)
Pulmonary	Pleuritis
	Pulmonary edema

Continued

■ **TABLE 5-2**
■ ■ **Clinical Findings in Uremic Syndrome—Cont'd**

System	Findings
Pulmonary—cont'd	Deep, rapid respirations; Kussmaul's respirations
	Recent respiratory infections (Goodpasture's syndrome or recent streptococcal infection), antineutrophil cytoplasmic antibody–related or Wegener's granulomatosis
Psychosocial	Altered self-image
	Diminished body image
	Depression to suicidal ideation
Other	Deafness (Alport's syndrome)

    b. Goals of care: BUN level is maintained below 100 mg/dl or at a level that minimizes uremic symptoms

    c. Collaborating professionals on health care team: See Overhydration

    d. Interventions: Based on minimizing azotemia and preventing dehydration

       i. Restrict oral protein intake.

       ii. Remove blood if it is present in the GI tract because this is another protein source that can be metabolized to ammonia and urea. These metabolites cannot be handled by diseased kidneys.

       iii. Consider dialysis to maintain BUN level below 100 mg/dl. In each patient, uremic symptoms develop at individual levels of BUN and creatinine. Identify these values, then strive to maintain BUN and creatinine below those levels.

    e. Evaluation of patient care

       i. BUN is below 100 mg/dl.

       ii. Uremic symptoms are absent or minimized.

8. Infection

    a. Description of problem: Major cause of death in patients with ARF and can seriously compromise patients with CRF (see Chapter 7)

    b. Interventions: See Chapter 7

       i. Keep in mind: patients with renal failure have an impaired immune response from uremic toxins and reduced phagocytosis by the reticuloendothelial system.

       ii. Implement the following precautions:

         (a) Obtain a urine specimen for culture on admission: UTI may be asymptomatic.

         (b) Prevent introduction of microorganisms; avoid indwelling urinary catheters and unnecessary invasive monitoring procedures.

         (c) Use an aseptic technique for urinary and IV catheter care.

         (d) Maintain the BUN level at 80 to 100 mg/dl or lower to minimize susceptibility to infection.

         (e) Implement isolation techniques for hepatitis antigen–positive patients receiving hemodialysis.

    c. Evaluation of patient care: See Chapter 7

9. Altered metabolism and excretion of pharmacologic agents related to renal failure

    a. Description of problem

       i. Kidneys unable to metabolize or excrete pharmacologic agents

       ii. Unusual untoward effects may include enhanced sensitivity to drugs.

       iii. Active or toxic metabolites of a medication retained

       iv. Increased azotemia due to elevation in metabolic wastes from drug usage

    b. Goals of care

       i. Patient tolerates pharmacologic therapy with no untoward drug effects.

       ii. Prescribed serum drug levels are adequate.

    c. Collaborating professionals on health care team: See Overhydration; also pharmacologist

    d. Interventions

        i. Recognize alterations in the body's use of drugs during renal failure.

           (a) Distribution of drugs in a uremic state

              (1) Decreased stores of body fat affect distribution of lipid-soluble drugs.

              (2) Low cardiac output states reduce renal metabolism or excretion of drugs.

              (3) Acidemia alters tissue uptake of drugs.

              (4) Increased body water has a dilutional effect.

              (5) Decreased protein binding causes competition by various drugs for tissue binding sites, leading to a higher concentration of unbound drugs.

           (b) Uremic effects that can alter drug absorption

              (1) Decreased GI motility and altered gastric pH

              (2) Electrolyte imbalances, which may affect GI tract

              (3) Inability of the kidney to excrete or metabolize drugs

              (4) Diminished protein binding

        ii. Follow general principles for drug administration during renal insufficiency.

           (a) Reduce drug dosage.

           (b) Increase intervals between doses.

           (c) Question orders for nephrotoxic agents (i.e., NSAIDs, meperidine).

           (d) Closely observe patients to recognize toxicosis due to drug accumulation.

           (e) Report any untoward signs, especially elevated serum creatinine level, so that the drug can be reconsidered, reduced in dosage, or discontinued.

           (f) Monitor serum drug levels, especially in situations requiring a specific drug concentration (e.g., antibiotics, digoxin, procaine).

           (g) To ensure a more stable serum concentration, administer initial loading doses of drugs that have a long half-life (e.g., digoxin).

    e. Evaluation of patient care: Patient tolerates pharmacologic therapy with no untoward drug effects

10. Ineffective patient and family coping (see also Chapter 10)

    a. Description of problem

        i. Insufficient, ineffective, or compromised support, comfort, assistance, or encouragement, usually by a supportive primary person (family member or close friend). The patient may need to manage adaptive tasks related to the stress of renal failure on the patient and the family.

        ii. Signs of maladaptive patient coping

           (a) Verbalization of the inability to cope or to ask for help

           (b) Inability to meet role expectations and solve problems

           (c) Diminished communication and socialization

           (d) Destructive behavior toward self or others (i.e., suicide attempt)

           (e) Failure to comply with the treatment regimen

        iii. Signs of maladaptive family coping

           (a) Patient communicates concern about the family's response to his or her disease.

           (b) Family members demonstrate preoccupation with their own personal reactions—fear, anticipatory grief, guilt, anxiety.

           (c) Family has inadequate understanding of the patient's condition, or therapy interferes with effective supportive behaviors.

           (d) Family withdraws from communication with the patient or demonstrates overprotective or underprotective behaviors.

    b. Goals of care

        i. Patient demonstrates increased functional independence, compliance with treatment regimen, and participation in programs that enhance quality of life (e.g., exercise or rehabilitation program).

        ii. Patient appropriately expresses ideas, feelings, and needs, participates in family activities, and accepts family support, as appropriate.

        iii. Patient and family adjust to any necessary role changes.

        iv. Patient resumes employment.

    c. Collaborating professionals on health care team (see also Overhydration)

         i.   Psychiatrist or psychologist

         ii.   Social worker

    d. Interventions

         i.   Identify common causes of stress in the patient and family.

            (a) Life-threatening nature of renal disease

            (b) Inability to perform activities of daily living

            (c) Restrictions caused by a shunt, a fistula, or a Tenckhoff catheter; demands of dialysis schedule and other treatments

            (d) Reversal in family roles, effects on sexual behavior and sexuality, and questions regarding ability to maintain or return to work

         ii.   Recognize that psychologic consequences of renal disease and its treatment include denial, depression, and dependency and that the suicide rate among patients maintained with hemodialysis is believed to be 100 times that of the general population.

         iii. Assess the patient's ability to cope with renal disease (see Chapter 10).

         iv. Specific nursing interventions to support adaptation of the patient with renal failure include the following:

            (a) Teach the patient about the various treatment alternatives and encourage participation in selection of the treatment method.

            (b) Link with support systems.

                (1) Visits with successfully adjusted patients

                (2) Support for family members; patients with supportive families tend to have fewer physical complications, survive longer, and adjust more readily

    e. Evaluation of patient care

         i.   Patient demonstrates the following:

            (a) Participation in self-care, social and family activities, and use of adaptive coping mechanisms such as functional denial

            (b) Increased self-esteem with acceptance of body image changes

            (c) Cooperation with health care staff and compliance with treatment plan

         ii.   Family demonstrates the following:

            (a) Decreased levels of anxiety, adaptive changes in family roles, and appropriate use of health care and community support systems

            (b) Participation in patient care

SPECIFIC PATIENT HEALTH PROBLEMS

Acute Renal Failure

The ARF syndrome affects 5% to 7% of all hospitalized patients and 20% of the critically ill. Oliguria with ARF is associated with a 50% mortality rate in the critically ill and a 50% to 70% mortality rate in trauma or postoperative patients. Nonoliguria with ARF carries a better prognosis and a lower mortality rate of 26%. A mortality rate of 87% is seen in patients with ARF 24 hours after cardiogenic shock due to acute MI. These mortality rates in the critically ill have not improved in the last 45 years, so prevention of ARF remains the best intervention.

  1. **Pathophysiology**

    a. Prerenal conditions

         i.   Physiologic states diminish renal perfusion without renal tubular damage.

         ii.   Effects of diminished kidney perfusion include the following:

            (a) Decreased renal arterial pressure

            (b) Decreased afferent arterial pressure (<100 mm Hg), which diminishes forces favoring filtration

    b. Intrarenal conditions

         i.   Cortical involvement of vascular, infectious, or immunologic processes

            (a) Causes renal capillary swelling and cellular proliferation, which eventually decrease the GFR

            (b) Edema and cellular debris obstruct the glomeruli, which results in oliguria.

ii. Medullary involvement after prolonged ischemia or hypoperfusion or nephrotoxic injury to the tubular portion of the nephrons (Figure 5-4, *A*)

(a) Medullary hemodynamics: Hypoperfusion states and oxygen insufficiency disrupt the fine balance between limited oxygen supply and high oxygen consumption in the outer medullary region; may contribute to ARF from hypoxic medullary damage

(1) Conditions predisposing to hypoperfusion

a) Presence of endotoxin

b) Rhabdomyolysis

c) Hypercalcemia

d) NSAID use

e) Exposure to radiologic contrast agents

f) Antibiotic use (i.e., amphotericin, cyclosporine)

(2) Pharmacologic agents can also alter medullary hemodynamics, especially if administered in absence of volume depletion (i.e., furosemide, mannitol, dopamine). Other substances suspected of improving medullary hemodynamics are nitric oxide, which is normally produced by the macula densa to control glomerular blood flow and renin release, and ANP, an endogenous vasodilator.

(b) Tubular necrosis produced as localized damage in patchy pattern (actual necrosis) or in apoptosis as disruption of cellular function (usually in the distal tubules): Extent of the damage differs in nephrotoxic injury, ischemia or hypoperfusion, sepsis-associated states, and multiple organ failure

(1) Nephrotoxic injury affects the epithelial cellular layer (can regenerate).

(2) Ischemia and hypoperfusion alter renal tubular cells and damage the tubular basement membrane (cannot regenerate).

a) Cellular injury may involve several factors: ATP depletion, oxygen free radical formation, loss of epithelial cell polarity, and increased calcium levels; apoptosis causes DNA fragmentation and cytoplasmic condensation.

b) ATP depletion: Begins 30 seconds after the kidney is hypoperfused; normal homeostatic benefits of cellular ATP (preservation of cellular volume, ionic composition, membrane integrity) are lost

c) Oxidative metabolism produces oxygen free radicals.

1) Because these substances are highly reactive and volatile, intracellular mechanisms (enzyme systems and antioxidants) exist for their rapid breakdown and destruction.

2) Left unopposed, as during ischemic events, these radicals disrupt cellular functioning (e.g., during ischemia, the renal cell is unstable and unable to protect itself from oxygen free radicals, which results in renal cell injury).

d) Loss of epithelial cell polarity: Ischemia alters the passage of water, electrolytes, and other charged elements through the tubule's epithelial wall, which leads to a concentration defect

e) Increased calcium levels: Ischemic and hypoperfusion states lead to a rise in intracellular calcium levels that causes renal vasoconstriction and a decrease in GFR

(3) Systemic inflammatory response syndrome (SIRS): Released endotoxins significantly reduce renal perfusion, and renal vasoactive substances alter renal cellular metabolism and constrict renal vasculature (see Chapter 9)

(4) Multiorgan dysfunction syndrome results in rapid and progressive deterioration of renal function (see Chapter 9).

(c) Phases of recovery: Classic form of ARF has four phases, whereas nonoliguric form has only three; the nonoliguric phase seems to be synonymous with the diuretic phase, which suggests that nonoliguric ARF reflects less tubular damage so recovery is more rapid

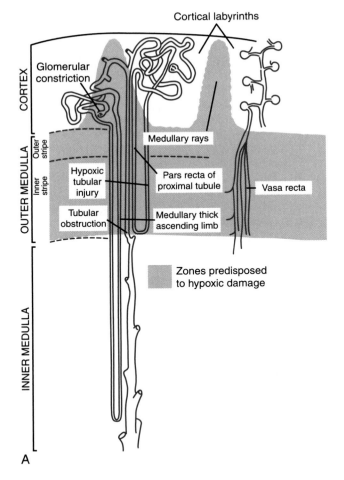

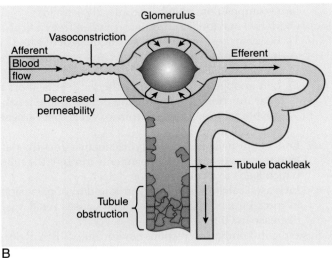

FIGURE 5-4 ■ **A,** Anatomy of intrarenal zones predisposed to hypoxic injury in acute renal failure. (From Heyman SN, Fuch S, Brezis M. The role of indwelling ischemia in ARF. *New Horiz.* 1995;3[4]:597.) **B,** Potential mechanisms causing oliguria in patients with acute renal failure. (From Goldman L, Ausiello D, eds. *Cecil Textbook of Medicine.* 22nd ed. Philadelphia, PA: Saunders; 2004:706.)

(d) Onset, or initial phase, precedes the actual necrotic injury and correlates with a major alteration in renal hemodynamics.
    (1) Associated with a decrease in RBF and GFR
    (2) Most important factor altering RBF is decrease in cardiac output.
    (3) Other mechanisms contributing to decreased renal perfusion are increased sympathetic activity and renal vascular resistance.
    (4) A consistent increase in cardiac output during this phase will maintain an increase in RBF and protect the patient from impending ARF.
(e) Oliguric phase reflects four processes (Figure 5-4, *B*).
    (1) Obstruction of tubules by cellular debris, tubular casts, or tissue swelling
    (2) Reabsorption or back-leak of urine filtration through the damaged tubular epithelium and into circulation
    (3) Tubular cell damage with development of necrotic, patchy areas; the cell leaks ATP and K^+, edema is present, mitochondria are altered, and calcium leaks into the cell
    (4) Renal vasoconstriction continues and may contribute to the decreased GFR.
(f) Nonoliguric phase reflects less tubular damage; symptomatology resembles that of the diuretic phase.
    (1) Urine output may exceed 1 L/hr.
    (2) Solute is present in urine at approximately 350 mOsm/L.
    (3) Creatinine clearance is as high as 15 ml/min, and Na^+ excretion is low.
    (4) Hyperkalemia remains a significant problem.
    (5) Phase is of short duration; recovery phase is reached in 5 to 8 days.
(g) Diuretic phase signifies that tubular function is returning.
    (1) Tubular obstruction relieved, but cellular edema remains as scar tissue forms on necrotic areas
    (2) Large daily urine output, sometimes exceeding 3 L; output due to the osmotic-diuretic effect of elevated BUN level and impaired ability of tubules to conserve Na^+ and water
    (3) Recovery phase
        a) Occurs after gradual improvement of kidney function extending over a 3- to 12-month period
        b) Residual renal impairment in GFR may result, with serum creatinine level remaining higher than previously.
  c. Postrenal conditions: Associated with obstruction of the urinary collecting system
    i. Partial obstruction: Can increase renal interstitial pressure, increasing opposing forces of glomerular filtration; result is diminished urine output
    ii. Complete obstruction: Impediment to urine flow accompanies bilateral kidney involvement; the "backup" pressure of urine compresses the kidneys
2. Etiology and risk factors: See Table 5-3
3. Signs and symptoms
  a. Malaise, fatigue, lethargy, confusion
  b. Twitching and/or weakness resulting from metabolic acidosis
  c. Impaired mobility
  d. Change in urine color and/or volume: Oliguria (<400 ml/24 hr); nonoliguria (excess, dilute urine); anuria (no urine output or <100 ml/24 hr); or hematuria
  e. Cardiac involvement
    i. Dysrhythmias resulting from electrolyte imbalance or heart failure
    ii. Change in pulse rate (either tachycardia or bradycardia)
    iii. Hypertension
    iv. Cardiac friction rub, indicative of pericarditis
  f. Skin changes: Dry skin, edema, pallor, bruising, uremic frost (rare), pruritus
  g. Flank pain
  h. Local or systemic infection presenting with shaking, chills, and fever
  i. Abdominal distention caused by enlarged bladder, obstruction
  j. Uremic signs and symptoms: See Table 5-2

■ **TABLE 5-3**
■ ■ **Common Causes of Acute Renal Failure**

Type of Renal Failure	Causes
Prerenal failure	Hypovolemia secondary to hemorrhage, gastrointestinal losses, third-spacing phenomena
	Excessive use of diuretics
	Impaired myocardial contractility (such as heart failure, pericardial tamponade)
	Sepsis, such as gram-negative shock with vasodilatation
	Increased renal vascular resistance from anesthesia or surgery
	Bilateral renal vascular obstruction caused by embolism or thrombosis
Intrarenal failure	
Cortical involvement	Acute poststreptococcal glomerulonephritis
	Acute cortical necrosis
	Systemic lupus erythematosus (lupus nephritis)
	Goodpasture's syndrome, antineutrophil cytoplasmic antibody disease such as Wegener's granulomatosis
	Bilateral endocarditis
	Pregnancy (i.e., abruptio placentae and abortion)
	Malignant hypertension
	Human immunodeficiency virus–related nephropathy
Medullary involvement	Nephrotoxic injury: Occurs after exposure to nephrotoxic agents; the effects are accentuated by dehydration, which leads to more extensive tubular damage; nephrotoxic damage may also compound the clinical picture of any type of existing renal deterioration
	• Antibiotics: Aminoglycosides, tetracyclines, penicillins, cephalosporins, pentamidine
	• Antiviral agents: Acyclovir
	• Nonsteroidal anti-inflammatory drugs (e.g., ibuprofen)
	• Immunosuppressive drugs: Cyclosporine, tacrolimus
	• Angiotensin-converting enzyme inhibitors (e.g., captopril) or angiotensin II receptor blockers (e.g., losartan)
	• Carbon tetrachloride (found in cleaning agents)
	• Heavy metals: Lead, arsenic, mercury, uranium
	• Pesticides and fungicides
	• Radiocontrast dye (e.g., in angiography or computed tomography)
	• Chemotherapeutic agent toxicity (e.g., cisplatin, uric acid crystals)
	Ischemic injury: During ischemia injury may occur if mean arterial pressure drops below 60 mm Hg for over 40 min; causes include massive hemorrhage, transfusion reaction (tubules are obstructed with hemolyzed erythrocytes), and cardiogenic shock
	Multiple organ dysfunction syndrome: Triggered by the inflammatory or immune response, leading to the progressive deterioration of organs, with the kidneys as a prime target
	Systemic inflammatory response syndrome: Renal injury can result from endotoxins, an inflammatory or immune response, or renal hypoperfusion
Postrenal failure	Ureteral obstruction (e.g., stone, tumor, fibrosis, or clot)
	Abscess
	Prostate hypertrophy
	Crystal deposition (e.g., uric acid, calcium oxalate, acyclovir)

4. **Diagnostic study findings**
   a. Laboratory
      i. Prerenal
         (a) Urinalysis
             (1) Urinary sodium level less than 10 mEq/L
             (2) SG greater than 1.020
             (3) Minimal or no proteinuria
             (4) Normal urinary sediment
             (5) Urine osmolality higher than 400 mOsm/kg

(b) Serum BUN/creatinine ratio higher than 25:1
ii. Intrarenal—Cortical disease
    (a) Urinalysis
        (1) Urinary sodium level less than 10 mEq/L
        (2) SG variable
        (3) Moderate to heavy proteinuria
        (4) Hematuria
        (5) Urinary sediment with erythrocyte casts, leukocytes
        (6) Urine osmolality less than 350 mOsm/kg
    (b) Serum BUN and creatinine levels elevated but remain in 10:1 ratio
iii. Intrarenal—Medullary disease
    (a) Urinalysis
        (1) Urinary sodium level greater than 20 mEq/L
        (2) SG 1.010
        (3) Minimal to moderate proteinuria
        (4) Urinary sediment with numerous renal tubular epithelial cells, tubular casts, and a rare erythrocyte
    (b) Serum BUN and creatinine levels elevated
iv. Postrenal
    (a) Serum BUN and creatinine levels elevated with complete obstruction
    (b) Bacteriologic report showing significant positive results for a specific organism
v. Special
    (a) Antistreptolysin O titer: To diagnose recent streptococcal infection (may cause poststreptococcal glomerulonephritis)
    (b) Antiglomerular basement membrane titers: To diagnose Goodpasture's syndrome, a devastating disease of pulmonary hemorrhage and renal failure
    (c) Antineutrophil cytoplasmic antibody test for pulmonary and renal failure
    (d) Serum studies for complement components: A fall in complement levels is seen in active complement-mediated glomerulonephritis (e.g., lupus nephritis)
    (e) Serum electrophoresis for immunoglobulin levels: Abnormal proteins (as in multiple myeloma) can damage kidneys
    (f) Hepatitis serologic tests: Hepatitis B and C cause kidney disease
b. Radiologic: To rule out obstruction as a cause of oliguria or anuria, because immediate treatment may reverse renal failure. Kidney size provides diagnostic information, because small kidneys imply chronic rather than acute renal failure (see Diagnostic Studies under Patient Assessment).

5. Goals of care
  a. ARF is resolved.
  b. Normal renal function and urine output resume.

6. Collaborating professionals on health care team
  a. Progressive care nurse, clinical specialist or physician assistant, case manager, hemodialysis nurse
  b. Physicians: Nephrologist (higher mortality when renal consult delayed >48 hours), hematology consult (if blood dyscrasias accompany ARF), vascular surgery consultant
  c. Dietitian
  d. Social worker
  e. Pharmacologist

7. Management of patient care
  a. Anticipated patient trajectory: Patients with ARF experience rapid decline, with recovery from 8 days for nonoliguric ATN and from 2 weeks to 3 months for oliguric ATN. Transfer or discharge varies with the stage of renal recovery. Expect patients with ARF to have needs in numerous areas:
    i. Skin care: Impaired skin integrity due to uremia, malnutrition, immobility
      (a) Assess for uremic effects on skin integrity (see Table 5-2).
      (b) Keep skin clean, dry, and intact to prevent infection.
      (c) Use aseptic technique during wound care.

ii.   Nutrition: ARF is associated with accelerated protein catabolism that contributes to negative nitrogen balance and uncontrollably high BUN levels usually indicative of a hypercatabolic state. Repeated elevations of BUN over 100 mg/dl despite routine dialysis correlate with evidence of rapid muscle wasting and indicate the need for higher levels of protein consumption, together with a continuous form of dialysis.

   (a) Maintain protein intake at a minimum of 0.6 to 0.8 g/kg of body weight; administer higher amounts of protein during hypercatabolism.
   (b) Provide total calories of 30 to 35 kcal/kg/day of a carbohydrate and lipid combination while controlling glucose and triglyceride intake.
   (c) Be aware that hyperalimentation and daily dialysis have been associated with increased survival rates in ARF as well as promotion of renal tubular cell regeneration. Hyperalimentation requirements include consumption of large amounts of both essential and nonessential amino acids.
   (d) Give IV glucose and lipid solution to augment caloric and nutritional intake, thereby reducing the need for protein in hypercatabolic states.
   (e) Maintain fluid restriction by limiting non–electrolyte-containing fluids.
   (f) Administer water-soluble vitamins. Avoid excessive doses of vitamin C (not exceeding 250 mg/day), which may exacerbate ARF. Be cautious with vitamin A, because excessive intake in the absence of renal excretion can lead to vitamin A toxicity.
   (g) Monitor serum protein, albumin, hematocrit, and urea levels and weigh daily to assess the effectiveness of nutritional therapy.

iii. Infection control: Uremia increases patient susceptibility to infection
   (a) Assess for BUN levels over 80 to 100 mg/dl because these are associated with an increased risk of infection.
   (b) Monitor for early signs of septic shock (SIRS).
   (c) Monitor serum protein and albumin levels, because inadequate levels have an immunosuppressive effect.

iv.   Discharge planning and patient education
   (a) Teach patient and family members or significant others the following:
       (1) Etiology and course of the disease
       (2) Dietary and fluid restriction requirements
       (3) Dialysis machine operation, procedure, and schedule
       (4) Prospects for recovery
   (b) Assess and prepare the home for patient care and, if appropriate, for dialysis.
   (c) Make the patient and family aware of community resources (e.g., national or local kidney foundation [http://www.kidney.org], local dialysis center).
   (d) Assist in patient transition to rehabilitation and/or home care.

v.   Pharmacology
   (a) Use pharmacologic agents with adequate fluid replacement to reestablish or augment RBF. This does not protect the tubules from damage but may limit the extent of damage, creating nonoliguric ATN.
       (1) Renal-dose dopamine: No longer the therapy of choice for prevention or treatment.
       (2) Diuretics:
           a) Commonly used agents
               1) Traditional diuretics (mannitol, loop diuretics): Used to convert oliguria to nonoliguria
               2) Mannitol: Protects the kidney by preventing the buildup of cellular debris, reducing tubular obstruction, and augmenting blood flow. Preserves mitochondrial function via osmotic effect; limits recovery ischemia and free radical production. Administer with caution; may precipitate pulmonary edema.
               3) Furosemide (Lasix): Acts as both a diuretic and an augmentor of RBF; maximum dosage should not exceed 4 mg/kg/min

b) Diuresis encourages removal of sloughed tubular cells, eliminating tubular obstruction.

c) Volume replacement needs to be a priority before administering diuretics; a trial of diuretics can be attempted but should be limited when effectiveness is in question.

d) Monitor and report changes in urine output (onset of oliguria, nonoliguria, or anuria).

e) Obtain urine and blood specimens, analyze results.

(b) Metabolism and excretion of pharmacologic agents may be altered in ARF (see Patient Care).

vi. Treatments

(a) Prevention modalities for ARF: Remain the best intervention; preservation of renal function is the desired outcome

(1) Identify patients at higher risk for ARF.

a) Hemodynamic instability; blood loss or hypotension in surgical patients

b) Multiple trauma, multiorgan dysfunction syndrome, rhabdomyolysis

c) Systemic and/or renal intravascular hemolysis

d) Receipt of nephrotoxic drugs

(2) Monitor for prerenal or onset stage of ATN (see Diagnostic Study Findings for prerenal failure).

a) Renal hypoperfusion from any cause diminishes the GFR as the MAP drops to 70 mm Hg or below.

b) Hypotension can eliminate renal autoregulation.

(b) Correct hypotension and/or renal hypoperfusion by fluid administration and/or pharmacologic agents.

(1) Fluid administration: The single best modality for reinstating renal perfusion is to increase cardiac output through the administration of fluids, especially in preventing radiocontrast-associated ARF

a) Consider the following fluids: normal saline, colloids (either albumin or dextran), and/or blood products.

b) Monitor patient response to administration of as much as 1 to 2 L normal saline over 2 or more hours; observe for nonresponse to volume expansion or pulmonary edema.

(2) Pharmacologic agents: Include calcium channel blockers, ANP

a) Dopamine not proven to be clinically useful

b) Calcium channel blockers vasodilate renal vasculature and augment renal function; found to be useful in ARF secondary to renal transplantation, radiocontrast nephrotoxicity, and cyclosporine use.

c) ANP use associated with improvement in oliguric rather than nonoliguric ARF; beneficial in management of heart failure

d) Mucomyst (*N*-acetylcysteine) beneficial in the prevention of ARF secondary to IV radiocontrast nephrotoxicity; consider 600 mg by mouth twice daily

(c) Determine the need for hemodialysis: early initiation of any form of dialysis is beneficial for the prevention and management of acute and chronic renal failure.

(1) Indications for which hemodialysis remains the initial treatment of choice

a) ARF

b) CRF when medications and diet no longer provide effective therapy

c) Symptomatic uremia (e.g., acidosis, hyperkalemia, pericardial friction rub)

d) To keep BUN level lower than 100 mg/dl and improve survival rate

(2) Contraindications

a) Intolerance to systemic heparinization (i.e., heparin-induced thrombocytopenia); consider nonheparin anticoagulant such as lepirudin (Refludan)

b) Hemodynamic instability: Labile cardiovascular status incompatible with rapid changes in ECF volume

(d) Initiate hemodialysis (Figure 5-5).

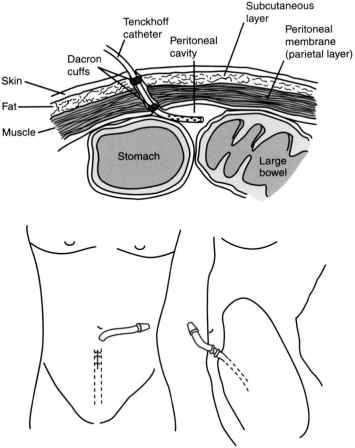

FIGURE 5-5 ■ Permanent peritoneal catheter in place, showing its position with respect to the different layers of the abdominal wall *(top)*, its anteroposterior position *(lower left)*, and the catheter angle with respect to the abdominal wall *(lower right)*. (From Levine DZ. *Care of the Renal Patient*. 3rd ed. Philadelphia, PA: Saunders; 1997.)

    (1) Principles of hemodialysis: Include osmosis (optional), diffusion, and convection-ultrafiltration

        a) Osmosis: Movement of water across a semipermeable membrane from an area of lesser to an area of greater osmolality

        b) Diffusion: Movement of molecules from area of higher to an area of lower concentration

        c) Ultrafiltration and convection: Movement of particles through a semipermeable membrane by hydrostatic pressure

    (2) Hemodynamics: By means of vascular access and a blood pump, about 300 ml of blood travels through an extracorporeal dialyzer, which removes wastes, toxic substances, excess electrolytes, metabolic products, and pharmacologic agents and then returns the blood to the systemic circulation

    (3) Anticoagulation

        a) Before the procedure, heparinization is performed to keep blood anticoagulated within the hemodialysis machine (regional heparinization).

        b) Nonheparin hemodialysis is available at some facilities.

        c) Patient must be monitored closely for signs of bleeding.

    (4) Vascular access for dialysis

        a) Central venous access (i.e., dual-lumen internal jugular, femoral, or subclavian catheter): For emergent dialysis or temporarily after failure of a permanent catheter while awaiting repair or replacement

1) Blood flow must range from 200 to 500 mL/min to accommodate hemodialysis.
2) Double- or triple-lumen catheter requires the use of a large vein, such as the femoral vein, which limits ambulation and carries the risk of dislodgment, infection, and kinking; other sites include the right or left subclavian and right or left jugular vein.
3) Palpate peripheral pulses in the cannulated extremity.
4) Observe for bleeding or hematoma formation; if it occurs, apply pressure dressing and notify the physician.
5) Properly position the catheter to avoid dislodgment during the dialysis procedure.
6) If the femoral vein catheter is to be maintained after dialysis, connect it to a pressurized IV flow system. Add a low dose of heparin (500 U/L) to the solution. Maintain a secure aseptic dressing to minimize the risk of infection. No standing or ambulation is allowed while the catheter is in place.
7) On removal of a femoral catheter, apply direct pressure to the puncture site for 5 to 10 minutes (or the time needed to stop the bleeding after dialysis and after the period of heparinization). Complete this procedure with the application of a pressure dressing and a period of bed rest.

b) Permanent vascular access: An arteriovenous fistula is usually placed in an upper rather than a lower extremity
1) Surgical procedure with anastomosis of an artery to a vein, or an artificial vascular graft is used.
2) Do not perform venipuncture, start IV therapy, give injections, or take BP with a cuff on the arm with a fistula; post this information on signage above bed.
3) Palpate the thrill or auscultate the bruit to confirm patency.
4) Avoid circumferential dressings and restrictive clothing.
5) Report bleeding, skin discoloration, drainage, and other signs of infection; culture the drainage.
6) For profuse bleeding, apply a pressure dressing.

c) External permanent vascular access: An arteriovenous shunt is rarely selected
1) Auscultate for the bruit or palpate for the thrill to assess shunt patency.
2) Promptly report any suspicion of clotting (color change of blood, separation of serum from erythrocytes, absence of pulsations in tubing).
3) Hydrate adequately to minimize clotting.
4) Change the sterile dressing over the shunt at least daily; reinforce the dressing as necessary.
5) Do not perform venipuncture, give IV therapy, give injections, or take BP with a cuff on the shunt arm.
6) Instruct the patient in the care of the shunt site.

(5) Hemodialysis membrane compatibility
(6) Frequency: ARF may require daily dialysis or a one-time dialysis treatment to resolve an acute problem, such as a hyperkalemic episode
(7) Complications
a) Muscle cramps, nausea, vomiting
b) Bleeding
c) Infection (e.g., hepatitis C or infection related to catheter placement or skin flora)
d) Hypertension, anaphylactic reactions
e) Technical error (dialyzer rupture)

(e) Peritoneal dialysis (PD): Effective in maintaining homeostasis

          (1) Indications
             a) Fluid overload
             b) Electrolyte or acid-base imbalance
             c) Acute or chronic renal failure
             d) Intoxication from dialyzable drugs and poisons
             e) Peritonitis or pericarditis
             f) Unavailability of vascular access for hemodialysis
          (2) Contraindications: Bleeding disorder, abdominal adhesions, recent peritoneal surgery
          (3) Principles of PD: Primarily osmosis and diffusion
          (4) Description: Dialysate is instilled into the peritoneal cavity through a catheter, allowed to "pool" (usually for a minimum of 30 minutes), then drained. New dialysate is infused, which initiates the next cycle.
          (5) Anticoagulation: Minimal amount of heparin required
          (6) Frequency: Continuous form of dialysis; dialysis sessions can last 3 to 4 days or longer depending on the needs of the patient
          (7) Hemodynamics: No direct impact on hemodynamics
          (8) Complications
             a) Bladder or bowel perforation caused by catheter placement
             b) Peritonitis, abdominal bleeding
             c) Respiratory impairment caused by increased abdominal size

b. Potential complications
  i. Pulmonary edema
    (a) Mechanism: Volume overload resulting from volume retention secondary to ARF or excess IV fluids administered to prevent ARF
    (b) Management: See Chapters 2 and 3
  ii. Uremic pericarditis with effusion
    (a) Mechanism: Uremic toxins on myocardium result in pericarditis with or without pericardial effusion
    (b) Management (see also Chapter 3)
      (1) Maintain BUN levels below 80 mg/dl.
      (2) Consider pericardiocentesis for large effusions over 250 ml.
      (3) Pericardiectomy necessary for repeated episodes or those causing cardiac tamponade
  iii. Anemia
    (a) Mechanism: Actual bleeding resulting from primary cause or uremia, septic shock, or SIRS, which is commonly associated with the onset of disseminated intravascular coagulation. Lack of erythropoietin observed at onset of ARF.
    (b) Management (see also Chapter 7)
      (1) Differentiate between anemia due to actual blood loss and that due to lack of erythropoietin.
      (2) Administer packed RBCs to maintain hematocrit per physician order.
  iv. Electrolyte imbalances
    (a) Mechanism: Inability of kidneys to excrete electrolytes and concentrate urine in ARF
    (b) Management: See later sections on hyperkalemia, hypocalcemia, hyperphosphatemia, and hypermagnesemia, which are the most common imbalances
  v. Metabolic acidosis
    (a) Mechanism: Inability of the kidney to secrete hydrogen ions in urine
    (b) Management (see also Chapter 2): Dialysis to correct or minimize acidosis
  vi. Sleep-pattern disturbance
    (a) Mechanism: During ARF, sleep is interrupted by the intensity of care, the hospital environment, sleep apnea, and uremic condition (e.g., tremors, restless leg syndrome). Nursing research reveals an increase in the number of recalled nightmares the night before dialysis at the uremic peak, which results in a disturbed sleep pattern. Disruption of sleep interferes with the healing process and quality of life.

(b) Management

    (1) Obtain a sleep history (i.e., day or night sleeper).

    (2) Organize care to minimize patient interruptions.

    (3) Limit noise in the environment.

    (4) Provide three to four 90-minute sleep cycles in each 24-hour period.

  vii. Altered metabolism and excretion of pharmacologic agents: See Patient Care

8. Evaluation of patient care

  a. Renal perfusion is improved to prevent prerenal failure and ATN.

  b. Urine output exceeds 30 ml/hr with normal concentration and volume; balanced 24-hour I&O record coincides with daily weight.

  c. Weight is stable, with no evidence of muscle wasting; nutrition is adequate.

  d. Electrolyte balance and metabolic acidosis are WNL or minimized at asymptomatic levels.

  e. Dialysis is tolerated and corrects or maintains asymptomatic fluid, electrolyte, and acid-base balance.

  f. Infection-free skin is dry, clean, and intact with no itching; wound healing is progressing.

  g. Patient is free of major anxiety, coping satisfactorily with illness, participating in care, using effective support systems, and not suffering from sleep deprivation.

  h. Patient has knowledge of ARF and treatment and is compliant with disease management expectations.

Chronic Renal Failure

CRF is a slowly progressive renal disorder culminating in end-stage renal disease (ESRD). The decline in kidney function correlates with the degree of nephron loss.

1. Pathophysiology: Systemic changes occur when overall renal function is less than 20% to 25% of normal

  a. The kidney has a unique ability to compensate and preserve homeostasis despite a significant (80%) loss of nephron function. During CRF, injury occurs to the nephrons in a progressive manner. The remaining intact nephrons compensate for loss of functioning nephrons by cellular hypertrophy, which enables these nephrons to accept larger blood volumes for clearances and results in excretion of more solute.

  b. Four stages of CRF: Each stage is associated with a certain degree of nephron loss, which can be correlated with the serum creatinine level

    i. Diminished renal reserve: 50% nephron loss

      (a) Kidney function is mildly reduced, but the excretory and regulatory functions are sufficiently maintained to preserve a normal internal environment; the patient usually is problem free.

      (b) The serum creatinine value usually doubles; a normal value of 0.6 mg/dl rises to 1.2 mg/dl, which is still WNL.

    ii. Renal insufficiency: 75% nephron loss

      (a) Evidence of impaired renal capacity appears in the form of mild azotemia, slightly impaired urinary concentrating ability, increasing serum phosphorus level, anemia, decreasing serum calcium and bicarbonate levels; hyperkalemia may occur.

      (b) Factors that exacerbate renal disease at this stage by increasing nephron damage are infection, dehydration, drugs, cardiac failure, and instability of the primary disease.

      (c) Serum creatinine level usually ranges from 4.0 to 9.9 mg/dl.

    iii. ESRD: 90% of nephrons damaged; GFR is usually less than 15 ml/min

      (a) Renal function has deteriorated so that persistent abnormalities exist.

      (b) Patient requires artificial support to sustain life (dialysis or transplantation).

      (c) Serum creatinine level is 10 mg/dl or higher.

    iv. Uremic syndrome: Complete nephron loss

      (a) The body's systemic responses to the buildup of uremic waste products and the results of the failed organ system

      (b) Usually described as the constellation of signs and symptoms exhibited in renal failure

      (c) Symptoms may be avoided or diminished by the initiation of early dialysis treatment or renal transplantation.

■ **TABLE 5-4**
■ ■ **Common Causes of Chronic Renal Failure**

Disorder	Underlying Cause
Tubulointerstitial disease or interstitial nephritis	Chronic pyelonephritis (most common cause)
	Analgesic-abuse nephropathy
	Immunologic mechanisms (transplant rejection, allergic response, hypersensitivity)
Glomerulonephropathies	Focal glomerulosclerosis
	Crescentic glomerulonephritis (rapid and progressing)
	Chronic glomerulonephritis
	Systemic lupus erythematosus (lupus nephritis)
	Bacterial endocarditis
Nephrotic syndrome	Glomerular disease
Renal vascular disorders	Systemic vasculitis (i.e., polyarteritis nodosa, hypersensitivity vasculitis)
	Scleroderma
	Coagulopathies such as hemolytic uremic syndrome
	Thromboembolic renal disease
	Sickle cell nephropathy
	Hypertensive nephrosclerosis: Benign, malignant, or accelerated
Renal cancer	Renal cell carcinoma, the most common renal neoplasm

2. **Etiology and risk factors: See Table 5-4**
3. **Signs and symptoms of uremia: See Table 5-2**
4. **Diagnostic study findings: See also Diagnostic Studies under Patient Assessment**
   a. Laboratory
      i.   Urinalysis: The following abnormalities may be the first indicators of renal disease. See later for specific findings for CRF.
         (a) Proteinuria: May exceed $3\,g/24\,hr$ in patients with glomerulonephropathies and nephrotic syndrome
         (b) Leukocyte casts and pyuria: Indicate infection in the urinary tract; suspect renal disease when pyuria occurs in conjunction with hematuria, casts, and proteinuria
         (c) Eosinophiluria: May occur in allergic interstitial nephritis
         (d) Epithelial cells: Renal tubular cells with lipid droplets in the cytoplasm suggest nephrotic syndrome; large numbers of these cells are present in glomerulonephritis and pyelonephritis
         (e) Casts: Provide important diagnostic clues (see section on casts in Diagnostic Studies under Patient Assessment)
            (1) Mixed leukocyte and erythrocyte casts may be prominent in acute exudative glomerulonephritis.
            (2) Fatty casts are seen in glomerular diseases in conjunction with moderate to heavy proteinuria.
            (3) Waxy, broad casts are seen in the final stages of renal failure.
         (f) Urine osmolality: Varies with the stage of CRF
         (g) Creatinine clearance or GFR
            (1) A decrease of 10 to $50\,ml/min$ or a renal reserve of 25% is associated with the onset of renal insufficiency.
            (2) A creatinine clearance of 10 to $15\,ml/min$ is consistent with ESRD.
      ii. Serum studies
         (a) Creatinine: An inverse relationship exists between serum creatinine level and GFR, and the stage of CRF
            (1) Diminished renal reserve: A 50% nephron loss is reflected by either a normal creatinine level of $1.4\,mg/dl$ or a twice-normal creatinine level of $2.8\,mg/dl$
            (2) Renal insufficiency: A 75% nephron loss causes the serum creatinine level to quadruple

(3) ESRD: A 90% nephron loss correlates with a serum creatinine value of 10 mg/dl or higher

(4) Uremic syndrome: A creatinine value of 10 mg/dl or higher is maintained by some form of dialysis

(b) BUN: In CRF, BUN levels above 100 mg/dl are usually associated with uremic symptoms; therefore, BUN level is used to determine the frequency and duration of dialysis treatments

(c) Uric acid: Increased serum levels may suggest gout or gouty nephropathy when the elevation is out of proportion to the degree of renal failure

(d) Serum triglyceride level: May be elevated

(e) Glucose tolerance test: Identifies the presence of carbohydrate intolerance

(f) Serum protein and albumin levels: Decreased values indicate malnutrition associated with a restricted-protein diet, anorexia, or chronic infection

b. Radiologic

i. IVP

(a) Small kidneys, or one atrophied and one normal-sized kidney, may indicate bilateral disease; unilateral disease always causes compensatory hypertrophy of the contralateral kidney.

(b) Enlarged kidneys suggest polycystic disease or obstruction.

(c) Scarring and altered calices can suggest chronic pyelonephritis or analgesic nephropathy.

ii. Ultrasonography: Identifies renal parenchymal disease and rules out obstruction; generally lacks the ability to differentiate between renal diseases

iii. CT: May reveal renal perfusion defects, pyelonephritis, renal cystic disorders, or renal colic

iv. MRI: Used to diagnose renovascular lesions

v. Special: Baseline motor nerve conduction velocity studies and long-bone x-ray films of the skull, hands, and feet identify the development of uremic neuropathy and bone disease

5. Goals of care

a. Uremic symptoms are avoided or minimized.

b. Effective renal replacement therapy is provided (e.g., dialysis, renal transplantation).

6. Collaborating professionals on health care team (see also disciplines for ARF)

a. Cardiologist consult

b. Renal transplant surgeon

7. Management of patient care

a. Anticipated patient trajectory: Patients with CRF, especially ESRD, face complex self-care expectations on discharge and the need for lifelong compliance with an intricate health care regimen. Throughout the course of recovery and discharge, patients with CRF may be expected to have needs in the following areas:

i. Skin care (see Management of Patient Care under Acute Renal Failure)

ii. Nutrition: Critical element in care; modification of diet in renal disease is implemented during the early stages of CRF for prevention and prolongation of renal health and in ESRD for moderation of uremic symptoms (National Kidney Foundation K/DOQI clinical practice guidelines for nutrition [National Kidney Foundation, 2003])

(a) General CRF diet: Restricted-protein diet of 0.6 to 0.8 g protein/kg/day with a total caloric intake of 35 mg/kcal/kg body weight and 2 g each of sodium and potassium. High-quality biologic protein (such as eggs, fish, meat) should account for two thirds of daily total protein intake.

(b) Dietary modifications for CRF: In the early stages of CRF, 0.6 g protein/kg/day plus 0.3 g protein/kg/day of high-quality biologic protein

(c) Dietary modifications for ESRD: 0.8 g protein/kg/day with a caloric intake of 35 mg/kcal/kg body weight

(d) Adjustments are made to the standard CRF diet depending on the type of dialysis and appetite; in many instances, protein intake is increased.

(1) Hemodialysis or PD: Increased protein requirements. Hemodialysis patients need 1.1 to 1.2 g protein/kg/day; PD patients, 1.3 to 1.4 g protein/kg/day.

(2) Continuous ambulatory peritoneal dialysis (CAPD): 1.1 to 1.4 g protein/kg/day

(3) Diminished appetite: Administer unlimited-protein diet to prevent malnutrition

(e) Be aware that the presence of hypoalbuminemia is associated with increased mortality in CRF.

(f) Low BUN value is another predictor of mortality, because it suggests reduced protein intake, reduced muscle mass, chronic illness, and cachexia.

(g) Sodium: Restrict to minimize hypertension, thirst, and weight gain

(h) Potassium: Restrict for most hemodialysis patients, but PD patients may not require restriction

(i) Lipids: Hyperlipidemia occurs in 20% to 75% of patients with CRF and dialysis

(1) Most common types
a) Hypertriglyceridemia
b) Elevated levels of low-density lipoproteins
c) Normal or reduced levels of high-density lipoproteins

(2) Increased risk of atherosclerosis

(3) Lack of conclusive evidence on treatment. Proponents of treatment can utilize dietary guidelines (e.g., National Cholesterol Education Program and American Heart Association diet).

(j) Vitamins: Water-soluble vitamins (i.e., vitamin B complex and C) are prescribed specifically for patients having dialysis

iii. Infection control: Infections are responsible for 15% of the yearly mortality

(a) Common infections include peritonitis resulting from PD catheterization and infection at hemodialysis vascular catheter site. Septicemia related to these infections is associated with a high mortality rate.

(b) Immunocompromise accompanies uremia (see Patient Care).

iv. Discharge planning

(a) General patient and family teaching: Be aware that the uremia of CRF impairs cognition and memory. In addition, the complexity of the renal replacement therapies demands multiple patient and family teaching sessions. Patient compliance is essential to minimize uremic symptoms as well as to ensure patient safety.

(1) Assess knowledge related to CRF, treatments, medications.

(2) Assess the effects of uremia on the patient's learning abilities (e.g., decreased attention span and memory, altered cognition).

(3) Develop a teaching plan including reinforcement, self-care activities, treatment, and compliance expectations.

(4) Instruct the patient and family or significant others about all aspects of CRF.
a) Normal renal function and renal disease state
b) Management of diet, fluids, medications, skin, rest
c) Avoidance of infection
d) Treatment alternatives and benefits and disadvantages of each; support the patient's and family's decision

(5) Instruct the patient and family about general features and elements of care for dialysis treatments.
a) Dynamics of hemodialysis or PD
b) Special diet and fluid allowances
c) Care of the dialysis access
d) Need for weight control
e) Signs and symptoms of complications such as an electrolyte imbalance
f) Transportation to the dialysis center

(b) Outcomes specific to various renal replacement therapies: See Box 5-1

v. Pharmacology

▓ BOX 5-1
▓ OUTCOMES OF RENAL REPLACEMENT THERAPIES

HEMODIALYSIS
- Circulatory access is maintained.
- Patient has hemodialysis treatment, usually three times a week (3 to 5 hours for each treatment).
- Patient complies with rigid diet and fluid restrictions.

HOME HEMODIALYSIS
- Proper environment is available: adequate space, plumbing, and hygiene.
- Patient demonstrates signs of compliance with the medical regimen and adaptation to the disease process.
- Patient demonstrates ability to physically tolerate dialysis procedure.
- There is evidence of established family support system or acceptance of surrogate dialyzer.
- Patient demonstrates ability to learn technical and aseptic skills.

CHRONIC PERITONEAL DIALYSIS
- Follows same principles and procedures as acute peritoneal dialysis; differences relate to patient expectations and use of automated peritoneal dialysis machine.
- Patient expectations for peritoneal dialysis:
  1. Maintenance of Tenckhoff catheter
  2. Use of aseptic technique throughout the procedure
  3. Treatment three to four times a week for 10 hours each treatment in hospital or 7 days, four times per day or every night with cycler
  4. Adherence to dietary and fluid restrictions
- Expectations for home peritoneal dialysis:
  1. Proper environment: Treatment requires space and storage area for equipment
  2. Cardiovascular stability: Not as necessary for home peritoneal dialysis because rapid fluid shifts and dramatic cardiovascular effects are not associated with this treatment
  3. Family support systems: Helpful but not essential because most patients use dialysis at night, and the family routine may not be disrupted
  4. Cognitive ability: Moderate technologic skill is required, but aseptic technique is essential

CONTINUOUS AMBULATORY PERITONEAL DIALYSIS
- Patient demonstrates ability to perform procedure.
- Patient recognizes that exchanges are four times a day, 7 days a week. Each exchange is 4 to 8 hours.
- Patient completes a rigorous training program.
- Patient demonstrates proper care of the Tenckhoff catheter.
- Patient adheres to the treatment schedule.
- Patient stores the dialysis equipment appropriately.
- Patient demonstrates measures to avoid complications such as peritonitis, back strain, visceral herniation, obesity, fluid excess.

RENAL TRANSPLANTATION
- Patient and family demonstrate knowledge of diet and fluid regimen, signs and symptoms of rejection.
- Patient demonstrates ability to obtain and record daily weight and administer medications.
- Patient reports for frequent clinic and other follow-up outpatient visits.
- Patient adheres to activity limitations and rehabilitation program.

    (a) Average CRF patient takes 8 to 10 medications.
    (b) Impact of CRF on pharmacologic agents: See Patient Care
    (c) Compliance necessary to receive optimal effect of pharmacologic therapy; noncompliance is associated with exaggerated uremic symptoms, exacerbation of coexisting disease (i.e., cardiac disease, diabetes, hypertension), and increased morbidity
  vi. Psychosocial issues: ESRD and dialysis or transplantation require adaptation and coping; adjustment is difficult and may contribute to depression

(a) Body image disturbance: Results from the effects of uremia, dependency on treatments, and primary illness other than renal disease (see Chapter 10)

(b) Sexual dysfunction: An experience of change in sexual function viewed as unsatisfying, unrewarding, or inadequate; results from uremia, its complications, and/or its treatment (see Chapter 10)

vii. Treatments: Renal replacement therapies include hemodialysis, CAPD, and renal transplantation. Continuous renal replacement therapy (CRRT) is a form of dialysis usually reserved for patients with ARF and performed in the critical care unit. (See Treatments under Acute Renal Failure.)

(a) Chronic hemodialysis
(1) Patient usually has hemodialysis treatment three times a week (3 to 5 hours per treatment) via a permanent or temporary vascular access.
(2) Temporary measure to replace renal function; thus, the patient must be compliant with diet and fluid restrictions
(3) Anticoagulation (heparin) usually required. A minimum heparin dosage can be used for patients at risk (i.e., postoperatively). In rare situations (e.g., patient has coagulopathy), heparin-free hemodialysis may be possible. For heparin-induced thrombocytopenia, use lepirudin or argatroban.
(4) Availability of chronic hemodialysis: Hospital, satellite center, or home performed by a surrogate or the patient

(b) Chronic PD: Follows the same principles and procedures as acute PD; differences relate to the patient's expectations and the use of an automated PD machine
(1) Frequency of treatment varies with the PD approach.
   a) Hospital based or at home: Usually dialyze four times per week for 10 hours
   b) Nighttime home PD: Dialyze all night every night
   c) CAPD: A continuous form; dialyze 24 hours a day, 7 days a week
(2) Tenckhoff catheter is permanent access placed surgically.
(3) Dietary and fluid restrictions vary.
(4) Anticoagulation is performed with use of heparin (low dose).

8. **Evaluation of patient care**
   a. No uremic symptoms are present (see Table 5-2).
   b. Effective dialysis treatment or successful renal transplantation is accomplished.
   c. Patient is able to complete the activities of daily living and participate in rehabilitation activities.
   d. Patient verbalizes achievement and acceptance of a satisfactory level of sexual functioning.
   e. Patient demonstrates the ability to cope with CRF, renal replacement therapy, and pharmacologic therapy.
   f. Family members or significant others actively support and participate in the patient's care.

Electrolyte Imbalances—Potassium Imbalance: Hyperkalemia

The serum potassium level in hyperkalemia is above 5.5 mEq/L.
1. **Pathophysiology**
   a. Inability of the kidney tubules to excrete K^+ because of tubular damage, salt depletion, or increased potassium load from injured tissues; or may be induced by drugs such as potassium-sparing diuretics (e.g., spironolactone), which inhibit aldosterone, or amiloride and triamterene, which block the sodium channel and thereby inhibit Na^+ reabsorption and promote K^+ retention
   b. Reduction in K^+ excretion caused by decreased renal perfusion because less Na^+ is available for exchange with K^+ (e.g., in cardiac failure)
   c. Alteration in K^+ release (rhabdomyolysis) or distribution (insulin deficiency)
2. **Etiology and risk factors**
   a. Acute and chronic renal failure or renal disease associated with distal tubule dysfunction (i.e., sickle cell anemia)

b. Increased cellular destruction with potassium release such as occurs in burns, trauma, crash injuries, severe catabolism, acute acidosis, intravascular hemolysis, rhabdomyolysis, and thrombocytosis

c. Excessive administration or ingestion of potassium chloride

d. Adrenal cortical insufficiency: Hypoaldosteronism or Addison's disease

e. Aldosterone deficiency

f. Low cardiac output or sodium depletion

g. Metabolic acidosis: Precipitates the movement of intracellular K^+ to the extracellular space

h. Certain drugs

   i. Potassium-sparing diuretics, which block Na^+ reabsorption, thereby facilitating K^+ retention

   ii. The antibiotics pentamidine and trimethoprim, which also promote K^+ retention via the same mechanism

   iii. Drugs that inhibit aldosterone production (e.g., ACE inhibitors, NSAIDs, heparin, cyclosporine, tacrolimus) and angiotensin II antagonists (e.g., losartan)

   iv. Drugs that inhibit extrarenal K^+ disposal (nonselective β-blockers, propranolol, nadolol, timolol)

i. Release of K^+ from injured cells: Seen in cocaine ingestion, rhabdomyolysis, and chemotherapy-induced tumor lysis syndrome

3. **Signs and symptoms: Detection of electrolyte imbalances is difficult. Suspect imbalances with renal or endocrine disease, with excessive loss of body fluids (e.g., vomiting, diarrhea), in some drug intoxications (e.g., indiscriminate use of electrolyte replacement, hormonal therapy, or vitamins), and with acute changes in mental status (confusion, agitation, coma) (Table 5-5).**

▓ TABLE 5-5
▓ ▓ Signs and Symptoms of Potassium Imbalance

System	Hyperkalemia	Hypokalemia
Cardiovascular	Bradycardia Dysrhythmias Hypotension	Diminished, irregular pulses Increased myocardial excitability or irritability Dysrhythmias: Premature atrial contractions, premature ventricular contractions, sinus bradycardia, paroxysmal atrial tachycardia, atrioventricular blocks, atrioventricular or ventricular tachycardia Enhanced digoxin effect to the point of digoxin toxicity
Neurologic	Lethargy Apathy Confusion	Drowsiness to coma, malaise, and confusion Muscle cramping (commonly in calf muscle) Muscular weakness progressing to paralysis
Pulmonary	Deep rapid respiration (Kussmaul's respirations) when hyperkalemia accompanied by acidosis Shallow respirations if muscle paralysis present	Shallow respirations secondary to muscle weakness
Gastrointestinal	Abdominal cramping and diarrhea	Vomiting Paralytic ileus
Musculoskeletal	Irritability to flaccid paralysis and numbness of extremities Fatigue associated with diminished exercise tolerance Diminished mobility to paralysis	Pain in calf similar to that of deep venous thrombosis
Genitourinary	Oliguria	Polyuria

4. **Diagnostic study findings**
   a. Laboratory: Serum potassium level exceeds 5.5 mEq/L
   b. Electrocardiogram (ECG): Progressive changes reveal peaked and elevated T waves → widened QRS → prolonged PR interval → flattened or absent P wave and ST segment depression → idioventricular rhythm → asystolic cardiac arrest
5. **Goals of care**
   a. Symptomatic hyperkalemia is eliminated.
   b. Cardiac function is restored to WNL for the patient.
6. **Collaborating professionals on health care team**
   a. Progressive care nurse
   b. Physician or intensivist
   c. Nurse practitioner, clinical nurse specialist, or physician assistant
   d. Case manager
   e. Dietitian
   f. Nephrology consult (if cause is associated with renal failure or to advise on treatments)
   g. Cardiologist (for cardiac emergencies)
   h. Endocrinology consult
7. **Management of patient care**
   a. Anticipated patient trajectory: Patients with acute symptomatic hyperkalemia face a life-threatening condition requiring urgent intervention and resolution. Recovery requires compliance with a treatment plan to prevent repeat episodes. Patients may be expected to have needs in the following areas:
      i. Positioning: Position to promote comfort; hyperkalemia can cause fatigue, muscle irritability, numbness, and flaccid paralysis
      ii. Nutrition: After K^+ stabilized to a safe, asymptomatic level, restrict dietary potassium (e.g., orange juice, cola, banana)
      iii. Discharge planning: Include discharge teaching to promote dietary compliance to avoid hyperkalemia
      iv. Pharmacology
         (a) Provide cardiac monitoring before and during pharmacologic therapy; monitor potassium levels frequently.
         (b) In emergency situations (e.g., if serum K^+ >6.5 mEq/L or ECG change indicates symptomatic hyperkalemia)
            (1) Administer regular insulin and dextrose IV with β-agonist inhalant to temporarily shift K^+ into cells.
               a) Insulin can rapidly lower serum potassium level.
               b) Dextrose must accompany insulin; patients who lack endogenous insulin production can experience a paradoxical increase in potassium or hypoglycemia.
            (2) Use sodium bicarbonate IV when severe metabolic acidosis complicates the hyperkalemia.
            (3) Essential to follow aforementioned temporary measures with a therapeutic measure to permanently remove potassium from the body (e.g., sodium polystyrene sulfonate [Kayexalate], hemodialysis)
            (4) Kayexalate with sorbitol administered orally or per rectum for the exchange of Na^+ into the intestinal cell and K^+ into the bowel space; when administered in combination with sorbitol, enhances a diarrhea stool for actual K^+ loss
               a) With Kayexalate, Na^+ ion is exchanged 1:1 for a K^+ ion in the bowel cell wall; therefore, assess the amount of sodium retained as well as the potassium loss.
               b) Ensure that the Kayexalate and sorbitol mixture is expelled, especially postoperatively, because retained Kayexalate can cause bowel obstruction and perforation.
               c) Rectal route of administration is rapid and produces a predictable outcome.

    v. Treatment: Hemodialysis is a rapid form of dialysis for serum potassium reduction (see Acute Renal Failure and Chronic Renal Failure)

  b. Potential complications

    i. Cardiac dysrhythmia: Bradycardia to asystole

      (a) Mechanism: Hyperkalemia depresses myocardial contractility and conductivity

      (b) Management: Treat hyperkalemia; if warranted, institute cardiopulmonary resuscitation for asystolic cardiac arrest

8. Evaluation of patient care

  a. Serum potassium level is between 3.5 and 5.5 mEq/L or in an asymptomatic range.

  b. No cardiac complications of hyperkalemia are present.

Electrolyte Imbalances—Potassium Imbalance: Hypokalemia

The serum potassium level in hypokalemia is below 3.5 mEq/L.

1. Pathophysiology

  a. Potassium loss exceeding intake

  b. Alkalosis: Stimulates the secretion of K^+ in the distal tubule

  c. Intracellular shifting of K^+

2. Etiology and risk factors

  a. Alkalosis: Causes K^+ to shift into the cell

  b. Abnormal GI losses: Nasogastric suction and drainage, laxative abuse, diarrhea, prolonged episode of vomiting

  c. Starvation or malnutrition (including hyperalimentation without adequate potassium replacement)

  d. Diuretic therapy (loop diuretics, thiazides, acetazolamide), renal tubular acidosis

  e. Increased adrenal corticosteroid secretion or corticosteroid therapy

  f. Liver disease

  g. Severe stress (K^+ shifts into cells)

3. Signs and symptoms: See Table 5-5

4. Diagnostic study findings

  a. Laboratory: Serum potassium levels below 3.5 mEq/L

  b. ECG: Depressed ST segments, flat or inverted T wave, presence of U wave, and ventricular dysrhythmias

5. Goals of care

  a. Serum potassium level is above 3.5 mEq/L and WNL or within asymptomatic range.

  b. Cardiac function is WNL.

6. Collaborating professionals on health care team: See Electrolyte Imbalances—Potassium Imbalance: Hyperkalemia

7. Management of patient care

  a. Anticipated patient trajectory: Patients with acute hypokalemia face serious cardiac symptomatology that requires immediate resolution in the clinical setting. Recovery and discharge require compliance with a treatment regimen that prevents repeated episodes. Patients may be expected to have needs in the following areas:

    i. Positioning: Place in a position of comfort to minimize muscle cramping and weakness, as well as to promote adequate respirations

    ii. Nutrition: Provide foods containing potassium (e.g., orange juice, raisins, milk, green vegetables)

    iii. Discharge planning: Include discharge teaching to promote sufficient potassium intake and compliance with the dietary regimen

    iv. Pharmacology: Provide cardiac monitoring before and during pharmacologic therapy

      (a) Administer oral potassium supplements when indicated; dilute to prevent GI irritation and to facilitate absorption.

      (b) Observe for ECG changes and the presence of dysrhythmias.

      (c) Monitor serum potassium levels.

      (d) Record the amount of urine output and other drainage (gastric aspirate, diarrhea) to aid in calculating total body potassium balance.

(e) Recognize and treat signs of alkalosis.
(f) Administer oral potassium supplements when indicated; dilute to prevent GI irritation and to facilitate absorption.
(g) Never give IV potassium chloride rapidly; large concentrations can precipitate hyperkalemia, producing necrosis of the vessel wall, and possibly inducing ventricular fibrillation. *Never administer an IV push.*
(h) Determine whether the patient is receiving digitalis or diuretics; correct potassium losses, because these can precipitate digitalis toxicity and decrease the effectiveness of most diuretics.
(i) Emergency treatment
  (1) Slowly administer IV potassium chloride while the patient is monitored with ECG for dysrhythmias.
  (2) Monitor for signs and symptoms of hyperkalemia.
  (3) Maintain a record of serum potassium levels to assess the adequacy of replacement therapy.
(j) Follow-up: If the patient is receiving digitalis and diuretics, consider the use of potassium chloride supplements or potassium-sparing diuretics
  b. Potential complications
    i. Digoxin toxicity
      (a) Mechanism: Hypokalemia enhances the effect of digoxin
      (b) Management: IV potassium on medication pump with cardiac monitoring
    ii. Dysrhythmias
      (a) Mechanism: Hypokalemia decreases the cardiac threshold, increasing the risk of dysrhythmia
      (b) Management: IV potassium on medication pump with cardiac monitoring
8. **Evaluation of patient care**
  a. Serum potassium levels are above 3.5 mEq/L or within asymptomatic range.
  b. No cardiac complications of hypokalemia are present.

Electrolyte Imbalances—Sodium Imbalance: Hypernatremia

The serum sodium level in hypernatremia is above 145 mEq/L.
1. **Pathophysiology**
  a. Increased ECF volume: Sodium and water retention
  b. Decreased ECF volume: Sodium retention without water retention; greater water loss compared with sodium loss (e.g., diuresis of water without excretion of equal amounts of sodium)
2. **Etiology and risk factors**
  a. Normal kidneys: Lack of ADH or neurohypophyseal insufficiency (e.g., diabetes insipidus, water loss in excess of sodium loss)
    i. Potassium depletion: Creates a concentrating defect in the kidney, causing polyuria
    ii. Hypercalcemia: Polyuria and dehydration
    iii. Drugs (e.g., osmotic diuretics or sodium bicarbonate, or NaCl solution); also mineralocorticoids, laxatives, and antacids
    iv. Excessive adrenocortical secretion
    v. Loss of the thirst mechanism (e.g., in a comatose patient)
    vi. Uncontrolled diabetes mellitus with osmotic diuresis due to hyperglycemia
    vii. Head injury
    viii. Post central nervous system surgery: Causes fluctuation (increase and decrease) in ADH release
  b. Impaired renal function: Inability of renal tubules to respond to ADH (e.g., nephrogenic diabetes insipidus)
3. **Signs and symptoms: Findings relate to "edematous states" and/or hypoproteinemia (Table 5-6)**
4. **Diagnostic study findings**
  a. Serum Na^+ level above 145 mEq/L, elevated hematocrit with volume depletion
  b. Serum osmolality greater than 295 mOsm/L

■ **TABLE 5-6**
■ ■ **Signs and Symptoms of Sodium Imbalance**

System	Hypernatremia	Hyponatremia
General	Excessive weight gain Dehydration—extreme thirst, fever, decreased urine output, dry mucous membranes	Weight loss or gain Malaise Headache Decreased hematocrit and blood urea nitrogen level (dilutional effect)
Cardiovascular	Weak, thready pulse with increased ECF Tachycardia with decreased ECF often progressing to bradycardia Hypertension with increased ECF Hypotension with or without postural changes with decreased ECF	Rapid pulse with overhydration Hypotension or hypertension Decreased central venous pressure and jugular venous pressure with overhydration
Neurologic	Restlessness Irritability Lethargy Confusion to coma Twitching to seizures Muscle tension	Confusion to coma Muscle weakness
Pulmonary	Labored breathing (dyspnea) associated with pulmonary edema	Dyspnea with crackles Pulmonary edema
Gastrointestinal	Anorexia Edematous tongue	Abdominal cramps Nausea
Musculoskeletal	Muscle weakness	
Integumentary	Dry, flushed skin Dry mucous membranes Pitting edema	Poor skin turgor
Genitourinary	Oliguria or anuria with dehydration Polyuria with osmotic diuresis	Thirst Normal urine output to polyuria Urine sodium level <20 mEq/L

ECF, Extracellular fluid.

    c. Urine SG may be greater than 1.030, except in diabetes insipidus, in which SG can be as low as 1.005.

    d. Urine osmolality 800 to 1400 mOsm/L; lower with diabetes insipidus

    e. Urine Na^+ level higher than 40 mEq/L when hypernatremia is due to sodium excess and normal to low value during a water deficit

5. Goals of care

    a. Serum and urine Na^+ levels are in a normal range or in a high, asymptomatic range.

    b. Normal fluid status is maintained.

6. Collaborating professionals on health care team: See Electrolyte Imbalances—Potassium Imbalance: Hyperkalemia

7. Management of patient care

    a. Anticipated patient trajectory: Patients with hypernatremia are experiencing a hyperosmolar state usually secondary to a serious previously existing condition. Both conditions need to be treated and resolved before discharge. Recovery and discharge require compliance with a treatment regimen that prevents repeat episodes. Patients may be expected to have needs in the following areas:

        i. Positioning: Initiate fall prevention protocol if patient exhibits neurologic signs and symptoms

        ii. Skin care

            (a) Dehydration: Hydrate patient and lubricate skin

            (b) Overhydration: Protect bony prominences; change position often

   iii.   Nutrition: Dietary and fluid restrictions with restricted sodium; I&O
   iv.   Pharmacology: Medication adjustments
      (a) Avoid laxatives and antacids (e.g., sodium bicarbonate) containing high-sodium ingredients.
      (b) Utilize diuretics: promote a greater loss of water than Na^+.
      (c) Administer corticosteroids to stimulate reabsorption of Na^+ and excretion of K^+.
   v.   Treatments
      (a) Monitor serum sodium levels, serum osmolality, urine osmolality, I&O, and body weight.
      (b) Perform neurologic assessments and correlate with serum Na^+ levels.
      (c) Administer water in excess of sodium if the patient requires volume expansion (5% dextrose in water or 0.45 normal saline or both).
      (d) Avoid rapid correction of sodium level, because this may precipitate acute pulmonary edema or cerebral edema; reduce sodium level gradually by encouraging Na^+ losses via diuretics or administration of fluids.
      (e) Determine precipitating factors and treat as ordered.
      (f) For patients in renal failure, treat via dialysis.
   b. Potential complications
      i.   Dyspnea, labored respirations related to pulmonary edema
      ii.   Seizures
         (a) Mechanism: Disruption of sodium pump dynamics in cerebral tissues, which leads to electrical instability
         (b) Management: Seizure precautions and correction of hypernatremia
8. **Evaluation of patient care**
   a. Sodium level is WNL and patient is asymptomatic.
   b. Serum osmolality is 280 to 295 mOsm/L.
   c. Urine osmolality is within the normal range.
   d. Hydration status is normal.

Electrolyte Imbalances—Sodium Imbalance: Hyponatremia

The serum sodium level in hyponatremia is below 136 mEq/L.
1. **Pathophysiology**
   a. Excess of water relative to the amount of sodium in the body, producing a dilutional effect on the sodium concentration
   b. Na^+ loss exceeds water loss.
2. **Etiology and risk factors**
   a. Water excess: Excessive water intake without sodium intake; SIADH
   b. Sodium depletion
      i.   Abnormal losses via diaphoresis, diuretics, nasogastric suction, diarrhea
      ii.   Hyperglycemia (glucose-induced diuresis)
      iii.   Salt-losing renal diseases: Interstitial nephritis
   c. Heart failure and cirrhosis of the liver: Decreased cardiac output increases water retention by the kidneys
3. **Signs and symptoms: Permanent neurologic changes with a serum sodium level below 110 mEq/L (see Table 5-6)**
4. **Diagnostic study findings**
   a. Serum Na^+ level below 136 mEq/L and low hematocrit caused by water excess
   b. Urine volume and SG can be normal.
   c. Urine Na^+ level less than 20 mEq/L (if due to Na^+ deficit) and normal to elevated (if due to water excess)
   d. Serum osmolality below 280 mOsm/L
5. **Goals of care**
   a. Serum sodium level is WNL or at an asymptomatic level.
   b. Normal fluid status is maintained.
6. **Collaborating professionals on health care team: See Electrolyte Imbalances—Potassium Imbalance: Hyperkalemia**

7. **Management of patient care**
   a. Anticipated patient trajectory: Patients with hyponatremia experience a hypo-osmolar condition. Recovery requires compliance with a treatment plan that prevents repeat episodes. Patients may be expected to have needs in the following areas:
      i. Skin care: See Electrolyte Imbalances—Sodium Imbalance: Hypernatremia
      ii. Nutrition and fluid balance
         (a) For sodium and water losses: Provide high-sodium diet and adequate fluid intake
         (b) For water intoxication: Restrict fluid intake (limit of 500 ml/day)
         (c) For water intoxication related to SIADH: Restrict water intake, because decreased sodium is due to the inability to excrete water normally
      iii. Pharmacology
         (a) Discontinue medications that cause loss of Na^+ (e.g., diuretics, laxatives).
         (b) Administer NaCl tablets orally as indicated.
         (c) Administer diuretics to treat water intoxication.
      iv. Treatments
         (a) Monitor neurologic signs.
         (b) For Na^+ and water losses:
            (1) Replace fluids with normal (0.9%) or hypertonic (3%) saline.
            (2) Administer hypertonic saline via an infusion pump; measure serum sodium levels frequently; observe for pulmonary edema; monitor I&O.
            (3) Monitor effectiveness of nutrition and other therapies by measuring serum and urine sodium levels and osmolality concentrations.
         (c) For water intoxication:
            (1) Restrict fluid intake.
            (2) Monitor serum sodium levels to determine whether sodium replacement is indicated.
            (3) Do not give normal saline in SIADH; normal saline does not correct the basic cause of SIADH.
   b. Potential complications: See Electrolyte Imbalances—Sodium Imbalance: Hypernatremia
8. **Evaluation of patient care**
   a. Sodium levels are WNL or patient is asymptomatic (see Electrolyte Imbalances—Sodium Imbalance: Hypernatremia).
   b. Urinary sodium level is above 30 to 40 mEq/L.
   c. Normal hydration status is maintained.

Electrolyte Imbalances—Calcium Imbalance: Hypercalcemia

The serum calcium level in hypercalcemia is above 10.5 mg/dl.
1. **Pathophysiology**
   a. Increased mobilization of calcium from bone
   b. Increased intestinal reabsorption of calcium ion (Ca^{2+}): May occur with large dietary intake or excessive vitamin D supplementation, or in granulomatous disease (e.g., sarcoidosis)
   c. Altered renal tubular reabsorption of Ca^{2+}
2. **Etiology and risk factors**
   a. Primary hyperparathyroidism: Causes increased tubular reabsorption of Ca^{2+} and Ca^{2+} release from bone
   b. Metastatic carcinoma with "osteolytic lesions" that release calcium into plasma and multiple myeloma
   c. Prolonged bed rest: Causes calcium to be mobilized from the bones, teeth, and intestines
   d. Alkalosis: Increases calcium binding to protein; decreases serum calcium levels
   e. Thyrotoxicosis
   f. Excessive intake of vitamin D: Increases Ca^{2+} reabsorption from intestines
   g. Drugs: Thiazide diuretic therapy inhibits Ca^{2+} excretion
   h. Renal tubular acidosis
3. **Signs and symptoms: See Table 5-7**
4. **Diagnostic study findings**

■ **TABLE 5-7**
■ ■ **Signs and Symptoms of Calcium Imbalance**

System	Hypercalcemia	Hypocalcemia
Cardiovascular	Hypertension (33% of all cases)	Dysrhythmias Irregular pulse
Neurologic	Lethargy Increased fatigue Confusion to coma Subtle personality changes	Lethargy Generalized tonic-clonic seizures
Pulmonary		Labored and shallow breathing Wheezing Bronchospasm when respiratory muscles involved
Gastrointestinal	Anorexia Nausea and vomiting Abdominal pain and constipation	Paralytic ileus with absent bowel sounds Constipation with or without distended abdomen or diarrhea
Renal	Acute or chronic renal failure Renal vascular constriction Polyuria Renal calcium deposits Flank and thigh pain associated with renal calculi	Oliguria or anuria
Musculoskeletal	Hypotonicity and weakness of muscles Pathologic fractures Metastatic calcifications Bone pain	Muscle cramps Muscle tremors Functional and physical limitations on ambulation and exercise Bone pain and fractures

    a. Laboratory
       i. Serum calcium level: Above 10.5 mg/dl
       ii. Other serum studies: Thyroid-stimulating hormone, PTH, PTH-related peptide, vitamin D levels
    b. Radiologic
       i. Nephrocalcinosis: Calcium deposits in renal parenchyma, renal calculi
       ii. Calcium deposits visible on bone films
    c. ECG: Shortening of the ST segment
5. Goals of care
    a. Calcium stays WNL or in an asymptomatic range.
    b. Cardiac and neurologic function is normal.
6. Collaborating professionals on health care team: See Electrolyte Imbalances—Potassium Imbalance: Hyperkalemia
7. Management of patient care
    a. Anticipated patient trajectory: Clinical course, recovery, and discharge planning for patients with hypercalcemia vary depending on whether the condition is acute or chronic. Patients may be expected to have needs in the following areas:
       i. Nutrition: Restrict dietary calcium (e.g., milk, cheese, yogurt)
       ii. Discharge planning: Teach the patient how to comply with the dietary regimen to avoid hypercalcemia
       iii. Pharmacology
          (a) Administer digitalis cautiously; hypercalcemia enhances the action of digitalis, and toxicosis can result.
          (b) Administer NaCl infusion and diuretics to reduce Ca^{2+} absorption.
          (c) Be aware that corticosteroids reduce GI absorption of Ca^{2+}.

(d) Institute mithramycin therapy to stimulate bone uptake of calcium.
(e) Consider the administration of bisphosphonates (e.g., pamidronate), calcitonin, or corticosteroids for the treatment of moderate to severe hypercalcemia associated with malignancy to reduce the rate of bone turnover.
    iv. Treatments
       (a) Monitor I&O status and renal function parameters.
       (b) If the patient is in renal failure, utilize dialysis.
       (c) Administer bisphosphonates.
  b. Potential complications
    i. Cardiac arrest
       (a) Mechanism: Enhanced digoxin effect, dysrhythmias (particularly atrioventricular blocks) may progress to cardiac arrest
       (b) Management: Cardiopulmonary resuscitation
8. Evaluation of patient care
  a. Calcium level is WNL or patient is asymptomatic.
  b. Cardiac and neuromuscular function is normal.

Electrolyte Imbalances—Calcium Imbalance: Hypocalcemia

The serum calcium level in hypocalcemia is below 8.5 mg/dl.
1. Pathophysiology
  a. Excessive GI losses of calcium resulting from diarrhea, diuretic use, and increased levels of lipoproteins
  b. Malabsorption syndromes, such as vitamin D deficiency and hypoparathyroidism
2. Etiology and risk factors
  a. Hypoparathyroidism or hypomagnesemia (Mg^{2+} needed for effective action of PTH)
  b. CRF
    i. Hyperphosphatemia due to CRF: Potentiates the peripheral deposition of calcium
    ii. Vitamin D deficiency due to CRF, hepatic failure, rickets: Lack of activated vitamin D (1,25-dihydroxycholecalciferol or 25-hydroxycholecalciferol) necessary for Ca^{2+} absorption
  c. Vitamin D resistance: Inability to absorb Ca^{2+} from the intestine; vitamin D mediated
  d. Chronic malabsorption syndrome resulting from magnesium depletion, gastrectomy, high-fat diet (fat impairs Ca^{2+} absorption), small-bowel disorder that prevents absorption of vitamin D
  e. Increased thyrocalcitonin: Stimulates osteoblasts to prevent Ca^{2+} entry into serum
  f. Malignancy
    i. Osteoblastic metastasis: Calcium is consumed for abnormal bone synthesis
    ii. Medullary carcinoma of the thyroid: Secretion of thyrocalcitonin is abnormal
  g. Acute pancreatitis: Calcium precipitates in an inflamed pancreas
  h. Hyperphosphatemia: Calcium and phosphate bind together and precipitate in tissues
    i. Cytotoxic drugs (cytolysis of bone)
    ii. Increased oral intake of phosphates
    iii. CRF (decreased excretion of phosphate)
3. Signs and symptoms: See Table 5-7
4. Diagnostic study findings
  a. Serum calcium level below 8.5 mg/dl
  b. ECG: Prolonged ST segment and QT interval
  c. Trousseau's sign
    i. Apply a BP cuff to the upper arm and inflate.
    ii. If carpopedal spasm occurs, the test result is positive.
    iii. If no spasm appears in 3 minutes, the test result is negative.
    iv. Remove the cuff and tell the patient to hyperventilate (30 times per minute).
    v. Respiratory alkalosis that develops can also produce a carpopedal spasm (a positive result if it occurs).

       d. Chvostek's sign: Tap on the supramandibular portion of the parotid gland; observe for twitches in the upper lip on the side tapped; muscle spasm indicates a positive test result

5. Goals of care
    a. Serum calcium level is WNL, and the patient is asymptomatic.
    b. There is no evidence of complications from hypocalcemia.

6. Collaborating professionals on health care team: See Electrolyte Imbalances—Potassium Imbalance: Hyperkalemia

7. Management of patient care
    a. Anticipated patient trajectory: Patients with hypocalcemia face a life-threatening condition requiring urgent pharmacologic intervention. Recovery and discharge focus on preventing repeat episodes. Patients can be expected to have needs in the following areas:
       i. Nutrition
          (a) Assess for a history of starvation, dietary abuse, or malabsorption.
          (b) Administer a diet high in calcium.
       ii. Discharge planning
          (a) Provide discharge teaching to promote dietary intake of calcium.
          (b) Instruct on the warning signs of tetany or seizures.
       iii. Pharmacology
          (a) Administer 10% calcium gluconate or calcium chloride slowly IV (1 ml/min) for emergency intervention; monitor for decreased cardiac output, enhanced digitalis effects, and dysrhythmias.
          (b) Chronic hypocalcemia necessitates daily oral doses of calcium, usually administered in the range of 1.5 to 3 g/day.
          (c) Administer correct vitamin D supplement (1,25-dihydroxycholecalciferol or 25-hydroxycholecalciferol) as ordered.
          (d) With phosphate deficiency, replace phosphates before administering calcium; hyperphosphatemia usually accompanies hypocalcemia.
       iv. Treatments
          (a) Monitor serum calcium and phosphate levels.
          (b) Institute cardiac monitoring; monitor therapeutic effectiveness via Chvostek's and Trousseau's signs plus ECG.
          (c) Implement seizure precautions; provide a quiet environment.
          (d) Monitor respiratory function; bronchospasm may precipitate respiratory arrest.
          (e) In renal failure, utilize dialysis and activated vitamin D.
    b. Potential complications
       i. Tetany, seizures
          (a) Seizure precautions
          (b) Calcium bolus at bedside
          (c) Treat cause of hypocalcemia; replace calcium.

8. Evaluation of patient care
    a. Patient is asymptomatic, and calcium level is WNL.
    b. There is no neuromuscular or cardiac involvement related to hypocalcemia or its treatment.

Electrolyte Imbalances—Phosphate Imbalance: Hyperphosphatemia

The serum phosphate level in hyperphosphatemia is above 4.5 mg/dl.

1. Pathophysiology
    a. Inability to excrete phosphate (HPO_4^-) via the kidney because of a decrease in GFR to one tenth of normal or because of renal failure
    b. Excessive intake due to diet, or cathartic abuse or drugs (cytotoxic agents)

2. Etiology and risk factors
    a. Acute or chronic renal failure (inability to excrete HPO_4^-)

▨ **TABLE 5-8**
▨ ▨ **Signs and Symptoms of Phosphate Imbalance**

System	Hyperphosphatemia	Hypophosphatemia
General Other	Vague, like those of hypocalcemia Seizures Muscle cramping Joint pain Pruritus	Vague Fatigue Confusion and malaise Lack of appetite, changes in weight Muscle weakness and wasting with or without impaired ambulation Dyspnea Tachycardia Hypotension Decreased urine output

    b. Hypoparathyroidism: PTH causes hypophosphatemia and lowers body phosphate levels

    c. Cathartic abuse or use of phosphate-containing laxatives or enemas

    d. Use of cytotoxic agents for neoplasms: Serum phosphate level increases as a result of cytolysis

    e. Overadministration of IV or oral phosphates

3. **Signs and symptoms: Vague symptomatology similar to that of hypocalcemia (Table 5-8)**

4. **Diagnostic study findings**

    a. Laboratory: Serum phosphate level higher than 4.5 mg/dl

    b. ECG: Changes comparable with those seen in hypocalcemia

5. **Goals of care**

    a. Phosphate level stays WNL or within a safe asymptomatic range.

    b. There are no episodes of tetany or seizures.

6. **Collaborating professionals on health care team: See Electrolyte Imbalances—Potassium Imbalance: Hyperkalemia**

7. **Management of patient care**

    a. Anticipated patient trajectory: Patients with hyperphosphatemia differ in clinical course depending on whether it is an acute or chronic problem. Recovery and discharge focus on preventing repeat episodes. Patients may be expected to have needs in the following areas:

        i. Nutrition: If hypocalcemia accompanies hyperphosphatemia, administer a diet high in calcium and low in phosphorus

        ii. Discharge planning

            (a) Provide discharge teaching to promote dietary compliance to avoid hyperphosphatemia (e.g., compliance with use of HPO_4^- binders).

            (b) Instruct on the warning signs of seizures.

        iii. Pharmacology

            (a) Administer phosphate binders, which act on the intestines to limit phosphate absorption, thereby reducing the serum phosphate level (e.g., calcium carbonate).

            (b) Administer acetazolamide to increase urinary phosphate excretion via the normal kidney.

            (c) Monitor serum phosphate and calcium levels to determine the effectiveness of therapy.

        iv. Treatment: Institute dialysis for rapid correction of hyperphosphatemia

    b. Potential complications: See Electrolyte Imbalances—Calcium Imbalance: Hypocalcemia

8. **Evaluation of patient care**

    a. Serum phosphate level is WNL.

    b. No neuromuscular symptomatology related to phosphate level is present.

Electrolyte Imbalances—Phosphate Imbalance: Hypophosphatemia

The serum phosphate level in hypophosphatemia is below 3.0 mg/L.

1. **Pathophysiology**
   a. Increased cell uptake to form sugar phosphates: Occurs during hyperventilation or glucose administration
   b. Decreased phosphate absorption from the bowel
   c. Renal phosphate wasting (loss of proximal tubular function): Seen in Fanconi's syndrome and vitamin D–resistant rickets
2. **Etiology and risk factors**
   a. Inadequate phosphate intake (seen in chronic alcoholism)
   b. Chronic phosphate depletion: Occurs in osteomalacia and rickets
   c. Long-term hyperalimentation without adequate phosphate replacement; glucose phosphorylation uses phosphate and can lead to phosphate depletion if no replacement is available
   d. Hyperparathyroidism: Causes renal phosphaturia
   e. Malabsorption syndrome
   f. Abuse or overadministration of phosphate-binding gels
   g. Fanconi's syndrome: Loss of phosphates in urine leading to osteomalacia (adults)
3. **Signs and symptoms: Vague presentation (see Table 5-8)**
4. **Diagnostic study findings**
   a. Laboratory
      i. Serum phosphate level below 3.0 mg/dl, low serum alkaline pyrophosphate level, and high serum pyrophosphate level
      ii. Hypercalcemia and hypophosphatemia: Indicators of acute phosphate depletion in hyperparathyroidism; PTH increases the serum calcium level by promoting the release of Ca^{2+} from bone and decreases serum phosphate level by promoting excretion of HPO_4^- into urine
   b. Radiologic: Skeletal abnormalities resembling osteomalacia (i.e., pseudofractures characterized by thickened periosteum and new bone formation over what appears to be an incomplete fracture)
5. **Goals of care**
   a. Serum phosphate level is in an asymptomatic range.
   b. No neuromuscular signs of hypophosphatemia are present.
6. **Collaborating professionals on health care team: See Electrolyte Imbalances—Potassium Imbalance: Hyperkalemia**
7. **Management of patient care**
   a. Anticipated patient trajectory: Patients with hypophosphatemia differ in their clinical course depending on whether the condition is acute or chronic. The treatment regimen aims to prevent repeat episodes. Patients may have needs in the following areas:
      i. Nutrition: If hypercalcemia accompanies hypophosphatemia, use a calcium-restricted diet
      ii. Discharge planning
         (a) Provide teaching to promote the proper use of phosphate binders.
         (b) Instruct on the warning signs of seizures; numbness and tingling around the month can occur immediately before a seizure.
      iii. Treatments
         (a) Treat the primary cause of hypophosphatemia.
         (b) Monitor phosphate and calcium levels.
         (c) Administer oral phosphate (potassium phosphate) or IV phosphorus.
         (d) Dialysis is an option in renal failure for acute episodes and/or for maintenance once the imbalance is corrected.
   b. Potential complications: See Electrolyte Imbalances—Calcium Imbalance: Hypocalcemia
8. **Evaluation of patient care**
   a. Phosphate level is within an asymptomatic range.
   b. No neuromuscular involvement is present.

Electrolyte Imbalances—Magnesium Imbalance: Hypermagnesemia

The serum magnesium level in hypermagnesemia is above 2.5 mEq/L.

1. **Pathophysiology**
   a. Mg^{2+} regulates nerve and muscle tone by preventing their activation by Ca^{2+}. Elevated level of Mg^{2+} can lead to excessive relaxation of nerves and muscles, including the myocardium and respiratory muscles.
   b. Magnesium is required for more than 300 enzymes to work, including those involved in protein, fat, and carbohydrate metabolism. Elevated Mg^{2+} levels can disrupt numerous metabolic interactions.

2. **Etiology and risk factors**
   a. Renal failure: Decreases excretion of Mg^{2+}
   b. Adrenal insufficiency
   c. Excessive intake or administration of Mg^{2+}-containing antacid gels or laxatives
   d. Acidotic states (e.g., diabetic ketoacidosis)

3. **Signs and symptoms: Vague presentation (Table 5-9)**

4. **Diagnostic study findings**
   a. Laboratory: Serum magnesium level over 2.5 mEq/L
   b. ECG: Peaked T wave similar to that seen in hyperkalemia

5. **Goals of care**
   a. Serum magnesium level is WNL.
   b. There is no neuromuscular or cardiac involvement.

6. **Collaborating professionals on health care team: See Electrolyte Imbalances—Potassium Imbalance: Hyperkalemia**

7. **Management of patient care**
   a. Anticipated patient trajectory: Patients with acute hypermagnesemia have a clinical course complicated by dramatic shifts in neurologic status. Emergent therapies are followed by preventive measures before discharge. Patients may have needs in the following areas:
      i. Nutrition: Eliminate or avoid magnesium-containing nutritional supplements (e.g., total parenteral nutrition, tube feeding, or oral protein drinks)
      ii. Discharge planning: Teach dietary and pharmacologic restrictions
      iii. Pharmacology
         (a) Teach the patient to avoid medications containing magnesium (e.g., laxatives, antacids).
         (b) If renal function is normal, administer diuretics or induce diuresis with saline to encourage magnesium loss.
         (c) Consider calcium gluconate administration to minimize symptoms of increased magnesium.

▧ **TABLE 5-9**
▧ ▧ **Signs and Symptoms of Magnesium Imbalance**

System	Hypermagnesemia	Hypomagnesemia
General	Lethargy to coma	Dizziness
	Fatigue	Lethargy
	Muscle weakness with or without loss of deep tendon reflexes	Confusion to psychosis
		Muscle weakness or tremors to tetany
	Bradycardia	Seizures
	Decreased respiration to apnea	Irregular pulse
	Hypotension secondary to depressed myocardial contractility, may lead to cardiac arrest	Dysrhythmias
		Enhanced digitalis effect
		Normal to decreased blood pressure
		Positive Chvostek's sign
		Positive Trousseau's sign

       iv. Treatments
          (a) Determine the primary cause of hypermagnesemia and intervene.
          (b) Consider dialysis if excesses are due to renal failure.
          (c) Monitor ECG and neurologic signs.
          (d) Monitor serum magnesium levels.
  b. Potential complications: See Electrolyte Imbalances—Potassium Imbalance: Hyperkalemia
8. Evaluation of patient care
  a. Magnesium levels are WNL or patient is asymptomatic.
  b. There is no evidence of neuromuscular or cardiac complications.

Electrolyte Imbalances—Magnesium Imbalance: Hypomagnesemia

The serum level in hypomagnesemia is below 1.5 mEq/L.
1. Pathophysiology
  a. Decreased intake, diminished intestinal reabsorption, or excess losses of magnesium in urine, wounds, or extracellular drainage
  b. Diminishes ability to relax muscular and neural tone
  c. Disrupts numerous physiologic and metabolic enzyme reactions
2. Etiology and risk factors
  a. Starvation, malabsorption syndrome, hypocalcemia, prolonged hyperalimentation without adequate Mg^{2+} replacement; excessive fistula or GI losses of Mg^{2+} (e.g., severe diarrhea, nasogastric suction) without sufficient replacement
  b. Bartter's syndrome
  c. Excessive diuretic therapy or excessive corticosteroid administration
  d. Chronic alcoholism
  e. Alkalotic states (in some instances)
  f. Hypocalcemia, hypoparathyroidism, hyperaldosteronism, hyperthyroidism
  g. Drugs: Cisplatin, cyclosporine, amphotericin, gentamicin
  h. Acute or chronic pancreatitis
3. Signs and symptoms: Vague presentation (see Table 5-9)
4. Diagnostic study findings
  a. Laboratory: Serum magnesium levels below 1.5 mEq/L
  b. ECG: Flat or inverted T waves, possible ST-segment depression, and prolonged QT interval
5. Goals of care
  a. Serum magnesium level returns to normal.
  b. There are no significant cardiac or neuromuscular symptoms.
6. Collaborating professionals on health care team: See Electrolyte Imbalances—Potassium Imbalance: Hyperkalemia
7. Management of patient care
  a. Anticipated patient trajectory: Patients with acute hypomagnesemia can experience serious neuromuscular symptoms. Emergent therapies are followed by a preventive regimen. Patients may be expected to have needs in the following areas:
    i. Nutrition
      (a) Provide magnesium-containing supplements and foods (e.g., seafood, green vegetables, whole grains, nuts).
      (b) Observe for coexisting electrolyte imbalances (e.g., hypocalcemia).
    ii. Discharge planning
      (a) Teach dietary measures to increase magnesium intake.
      (b) Teach diuretic regimen.
    iii. Pharmacology
      (a) Administer magnesium sulfate 50% intramuscularly or IV; in acute MI, IV infusion rates vary, and the dose of magnesium may range from 33 to 91.6 mmol.
      (b) Calcium gluconate may be given when replacing with large boluses of magnesium, because calcium retards the effects of a sudden reversal to hypermagnesemia.
      (c) If hypokalemia occurs simultaneously with hypomagnesemia, correct the magnesium deficit first.
      (d) Be aware that hypomagnesemia enhances digitalis toxicity.

iv. Treatments
    (a) Establish seizure precautions.
    (b) Correct alkalosis if present.
    (c) Monitor ECG changes.
    (d) Monitor serum magnesium levels.
  b. Potential complications: See Electrolyte Imbalances—Potassium Imbalance: Hypokalemia
8. Evaluation of patient care
  a. Level of magnesium is in an asymptomatic range.
  b. There are no significant cardiac or neuromuscular symptoms.

REFERENCES AND BIBLIOGRAPHY

Physiologic Anatomy

Brenner BM. *Brenner and Rector's the Kidney.* 8th ed. Philadelphia, PA: Elsevier; 2008.

Massry SG, Glassuck RS. *Textbook of Nephrology.* 4th ed. Philadelphia, PA: Lippincott Williams & Wilkins; 2001.

Schira M. Renal anatomy and physiology. In: Urden LD, Stacy KM, Lough ME, eds. *Thelan's Critical Care Nursing.* St Louis, MO: Mosby; 2006.

Schrier RW. *Diseases of the Kidney and Urinary Tract.* 8th ed. Philadelphia, PA: Lippincott Williams & Wilkins; 2006.

Tanagho EA, McArich JW. *Smith's General Urology.* New York, NY: Lange Medical Books/McGraw-Hill; 2007.

Wein AJ, Kavoussi LR, Novick AC, et al. *Campbell-Walsh Urology.* 9th ed. Philadelphia, PA: Saunders; 2007.

Patient Assessment

Barozzi L, Valentino M, Santoro A, et al. Renal ultrasonography in critically ill patients. *Crit Care Med.* 2007;35(5 Suppl):S198-S205.

Finfer S, Bellomo R, Boyce N, et al. A comparison of albumin and saline for fluid resuscitation in the intensive care unit. *N Engl J Med.* 2004;350(22):2247-2256.

Lough ME. Renal clinical assessment and diagnostic procedures. In: Urden LD, Stacy KM, Lough ME, eds. *Thelan's Critical Care Nursing.* St Louis, MO: Elsevier; 2006.

Luckey AE, Parsa CJ. Fluid and electrolysis in the aged. *Arch Surg.* 2003;138(10):1055-1060.

Sherman DS, Fish DN, Tertelbaum I. Assessing renal function in cirrhotic patients: problem and pitfalls. *Am J Kidney Dis.* 2003;41:269-278.

Acute Renal Failure

Abay MC, Delos Reyes J, Everts K, et al. Current literature questions the routine use of low-dose dopamine. *AANA Journal.* 2007;75(1):57-63.

Agraharkar M, Safirstein RL. The pathophysiology of acute renal failure. In: Greenberg A, ed. *Primer on Kidney Diseases.* National Kidney Foundation. 4th ed. Philadelphia, PA: Saunders; 2005.

Anderson AL, Smith KM. Prevention of contrast-induced nephropathy: a pharmacological overview. *Orthopedics.* 2006;29(10):893-895.

Bagshaw SM, Berthiaume LR, Delaney A, et al. Continuous versus intermittent renal replacement therapy for critically ill patients with acute kidney injury: a meta-analysis. *Crit Care Med.* 2008;36(2):610-617.

Bartorelli AL, Marenzi G. Contrast-induced nephropathy. *J Intervent Cardiol.* 2008;21(1):74-85.

Bouman CS, Oudemans-van Straaten HM. Timing of renal replacement therapy in critically ill patients with acute kidney injury. *Curr Opin Crit Care.* 2007;13(6):656-661.

Brenner BM. *Brenner and Rector's the Kidney.* 8th ed. Philadelphia, PA: Elsevier; 2008.

Cartin-Ceba R, Afessa B, Gajic O. Low baseline serum creatinine concentration predicts mortality in critically ill patients independent of body mass index. *Crit Care.* 2007;35(10):2420-2423.

Criddle L. Rhabdomyolysis: pathophysiology, recognition and management. *Crit Care Nurse.* 2003;23(6):14.

Dirkes S, Hodge K. Continuous renal replacement therapy in the adult intensive care unit: history and current trends. *Crit Care Nurse.* 2007;27:61-80.

Debaveye YA, Vanden Berghe GH. Is there still a place for dopamine in the modern ICU? *Anesth Analg.* 2004;98(2):461-468.

Landreneau KJ, Ward-Smith P. Perceptions of adult patients on hemodialysis concerning choice among renal replacement therapies. *Nephrol Nurs J.* 2007;34(5):513-520, 525.

Lough ME. Renal disorders and therapeutic management. In: Urden LD, Stacy KM, Lough ME, eds. *Thelan's Critical Care Nursing.* St Louis, MO: Mosby; 2006.

Liu Y, Coresh JA, Eustace JC, et al. Association between cholesterol level and mortality in dialysis patients: rule of inflammation and malnutrition. *JAMA.* 2004;291(4):451-459.

Sumnall R. Fluid management and diuretic therapy in acute renal failure. *Nurs Crit Care.* 2007;12(1):27-33.

Uchino S. Choice of therapy and renal recovery. *Crit Care Med.* 2008;36(4 Suppl):S239-S242.

Uchino S, Doig GS, Bellomo R, et al: Beginning and Ending Supportive Therapy for the Kidney (B.E.S.T. Kidney) Investigators. Diuretics and mortality in acute renal failure. *Crit Care Med.* 2004;32(8):1669-1677.

Venkataraman R, Kellum JA. Defining acute renal failure: the RIFLE criteria. *J Intensive Care Med.* 2007;22(4):187-193.

Chronic Renal Failure

Barrantes F, Tian J, Vazquez R, et al. Acute kidney injury criteria predict outcomes of critically ill patients. *Crit Care Med.* 2008;36(5):1397-1403.

Breiterman-White R. Infection and inflammation in patients on dialysis: an underlying contributor to anemia and epoetin alfa hyporesponse. *Nephrol Nurs J.* 2006;33(3):319-324.

Broscious SK, Castagnola J. Chronic kidney disease: acute manifestations and role of critical care nurses. *Crit Care Nurse.* 2006;26(4):17-20, 22-28

Cherton GM. A 43-year-old woman with chronic renal insufficiency. *JAMA.* 2004;291(10):1252.

Denhaerynck K, Manhaeve D, Dobbels F, et al. Prevalence and consequences of nonadherence to hemodialysis regimens. *Am J Crit Care.* 2007;16(3):222-236.

Goodman WG. Medical management of secondary hyperparathyroidism in chronic renal failure. *Nephrol Dial Transplant.* 2003;18(suppl 3):2-8.

Liu Y, Coresh J, Eustace JA, et al. Association between cholesterol level and mortality in dialysis patients: role of inflammation and malnutrition. *JAMA.* 2004;291(4):451-459.

Lough ME. Renal disorders and therapeutic management. In: Urden LD, Stacy KM, Lough ME, eds. *Thelan's Critical Care Nursing.* St Louis, MO: Elsevier; 2006.

★ Medicare Payment Advisory Commission. Report to the Congress: blood safety in hospitals and Medicare inpatient payments. Washington, DC: Medicare Payment Advisory Commission; 2001.

National Kidney Foundation. K/DOQI clinical practice guidelines for managing dyslipidemias in chronic kidney disease. *Am J Kidney Dis.* 2003;41 (4 suppl 3):522-559.

Rabindranath KS, Adams J, Ali TZ, et al. Continuous ambulatory peritoneal dialysis versus automated peritoneal dialysis for end-stage renal disease. *Cochrane Database Syst Rev.* 2007;CD006515.

Riegersperger M, Sunder-Plassmann G. How to prevent progression to end stage renal disease. *EDTNA/ERCA J.* 2007;33(3):105-107.

Uchino S, Doig GS, Bellomo R, et al. Beginning and Ending Supportive Therapy for the Kidney (B.E.S.T. Kidney) Investigators. Diuretics and mortality in acute renal failure. *Crit Care Med.* 2004;32(8):1669-1677.

US Renal Data System. *USRDS 2007 Annual Report.* Bethesda, MD: National Institutes of Health, National Institute of Diabetes and Digestive and Kidney Disease; 2007.

Electrolyte Imbalances

Akizawa T, Kamimura M, Mizobuchi M, et al. Management of secondary hyperparathyroidism of dialysis patients. *Nephrology.* 2003;8(suppl 2):S53.

Ariyan CE, Susa JA. Assessment and management of patients with abnormal calcium. *Crit Care Med.* 2004;32(4):S146.

Armstrong LE. Exertional hyponatremia. *J Sports Sci.* 2004;22(1):144.

Astle SM. Restoring electrolyte balance. *RN.* 2005;68(5):34-40.

Babatin DM, Lee SS. Vasopressin antagonists and dilutional hyponatremia. *Can J Gastroenterol.* 2004;18(2):117.

David K. IV fluids: Do you know what's hanging and why? *RN.* 2007;70(10):35-40, 41.

Dickerson RN. Hyperkalemia in the patient receiving specialized nutrition support. *JPEN J Parenter Enteral Nutr.* 2004;28(2):124.

Hajjar I, Graves JW. Hyponatremia in older women. *J Clin Hypertens.* 2004;6(1):37.

Hsieh M. Recommendations for treatment of hyponatremia at endurance events. *Sports Med.* 2004;34(4):231.

Humphreys M. Potassium disturbances and associated electrocardiogram changes. *Emerg Nurse.* 2007;15(5):28-34.

Katapodis KP, Kolious EL, Andrikos EK, et al. Magnesium homeostasis in patient undergoing continuous ambulatory peritoneal dialysis: role of dialysate magnesium concentration. *Artif Organs.* 2003;27(9):853-857.

Kraft MD, Btaiche IF, Sacks GS, et al. Treatment of electrolyte disorders in adult patients in the intensive care unit. *Am J Health Syst Pharm AJHP.* 2005;62(16):1663-1682.

Lough ME. Renal disorders and therapeutic management. In: Urden LD, Stacy KM, Lough ME, eds. *Thelan's Critical Care Nursing.* St Louis, MO: Mosby; 2006.

Malinoski DJ, Slater MS, Mullins RJ. Crush injury and rhabdomyolysis. *Crit Care Clin.* 2004;20(1):171.

Miller W, Graham MG. Life-threatening electrolyte abnormalities. *Patient Care.* 2006;40(12):19-27.

Miltiadons G, Mikhailidis DP, Elisaf M. Acid-base and electrolyte abnormalities observed in patient receiving cardiovascular drugs. *J Cardiovasc Pharmacol Ther.* 2003;8(4):267.

Nanovic L. Electrolytes and fluid management in hemodialysis and peritoneal dialysis. *Nutr Clin Pract.* 2005;20(2):192-201, 286.

Rivard AL, Raup RM, Berlman GJ. Sodium polystyrene sulfonate used to reduce the potassium content of a higher protein internal formula: a quantitative analysis. *JPEN J Parenter Enteral Nutr.* 2004;28(2):76.

Sirken G, Raja R, Garcus J, et al. Contrast-induced translocational hyponatremia and hyperkalemia in advanced kidney disease. *Am J Kidney Dis.* 2004;43(2):E31.

Stark J. A comprehensive analysis of the fluid and electrolytes system: an interactive system. *Crit Care Clin North Am.* 1998;10(4):471.

Uribarri J, Prabhakas S, Kahn T. Hyponatremia in peritoneal dialysis patients. *Clin Nephrol.* 2004;61(1):54.

Yeates KE, Singer M, Morton AR. Salt and water: a simple approach to hyponatremia. *CMAJ.* 2004;170(3):365.

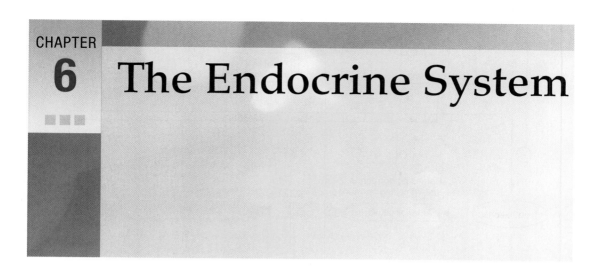

SYSTEMWIDE ELEMENTS

Physiologic Anatomy

1. **Definition of a hormone**
   a. Hormones are molecules that are synthesized and secreted by specialized cells and released into the blood, exerting biochemical effects on target cells away from the site of origin.
   b. Hormones control metabolism, transport of substances across cell membranes, fluid and electrolyte balance, growth and development, adaptation, and reproduction.
2. **Chemically categorized by physiologic action**
   a. Peptide or protein hormones: Vasopressin (antidiuretic hormone [ADH]) thyrotropin-releasing hormone (TRH), insulin, growth hormone (somatotropin [GH]), follicle-stimulating hormone (FSH), luteinizing hormone (LH), corticotropin (adrenocorticotropic hormone [ACTH]), calcitonin
   b. Steroids: Glucocorticoids (cortisol), mineralocorticoids (aldosterone), estradiol, progesterone, testosterone
   c. Amines and amino acid derivatives: Norepinephrine, epinephrine, triiodothyronine (T_3), thyroxine (T_4)
3. **Hormone receptors**
   a. Specificity of hormone action is determined by the presence of a specific hormone receptor on or in the target cell.
      i.   Protein hormones react with receptors on the cell surface.
      ii. Steroid hormones react with receptors inside the cell.
   b. Receptors distinguish hormones from each other and translate the hormonal signal into a cellular response.
   c. The hormone-receptor complex initiates intracellular events that lead to the biologic effects of the hormone acting on the target cell.
4. **Mechanisms of hormone action**
   a. Activation of cyclic adenosine monophosphate (cAMP): Thyrotropin (thyroid-stimulating hormone [TSH]), ACTH, parathyroid hormone (PTH), and ADH
   b. Activation of genes: Steroid hormones and gonadal hormones
5. **Feedback control of hormone production (Figure 6-1)**
   a. Feedback control can be positive (low levels of hormone stimulate the release of its controlling hormone) or negative (high levels of hormone inhibit the release of its controlling hormone).
   b. Feedback control systems allow self-regulation and prevent hormonal overproduction.

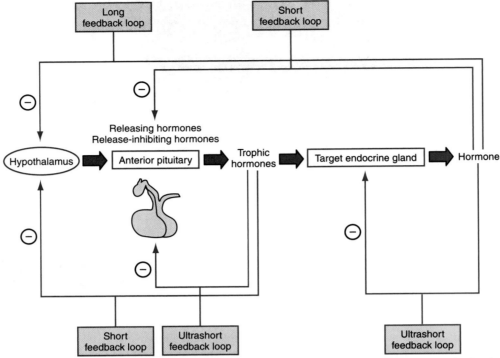

FIGURE 6-1 ■ Negative feedback in the hypothalamic-pituitary axis. Three levels of negative feedback regulate secretion in the hypothalamic-pituitary axis. In the *long feedback loop*, circulating levels of the target endocrine gland hormone influence hypothalamic secretion of releasing and release-inhibiting hormones. In a *short feedback loop*, levels of target gland hormones or tropic hormones feed back to the anterior pituitary or hypothalamus, respectively. In an *ultrashort feedback loop*, hormone levels signal the gland from which they were secreted. (From Hansen M. *Pathophysiology: Foundations of Disease and Clinical Intervention.* Philadelphia, PA: Saunders; 1998:802.)

Pituitary Gland

1. **Location: Base of the skull in the sphenoid bone; connected to the hypothalamus by the pituitary stalk (infundibulum), which links the nervous and endocrine systems**
2. **Composition**
   a. Anterior lobe (adenohypophysis—75% of gland): Hormones are controlled by hypothalamic releasing or inhibiting hormones in response to stimuli received in the central nervous system
   b. Posterior lobe (neurohypophysis—25% of gland)
      i. Hormones are controlled by nerve fibers originating in the hypothalamus and terminating in the posterior pituitary gland.
      ii. Hormones are synthesized in the hypothalamus, stored in the posterior pituitary, and released after activation of the cell bodies in the nerve tract.
3. **Anterior pituitary hormones**
   a. GH
      i. Regulation of secretion
         (a) Stimulation: GH-releasing hormone (GRH) in response to physical and/or emotional stress, starvation, hypoglycemia, other protein-depleted states
         (b) Inhibition: Somatostatin from the hypothalamus, postprandial hyperglycemia, and pharmacologic doses of corticosteroids
      ii. Physiologic activity
         (a) Increases rate of protein synthesis
         (b) Increases lipolysis
         (c) Decreases protein catabolism

(d) Decreases carbohydrate use

(e) Stimulates bone and cartilage growth

(f) Works with insulin, thyroid hormones, and sex steroids to promote growth

iii. Disorders resulting from dysfunction: Not of significance in critical care

(a) Excess: Gigantism (prepubertal), acromegaly (postpubertal)

(b) Deficiency: Dwarfism (prepubertal)

b. ACTH

i. Regulation of secretion

(a) Stimulation: Corticotropin-releasing hormone (CRH) in response to physical or emotional stress, trauma, hypoglycemia, hypoxia, surgery, decreased plasma cortisol levels

(b) Inhibition: Increased plasma cortisol levels exert negative feedback on CRH and thus ACTH; stress can overcome this negative feedback

ii. Physiologic activity: Production and release of adrenocortical hormones (glucocorticoids, adrenal androgens, and mineralocorticoids)

iii. Disorders resulting from dysfunction

(a) Excess: Cushing's disease

(b) Deficiency: Adrenal insufficiency (chronic), adrenal crisis (acute)

c. TSH

i. Regulation of secretion

(a) Stimulation: TRH in response to low concentration of thyroid hormones

(b) Inhibition: Somatostatin from the hypothalamus, increased thyroid hormone levels

ii. Physiologic activity

(a) Increases synthesis of thyroid hormones

(b) Releases stored thyroid hormones

(c) Stimulates iodide uptake into thyroid cells

(d) Increases size, number, and secretory activities of thyroid cells

iii. Disorders resulting from dysfunction: See Thyroid Gland

d. Other anterior pituitary hormones under hypothalamic control

i. LH

ii. FSH

iii. Prolactin

4. Posterior pituitary hormones

a. ADH

i. Regulation of secretion

(a) Stimulation: Increase in plasma osmolality, hypoxia, reduction in blood volume or blood pressure

(b) Inhibition: Decrease in plasma osmolality

ii. Physiologic activity

(a) Increases water permeability in renal collecting duct epithelial cells, thereby controlling extracellular fluid osmolality

(b) In pharmacologic amounts, constricts arterioles to increase blood pressure

iii. Disorders resulting from dysfunction

(a) Primary: Pituitary dysfunction (syndrome of inappropriate ADH secretion [SIADH])

(b) Secondary: Renal dysfunction (diabetes insipidus)

b. Oxytocin

i. Dilatation of the cervix and stimulation of the vagina, lower segment of the uterus, and nipple cause reflex release of oxytocin.

ii. Oxytocin stimulates uterine contractions and milk ejection during lactation.

Thyroid Gland

1. Location: Immediately below the larynx laterally and anterior to the trachea

2. Composition: Two lobes connected by an isthmus

a. Follicular cells: Produce T_3 (20%) and T_4 (80%); T_4 converted in periphery to T_3

b. Parafollicular cells (C cells): Produce thyrocalcitonin

3. **Regulation of secretion (thyroid hormones)**
   a. Stimulation: TSH stimulates thyroid hormone release, which is regulated by TRH from the hypothalamus; decreased levels of thyroid hormones stimulate the release of TSH and TRH
   b. Inhibition: Elevated levels of thyroid hormones inhibit TSH and TRH
4. **Physiologic activity**
   a. Increases the metabolic activity of cells, which results in increased oxygen consumption, increased rate of chemical reactions, and heat production
   b. Stimulates carbohydrate, fat, and protein metabolism
   c. Works with insulin, GH, and sex steroids to promote growth
   d. Critical for fetal neural and skeletal system development (intrauterine hypothyroidism causes cretinism)
   e. Positive chronotropic and inotropic effects on the heart
   f. Required for a normal hypoxic and hypercapnic drive in respiratory centers
   g. Increases erythropoiesis
   h. Increases metabolism and clearance of steroid hormone and insulin
5. **Disorders resulting from dysfunction**
   a. Thyroid enlargement (goiter)
   b. Excess: Hyperthyroidism (chronic), thyroid storm (acute)
   c. Deficiency: Hypothyroidism (chronic), myxedema coma (acute)
6. **Thyrocalcitonin (calcitonin)**
   a. Regulation of secretion
      i. Stimulation: Increase in calcium levels
      ii. Inhibition: Decrease in calcium levels
   b. Physiologic activity
      i. Decreases blood calcium levels by inhibiting calcium mobilization from bone and decreasing calcium resorption in the kidney
      ii. Decreases phosphate levels by inhibiting bone remodeling and by increasing phosphate loss in urine

Parathyroid Glands

1. **Location: Four glands on the posterior surface of the thyroid gland**
2. **Composition: Chief cells release PTH**
3. **Regulation of secretion**
   a. Stimulation: Decrease in serum calcium level
   b. Inhibition: Increase in serum levels of calcium and vitamin D metabolites, hypermagnesemia, and hypomagnesemia
4. **Physiologic activity**
   a. Kidney
      i. Increases renal tubular reabsorption of calcium and magnesium
      ii. Decreases renal tubular reabsorption of phosphate and bicarbonate
      iii. Stimulates the formation of the fat-soluble form of vitamin D
   b. Gastrointestinal tract: Increases calcium absorption
   c. Bone: Larger amounts increase calcium reabsorption
5. **Disorders resulting from dysfunction**
   a. Excess: Hypercalcemia (not significant in critical care)
   b. Deficiency: Hypoparathyroidism leads to hypocalcemia (in critical care, most hypocalcemia is due to renal disease, not hypoparathyroidism)

Adrenal Glands

1. **Location: Retroperitoneal, superior to the kidney**
2. **Composition: Two separate endocrine tissues that produce distinct hormones**
   a. Cortex (90% of gland) produces aldosterone, glucocorticoids, and adrenal androgens.
   b. Medulla (10% of gland) produces catecholamines.

3. **Cortical hormones**
   a. Glucocorticoids (cortisol is the major hormone)
      i. Regulation of secretion
         (a) Stimulation: ACTH (diurnal variation—increased 1 hour after awakening, incidence of myocardial infarction increased in the morning)
         (b) Inhibition: Cortisol exerts negative feedback on the anterior pituitary and hypothalamus
      ii. Physiologic activity
         (a) Carbohydrate metabolism
            (1) Increases gluconeogenesis
            (2) Decreases glucose uptake in muscle and adipose tissue (insulin-antagonistic effect)
         (b) Protein metabolism
            (1) Decreases protein stores and protein synthesis in all cells except liver cells
            (2) Increases protein catabolism
            (3) Promotes gluconeogenesis
         (c) Promotes lipolysis
         (d) Increases tissue responsiveness to other hormones, such as glucagon and the catecholamines
         (e) Anti-inflammatory effects
            (1) Decreased migration of inflammatory cells to sites of injury
            (2) Inhibition of production and/or activity of vasoactive substances
            (3) Prevention of immune response to tissue antigens released by injury
      iii. Disorders resulting from dysfunction
         (a) Excess: Cushing's syndrome
         (b) Deficiency: Adrenal insufficiency (common in the intensive care unit), adrenal crisis (acute)
   b. Mineralocorticoids (aldosterone is the major hormone)
      i. Regulation of secretion
         (a) Stimulation: Renin-angiotensin system as well as hyponatremia, hyperkalemia, and ACTH
         (b) Inhibition: Hypokalemia, sodium loading, and increased plasma volume
      ii. Physiologic activity
         (a) Increases sodium reabsorption, indirectly increasing extracellular fluid volume
         (b) Increases potassium excretion
      iii. Disorders resulting from dysfunction
         (a) Excess: Primary aldosteronism, characterized by potassium depletion, extracellular fluid volume expansion, and nephrosclerotic hypertension
         (b) Deficiency: Adrenal insufficiency (chronic), adrenal crisis (acute)
         (c) Adrenal androgens: Not of significance in critical care
4. **Medullary hormones: Epinephrine and norepinephrine**
   a. Regulation of secretion: Stimulated by fear, anxiety, pain, trauma, fluid loss, hemorrhage, extremes in temperature, surgery, hypoxia, hypoglycemia, hypokalemia, hypernatremia, hypotension
   b. Physiologic activity (Table 6-1)
      i. Fight or flight (stress) response
      ii. Critical in the recovery from insulin-induced hypoglycemia
      iii. Major insulin antagonists
   c. Disorders resulting from dysfunction
      i. Excess: Pheochromocytoma; tumor produces epinephrine and/or norepinephrine, causing hypertension
      ii. Deficiency: Persons with an intact sympathetic nervous system manifest no clinically significant disability

■ **TABLE 6-1**
■ ■ **Adrenergic Responses of Selected Organs**

Organ	Receptor Type	Effect
Heart		
Sinoatrial node	β_1	Inotropic effect ($\uparrow$ rate)
Atrioventricular node	β_1	$\uparrow$ Automaticity and conduction speed
Ventricle	β_1	$\uparrow$ Automaticity, conduction speed, and contractility
Arterioles	α	Vasoconstriction
	β_2	Vasodilation
Kidney	β	$\uparrow$ Renin release
Lung: Bronchial muscle	β_2	Relaxation (dilatation)
Liver	α, β	$\uparrow$ Glycogenolysis
Pancreas	α	$\downarrow$ Insulin and glucagon release
	β	$\uparrow$ Insulin and glucagon release
Uterus	α	Contraction
	β_2	Relaxation

Pancreas

1. **Location:** Lies transversely behind the peritoneum and stomach
2. **Composition:** Exocrine and endocrine components. Endocrine functions originate from the islet cells, which constitute less than 2% of the total pancreatic volume; 65% of the islet cells are beta cells, which produce insulin. Glucagon is produced by the alpha cells; somatostatin and gastrin are produced by the delta cells.
3. **Insulin**
   a. Regulation of secretion
      i. Stimulation: Increases in blood glucose, gastrin, secretin, cholecystokinin, and gastrointestinal hormone levels, and β-adrenergic stimulation
      ii. Inhibition: α-adrenergic effects of somatostatin, catecholamines, and drugs, including diazoxide, phenytoin, and vinblastine
   b. Physiologic activity
      i. Carbohydrate metabolism
         (a) Increases glucose transport across the cell membrane in muscle and fat
         (b) Increases glycogenesis
         (c) Inhibits gluconeogenesis
      ii. Protein metabolism
         (a) Increases amino acid transport across the cell membrane
         (b) Increases protein synthesis
         (c) Decreases protein catabolism
      iii. Fat metabolism
         (a) Increases triglyceride synthesis
         (b) Increases fatty acid transport across the cell membrane
         (c) Inhibits lipolysis
      iv. Works with thyroid hormones, the sex steroids, and GH
         to promote growth
   c. Disorders resulting from dysfunction
      i. Excess: Hypoglycemia
      ii. Deficiency: Diabetes mellitus
         (a) Type 1: Absolute deficiency of insulin due to islet cell antibodies; genetic link, autoimmune disorder
         (b) Type 2: Relative deficiency of insulin caused by decreased sensitivity of receptors to insulin, decreased production, premature destruction of insulin or receptors, and/or hyperinsulinemia; polygenetic etiologies, dietary link

4. Glucagon
  a. Regulation of secretion
     i. Stimulation: Hypoglycemia, catecholamines, gastrointestinal hormones, and gluco-corticoids
     ii. Inhibition: Hyperglycemia and somatostatin
  b. Physiologic activity
     i. Increases blood glucose via glycogenolysis and gluconeogenesis
     ii. Increases lipolysis
     iii. Increases amino acid transport to the liver and the conversion of amino acids to glucose precursors
     iv. Is a major insulin-antagonistic hormone
     v. Critical hormone in the recovery from insulin-induced hypoglycemia
  c. Deficient glucagon production is thought to play a role in defective glucose counter-regulation in insulin-induced hypoglycemia in type 1 diabetes mellitus.
  d. Available as a pharmacologic agent to correct insulin-induced hypoglycemia (all patients with diabetes should have a readily available source)
5. Somatostatin
  a. Present in islet cells, the hypothalamus, and the gastrointestinal tract
  b. Physiologic activity: Inhibits the secretion of insulin, glucagon, GH, TSH, and gastrointestinal hormones (gastrin, secretin)

Gonadal Hormones (Testosterone, Estrogen, Progesterone)

Not significant in critical or progressive care

PATIENT ASSESSMENT

1. Nursing history
  a. Patient health history
     i. Presence of pathophysiologic processes that can result in endocrine dysfunction
        (a) Adrenal gland hypoperfusion
        (b) Infection, inflammation, autoimmune processes
        (c) Neoplasms and exposure to the chemotherapeutic agents and radiotherapy used to treat the neoplasms
        (d) Infiltrative disorders
        (e) Acquired immunodeficiency syndrome (AIDS)
     ii. Pregnancy, postpartum state
     iii. Presence of preexisting chronic endocrine disorder (diagnosed or undiagnosed)
     iv. Poor compliance with pharmacologic therapy for a preexisting endocrine disorder
     v. Presence of an unrelated critical illness in a patient with a preexisting chronic endocrine disorder
     vi. Positive family history of an endocrine disorder
     vii. Use of systemic steroids
     viii. Indicators of altered health patterns
        (a) Cognition and perception
           (1) Personality changes, lethargy, emotional lability, attention span deficit, memory impairment
           (2) Visual disturbances
           (3) Changes in level of consciousness
           (4) Depression, paranoia, delusions, delirium
           (5) Verbalizations that indicate lack of knowledge or misconceptions regarding self-care management
        (b) Nutrition and metabolism
           (1) Change in weight (increase or decrease)
           (2) Nausea, anorexia, vomiting
           (3) Polydipsia
           (4) Heat or cold intolerance
           (5) Edema

      (c) Elimination
        (1) Diarrhea or constipation
        (2) Polyuria, anuria, oliguria, nocturia
        (3) Excessive perspiration
      (d) Activity and exercise
        (1) Fatigue, weakness
        (2) Impairment in performance of the activities of daily living
      (e) Sleep and rest: Restlessness, inadequate sleep
      (f) Sexual function
        (1) Menstrual irregularities
        (2) Impotence
        (3) Decreased libido
        (4) Infertility
      (g) Roles and relationships
        (1) Discord in previously stable relationships
        (2) Physical and emotional inability to engage in usual role activity
      (h) Coping and stress tolerance
        (1) Inability to cope
        (2) History of a past or present psychiatric disorder
      (i) Health perception and health management: Evidence of noncompliance with the prescribed medical regimen
  b. Family history: Endocrine disorders in other family members
  c. Social history
    i. Elderly persons may be at special risk for the development of an endocrine crisis because of changes associated with aging and a diminished thirst mechanism.
    ii. Economically disadvantaged persons may be at risk for the development of an endocrine crisis because many of the regimens for treating chronic endocrine disorders are costly and necessitate regular medical follow-up.
    iii. Teenagers with poor compliance with a prescribed medical regimen, particularly patients with diabetes, are at increased risk of crisis.
  d. Medication history
    i. Use of pharmacologic agents to treat chronic endocrine disorders
    ii. Use of pharmacologic agents that may stimulate or inhibit hormone release, or interfere with hormone action at target tissue
    iii. Exposure to radiographic contrast dyes
2. Nursing examination of patient
  a. Physical examination data
    i. Inspection
      (a) Excessive or diminutive stature
      (b) Fat distribution in relation to gender and maturational level
      (c) Mobility, tremor, hyperkinesis
      (d) Scars, especially in the neck area
      (e) Hair distribution and texture relative to gender and maturational level
      (f) Edema
      (g) Goiter
      (h) Seizure activity
      (i) Presence of medical alert identification
      (j) Hydration status of oral cavity
      (k) Periorbital edema, ptosis, eye protrusion, stare, dry eyes
      (l) Unusual pigmentation, temperature, turgor, striae, or thinning of the skin
    ii. Palpation: Enlarged or nodular thyroid gland, often painful
    iii. Percussion: Abnormal deep tendon reflexes (may be hyperreflexic or hyporeflexic)
    iv. Auscultation
      (a) Neck: Bruits over the thyroid gland
      (b) Heart: Distant heart sounds, third heart sound (due to pericardial effusion, heart failure)

   (c) Blood pressure: Hypotension, hypertension
   (d) Heart rate and rhythm disturbances
   (e) Altered respiratory pattern
   (f) Altered bowel sounds
   (g) Pericardial and/or pleural friction rub (due to effusion)
   b. Monitoring data
   i. Pulse oximetry
   ii. Electrocardiography
   iii. Blood pressure monitoring
   iv. Temperature monitoring
   v. Electrolyte analysis
   vi. Arterial blood gas (ABG) analysis
   vii. Hormonal assays
3. Appraisal of patient characteristics
   a. Resiliency
   i. Level 1—*Minimally resilient*: An 83-year-old man admitted with hypoglycemia who reports feeling sweaty, agitated, and slightly disoriented after 3 days of vomiting
   ii. Level 3—*Moderately resilient*: A 32-year-old man admitted in diabetic ketoacidosis after an episode of the flu
   iii. Level 5—*Highly resilient*: A 74-year-old woman with a history of diabetes who is on postoperative day 2 after cardiac surgery
   b. Vulnerability
   i. Level 1—*Highly vulnerable*: A 49-year-old woman admitted with severe dehydration and hypotension due to nephrogenic diabetes insipidus resulting from repeated episodes of pyelonephritis with scarring
   ii. Level 3—*Moderately vulnerable*: A 44-year-old man admitted after transsphenoidal removal of a pituitary tumor in whom diabetes insipidus develops, which responds immediately to administration of vasopressin
   iii. Level 5—*Minimally vulnerable*: A 56-year-old woman with a history of diabetes insipidus, immediately after cardiac catheterization with percutaneous coronary intervention
   c. Stability
   i. Level 1—*Minimally stable*: A 78-year-old woman admitted with SIADH with hyponatremia, vomiting, and confusion
   ii. Level 3—*Moderately stable*: A 63-year-old man admitted with SIADH with complaints of severe thirst and nausea
   iii. Level 5—*Highly stable*: A 72-year-old woman with a history of SIADH who is on postoperative day 1 after a thoracotomy
   d. Complexity
   i. Level 1—*Highly complex*: An 85-year-old man admitted in diabetic ketoacidosis from a board and care facility with two necrotic toes and an open wound on his hip from a fall. Patient is confused, does not speak English, and does not have any family immediately available.
   ii. Level 3—*Moderately complex*: A 44-year-old man admitted in diabetic ketoacidosis after inability to obtain insulin. Patient recently became unemployed and lost health insurance and prescription coverage.
   iii. Level 5—*Minimally complex*: A 79-year-old man with newly diagnosed diabetes who has a blood glucose level of 200 mg/dl and a hemoglobin A_1c fraction of 8.6%. Patient shows cardiovascular and neurologic stability. Has good family support and insurance. Is well educated.
   e. Resource availability
   i. Level 1—*Few resources*: A patient with newly diagnosed diabetes who has no insurance and no family, is unemployed, is new to the area, and is homeless
   ii. Level 3—*Moderate resources*: A patient with newly diagnosed diabetes who has Medicare coverage and a niece who lives an hour away and who currently resides in an assisted living facility

        iii.   Level 5—*Many resources*: A patient with newly diagnosed diabetes who has insurance and prescription coverage. Patient is well educated and has strong family support. Independent in care and finances.

   f. Participation in care

        i.   Level 1—*No participation*: A 68-year-old woman admitted from a nursing home with diabetes insipidus after a head injury. She is in a persistent vegetative state. No family nearby.

        ii.   Level 3—*Moderate level of participation*: A 68-year-old woman admitted with tachycardia and elevated blood sugar who confesses to having stopped insulin therapy because she could not afford to visit her physician for a new prescription

        iii.   Level 5—*Full participation*: A 21-year-old man who is treated successfully for diabetic ketoacidosis and who, with his family, requests assistance in learning more about his disease and its management

   g. Participation in decision making

        i.   Level 1—*No participation*: A fiftyish homeless man admitted in diabetic ketoacidosis. Patient is alcoholic with a history of mental health problems requiring hospitalization. No known family.

        ii.   Level 3—*Moderate participation*: A 78-year-old patient with newly diagnosed diabetes who has a history of prostate cancer. Has a sister who is also diabetic. Asks for information to access home nursing care for assistance.

        iii.   Level 5—*Full level of participation*: An 86-year-old patient admitted in diabetic ketoacidosis. Patient has durable power of attorney for health care and living will. Patient's family is present with the patient and fully knowledgeable about the disease. Family provides history and treatment authorization and will be available to aid in care after discharge.

   h. Predictability

        i.   Level 1—*Not predictable*: A 44-year-old patient with brittle diabetes admitted in diabetic ketoacidosis for the fourth time this year. Poorly compliant with the medical regimen, smokes; chronic obstructive pulmonary disease has been newly diagnosed.

        ii.   Level 3—*Moderately predictable*: A 32-year-old patient with diabetes admitted in diabetic ketoacidosis. Responds well to administration of insulin and fluids. Aware that her triggers for diabetic ketoacidosis are infection, particularly bladder infections, and the flu.

        iii.   Level 5—*Highly predictable*: An 88-year-old woman admitted from a nursing home in hyperosmolar, nonketotic coma after dehydration caused by the flu. Responds well to rehydration and insulin.

4. Diagnostic studies

   a. Laboratory: Blood and urine

        i.   Electrolyte levels

        ii.   Glucose, ketoacid, blood urea nitrogen, cholesterol, creatinine, serum creatine phosphokinase levels

        iii.   Plasma osmolality, hematocrit, white blood cell count with differential

        iv.   ABG levels

        v.   Specific hormone assays

        vi.   Urine specific gravity, osmolality, pH

   b. Radiologic (to identify precipitating factor)

        i.   Radiography (skull, chest, abdomen)

        ii.   Scans (thyroid, pancreas)

        iii.   Computed axial tomography

        iv.   Magnetic resonance imaging

        v.   Arteriography

        vi.   Bone mineral densitometry

   c. Other

        i.   Electrocardiography

        ii.   Visual field testing

        iii.   Temperature monitoring

PATIENT CARE

1. **Fluid volume deficit (hypovolemia)**
   a. Description of problem
      i.   Dry skin and mucous membranes, decreased skin turgor
      ii.   Hypertension, orthostasis, tachycardia
      iii. Hypernatremia
      iv.   Weight loss
      v.   Polyuria
      vi.   Negative intake and output (I&O) balance
   b. Goals of care
      i.   Fluid and electrolyte balance are achieved and maintained.
      ii.   Cardiovascular stability is maintained.
   c. Collaborating professionals on health care team
      i.   Nurse
      ii.   Physician
   d. Interventions
      i.   Administer fluids and hormone therapy as prescribed.
      ii.   Monitor and document I&O, electrolyte levels, vital signs, urine specific gravity, weight, laboratory test results on flow sheet.
      iii. Provide oral care and skin care.
   e. Evaluation of patient care
      i.   Fluids, electrolytes, and I&O in balance
      ii.   Cardiovascular stability
      iii. No skin or mucous membrane breakdown
2. **Fluid volume excess (hypervolemia)**
   a. Description of problem
      i.   Intake exceeding output
      ii.   Weight gain
      iii. Third heart sound
      iv.   Pulmonary congestion and dyspnea
      v.   Deterioration of mental status
      vi.   Hemodilution
      vii. Abnormal electrolyte values
      viii. Edema
   b. Goals of care: Fluid and electrolyte balance is achieved and maintained
   c. Collaborating professionals on health care team
      i.   Nurse
      ii.   Physician
      iii. Respiratory therapist
   d. Interventions
      i.   Monitor I&O, electrolyte levels.
      ii.   Use flow sheet to document I&O, vital signs, urine specific gravity, weight, and laboratory test results.
      iii. Identify patients at risk for fluid overload.
      iv.   Monitor pulmonary status and function.
      v.   Administer prescribed diuretics.
   e. Evaluation of patient care
      i.   I&O and electrolytes in balance
      ii.   Cardiovascular and pulmonary stability
      iii. ABG levels and pulse oximetry within normal limits
3. **Altered carbohydrate, fat, and/or protein metabolism**
   a. Description of problem
      i.   Hyperglycemia with or without ketosis
      ii.   Decreased serum albumin level

   iii. Weight loss of 10% to 20%
   iv. Generalized fatigue and weakness
   b. Goals of care
   i. Body weight normalizes and stabilizes.
   ii. No evidence of ketosis is present.
   iii. Nitrogen balance is positive.
   iv. Serum albumin level is within normal limits.
   c. Collaborating professionals on health care team
   i. Nurse
   ii. Physician
   iii. Dietitian
   d. Interventions
   i. Provide sufficient calories and vitamins.
   ii. Administer hormone or antihormone therapy as prescribed.
   iii. Monitor ABG, serum albumin, electrolyte levels.
   e. Evaluation of patient care
   i. Stable body weight
   ii. No ketosis
   iii. Normal serum albumin level
4. **Need for patient and family education and discharge planning**
   a. Description of problem
   i. Lack of knowledge or skills may seriously compromise self-care.
   ii. Patient and/or family is unable to explain or follow instructions correctly.
   iii. Patient and/or family raises questions and requests information.
   b. Goals of care: Patient demonstrates knowledge and skills needed for providing self-care and contacting health care resources
   c. Collaborating professionals on health care team
   i. Nurse, clinical nurse specialist, nurse practitioner
   ii. Physician
   iii. Diabetes educator
   iv. Dietitian
   v. Care manager
   d. Interventions
   i. Assess patient and family knowledge of the health disorder and the required self-care.
   ii. Provide appropriate information about the health disorder and self-care.
   iii. Provide an opportunity for the patient and family to demonstrate needed skills.
   iv. Provide appropriate resources for additional information and support.
   e. Evaluation of patient care: Ability of the patient and family to explain and demonstrate optimal self-care management

SPECIFIC PATIENT HEALTH PROBLEMS

Diabetic Ketoacidosis

1. **Pathophysiology: Diabetic ketoacidosis (DKA) is the most serious metabolic complication of insulin-dependent, or type 1, diabetes mellitus. DKA is a state of insulin deficiency combined with an increase in the level of insulin-antagonistic hormones (glucagons, cortisol, catecholamines, and GH). The result is altered metabolism of carbohydrate, fat, and protein (Figure 6-2) and hyperglycemia.**
   a. Decreased insulin level with gluconeogenesis and increased insulin resistance result in exaggerated hepatic glucose production.
   b. Ketosis and metabolic acidosis result from increased synthesis of ketones and lactic acidosis.
   c. Fluid and electrolyte imbalance and osmotic diuresis are caused by glycosuria; accompanied by loss of sodium, potassium, and chloride.
   d. Altered mental status results from hyperosmolality, cellular dehydration, acidosis, and possibly impaired oxygen dissociation, because glycosylated hemoglobin binds oxygen more tightly.

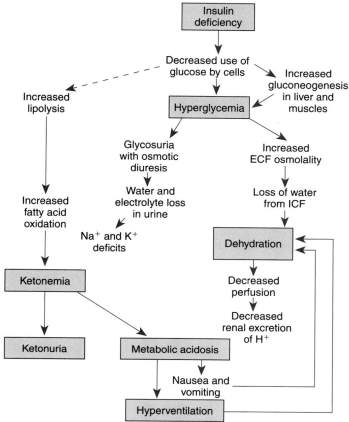

FIGURE 6-2 ■ Pathophysiology of acidosis in diabetes mellitus. *ECF*, Extracellular fluid; *ICF*, intracellular fluid. (From Hockenberry M. *Wong's Nursing Care of Infants and Children*. 7th ed. St Louis, MO: Mosby; 2003:1735.)

2. **Etiology and risk factors**
   a. Diagnosed diabetes mellitus
      i.   Insufficient exogenous insulin: Dose missed or insufficient for needs
      ii.   Infection or trauma
      iii. Poor compliance with established self-care regimen
            (a) Alcohol or drug use
            (b) Educational deficits
            (c) Psychosocial distress or disease
            (d) Adolescence
      iv.   Medication side effects
            (a) Glucocorticoids increase gluconeogenesis.
            (b) Thiazide diuretics, diazoxide, and phenytoin decrease insulin resistance.
   b. Undiagnosed diabetes mellitus: Positive family history of diabetes
3. **Signs and symptoms**
   a. Blurred vision, diminished level of consciousness
   b. Nausea, abdominal cramping, vomiting
   c. Polyphagia, polyuria, polydipsia
   d. Fatigue, weakness
   e. Muscle cramps
   f. Decreased skin turgor, dry mucous membranes
   g. Fruity odor to breath (ketosis)
   h. Tachycardia, orthostatic hypotension
   i. Tachypnea, Kussmaul's respirations

4. **Diagnostic study findings**
   a. Elevated plasma and urine glucose levels: Plasma glucose level above 250 mg/dl; presence of glucose in urine (normal = no trace)
   b. Metabolic acidosis: Arterial pH less than 7.3; serum HCO_3^- less than 18 mEq/dl
   c. Positive results for serum and urine ketones
   d. Azotemia
   e. Anion gap: $Na^+ - (Cl^- + HCO_3^-) > 10$ (other formulas may be used)
   f. Electrocardiogram: May reflect hypokalemia, although serum potassium level may be normal or elevated; flat T waves
   g. Hypocalcemia in 30% of patients
   h. Hyperosmolality
5. **Goals of care**
   a. Acid-base balance is restored.
   b. Blood glucose level is normalized and maintained.
   c. Fluid balance is restored.
   d. Any infection, if present, is resolved.
6. **Collaborating professionals on health care team**
   a. Nurse
   b. Physician, consulting physician
   c. Diabetes educator or diabetes case manager
   d. Dietitian
7. **Management of patient care**
   a. Anticipated patient trajectory: DKA can recur easily in patients with diabetes if medication compliance, diet, and sick-day management are not well understood. Recurrence is most common in teens and patients with newly diagnosed diabetes. Patients with DKA may have needs in the following areas:
      i. Delivery of care: Depending on the severity of the patient's signs and symptoms or the frequency or type of interventions required, the patient may need to be transferred to the intensive care unit for treatment
      ii. Discharge planning
         (a) For patients with newly diagnosed diabetes: Education about the disease, pathophysiology, and self-care management
         (b) For patients with previously diagnosed diabetes: Education about the self-care regimen, compliance, and sick-day management
      iii. Pharmacology
         (a) Administer intravenous (IV) fluids to correct dehydration based on *corrected* sodium.
            (1) Corrected $Na^+ =$ Measured serum $Na^+ + \{[(\text{Serum glucose in mg/dl} - 100)/100] \times 1.6\}$
            (2) 0.9% NaCl is recommended if the corrected Na^+ level is low.
            (3) 0.45% NaCl is recommended if the corrected Na^+ level is normal or high.
            (4) 5% Dextrose is added to prevent hypoglycemia when the glucose level is less than 250 mg/dl.
         (b) Administer regular insulin via IV bolus then continuous drip.
            (1) Change to subcutaneous insulin 1 to 2 hours before stopping the drip to prevent the recurrence of ketosis and accelerated hyperglycemia.
            (2) Monitor the serum glucose level hourly.
            (3) Measure urine ketone levels (insulin infusion may be stopped if the patient stops excreting ketones).
            (4) Insulin infusion is usually stopped when the serum glucose level is less than 250 mg/dl.
         (c) Administer sodium bicarbonate if the pH is less than 7.0.
            (1) Goal is cerebral and myocardial protection.
            (2) Monitor ABG levels.
         (d) Administer antibiotics if infection is present.
      iv. Psychosocial issues
         (a) For patients with newly diagnosed diabetes: Major lifestyle changes required

        (b) For patients with preexisting diabetes: Must address noncompliance and poor compliance with the medical regimen

    v. Treatments

        (a) Assess respiratory and neurologic status (a decline may signal cerebral edema).

        (b) Monitor electrolyte levels while acidosis and volume deficits are being corrected (K^+, Na^+, PO_4^-).

        (c) Monitor liver enzyme levels.

        (d) Record I&O, daily weights.

  b. Potential complications

    i. Metabolic acidosis

        (a) Mechanism: Ketosis resulting from insulin deficiency and stress hormone excess

        (b) Management: Administration of insulin and sodium bicarbonate as needed

    ii. Hyperglycemia

        (a) Mechanism: Resulting from insulin deficiency, ketosis, stress hormone excess, infection

        (b) Management: Insulin administration with reduction of serum glucose levels at rates not to exceed 100 mg/dl/hr

    iii. Dehydration

        (a) Mechanism: Due to osmotic diuresis induced by hyperglycemia; deficit worsened by vomiting and/or inadequate oral intake

        (b) Management: Fluid replacement

    iv. Hypoglycemia

        (a) Mechanism: Resulting from insulin therapy and a decrease in levels of circulating insulin-antagonist hormones (blood glucose level <50 mg/dl); hypoglycemia can precipitate dysrhythmias, extend infarcts

        (b) Management: Requires administration of a rapid-acting carbohydrate, 50% dextrose IV or glucose-containing solution orally if consciousness is not depressed

8. Evaluation of patient care

  a. Acid-base and potassium levels within normal limits

  b. Normal anion gap

  c. Blood glucose level stabilized at 150 to 200 mg/dl with no episodes of hypoglycemia

  d. Absence of ketosis

  e. Restoration of fluid balance as evidenced by I&O, laboratory values, and cardiovascular stability

  f. Resolution of any infection

  g. If the diabetes is newly diagnosed, referral of the patient for diabetic management teaching

  h. If the diabetes is preexisting, ability of the patient to identify precipitating factors and to modify self-care management as needed

Hypoglycemic Episode

1. Pathophysiology: Decrease in serum glucose level to 50 mg/dl or below. Glucose production (feeding and/or liver gluconeogenesis) lags behind glucose use. May be caused by decreased clearance of insulin or oral hypoglycemia agents or by drug interactions.

2. Etiology and risk factors

  a. Insulin therapy

    i. Insulin dose greater than the body's current needs

    ii. Sudden rotation of injection sites from a hypertrophied area to one with unimpaired absorption

    iii. Interruption of enteral tube feedings

  b. Oral hypoglycemic therapy, especially with sulfonylurea agents

  c. Insufficient caloric consumption—a meal or snack missed or delayed or intake compromised because of nausea, vomiting, or anorexia

  d. Strenuous physical exercise that is not compensated by increased food intake or decreased dose of insulin

  e. Potentiation of hypoglycemic medications

    i. Renal insufficiency (decreased creatinine clearance)

      ii. Use of medications that potentiate the action of the sulfonylureas (phenylbutazone, large doses of salicylates, sulfonamides)

  f. Excessive alcohol intake, which inhibits gluconeogenesis

  g. Decreased requirements for exogenous insulin resulting from

      i. Recovery from physiologic stress, which decreases the levels of insulin-antagonistic hormones and thus decreases the need for insulin

      ii. Weight loss, which decreases insulin resistance

      iii. Immediate postpartum period: Sudden reduction in anti-insulin effects of placental hormones

      iv. Decrease in steroid dose

  h. Presence of other health problems (e.g., severe liver disease, pancreatic islet cell tumor)

  i. Use of regular insulin can be associated with a rapid fall in glucose levels and may prompt more adrenomedullary symptoms. Use of intermediate-acting insulins or continuous insulin infusion devices may result in a more gradual drop in plasma glucose level and thus may produce central nervous system symptoms (neuroglycopenia).

  j. Patients taking β-adrenergic blocking agents (e.g., metoprolol) may not exhibit adrenomedullary symptoms; the use of β-adrenergic blocking agents can also impair recovery from hypoglycemia by inhibiting glycogenolysis.

3. Signs and symptoms

  a. Headache, fatigue, irritability

  b. Pallor

  c. Hunger

4. Diagnostic study findings: Serum glucose levels lower than 50 mg/dl

5. Goals of care: Hypoglycemia and its sequelae are corrected

6. Collaborating professionals on health care team

  a. Nurse

  b. Physician

  c. Diabetes educator

7. Management of patient care

  a. Anticipated patient trajectory: Hypoglycemia is a potential complication with a high likelihood of recurrence in patients in whom diabetes has been newly diagnosed or in whom an insulin-food-activity balance either has not been achieved or has been disrupted. Throughout their recovery and discharge, patients with hypoglycemia may be expected to have needs in the following areas:

      i. Pharmacology

        (a) Administer oral or IV glucose.

          (1) Remeasure serum glucose level 20 to 30 minutes after treatment.

          (2) Readminister glucose, if needed.

          (3) Discontinue insulin infusion if present.

  b. Potential complications

      i. Seizures

        (a) Mechanism: Due to hypoglycemia

        (b) Management: Administer IV glucose; protect the patient from injury

      ii. Dysrhythmias

        (a) Mechanism: Resulting from hypoglycemia; important to note that hypoglycemia has the potential to extend infarcts

        (b) Management: Administer oral or IV glucose and antiarrhythmic agent per advanced cardiac life support protocols

8. Evaluation of patient care

  a. Maintenance of serum glucose level at 80 to 110 mg/dl

  b. No subjective or objective evidence of hypoglycemia

  c. Patient use of medical alert identification indicating diabetes mellitus

Hyperglycemic, Hyperosmolar Nonketotic Syndrome

1. Pathophysiology: Life-threatening hyperglycemic emergency accompanied by hyperosmolality, severe dehydration, and alterations in neurologic status without ketosis. Pathophysiologic processes (Figure 6-3) include the following:

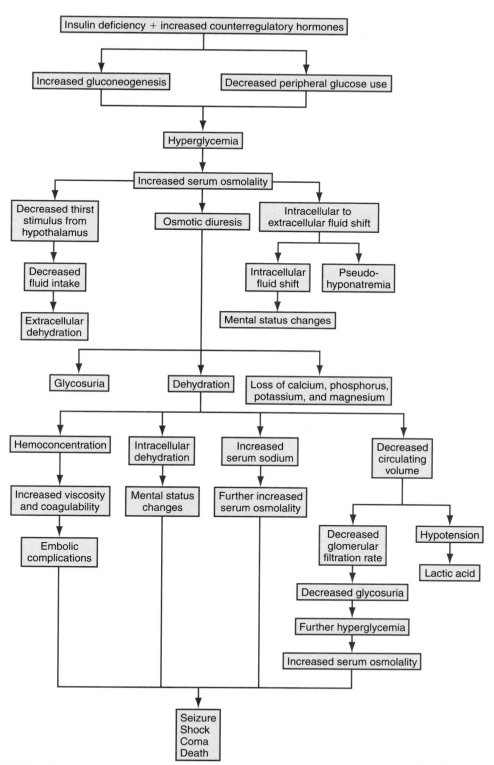

FIGURE 6-3 ■ Hyperosmolar, hyperglycemic nonketotic syndrome. (From Jakubauskas K. Hyperosmolar hyperglycemic nonketotic coma. *AACN News.* 2001;May:14-17.)

    a. Relative insulin deficiency that impairs glucose transport across the cell membrane. There may be sufficient insulin present to inhibit lipolysis or ketogenesis in the liver but not enough to control hyperglycemia. Not uncommon for some ketosis to be present, but pH is rarely lower than 7.3.

    b. Hyperosmolality resulting from hyperglycemia and hypernatremia may impair insulin secretion, promote insulin resistance, and inhibit free fatty acid release from adipose tissue.

    c. Fluid shifts from intracellular to extracellular space to offset hyperosmolality.

    d. Osmotic diuresis caused by hyperglycemia results in extracellular fluid volume depletion; fluid deficits usually are greater than those seen in DKA.

    e. Severe electrolyte losses (sodium, chloride, phosphate, magnesium, potassium) occur with osmotic diuresis.

    f. Volume depletion compromises glomerular filtration, diminishing urinary escape of glucose.

    g. Coma results from cellular dehydration.

2. Etiology and risk factors

    a. Inadequate insulin secretion and/or action (newly diagnosed type 2, or non–insulin-dependent, diabetes)

    b. Advanced age and severe dehydration (majority of patients)

    c. Concomitant illness that increases glucose production or contributes to dehydration, including sepsis, pancreatitis, stroke, uremia, burns, myocardial infarction, and gastrointestinal hemorrhage

    d. Lack of ready access to fluids or inability to recognize or express the need for fluids

    e. Use of insulin or oral hypoglycemic, disruption of an established medication regimen

    f. Use of medications known to elevate glucose levels and/or resist insulin action, including corticosteroids, thiazide diuretics, phenytoin, sympathomimetics

    g. Preadmission medication regimen that suggests cardiovascular or renal disease; crisis is more common in late-middle-aged patients and in elderly patients with preexisting renal or cardiovascular disease

3. Signs and symptoms

    a. Lethargy, fatigue, coma

    b. Polydipsia, polyuria, polyphagia

    c. Flushed skin and dry mucous membranes

    d. Tachycardia, hypotension

    e. Shallow, rapid respirations

4. Diagnostic study findings

    a. Severely elevated glucose levels (>1000 mg/dl)

    b. No ketosis

    c. Sodium and potassium levels vary with the state of hydration; often severely depleted as a result of osmotic diuresis; hypokalemia necessitates potassium replacement

    d. Plasma hyperosmolality (>330 mOsm/kg)

    e. Acidosis, if present, usually caused by lactic acid or renal dysfunction

5. Goals of care

    a. Dehydration is corrected.

    b. Hyperglycemia is corrected.

    c. Peripheral tissue perfusion is restored.

6. Collaborating professionals on health care team

    a. Nurse

    b. Physician, consulting physician

    c. Diabetes educator

    d. Home care coordinator or discharge planner

7. Management of patient care

    a. Anticipated patient trajectory: Hyperglycemic, hyperosmolar nonketotic coma (HHNKC) can develop rapidly in an elderly patient with type 2 diabetes who becomes ill and then dehydrated. These patients will require aggressive sick-day management to prevent recurrence. Throughout their course of recovery and discharge, patients with HHNKC may be expected to have needs in the following areas:

    i.   Delivery of care: Depending on the severity of the patient's signs and symptoms or the frequency or type of interventions required, the patient may need to be transferred to the intensive care unit for treatment.

    ii.   Pharmacology

       (a) Fluid replacement with 0.9% NaCl

       (b) IV insulin via infusion to correct hyperglycemia

    iii.   Treatments

       (a) Hourly serum glucose monitoring

       (b) Strict management and recording of I&O

b. Potential complications

    i.   Heart failure

       (a) Mechanism: Many of these patients are elderly or have preexisting heart disease. Rapid fluid replacement to treat severe fluid deficits may result in heart failure. The patient may require placement of a central venous catheter or pulmonary artery catheter.

       (b) Management: Provide inotropic support, administer diuretics, oxygen

    ii.   Hypoglycemia

       (a) Mechanism: As hyperglycemia resolves, the serum glucose level must be closely monitored to avoid hypoglycemia

       (b) Management: Stop insulin administration; give IV glucose if the patient is conscious or glucose (e.g., orange juice) by mouth if tolerated

    iii.   Thromboembolic event

       (a) Mechanism: Dehydration causes diminished tissue perfusion, hyperviscosity, and increased platelet activity and thereby increases the risk of thrombus formation

       (b) Management

          (1) Assess for decreased pulses, pallor in extremities, decreased blood pressure.

          (2) Assess for and report localized redness, swelling, tenderness, or increased warmth.

          (3) Replace fluids.

          (4) Have the patient perform active or passive range-of-motion exercises.

8. Evaluation of patient care

  a. Blood pressure stable at baseline

  b. No evidence of heart failure (edema, crackles, weight gain)

  c. Maintenance of blood glucose levels within normal limits

  d. No evidence of thrombus formation or embolization

  e. Correction of the underlying cause that precipitated the crisis

Diabetes Insipidus

1. Pathophysiology: Occurs when any organic lesion or chemical substance (e.g., alcohol) affecting the hypothalamus or posterior pituitary interferes with ADH synthesis and transport or release. Deficiency results in the inability to conserve water and the excretion of large amounts of dilute urine.

2. Etiology and risk factors

  a. Central or neurogenic diabetes insipidus (ADH sensitive)

    i.   Idiopathic (30%): Autoimmune (common), familial (rare)

    ii.   Trauma: Injury to hypothalamus or pituitary trauma (most common cause of polyuria after neurosurgery)

    iii.   Craniopharyngioma, pituitary tumor

    iv.   Infections: Meningitis, encephalitis

    v.   Vascular disorder: Aneurysm

    vi.   Infiltrative disorders (histiocytosis X, sarcoidosis)

    vii. Malignancy (lung cancer, leukemia, lymphoma)

    viii. History of an impaired thirst mechanism or a state in which the patient is confused, incapacitated, or otherwise unable to secure fluids

    b. Nephrogenic diabetes insipidus (ADH insensitive): Most common forms are the following:

        i.   Renal: Polycystic kidneys, pyelonephritis, congenital disorder

        ii. Multisystem disorders: Multiple myeloma, amyloidosis

        iii. Familial

    c. Pharmacologic agents: Ethanol, lithium, glyburide, and phenytoin inhibit ADH secretion and action

    d. Insufficient exogenous ADH in a person with diabetes insipidus

3. Signs and symptoms

    a. Polydipsia

    b. Polyuria (5 to 20 L/24 hr)

    c. Decreased skin turgor, dry mucous membranes

    d. Fatigue

    e. Tachycardia; hypotension if the patient has become dehydrated

4. Diagnostic study findings

    a. Elevated plasma osmolality (>295 mOsm/kg), decreased urine osmolality (<500 mOsm/kg; can be as low as 30 mOsm/kg)

    b. Hypernatremia

    c. Low urine specific gravity (1.001 to 1.005)

    d. Water deprivation test: With adequate stimulus for ADH release (simple dehydration), the kidneys cannot concentrate urine. Differentiates psychogenic polydipsia from diabetes insipidus; no response occurs in either neurogenic or nephrogenic diabetes insipidus.

    e. ADH test: To demonstrate that the kidneys can concentrate urine with exogenous ADH. Corrects central diabetes insipidus; no response in nephrogenic diabetes insipidus.

    f. Low plasma ADH levels in patients with central diabetes insipidus

5. Goals of care

    a. Tissue hypoperfusion is prevented.

    b. Fluid and electrolyte balance is maintained.

6. Collaborating professionals on health care team

    a. Nurse

    b. Physician

7. Management of patient care

    a. Anticipated patient trajectory: Patients with diabetes insipidus may experience the spontaneous resolution of symptoms or require lifetime medication. The success of pharmacologic therapy depends solely on patient compliance. Throughout their course of recovery and discharge, patients with diabetes insipidus may be expected to have needs in the following areas:

        i.   Pharmacology

            (a) Administer hormone replacement for central diabetes insipidus.

                (1) Desmopressin acetate (DDAVP)

            (b) Administer pharmacologic agents for nephrogenic diabetes insipidus.

                (1) Chlorpropamide: Stimulates ADH release and promotes renal response to ADH

                (2) Thiazide diuretics: Promote concentration of urine, improving specific gravity and urine osmolality

        ii. Discharge planning

            (a) Medication instruction

            (b) Signs and symptoms to report

        iii. Treatments

            (a) Monitor I&O, urine specific gravity, and osmolality.

            (b) Monitor serum osmolality.

    b. Potential complications

        i.   Dehydration

            (a) Mechanism: Resulting from fluid loss

            (b) Management: Fluid and hormone replacement

      ii. Hypoperfusion
        (a) Mechanism: From decreased intravascular volume
        (b) Management: Restoration of circulatory volume via fluid and hormone replacement
      iii. Electrolyte imbalance
        (a) Mechanism: Resulting from fluid loss
        (b) Management: Restoration of circulating volume

8. Evaluation of patient care
   a. Normalization of fluid balance
   b. Electrolyte levels within normal limits
   c. Patient's understanding of the purpose and dosing of medications

Syndrome of Inappropriate Antidiuretic Hormone

1. Pathophysiology: Syndrome characterized by plasma hypotonicity and hyponatremia that result from aberrant secretion of ADH, which in turn is caused by the failure of the negative feedback system. Dysfunction results in water intoxication.

2. Etiology and risk factors
   a. Central nervous system disorders
      i. Trauma: Skull fracture, subdural hematoma, subarachnoid hemorrhage, cerebral contusion, post neurosurgery
      ii. Neoplasms
      iii. Infections: Meningitis, encephalitis, brain abscess, Guillain-Barré syndrome, AIDS
      iv. Vascular disorders: Aneurysm, cerebral vascular accident
   b. Stimulation of ADH release via hypoxia and/or low left atrial filling pressure
      i. Pulmonary infections
      ii. Asthma
      iii. Heart failure
      iv. Positive pressure ventilation
   c. Pharmacologic agents: Either increase ADH secretion or potentiate its action
      i. Cancer chemotherapeutic agents: Cyclophosphamide, vincristine
      ii. Chlorpropamide, acetaminophen, amitriptyline, thiazide diuretics, carbamazepine, pentamidine
   d. Excessive exogenous ADH therapy
   e. Ectopic ADH production associated with bronchogenic, prostatic, or pancreatic cancers and with leukemia

3. Signs and symptoms
   a. Nausea, vomiting
   b. Confusion, impaired memory
   c. Muscle twitching or seizure activity, delayed deep tendon reflexes

4. Diagnostic study findings
   a. Hyponatremia
   b. Decreased plasma osmolality
   c. Elevated urine sodium level and osmolality
   d. Elevated plasma ADH levels

5. Goals of care
   a. Fluid balance is restored.
   b. Patient safety is ensured.

6. Collaborating professionals on health care team
   a. Nurse
   b. Physician, consulting physician

7. Management of patient care
   a. Anticipated patient trajectory: If the underlying cause of SIADH is treated, the symptoms will resolve. If the precipitating cause cannot be removed or treated, the patient will require ongoing electrolyte monitoring throughout recovery and discharge. Patients with SIADH may be expected to have needs in the following areas:
      i. Pharmacology: Fluid therapy based on urine output plus insensible losses
      ii. Treatments

(a) Monitor electrolyte levels, osmolality, weight.

(b) Initiate seizure and injury precautions.

b. Potential complications

   i. Fluid overload and congestive heart failure

     (a) Mechanism: Resulting from excess ADH secretion

     (b) Management: Administration of diuretics and inotropic support

   ii. Electrolyte imbalance

     (a) Mechanism: Resulting from fluid overload

     (b) Management: Monitor electrolyte levels during and with administration of diuretics

   iii. Seizures

     (a) Mechanism: Resulting from sodium and osmolality alterations

     (b) Management: Restore fluid balance; protect the patient

8. Evaluation of patient care

  a. Normalization of fluid and electrolyte balances

  b. Absence of seizures

  c. Absence of injury

REFERENCES AND BIBLIOGRAPHY

Physiologic Anatomy

Guyton AC, Hall JT. *Textbook of Medical Physiology.* 11th ed. Philadelphia, PA: Saunders; 2006.

Kronenberg H, Melmed S, Polonsky K, Larsen P. *Williams Textbook of Endocrinology.* 11th ed. Philadelphia, PA: Saunders; 2008.

McCance KL, Huether SE, eds. *Pathophysiology: The Biologic Basis for Disease in Adults and Children.* 5th ed. St Louis, MO: Mosby; 2006.

Patient Assessment

Ignatavicius DD, Workman L. *Medical-Surgical Nursing: Critical Thinking for Collaborative Care.* 5th ed. St Louis, MO: Elsevier; 2006.

Diabetic Ketoacidosis; Hypoglycemia; Hyperglycemic, Hyperosmolar Nonketotic Syndrome

★ American Diabetes Association. Position statement: hyperglycemic crisis in patients with diabetes mellitus. *Diabetes Care.* 2002;25(suppl 1):S100-S108.

Fonseca VA, Kulkarni KD. Management of type 2 diabetes: oral agents, insulin, and injectables. *J Am Diet Assoc.* 2008;108:S29-S33.

Guettier JM, Gorden P. Hypoglycemia. *Endocrinol Metab Clin North Am.* 2006;35(4):753-766.

Kitabchi AE, Nyenwe EA. Hyperglycemic crises in diabetes mellitus: diabetic ketoacidosis and hyperglycemic hyperosmolar state. *Endocrinol Metab Clin North Am.* 2006;35(4):725-751.

Kwon KT, Tsai VW. Metabolic emergencies. *Emerg Med Clin North Am.* 2007;25(4):1041-1060.

Nugent BW. Hyperosmolar hyperglycemic state. *Emerg Med Clin North Am.* 2005;23(3):629-648.

Scott A. Hyperosmolar hyperglycaemic syndrome. *Diabet Med.* 2006;23 (Suppl 3):22-24.

Turina M, Christ-Crain M, Polk HC. Diabetes and hyperglycemia: strict glycemic control. *Crit Care Med.* 2006;34(9 Suppl):S291-S300.

Diabetes Insipidus

Adler SM, Verbalis JG. Disorders of body water homeostasis in critical illness. *Endocrinol Metab Clin North Am.* 2006;35(4):873-894.

Arvanitis ML, Pasquale JL. External causes of metabolic disorders. *Emerg Med Clin North Am.* 2005;23(3):827-841.

Garofeanu CG, Weir M, Rosas-Arellano MP, Henson G, Garg AX, Clark WF. Causes of reversible nephrogenic diabetes insipidus: a systematic review. *Am J Kidney Dis.* 2005;45(4):626-637.

Loh JA, Verbalis JG. Disorders of water and salt metabolism associated with pituitary disease. *Endocrinol Metab Clin North Am.* 2008;37(1):213-234.

Mavrakis AN, Tritos NA. Diabetes insipidus with deficient thirst: report of a patient and review of the literature. *Am J Kidney Dis.* 2008;51(5):851-859.

Syndrome of Inappropriate Antidiuretic Hormone

Arvanitis ML, Pasquale JL. External causes of metabolic disorders. *Emerg Med Clin North Am.* 2005;23(3):827-841.

Lien YH, Shapiro JI. Hyponatremia: clinical diagnosis and management. *Am J Med.* 2007;120(8):653-658.

Lin M, Liu SJ, Lim IT. Disorders of water imbalance. *Emerg Med Clin North Am.* 2005;23(3):749-770.

Loh JA, Verbalis JG. Disorders of water and salt metabolism associated with pituitary disease. *Endocrinol Metab Clin North Am.* 2008;37(1):213-234.

Robertson GL. Regulation of arginine vasopressin in the syndrome of inappropriate antidiuresis. *Am J Med.* 2006;119:S36-S42.

Hematologic and Immunologic Systems

SYSTEMWIDE ELEMENTS

Physiologic Anatomy

1. **Hematologic system**
   a. Anatomic structures
      i. Bone marrow
         (a) Spongy center of the bones where the hematologic and immunologic cell lines originate and mature before being released into the circulation
         (b) Present throughout the bones of the body, although the majority of the cells are produced in the vertebrae, ribs, sternum, pelvis, and proximal epiphyses of the femur and humerus
      ii. Liver
         (a) Located in the upper right quadrant of the abdomen in the peritoneal space below the diaphragm and under the rib cage. The liver receives 27% of the resting cardiac output—approximately 1350 ml of blood flow each minute—via the hepatic artery and portal vein.
         (b) Synthesizes various plasma proteins, including clotting factors and albumin. In addition, the liver clears damaged and nonfunctioning red blood cells (RBCs), or erythrocytes, from circulation.
   b. Components: See Table 7-1 and Figure 7-1
   c. Functions: See Table 7-2 and Figure 7-2
2. **Immunologic system**
   a. Anatomic structures
      i. Bone marrow (see preceding description)
      ii. Thymus
         (a) The thymus is a bilobed lymphoid organ located in the mediastinum below the thyroid. Early in life, lymphocytes released from the bone marrow migrate to the thymus, where they mature into T cells before being released into the circulation.
         (b) During fetal development and throughout the first 2 years of life, the thymus grows rapidly. After puberty the thymus slowly involutes as the circulating, long-lived T-cell population is maximized.
      iii. The lymph system is a separate vessel system that collects plasma and leukocytes that are not returned to the circulatory system from the tissue capillary beds. This lymph fluid is filtered and returned to the circulatory system, so that appropriate tissue fluid pressures are maintained and edema is prevented. Lymph fluid is propelled along the system by the normal contraction of skeletal muscles.

■ **TABLE 7-1**
■ ■ **Components of the Hematologic System**

Component	Description
Pluripotent stem cell	The pluripotent stem cell is a self-renewing cell from which all the differentiated bone marrow cell lines derive. Various developmental cell lineages can be identified in the bone marrow before the mature cells are released into the circulation (Figure 7-1).
Red blood cells (RBCs)	RBCs are biconcave disk-shaped cells enveloped with a tough, flexible membrane. Erythropoiesis, or the production of RBCs, occurs in the bone marrow, where the pluripotent stem cell gives rise to the erythrocyte lineage, as shown in Figure 7-1. Erythropoiesis is regulated by the glycoprotein erythropoietin, which is produced primarily by the kidneys. In response to decreased oxygen levels in the blood, the kidney produces more erythropoietin, which acts on the bone marrow to increase and accelerate erythropoiesis. Iron, cobalamin (vitamin B$_{12}$), and folic acid are all needed for RBC production. RBCs have a life span of approximately 120 days, at the end of which they are filtered out of circulation by the spleen and liver. Iron released from the heme is transported by transferrin back to the bone marrow, where it is recycled to make new RBCs. The porphyrin ring of the heme is reduced to bilirubin and eliminated as bile through the intestine. Genetically determined antigens are located on the RBC cell membrane. The major antigens are designated A and B. On the basis of the presence or absence of these two antigens, four major blood groups are defined. Persons without a given antigen will form a naturally occurring antibody against the absent antigen shortly after birth. Rh is another type of RBC antigen that is different from A and B antigens. Persons without the Rh antigen (known as *Rh-negative* persons) form antibody against Rh only when exposed to Rh-positive blood. Rh-negative persons can be exposed to the Rh antigen if they receive Rh-positive blood through transfusion. An *Rh-negative* woman can be exposed to the Rh antigen if she delivers an Rh-positive baby.
Platelets (thrombocytes)	Platelets are nonnucleated cell fragments of megakaryocytes produced in the bone marrow (see Figure 7-1). Platelets activate the blood clotting system by going to sites of blood vessel or tissue injury, forming a platelet plug, and releasing cytokines that recruit more platelets and the clotting factors to the injury site. The life span of a platelet is approximately 10 days.
Clotting factors	Clotting factors are proteins and other substances, numbered I to XIII, that form a fibrin matrix at sites of blood vessel or tissue injury. Factors commonly referred to include the following: • Factor I, also known as *fibrinogen* • Factor II, also known as *prothrombin* • Factor III, also known as *tissue thromboplastin* or *tissue factor* • Factor IV, which is *calcium* • Factor V, also known as *AC-globulin* • Factor VII, also known as *prothrombin conversion accelerator* or *proconvertin* • Factor VIII, also known as *antihemophilic factor* • Factor IX, also known as *Christmas factor* • Factor X, also known as *Stuart-Prower factor* • Factor XI, also known as *thromboplastin antecedent factor* • Factor XII, also known as *Hageman factor* • Factor XIII, also known as *fibrin-stabilizing factor*
Plasma	Plasma is the straw-colored fluid that carries the blood components through the circulatory system and is made up primarily of water, proteins (albumin, globulins, and fibrinogen), small amounts of nutrients, electrolytes, hormones, enzymes, and metabolites. Serum is plasma without clotting factors.

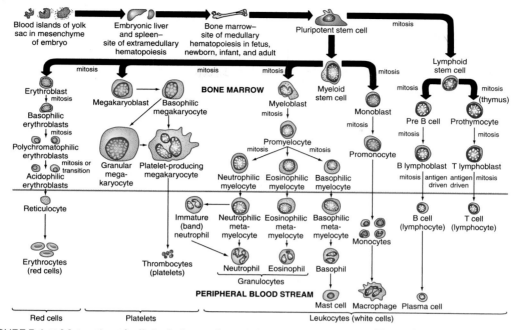

FIGURE 7-1 ■ Maturation of cells in the hematologic and immunologic systems. (From Copstead LC, Banasik JL. *Pathophysiology*. 3rd ed. St Louis, MO: Mosby; 2005:324.)

TABLE 7-2
Functions of the Hematologic System

Function	Description
Oxygenation	The red blood cells (RBCs) transport oxygen from the lungs to the tissues and carry carbon dioxide from the tissues to the lungs for excretion. Hemoglobin in the RBCs combines with oxygen, carbon dioxide, and nitric oxide. As hemoglobin transfers oxygen to the tissue, it also sheds small amounts of nitric oxide. The affinity of hemoglobin for oxygen and the mechanism by which oxygen is bound to hemoglobin in the lungs and released in the tissues is best described by the oxyhemoglobin dissociation curve (see Chapter 2).
Hemostasis	**Vascular constriction** Vessel spasm is initiated by endothelial cell injury caused by local and humoral mechanisms such as the release of the vasoconstrictor thromboxane A_2 from the cells and platelets as well as local myogenic contraction. The value of the vascular constriction is to reduce the blood flow and allow platelets to adhere to the exposed surfaces. **Platelet plug** 1. Platelets then degranulate, releasing serotonin, histamine, von Willebrand factor, adenosine diphosphate, fibrinogen, and thromboxane from cell vesicles into the surrounding environment, which constricts the blood vessel further to minimize blood loss and recruits more platelets and clotting factors to the area. The coagulation cascade is initiated through mechanisms dependent on phospholipids in the platelet membrane. 2. The platelets form an initial, unstable platelet plug.

Continued

■ **TABLE 7-2**
■ ■ **Functions of the Hematologic System—Cont'd**

Function	Description

	Coagulation
	1. At the same time the platelet plug is forming, the coagulation pathway is initiated.
	2. Two primary mechanisms activate the coagulation pathway (see Figure 7-2).
	   a. The extrinsic pathway is activated after tissue trauma when factor III released from the damaged tissues comes in contact with factor VII (proconvertin) circulating in the blood.
	   b. The intrinsic pathway is activated after endothelial damage when factor XII (Hageman factor) circulating in the blood comes in contact with subendothelial substances such as collagen exposed by vascular injury.
	   c. Division of the coagulation process into strictly defined extrinsic and intrinsic pathways has been modified because the cascade theory has been revised. These revisions include the fact that factor VIIa of the extrinsic pathway can directly activate factor IX of the intrinsic pathway and that factor VII can be activated by factors XIIa, IXa, Xa, and thrombin (see Figure 7-2).
	3. At each step in each pathway, an inactive proenzyme is converted into an active enzyme by proteolytic cleavage. Calcium, coenzymes, or phospholipids are required for some of the reactions to proceed.
	4. The activation of the pathway results in the conversion of factor I (fibrinogen) to factor Ia (fibrin), which forms a fibrin clot; in the presence of factor XIIIa, a stabilized fibrin clot is formed.
	5. The final step of hemostasis is clot retraction, in which the formed clot expels serum. Fibrin strands shorten; become denser and stronger, approximating the edges of the injured vessel; and seal the site of injury.
	Limiting and focusing of hemostasis to sites of blood vessel damage
	1. Platelet aggregation and the coagulation cascade are normally initiated only when blood comes in contact with nonvascular tissues, which thus localizes hemostasis to sites of injury.
	2. As the clot extends to areas where the blood vessel is intact, antithrombin III, a plasma protein normally circulating in the blood, inactivates thrombin. Heparin greatly improves the activity of antithrombin III.
	3. The fibrin clot is eventually removed by an enzyme called *plasmin*. Damaged endothelial cells secrete a protein that converts the inactive form of plasmin, plasminogen, to its active form so that degradation of the fibrin clot can begin. Like antithrombin III, plasminogen normally circulates freely in the blood. As the fibrin clot is degraded, fibrin split products can be detected in the blood.

(a) Lymph fluid is a pale yellow liquid made up of plasma, leukocytes, enzymes, and antibodies; it lacks clotting factors and thus coagulates very slowly.

(b) Lymphatic capillaries and vessels are a network of open-ended tubes with one-way valves that collect lymph fluid from the tissues and eventually return it to the venous system via both the right lymphatic duct, which drains into the right subclavian vein, and the thoracic duct, which drains into the left subclavian vein.

(c) Lymph nodes are small, flat, bean-shaped patches of tissue located along the length of the lymphatic system that filter microorganisms from the lymph fluid before it is returned to the bloodstream.

   (1) Lymph nodes can become swollen with white blood cells (WBCs), or leukocytes, that are responding to invading microorganisms if an infectious process is occurring in the area drained by the lymph node.

   (2) Lymph nodes can also become swollen with metastatic cancer cells that have migrated away from the primary site and become trapped in the network of the lymph node.

  iv. The spleen is a lymphoid organ located in the upper left quadrant of the abdomen that clears damaged or nonfunctioning RBCs and filters antigens from the blood for evaluation by lymphocytes.

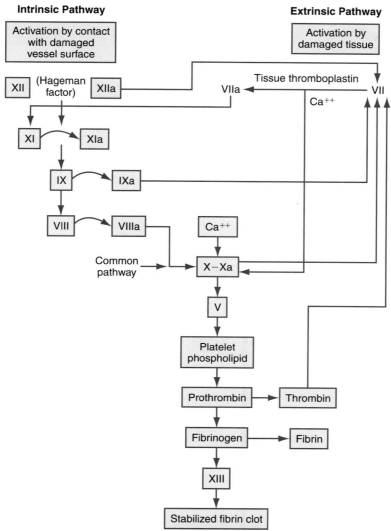

FIGURE 7-2 ■ Intrinsic and extrinsic coagulation cascades. (From McCance KL, Huether SE. *Pathophysiology: The Biologic Basis for Disease in Adults and Children.* 5th ed. St Louis, MO: Mosby; 2006.)

    b. Components: See Tables 7-3, 7-4, and 7-5, and Figure 7-3
    c. Functions: See Table 7-6

Patient Assessment

  1. Nursing history
    a. Patient health history
      i. Many times a hematologic or immunologic problem is identified when the patent seeks medical attention for some other reason.
      ii. Elements of the medical history indicating a potential or existing hematologic or immunologic problem include the following:
        (a) Recent, recurrent, or chronic infections
        (b) Cancer or prior treatment for cancer
        (c) Human immunodeficiency virus (HIV) infection
        (d) Liver disorder
        (e) Kidney disorder
        (f) Malabsorption disorder

Component	Description
Pluripotent stem cell	See description in Table 7-1.
WBCs	WBCs circulate throughout the body, detecting and destroying bacteria, viruses, fungi, parasites, and other proteins identified as foreign to the body. The pluripotent stem cell gives rise to all WBC lineages. The different WBCs mature primarily in the bone marrow before being released into circulation (Figure 7-1). The average life span of a WBC in circulation is 12 hr.

Granulocytes or myeloid series of leukocytes

1. Neutrophils
   - Because these cells are segmented polymorphonuclear neutrophils, they are also known as *segs, PMNs, polys,* or *neuts.* Because these cells are also granulocytes, they are also known as *grans.*
   - Neutrophils are the most numerous of the WBCs. They are efficient phagocytic cells that are able to migrate through endothelial cells to sites of microbial invasion.
   - Neutrophils are often destroyed during phagocytosis. Pus is the accumulation of cellular debris from the destruction of microorganisms and neutrophils at the site of infection.
2. Monocytes
   - Monocytes and macrophages compose the MPS.
   - Monocytes are released from the bone marrow into the peripheral circulation, where they mature. When they enter the tissue, they become highly efficient phagocytic macrophages.
   - Some macrophages move throughout the body, whereas others stay in one particular tissue and are named according to where they reside. For example, Kupffer cells are liver macrophages, Langerhans cells are skin macrophages, alveolar macrophages are lung macrophages, mesangial cells are kidney macrophages, and microglial cells are central nervous system macrophages.
   - Unlike neutrophils, which are often destroyed during phagocytosis, macrophages can phagocytose many foreign antigens, surviving months to years.
3. Eosinophils
   - Eosinophils are motile phagocytic cells that combat infection with multicellular parasites. They are also associated with allergic reactions and other inflammatory processes.
4. Basophils
   - Basophils are nonphagocytic cells that attract IgE antibodies to their cell membranes. When the IgE binds antigen, the basophils release histamine, bradykinin, serotonin, heparin, and slowly reacting substances of anaphylaxis, triggering a massive inflammatory response.
   - Basophils are involved in various inflammatory conditions.
5. Mast cells
   - Mast cells, like basophils, attract IgE antibodies to their cell membranes. Also like basophils, mast cells release histamine, bradykinin, serotonin, heparin, and slowly reacting substances of anaphylaxis when the IgE binds antigen, triggering a massive inflammatory response.
   - Mast cells and basophils differentiate along separate pathways. Basophils circulate in the blood and survive only days, whereas mast cells are located in the tissue and live weeks or months.
   - IgE-mediated mast cell degranulation is responsible for type I hypersensitivity reactions.

■ **TABLE 7-3**
■ ■ **Components of the Immunologic System—Cont'd**

Component	Description
	6. Lymphocytes
	• B cells or B lymphocytes
	a) B cells manufacture and express antigen-binding proteins called *immunoglobulins* on their cell membranes.
	b) When the B-cell immunoglobulin binds a particular antigen, the cell is stimulated to differentiate into two separate cells called *plasma cells* and *memory B cells*.
	1) Plasma cells are antibody factories that immediately produce and secrete large amounts of antibody to bind to the antigen.
	2) Memory B cells go into a resting state but can be quickly reactivated to produce plasma cells and antibody if exposed to the same antigen in the future.
	c) Antibodies are secreted protein immunoglobulins that can bind to more of the same antigen. There are five major types of antibodies:
	1) IgM is the first immunoglobulin to be secreted during the primary immune response to an antigen.
	2) IgG is secreted during the secondary immune response and is more specific to a particular antigen.
	3) IgA is present in secretions such as mucus and breast milk.
	4) IgE attaches to the cell membranes of basophils and mast cells. When IgE binds to antigen, it triggers the cell to release histamine.
	5) IgD is found primarily on the cell membrane of B lymphocytes and serves as an antigen receptor for initiating the differentiation of B cells.
	• T cells or T lymphocytes
	a) T cells mature in the thymus and recognize antigen in association with cell membrane proteins. The cell membrane proteins are known as *major histocompatibility complexes* (MHCs). There are two classes of MHC proteins (I and II) that work with different T cells as part of the immune system. Class I MHC proteins are found on all cells, whereas class II MHC proteins are found on B cells and macrophages.
	b) T_H, also called *CD4 cells* because they display the membrane glycoprotein antigen CD4, recognize class II MHC molecules on the cell surface of B cells and macrophages. In response to recognition of a foreign antigen–MHC II complex, T_H cells secrete hormones, called *cytokines,* that activate other components of the immune system (see also Acquired Immunity in Table 7-6).
	c) T_C, also called *CD8 cells* because they display the membrane glycoprotein CD8, recognize class I MHC molecules on the surface of cells. In response to recognition of a foreign antigen–MCH I complex, T_C cells secrete cytotoxic substances that directly destroy the cell (see also Acquired Immunity in Table 7-6).
	• NK cells are a type of null (neither T nor B) lymphocyte. NK cells do not express antigen-binding receptors but do have cytotoxic capabilities against bacteria-infected and virus-infected cells as well as against tumor cells.
Complement	Complement is a group of more than 20 serum proteins, designated C1 to C9, B, and D, that act through an enzymatic cascade against invading pathogens. These proteins act sequentially and in concert to lyse microorganisms and/or infected cells.
Cytokines	Cytokines are protein hormones secreted by cells to signal other cells and play an important role in mediating the process of inflammation. As can be seen in Table 7-4, cytokines can be released from both immune and nonimmune cell types and be either proinflammatory or anti-inflammatory depending on the response.
Eicosanoids	Eicosanoids such as prostaglandins, prostacyclin, thromboxanes, leukotrienes, and HETE and EET are short-lived compounds that signal cells in a paracrine fashion, some of which are listed in Table 7-5. Many commonly prescribed drugs, such as aspirin and other nonsteroidal anti-inflammatory agents, inhibit eicosanoid production but, in the process, affect other physiologic processes dependent on eicosanoid regulation (see Figure 7-3).

EET, Cis-epoxyeicosatrienoic acid; *HETE,* hydroxyeicosatetraenoic acid; *Ig,* immunoglobulin; *MPS,* mononuclear phagocyte system; *NK,* natural killer; T_C, cytotoxic T cells; T_H, helper T cells; *WBCs,* white blood cells.

■ **TABLE 7-4**
■ ■ **Examples of Cytokines**

Cytokine	Source	Major Activities/Comments
IL-1	IL-1α: Macrophages, endothelial cells, and fibroblasts; IL-1β: NK cells, macrophages, and monocytes	Generic name for two different proteins, IL-1α and IL-1β, which are regulatory and inflammatory cytokines. Important in up- and down-regulation of acute inflammation. IL-1 is associated with bone formation, appetite regulation, and fever induction.
IL-2	Primarily from activated helper T cells	IL-2 autocrine activity → differentiation of antigen-specific cells. Paracrine activity → stimulation of B cells and NK cells.
IL-3	T cells	Enhances production of a variety of hematopoietic precursor cells, mast cells, basophils, and NK cells. Regulates differentiation and growth of many cell types.
IL-4	T cells	Stimulates proliferation of activated B and T cells, enhances the production of specific immunoglobulin subclasses, and increases cytotoxic activity of lymphocytes.
IL-5	Eosinophils, NK cells, T cells, and mast cells	Has key role in coordinating inflammatory process originating with eosinophils.
IL-6	Fibroblasts, synoviocytes, adipocytes, osteoblasts, endothelial cells, cerebral cortex neurons, neutrophils, monocytes, and eosinophils	This is the archetypal pleiotropic cytokine as evidenced by the variety of names originally given to it (e.g., IFN-β2, hepatocyte-stimulating factor, and cytotoxic T-cell differentiation factor). Has both proinflammatory and antiinflammatory action. Modulates bone resorption and induces activation of plasma cells.
IL-7	Stromal cells	Pleiotropic in regulation of helper T cells. Necessary for T-cell memory. Early B- and T-cell differentiation.
IL-8	Monocytes, lymphocytes	Chemotactic for neutrophils and basophils.
IL-9	T helper cells	Pleiotropic cytokine involved in allergic response and mast cell response.
IL-10	T cells, monocytes, and macrophages	Pleiotropic immunosuppressive and immunostimulatory cytokine. Inhibits IL-2 synthesis in helper T cells. Inhibits cytokine synthesis in monocytes. Stimulates IL-3 and IL-4 production.
IL-11	Bone marrow stroma	Involved in lymphopoiesis, thrombopoiesis, and myelopoiesis.
IL-12	Antigen-presenting cells, monocytes	Stimulates T and NK cells. Regulates cell-mediated immunity. Induces the production of interferon γ.
IL-13	T cells	IL-13 and IL-4 are pleiotropic immunoregulatory cytokines. Induces vascular cell adhesion molecule-1 on endothelial cells. Inhibits the proinflammatory gene expression of IL-1, TNF, and IL-6.
IL-14	T cells	Enhances proliferation of activated B cells, inhibits immunoglobulin synthesis, and is involved in B-cell memory.
IL-15	Monocytes, epithelial cells	Stimulates T-cell proliferation.
IL-16	Mast cells, lymphocytes	Chemotactic for monocytes and eosinophils.
IFN-α	T cells, B cells, monocytes, macrophages, and fibroblasts	Antiviral. Stimulates macrophages and NK cell activity. Has antitumor properties.
IFN-β	Mast cells	Antiviral—similar activity to IFN-α.
IFN-γ	T, NK cells	Involved in regulation of immune and inflammatory responses. Weak antiviral activity. Increases the antiviral and antitumor action of IFN-α and IFN-β. Activates macrophages.

■ **TABLE 7-4**
■ ■ **Examples of Cytokines—Cont'd**

Cytokine	Source	Major Activities/Comments
TGF-β	Macrophages, lymphocytes, dendritic cells	TGF-β belongs to a family of TGF proteins. Pleiotropic immunoregulatory functions. Autocrine and paracrine function controls differentiation, proliferation, and level of activation of immune cells. Chemotactic for leukocytes during inflammatory response and inhibits the same cells once activated.
TNF-α	Monocytes, macrophages, T cells, B cells, fibroblasts, neutrophils, NK cells, LAK cells, endothelial cells	Paracrine and endocrine mediator of inflammation and immune system functions. B cell, T cell, macrophage, and neutrophil activity. Regulates growth and differentiation of a wide variety of cell types. Kills tumors.
TNF-β	T cells, B cells	Similar to TNF-β. Inflammation, tumor killing, and enhancement of phagocytosis.

From Rankin JA. Biological mediators of acute inflammation. *AACN Clin Issues.* 2004;15(1):6.
IFN, Interferon; *IL,* interleukin; *LAK,* lymphokine-activated killer; *NK,* natural killer; *TGF,* transforming growth factor; *TNF,* tumor necrosis factor.

■ **TABLE 7-5**
■ ■ **Functions of Eicosanoids**

Eicosanoid	Function
Prostaglandins	Cardiovascular: Vasodilation
	Pulmonary: Constriction of airways
	Gastrointestinal: Maintenance of mucosal barrier
	Endocrine: Temperature elevation
	Renal: Renin release, regulation of renal blood flow
	Genitourinary: Uterine contraction
	Hematologic: Antiplatelet aggregation
	Immunologic: Inflammatory response
Thromboxanes	Cardiovascular: Vasoconstriction
	Hematologic: Platelet aggregation
Leukotrienes	Pulmonary: Bronchial smooth muscle contraction
	Immunologic: Inflammatory response
Epoxygenase products (HETE and EET)	Vascular: HETE, potent vasoconstriction; EET, vasodilation and angiogenesis

Data from Boron W, Boulpaep EL. *Medical Physiology.* Philadelphia, PA: Saunders; 2003.
*EET, Cis-*epoxyeicosatrienoic acid; *HETE,* hydroxyeicosatetraenoic acid.

      (g) Any prolonged bleeding or delayed healing with prior surgeries and/or dental extractions

      (h) Receipt of a blood transfusion

      (i) Splenectomy

      (j) Placement of a prosthetic heart valve

      (k) Placement of an indwelling venous access device, which indicates that the patient needed long-term venous access

  iii. Review of systems with the patient and/or family for signs and symptoms

      (a) General: Fatigue, weakness, lethargy, malaise, fever, chills, night sweats, dyspnea, restlessness, apprehension, pain, altered mental status, vertigo, dizziness, confusion

      (b) Skin: Pruritus, change in skin color, rash, unusual bruising, ulcers, or other lesions

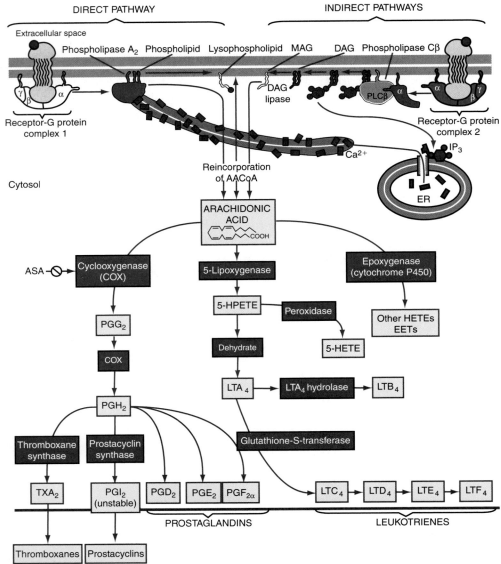

FIGURE 7-3 ■ Eicosanoid production. *AACoA,* Acetoacetyl coenzyme A; *ASA,* acetylsalicylic acid; *DAG,* diacylglycerol; *ER,* endoplasmic reticulum; *EET, cis-*epoxyeicosatrienoic acid; *HETE,* hydroxyeicosatetraenoic acid; *5-HETE,* 5-hydroxyeicosatetraenoic acid; *5-HPETE,* 5-hydroperoxyeicosatetraenoic acid; *IP$_3$,* inositol 1,4,5-triphosphate; *LTA$_4$, LTB$_4$, LTC$_4$, LTD$_4$, LTE$_4$, LTF$_4$,* leukotriene A$_4$, B$_4$, C$_4$, D$_4$, E$_4$, F$_4$; *MAG,* monoacylglycerol; *PGD$_2$, PGE$_2$, PGF$_{2\alpha}$, PGG$_2$, PGH$_2$, PGI$_2$,* prostaglandin D$_2$, E$_2$, F$_2$, G$_2$, H$_2$, I$_2$; *PLCβ,* phospholipase Cβ; *TXA$_2$,* thromboxane A$_2$. (From Boron W, Boulpaep EL. *Medical Physiology.* Philadelphia, PA: Saunders; 2003.)

(c) Head and neck: Headache, change in vision, sinus pain, epistaxis, gingival bleeding, sore throat, pain with swallowing, enlarged lymph nodes

(d) Respiratory: Cough, hemoptysis, dyspnea, orthopnea

(e) Cardiovascular: Palpitations, dizziness with position changes

(f) Gastrointestinal: Change in eating habits, anorexia, abdominal fullness, nausea, vomiting, hematemesis, change in bowel habits, hematochezia, melena, pain with defecation, change in weight

(g) Genitourinary: Hematuria, pain with urination, menorrhagia, enlarged inguinal lymph nodes

▦ TABLE 7-6
▦ ▦ Functions of the Immunologic System

Function	Description

Innate immunity	**Anatomic and physiologic barriers**
	1. Mechanical barrier of the skin and mucosa
	2. Acid pH on the skin and in the stomach
	3. Flushing or mechanical removal of pathogens (e.g., bladder emptying, gastrointestinal motility, coughing and sneezing, ciliary activity)
	4. Mucous secretions (e.g., saliva, tears) that contain enzymes and immunoglobulin A
	Inflammation
	1. The hallmarks of inflammation are rubor (erythema), tumor (edema), calor (heat), and dolor (pain) that occur as a result of the following:
	  a. Vasodilation of the capillary bed in the affected area
	  b. Increased capillary permeability, which allows fluid and immune competent cells into the area
	  c. An influx of phagocytic cells to attack microorganisms
	2. The eicosanoids thromboxane and leukotriene are potent mediators of inflammation that increase the migration of inflammatory cells to the area and increase capillary permeability.
	Phagocytosis
	1. Neutrophils and macrophages are capable of ingesting and digesting antigens such as microorganisms, dead cells, and cellular debris.
	2. Inside the phagocytic cell, lysozymes break down antigens, recycling usable products and displaying antigenic protein pieces on their class II MHC molecule for evaluation by T cells.
	Complement pathway
	1. The classical complement pathway is the major effector of the humoral branch of the immune response. The trigger for the classical pathway is either IgG or IgM bound to antigen. Binding of antibody to antigen exposes a site on the antibody that is a binding site for the first complement component, C1. The alternative complement pathway does not require antibody for activation. A variety of antigens such as bacteria lipopolysaccharide and components of viruses and other pathogens have the ability to activate this pathway.
	2. The complement pathway acts against invading pathogens by inducing inflammation, attracting neutrophils and monocytes, promoting phagocytosis, and building an MAC, which makes a hole in the microorganism's cell membrane and thereby kills it.

Acquired immunity	**Humoral or antibody-mediated immunity** is aimed primarily at extracellular microorganisms and is also responsible for immediate hypersensitivity reactions.
	1. Immunoglobulins on B cells bind antigen on the cell surface. The B cells internally process the antigen-antibody complex, redisplaying the antigen on the B cell's surface on a class II MHC molecule.
	2. A helper T CD4 cell then binds the antigen displayed on the class II MHC molecule of the B cell and, recognizing it as foreign, secretes cytokines that stimulate the B cell to both secrete IgM and differentiate into antibody-secreting plasma cells and memory B cells.
	3. When antibody binds to an antigen, it does not actually destroy the antigen, but it facilitates its neutralization, elimination, or destruction in the following ways:
	  a. Neutralization or binding of the antigen so that the function of the antigen is disrupted until the antigen can be phagocytized
	  b. Opsonization or coating of the invading microorganism so that it can be easily recognized as foreign and phagocytized
	  c. Activation of complement, which lyses the invader's cell membrane
	Cell-mediated or T-cell immunity is aimed primarily at intracellular microorganisms, viruses, and cancer and is also responsible for delayed hypersensitivity reactions and transplanted tissue rejection. When T_C CD8 cells recognize foreign antigen on a cell's surface on class I MHC molecules, the T_C cell secretes cytotoxic substances that destroy the foreign cell. This is particularly important in eliminating virus-infected cells, tumor cells, and cells of a transplanted tissue graft.

Continued

Function	Description
Tolerance	In addition to recognizing foreign antigens and initiating an immunologic response, the immune system must also be able to recognize its own proteins and not mount an immune response against self.
	This process of self-recognition occurs as part of normal neonatal growth and development.
	Autoimmune diseases occur when there is a breakdown of tolerance in which the immune system identifies its own proteins as foreign and inappropriately mounts a response to destroy these self proteins.
	Examples of autoimmune diseases include systemic lupus erythematosus, rheumatoid arthritis, acute rheumatic fever, Graves' disease, Hashimoto's thyroiditis, and type 1 diabetes mellitus.
Hypersensitivity reactions	Hypersensitivity reactions, or allergies, are exaggerated immune responses that can be uncomfortable and potentially harmful to the individual.
	There are four types of hypersensitivity reactions, classified according to the time between the exposure and the reaction, the immune mechanism involved, and the site of reaction.
	Hypersensitivity reactions to drugs, or drug allergies, are one of many possible adverse drug reactions. Drug-induced hypersensitivity reactions can be any of the four types of hypersensitivity reaction. See Anaphylactic Hypersensitivity Reactions in Chapter 9.

Ig, Immunoglobulin; *MAC*, membrane attack complex; *MHC*, major histocompatibility complex; T_C, cytotoxic T cells.

      (h) Musculoskeletal: Swelling of joints, tenderness or pain in the bones or joints
      (i) Endocrine: Heat or cold intolerance
  b. Family history indicating a potential hematologic or immunologic problem: Hemophilia, sickle cell anemia, cancer, or death of a relative at a young age for reasons other than trauma
  c. Social history and habits that may assist with the diagnosis and treatment of the underlying condition, including the following:
    i. Any unusual or excessive exposure to chemicals (e.g., gasoline, benzene, solvents, glues, paints, varnishes) or radiation (e.g., x-rays) at work or in pursuit of a hobby
    ii. Any unusual dietary preferences, pica
    iii. Excessive alcohol consumption
    iv. Sexual preference, number of partners, history of sexually transmitted diseases, current contraceptive method, use of safe sex practices
    v. Intravenous (IV) drug use
  d. Medication history
    i. Current medications or a recent change in medication may suggest an underlying hematologic or immunologic problem. Always ask about over-the-counter medication use, because many of these preparations contain aspirin or nonsteroidal anti-inflammatory drugs (NSAIDs).
    ii. Many medications used to treat nonhematologic and nonimmunologic problems can affect the hematologic and immunologic systems; examples of these drugs are the following:
      (a) Analgesics and anti-inflammatory drugs
        (1) Aspirin and aspirin-containing drugs, such as
          a) Oxycodone and aspirin (Percodan)
          b) Bismuth subsalicylate (Pepto-Bismol)
        (2) NSAIDs, such as
          a) Ibuprofen (Motrin)
          b) Indomethacin (Indocin)

        c) Ketoprofen (Orudis)

        d) Ketorolac (Toradol)

        e) Sulindac (Clinoril)

      (3) Steroids, such as

        a) Dexamethasone (Decadron)

        b) Prednisone

  (b) Antibiotics, such as

      (1) Chloramphenicol (Chloromycetin)

      (2) Isoniazid (INH)

      (3) Para-aminosalicylic acid (PAS)

      (4) Penicillin

      (5) Streptomycin

      (6) Trimethoprim-sulfamethoxazole (TMP-SMX, Bactrim, Septra)

      (7) Zidovudine (AZT, Retrovir)

  (c) Anticoagulants, such as

      (1) Heparin

      (2) Warfarin (Coumadin)

  (d) Anticonvulsants, such as

      (1) Carbamazepine (Tegretol)

      (2) Phenytoin (Dilantin)

  (e) Antidiabetic agents, such as chlorpropamide

  (f) Antineoplastic chemotherapy agents, such as

      (1) Cyclophosphamide (Cytoxan)

      (2) Cytosine arabinoside (ara-C)

      (3) Daunorubicin (daunomycin)

      (4) Doxorubicin (Adriamycin)

      (5) Etoposide (VP-16)

      (6) Hydroxyurea (Hydrea)

      (7) Methotrexate

      (8) Nitrogen mustard

      (9) Paclitaxel (Taxol)

    (10) Vinblastine (Velban)

  (g) Antipsychotic agents, such as clozapine (Clozaril)

  (h) Antirheumatic agents, such as

      (1) Gold

      (2) Methotrexate

  (i) Cardiovascular agents, such as

      (1) Digoxin

      (2) Methyldopa (Aldomet)

      (3) Procainamide (Pronestyl)

      (4) Quinidine sulfate

  (j) Diuretics, such as chlorothiazide (Diuril)

  (k) Hormones, such as

      (1) Estrogens

      (2) Androgens

  (l) Immunosuppressives, such as

      (1) Azathioprine (Imuran)

      (2) Cyclophosphamide

      (3) Cyclosporine

      (4) Methotrexate

      (5) Vincristine (Oncovin)

  (m) Oral contraceptives

2. Nursing examination of patient

  a. Physical examination data

    i. Inspection

      (a) Temperature: Exceeds 101° F (38.3° C)

        (b) Skin: Pallor, jaundice, flushing, rash, petechiae, purpura, ecchymoses, hematomas, urticaria, integrity

        (c) Head and neck: Integrity of mucosal membranes, tongue appearance (e.g., smooth, coated), conjunctival bleeding

        (d) Chest: Shortness of breath, hemoptysis

        (e) Abdomen: Vomiting, hematemesis, hematuria, diarrhea, melena

        (f) Musculoskeletal system: Swelling of joints

    ii. Palpation and percussion

        (a) Skin: Warm to touch

        (b) Neck: Enlarged lymph nodes

        (c) Abdomen: Hepatomegaly, splenomegaly, enlarged lymph nodes in the axilla or groin

        (d) Musculoskeletal system: Pain on palpation

    iii. Auscultation

        (a) Tachycardia

        (b) Hypotension

        (c) Orthostatic changes (pulse increases 20 beats/min and blood pressure decreases 20 mm Hg when the patient moves from lying to sitting or standing)

        (d) Tachypnea

        (e) Crackles, rhonchi

        (f) Decreased breath sounds

b. Monitoring data

    i. Fatigue related to hypoxemia

    ii. Pulse oximetry

    iii. Skin color

    iv. Skin turgor as an indicator of dehydration

    v. Overt and covert bleeding

    vi. Acute or persistent pain

    vii. Exposure to infection or disease

    viii. Body temperature

    ix. Development of unusual cancers

3. Appraisal of patient characteristics: Patients needing acute or life-saving care for hematologic disorders or for immunologic compromise come to progressive care units as a result of their comorbidities or primary complications. The need for progressive care may be brief or extended with quick to no recovery. Many hematologic and immunologic disorders are incurable. Occasionally, the focus is anticipated end-of-life care, although in no case is one able to predict with any certainty. Some patient characteristics that the nurse needs to assess for this population are the following:

a. Resiliency

    i. Level 1—*Minimally resilient:* A frail 27-year-old young man with acquired immunodeficiency syndrome (AIDS) dementia, severe stomatitis, and chronic diarrhea, who is unresponsive to antiretroviral therapy

    ii. Level 3—*Moderately resilient:* A 55-year-old woman with newly diagnosed acute lymphocytic leukemia after her second bone marrow transplant due to failed engraftment of the original donor stem cells

    iii. Level 5—*Highly resilient:* An 18-year-old man with a hemoglobin level of 8.0 g/dl recovering from a hypovolemic hemorrhage related to a table saw accident at his family's farm

b. Vulnerability

    i. Level 1—*Highly vulnerable:* A 45-year-old man with acute myelogenous leukemia who is neutropenic and has a lung abscess and thrombocytopenia

    ii. Level 3—*Moderately vulnerable:* A 36-year-old man, who is otherwise healthy, experiencing a type I hypersensitivity reaction to poison ivy hidden in the brush he was removing

    iii. Level 5—*Minimally vulnerable:* A petite 40-year-old woman with vitamin B_{12} deficiency anemia and alcoholism

   c. Stability

      i. Level 1—*Minimally stable:* A 78-year-old widowed retired Air Force colonel in whom viral pneumonia and confusion develop on the second day after admission for induction chemotherapy for acute lymphocytic leukemia

      ii. Level 3—*Moderately stable:* A 59-year-old housewife in whom thrombocytopenia has been diagnosed and who has a platelet count of $60,000/mm^3$

      iii. Level 5—*Highly stable:* A 28-year-old professor with lymphoma recovering in contact isolation from a methicillin-resistant *Staphylococcus aureus* toenail infection

   d. Complexity

      i. Level 1—*Highly complex:* A 48-year-old mother of four transferring to a critical care unit after heparin-induced thrombocytopenia developed 6 days after a bilateral mastectomy and transversus rectus abdominis myocutaneous flap surgical reconstruction

      ii. Level 3—*Moderately complex:* A 19-year-old man with a diagnosed HIV infection that he wishes to be kept confidential from his parents and siblings

      iii. Level 5—*Minimally complex:* A 35-year-old accountant in whom autoimmune thrombocytopenic purpura (ATP) is diagnosed after a prolonged case of the flu

   e. Resource availability

      i. Level 1—*Few resources:* A 47-year-old housekeeper with rheumatoid arthritis who provides the sole income for a family of six and receives a diagnosis of leukemia

      ii. Level 3—*Moderate resources:* A 32-year-old Spanish-speaking migrant worker who contracted hepatitis C after a blood transfusion and has a bilingual sister who is a United States citizen and a social worker

      iii. Level 5—*Many resources:* A 49-year-old chief executive officer of a major computer software company who is hospitalized for maintenance chemotherapy

   f. Participation in care

      i. Level 1—*No participation:* An obese 26-year-old woman in anaphylactic shock awaiting transfer to the critical care unit

      ii. Level 3—*Moderate level of participation:* A 67-year-old salesman who is learning about home care for a Hickman catheter

      iii. Level 5—*Full participation:* A 32-year-old woman with AIDS who is compliant with antiretroviral therapy, exercise, and diet recommendations

   g. Participation in decision making

      i. Level 1—*No participation:* A 30-year-old children's tennis coach who chooses to let God's will be done after the physician team decides not to render further treatment for advanced cancer of the thoracic spine

      ii. Level 3—*Moderate level of participation:* A 56-year-old Mediterranean man who defers to his wife for decisions about treating his blood disorder

      iii. Level 5—*Full participation:* A 37-year-old kindergarten teacher who asks to know platelet counts before consenting to each platelet transfusion

   h. Predictability

      i. Level 1—*Not predictable:* An elegant 82-year-old grandmother with newly diagnosed chronic myelocytic leukemia

      ii. Level 3—*Moderately predictable:* A 29-year-old day care worker receiving a second bone marrow transplant (BMT) after complete engraftment of the primary BMT stem cells

      iii. Level 5—*Highly predictable:* A 27-year-old man with cognitive and behavioral challenges from AIDS dementia

4. Diagnostic studies

   a. Laboratory: See Table 7-7 for normal values

      i. Blood: See Table 7-8

      ii. Sputum culture: Detects and identifies microorganisms in the sputum

      iii. Urine tests

         (a) Urinalysis can detect gross amounts of blood or protein in the urine.

         (b) Urine cultures detect and identify microorganisms in the urine.

         (c) Urine protein electrophoresis determines the levels of proteins excreted in the urine, particularly the levels of immunoglobulins.

      iv. Stool occult blood test (Hemoccult): Detects microscopic amounts of blood in the stool

■ **TABLE 7-7**
■ ■ **Normal Blood Values**

Laboratory Test	Reference Values	Description
WBC count	4500-10,000/mm^3	Total number of leukocytes
Differential WBC		Part of CBC; indicates distribution of five types of leukocytes
Neutrophils	2500-7000/mm^3	
Segments	2500-6500/mm^3	
Bands	0-500/mm^3	
Monocytes	200-600/mm^3	
Basophils	40-100/mm^3	
Eosinophils	100-300/mm^3	
Lymphocytes	1700-3500/mm^3	
RBC indices		Erythrocyte indicators for anemia
RBC count		
Men	4.6-6.0 million/mm^3	
Women	4.0-5.0 million/mm^3	
MCV	80-98 mm^3	Indicates size of RBC
MCH	27-31 pg	Indicates weight of hemoglobin in RBC
MCHC	32%-36%	Hemoglobin per volume RBC
RDW	11.5-14.5 Coulter S	Size (width) difference of RBCs
Hb level		Iron composition of RBC for oxygen-carrying capability
Men	13.5-17 g/dl	
Women	11.2-115 g/dl	
HCT of blood		Measure of the percentage of the total blood volume that is made up by RBCs
Men	40%-54%	
Women	36%-46%	
Panic value	<15% and >60%	
Reticulocyte count	0.5%-1.5%	Indicator of bone marrow activity
Erythrocyte sedimentation rate		Rate at which erythrocytes settle (sediment) in unclotted blood
Men	0-9 mm/hr (Wintrobe method)	
Women	0-15 mm/hr (Wintrobe method)	
Serum ferritin level		An indicator of protein stores of iron in the tissues, where 1 ng/ml ferritin = 8 mg stored iron
Men	15-445 ng/ml	
Women	10-235 ng/ml	
Postmenopausal	15-310 ng/ml	
TIBC	250-450 mg/dl	Total (maximum) iron-binding capacity of transferrin for transport of iron to marrow for hemoglobin synthesis
PLT	150,000-400,000/mm^3	Measure of thrombocytes available for coagulation of blood
FSP	2-10 mg/ml	Indicator of fibrin degradation products acting as anticoagulant in continuous bleeding associated with hemorrhage
Clotting times		
PT	10-13 sec	Measures clotting factor ability
PTT	60-70 sec	Detects deficiencies in clotting factors
INR	2.5-3.5	Standard for warfarin-sensitive PT

Data from Kee JL. *Laboratory Diagnostic Tests With Nursing Implications*. 5th ed. Stamford, CT: Appleton & Lange; 1999.
CBC, Complete blood cell count; *FSP,* fibrin split products; *Hb,* hemoglobin; *HCT,* hematocrit; *INR,* international normalized ratio; *MCH,* mean corpuscular hemoglobin; *MCHC,* mean corpuscular hemoglobin concentration; *MCV,* mean corpuscular volume; *PLT,* platelet count; *PT,* prothrombin time; *PTT,* partial thromboplastin time; *RBC,* red blood cell; *RDW,* RBC distribution width; *TIBC,* total iron-binding capacity; *WBC,* white blood cell.

■ **TABLE 7-8**
■ ■ **Blood Studies**

Study	Abbreviation	Comments
Complete blood cell count with differential	CBC	The total white blood cell (WBC) count measures the total number of WBCs found in 1 mm^3 of blood.
		The differential measures the contribution that each type of WBC (neutrophils, monocytes, basophils, eosinophils, and lymphocytes) makes to the total WBC count.
		A "shift to the right" on a CBC indicates that only a small percentage of the WBCs are neutrophils. The lower the neutrophil count, the greater the patient's risk of infection. To calculate the absolute neutrophil count (ANC), multiply the percentage of neutrophils indicated on the differential of the CBC by the total number of WBCs.
		A "shift to the left" on a CBC indicates that a large percentage of the WBCs are neutrophils. This usually implies that the bone marrow has been stimulated to produce more neutrophils to fight a severe infection.
Red blood cell	RBC	Total number of RBCs found in 1 mm^3 of blood count
Hemoglobin count	Hb	A measure of the amount of hemoglobin in 1 dl of blood and an indicator of the blood's oxygen-carrying capacity
Hematocrit	HCT	Percentage of RBCs in a volume of whole blood
Mean corpuscular volume	MCV	Average size (volume) of RBCs
Mean corpuscular hemoglobin concentration	MCHC	Average concentration of hemoglobin in the RBCs
Mean corpuscular hemoglobin	MCH	Average amount of hemoglobin per RBC
Platelet count		Total number of platelets per 1 mm^3 of blood
Reticulocyte count		Number or percentage of immature RBCs in the peripheral circulation
Erythrocyte sedimentation rate	ESR, or sed rate	Rate at which RBCs settle out of anticoagulated whole blood sample over a specified period of time. The ESR can be elevated in inflammatory conditions or anemia. ESR is best used for assessment of response to treatment, rather than as a diagnostic test.
Serum iron level		Amount of iron in serum
Total iron-binding capacity	TIBC	Reflects the body's ability to transport available iron
Ferritin level		A rough measure of the body's iron stores and a good indicator of the body's iron storage status
Bleeding time		The primary phase of hemostasis: How long it takes platelets to adhere to the broken blood vessel and form the platelet plug; a rough gauge of platelet function
Thrombin time	TT	Time it takes thrombin (factor IIa) to convert fibrinogen (factor I) to fibrin (factor Ia); it is markedly prolonged by the presence of heparin
Prothrombin time	PT	Clotting ability of the extrinsic coagulation cascade (factor VII) and the common pathway (factor X [Stuart-Prower factor], factor V [proaccelerin or AC-globulin], factor II [prothrombin], and factor I [fibrinogen]). PT is used to monitor warfarin (Coumadin) therapy.
Partial thromboplastin time	PTT	A more sensitive measure of the clotting ability and a test of the common pathway (factor X [Stuart-Prower factor], factor V [proaccelerin], factor II [prothrombin], and factor I [fibrinogen]). PTT is used to monitor heparin therapy.
International normalized ratio	INR	A comparative rating of PT ratios in which the measured PT is adjusted by the International Reference thromboplastin. It is a uniform way of monitoring warfarin therapy.

Continued

■ **TABLE 7-8**
■ ■ **Blood Studies—Cont'd**

Study	Abbreviation	Comments
Fibrin split products	FSP	The levels of fibrin degradation products
D-dimers level		Also reflects levels of fibrin degradation products but is a more specific test for disseminated intravascular coagulation because D-dimers are specific for fibrinolysis
Fibrinogen level		Blood level of fibrinogen (factor I)
Serum bilirubin level		Amounts of the various types of bilirubin in the blood; bilirubin is produced during the breakdown of hemoglobin in RBCs
		Conjugated or direct bilirubin circulates freely in the blood until it is cleared by the liver and excreted in bile; an increase in conjugated bilirubin level is indicative of a dysfunction or blockage of the liver.
		Unconjugated or indirect bilirubin is protein bound; an increase in unconjugated bilirubin often is evidence of increased RBC destruction.
		Total bilirubin level is a measure of both conjugated and unconjugated bilirubin.
Serum protein electrophoresis	SPEP	Determines the levels of serum proteins in blood, particularly levels of immunoglobulins
Coombs' test		The direct Coombs' test detects the presence of antibody on the RBC membrane.
		The indirect Coombs' test detects antibody in the serum.
T-cell count		Reflects the levels of T-cells in the blood
Human immunodeficiency virus (HIV)		Includes the enzyme-linked immunosorbent assay (ELISA) and the Western blot. Both of these tests are used to detect the presence of antibody to HIV. The Western blot is a more specific and sensitive test.
Blood and tissue typing		Blood typing detects ABO and Rh antigens present on RBCs and is necessary for compatibility testing before blood product transfusion.
		A more specific blood typing test detects human leukocyte antigens (HLAs) and is necessary for compatibility testing before some types of tissue transplantation (e.g., bone marrow transplantation)
Blood culture		Detects and identifies microorganisms in the blood

    b. Radiologic
       i. Spleen ultrasonography is used to estimate the size of the spleen.
       ii. In a liver-spleen scan, a radioactive tracer is used to evaluate the size as well as the function of the liver and spleen.
       iii. In a gallium scan, a radioactive tracer is used to detect the presence of malignant tissue, particularly malignant lymphoid tissues.
       iv. In a lymphangiogram, contrast dye is used to radiologically visualize the lymph system, particularly the size and architecture of lymph nodes.
    c. Biopsy
       i. Bone marrow biopsy includes aspiration of bone marrow fluid and removal of a needle core biopsy sample of the bone marrow tissue for pathologic examination.
       ii. In a lymph node biopsy, one or more lymph nodes are removed for pathologic examination.
    d. Skin tests: Barometers of immune functioning, pointing out hyposensitivities or hypersensitivities to a particular antigen. Examples of allergens used in skin testing are allergenic extracts (e.g., dust, pollen, animal dander); purified protein derivative (PPD) for tuberculin skin tests; mumps virus; *Candida albicans*; and skin fungi.

Patient Care

1. **Susceptibility to infection**
   a. Description of problem
      i. Immune compromise and/or coagulopathy increases patient risk for opportunistic and host infections.
      ii. Clinical findings include reports of fever, chills, night sweats, sore throat, cough, malaise, pain with swallowing, pain with urination, pain with defecation, diarrhea, reddened areas, sore areas, and swollen areas (these symptoms may not be present if the patient has neutropenia and is unable to mount a WBC response); flushing, lethargy, skin warm to touch; abnormal vital signs—temperature exceeding 101° F (38.3° C), hypotension, tachycardia; WBC count lower than 1500/mm³, absolute neutrophil count (ANC) lower than 500/mm³
   b. Goals of care
      i. Vital signs within normal limits for the patient
      ii. Absence of signs or symptoms of active infection
      iii. Maintenance of the WBC count within an acceptable range
      iv. Patient's and family's verbalization of an understanding of the underlying pathology and infection prevention
   c. Collaborating professionals on health care team
      i. Nurse
      ii. Pharmacist
      iii. Physician
      iv. Radiologist
      v. Laboratory technician
      vi. Blood bank specialist
   d. Interventions: See Table 7-9

▨ TABLE 7-9
▨ ▨ Leukocyte Intervention Activity Bundle

Root cause	**Protection from infection:** A proliferation of immature leukocytes or a chemotherapy-induced neutropenic state creates immunocompromise leading to a high alteration in patient's ability to fight infection.
Interventions to protect against and detect infection	1. Assess daily absolute neutrophil count, white blood cell count and differential for abnormal granulocyte levels.
	2. Bathe or assist the patient with bathing daily, because normal flora pose highest risk for infection.
	3. Inspect skin and mucous membranes every 4 hr for areas of redness or wound formation.
	4. Assess each invasive site (intravenous line, Hickman catheter, peripherally inserted central catheter, nasogastric tube, gastrostomy tube, Foley catheter, etc.) twice a shift for signs of portal infection.
	5. Obtain cultures immediately from any new sites with suspicious drainage.
	6. Administer antibiotics on schedule and as prescribed.
	7. Monitor and supplement nutritional intake of vitamins, proteins, and fats.
	8. Monitor, encourage, and supplement free water intake.
	9. Anticipate daily chest radiography for patients prone to pneumonia.
	10. Encourage deep breathing and coughing and change of position every 2-4 hr.
	11. Place fresh flower and plant gifts for patients outside of patient area, yet within patient's sight.
	12. Ensure that all persons entering room are free of communicable disease.
	13. Recommend private rooms for all patients at risk of infection.

From Schneider S. Interventions for clients with hematologic problems. In: Ignatavicius DD, Workman ML, eds. *Medical-Surgical Nursing: Critical Thinking for Collaborative Care.* 4th ed. Philadelphia, PA: Saunders; 2002.

    e. Evaluation of patient care
- **i.** Absence of fever
- **ii.** Maintenance of an ANC exceeding $1000/mm^3$
- **iii.** Ability of the patient and family to describe how to reduce the patient's risk of infection

2. Increased risk for hemorrhage
    a. Description of problem
- **i.** Disease and/or treatment creates an altered state of protection against bleeding.
- **ii.** Clinical findings include reports of unusual bruising, prolonged bleeding, hematemesis, hemoptysis, hematochezia, melena, hematuria, menorrhagia.

    b. Goals of care
- **i.** No evidence of spontaneous bleeding
- **ii.** Maintenance of platelet counts and levels of clotting factors within an acceptable range
- **iii.** Patient's and family's verbalization of an understanding of the underlying pathology and bleeding precautions

    c. Collaborating professionals on health care team
- **i.** Nurse
- **ii.** Pharmacist
- **iii.** Physician
- **iv.** Laboratory technician
- **v.** Blood bank specialist

    d. Interventions: See Table 7-10

    e. Evaluation of patient care
- **i.** No evidence of spontaneous bleeding
- **ii.** Maintenance of a platelet count of more than $50,000/mm^3$ and prothrombin time (PT) and partial thromboplastin time (PTT) within prescribed ranges
- **iii.** Ability of the patient and family to describe how to reduce the patient's risk of bleeding

3. Impaired respiratory gas transport: See Chapter 2
    a. Interventions: See Table 7-10

4. Impaired fluid volume regulation (see also Chapter 5)
    a. Description of problem
- **i.** Fever, vomiting, diarrhea, hemorrhage, and shock deplete body fluid volume.
- **ii.** Clinical findings include reports of thirst, sweating, vomiting, polyuria, diarrhea, lightheadedness; pallor, mucosal dryness, loss of skin turgor, decreased venous filling; abnormal vital signs—fever, tachycardia, hypotension, changes in orthostatic vital signs; decreased urine output and concentrated urine with a specific gravity exceeding 1.020; altered mental status.

    b. Goals of care
- **i.** Absence of dehydration, hypovolemia, and shock
- **ii.** Urine output greater than 30 ml/hr

    c. Collaborating professionals on health care team
- **i.** Nurse
- **ii.** Pharmacist
- **iii.** Physician
- **iv.** Blood bank specialist

    d. Interventions: See Table 7-11
- **i.** Administer IV fluids and blood products as prescribed.
  - (a) Transfuse blood products (Table 7-12).
  - (b) Keep in mind special considerations related to blood product administration (Table 7-13 and Box 7-1).
- **ii.** Treat underlying condition as prescribed.
- **iii.** Encourage oral fluid intake as the patient's condition allows.
- **iv.** Monitor fluid balance with recording of intake and output and daily weights.

▤ TABLE 7-10
▤ ▤ Erythrocyte Intervention Activity Bundle

Root causes	**Monitor oxygen transport:** Alterations in hemoglobin due to anemic states or profuse bleeding cause a lack of sufficient oxygen binding and oxygen-carrying capability, potentially leading to respiratory compromise and tissue ischemia. **Precautions for bleeding:** A proliferation of immature erythrocytes or a severe lack of platelets from idiopathic or induced thrombocytopenia prevents clot formation and induces bleeding.
Interventions to prevent and detect hypoxia	1. Monitor pulse oximetry every 2-4 hr or more often as indicated. 2. Assess ferritin and hemoglobin levels daily to predict oxygen-carrying capability. 3. Assess circumoral area and the nailbeds of fingers and toes every 4 hr for cyanosis. 4. Monitor for changes in mental status and difficulty breathing every 2-4 hr. 5. Administer prophylactic supplemental oxygen and/or hematopoietic growth factors as prescribed. 6. See Interventions to Protect Against and Detect Infection in Table 7-9.
Interventions to prevent hemorrhage	1. Monitor daily hematocrit, hemoglobin level, clotting times, and platelet counts. 2. Monitor temperature, heart rate, breathing pattern, and blood pressure every 2-4 hr and with every episode of bleeding. 3. Check expectorant, residuals from feedings, urine, and feces for frank blood. 4. Administer platelets, fresh frozen plasma, or clotting factors as prescribed using proper method. 5. Administer stool softeners, vitamin K supplements, and synthetic platelet aggregates as ordered. 6. Avoid administration of nonsteroidal antiinflammatory drugs and anticoagulants. 7. Protect patient from injury, constipation, falls, and trauma at all times. 8. Avoid damage to rectal mucosa; avoid intramuscular, subcutaneous, and venous or arterial cannulation. 9. Use a soft Toothette for oral care and an electric razor for shaving. 10. Instruct patient and family on risks and signs of bleeding. 11. Encourage patient to eat green leafy vegetables and fruits high in vitamin K.

From Schneider S. Interventions for clients with hematologic problems. In: Ignatavicius DD, Workman ML, eds. *Medical-Surgical Nursing: Critical Thinking for Collaborative Care.* 4th ed. Philadelphia, PA: Saunders; 2002.

▤ TABLE 7-11
▤ ▤ Dehydration Intervention Activity Bundle

Root cause	**Fluid volume deficit:** Nausea, vomiting, diarrhea, loss of appetite, loss of insensible water due to fever, and bleeding tendencies result in chronic phases of dehydration.
Interventions to prevent and detect dehydration	1. Monitor daily serum chemistry values for sodium, potassium, and chloride. 2. Monitor daily serum renal panel values, arterial blood gas levels, and liver panel values as indicated. 3. Determine patient's self-report of activities and interventions that contribute to fluid losses. 4. Monitor temperature, heart rate, breathing pattern, and blood pressure every 4 hr. 5. Assess daily LOC, skin turgor, appetite, and number, character, color, and frequency of emesis, diarrhea, urine, and bleeding. 6. Assess and manage treatable contributing factors (food odors or appearance, flavor, preference and availability of oral fluids, antiemetic choice, medication side effects, room temperature, air currents in room). 7. Administer prophylactic antiemetics as indicated. 8. Administer supplemental or maintenance intravenous fluids as ordered. 9. See Interventions to Prevent Hemorrhage in Table 7-10.

From Schneider S. Interventions for clients with hematologic problems. In: Ignatavicius DD, Workman ML, eds. *Medical-Surgical Nursing: Critical Thinking for Collaborative Care.* 4th ed. Philadelphia, PA: Saunders; 2002.
LOC, Level of consciousness.

■ **TABLE 7-12**
■ ■ **Indications for Treatment with Blood Components**

Component	Volume	Infusion Time	Indications
Packed red blood cells (PRBCs)	200-250 ml	2-4 hr	Anemia; hemoglobin level <6 g/dl, 6-10 g/dl, depending on symptoms
Washed red blood cells (white blood cell–poor PRBCs)	200 ml	2-4 hr	History of allergic transfusion reactions; bone marrow transplant clients
Platelets			
Pooled	Approximately 300 ml	15-30 min	Thrombocytopenia, platelet count<20,000/mm³; clients who are actively bleeding with a platelet count <80,000/mm³
Single donor	200 ml	30 min	History of febrile or allergic reactions
Fresh frozen plasma	200 ml	15-30 min	Deficiency in plasma coagulation factors; prothrombin or partial thromboplastin time 1.5 times normal
Cryoprecipitate	10-20 ml/U	15-30 min	Hemophilia VIII or von Willebrand's disease; fibrinogen levels <100 mg/dl
White blood cells	400 ml	1 hr	Sepsis, neutropenic infection not responding to antibiotic therapy

From Schneider S. Interventions for clients with hematologic problems. In: Ignatavicius DD, Workman ML, eds. *Medical-Surgical Nursing: Critical Thinking for Collaborative Care.* 4th ed. Philadelphia, PA: Saunders; 2002.

■ **TABLE 7-13**
■ ■ **Types of Blood Transfusion Reaction**

Reaction	Mechanism	Signs and Symptoms	Time of Occurrence	Treatment
Hemolytic	Type II antigen-complement reaction to transfusion of ABO- or Rh-incompatible blood	Fever, chills, headache, chest pain, low back pain, tachypnea, tachycardia, DIC, or circulatory collapse	Immediately or may not occur until subsequent units have been transfused	Stop the transfusion; notify the physician and blood bank immediately; provide supportive therapy to maintain blood pressure and urine output.
Allergic-urticaric-anaphylactic	Type I hypersensitivity to plasma proteins	Urticaria, wheezing, dyspnea, hypotension	Within 30 min of transfusion, but may also be up to 24 hr	Temporarily stop the transfusion; notify the physician and blood bank; be prepared to administer antihistamines or epinephrine orally or intramuscularly; use washed RBCs.
Febrile	Antibody to donor leukocyte	Fever, chills, tachycardia, tachypnea, hypotension	Within 30-90 min of the start of the transfusion	Administer antipyretics, white blood cell–poor RBCs, or single-donor human leukocyte antigen–matched platelets.

TABLE 7-13

Types of Blood Transfusion Reaction—Cont'd

Reaction	Mechanism	Signs and Symptoms	Time of Occurrence	Treatment
Bacterial	Blood contaminated with gram-negative organisms (endotoxin producing)	Fever, chills, tachycardia, shock, DIC, renal failure	Within 30 min of the start of the transfusion	Stop the transfusion; notify the physician and blood bank; give high-dose antibiotics, steroids, and blood pressure support.
Circulatory overload	Transfusion administered too quickly	Restlessness, confusion, dyspnea, bounding pulse, hypertension	Anytime during the transfusion	Slow the transfusion; provide supportive therapy and monitor.

Data from Hankins J, Lonsway RAW, Hedrick D, et al. *Infusion Therapy in Clinical Practice.* 2nd ed. St Louis, MO: Saunders; 2001; and Ignatavicius DD, Workman ML, eds. *Medical-Surgical Nursing: Critical Thinking for Collaborative Care.* 5th ed. Philadelphia, PA: Saunders; 2006.
DIC, Disseminated intravascular coagulation; *RBC,* red blood cell.

BOX 7-1

CONSIDERATIONS IN ADMINISTERING BLOOD PRODUCTS

1. **Alloimmunization** is a state in which the patient develops antibodies against human leukocyte antigen (HLA), granulocyte-specific antigens, red blood cell (RBC)–specific antigens, or platelet-specific antigens after repeated blood product transfusions. As a result, the transfused cells are destroyed and the transfusion is ineffective in correcting the patient's blood counts. Platelet destruction related to HLA antibodies accounts for 95% of cases of alloimmunization in patients who fail to respond to platelet transfusions. HLA matching and platelet cross-matching are two options for patients with alloimmunization. For both of these options, nearly 2 days can be required to provide a proper match.
2. **Pathogen contamination of blood products** has been reduced because of better screening of donors, viral nucleic acid testing of donor blood, purification of plasma and plasma-derived products, and recombinant factor concentrate production technology. Current estimated risk of transmission of viruses ranges from 0.5 to 7.0 per million transfusions. However, 1 in 500 to 2000 platelet transfusions has bacterial contamination. Consideration should be given to the rate at which new blood-borne pathogens are identified and the inability to outpace growth with appropriate screening tests. Pathogen inactivation technologies are actively being studied.
3. **Irradiation of blood products** incapacitates lymphocytes, with approximately 2500 rads of gamma radiation thus reducing the incidence of cytomegalovirus (CMV) infection, alloimmunization, and transfusion-associated graft-versus-host disease (GVHD). Cryoprecipitate and fresh frozen plasma are lymphocyte free and need not be irradiated. Irradiation of blood is beneficial for immunocompromised patients at risk for GVHD, hematopoietic stem cell donors, and transplant patients, and in cases of cellular (T-cell) immunodeficiency, intrauterine transfusion, transfusions from family members, matched platelet transfusions, Hodgkin's disease, neonatal exchange transfusions, acute myelogenous leukemia, acute lymphocytic leukemia, and lymphoma.
4. **CMV-negative blood products** are necessary for patients who need a bone marrow transplant and who have never been exposed to CMV. A CMV infection during transplantation could be life-threatening. Use of CMV-negative blood products benefits premature infants or infants younger than 4 weeks of age, fetuses undergoing intrauterine transfusions, and any CMV-negative patient who is pregnant, potentially a transplant candidate, or about to undergo splenectomy or has acquired immunodeficiency syndrome, human immunodeficiency virus infection, or a congenital immune deficiency.
5. **Leukocyte-reduced (LR) blood products** reduce the risk of development of a nonhemolytic transfusion reaction, alloimmunization, or GVHD, and potentially prevent the transmission of CMV. When administering LR blood

Continued

■ **BOX 7-1**
■ **CONSIDERATIONS IN ADMINISTERING BLOOD PRODUCTS—Cont'd**

products, be sure to use an appropriate blood filter at the bedside to trap the cellular debris accumulated since the original filtration process. Leukocyte reduction benefits patients with a history of more than one nonhemolytic febrile transfusion reaction, immunocompromised patients at risk for CMV, and patients who will potentially receive multiple transfusions and are at an increased risk for alloimmunization.

6. **Washing of blood** removes proteins, electrolytes, antibodies, and glycerol (from frozen RBCs) that could trigger severe reactions in some recipients. To wash blood, 0.9% normal saline is added to the unit and mixed, the mixture is centrifuged, and the saline is removed. Washing of blood benefits patients receiving RBCs frozen in glycerol and patients exhibiting severe hypersensitivity to donor plasma components such as immunoglobulin A or B.

7. **Blood substitutes** (hemoglobin solutions and perfluorocarbon emulsions) are currently under investigation, but common adverse effects have been identified. Increased systemic and pulmonary vascular resistance leading to a decreased cardiac index and impaired oxygen delivery is the primary adverse effect associated with hemoglobin solutions. Cell-free hemoglobin acts as a nitric oxide scavenger. Perfluorocarbon emulsions can immerse in water, are chemically inert, and are not metabolized in vivo. Both types of blood substitute have a half-life of hours to days versus a half-life of weeks for an RBC. The dark red color of blood substitutes makes ABO typing a challenge. Blood substitutes may be useful as a bridge to transfusion in patients difficult to transfuse.

Data from Fitzpatrick L. When to administer modified blood products. *Nursing.* 2002;32(5):36-42; Fung M, Triulzi D. Pathogen inactivation of blood products, *Transfusion Medicine Update,* 2003. http://www.itxm.org/tmu2002/issue7.htm. Accessed October 24, 2008; Nester T. Blood substitutes. *Transfusion Medicine Update,* 2000. http://www.itxm.org/tmu2000/tmu12-2000.htm. Accessed October 24, 2008; and Sepulveda J, Oren E. Alloimmunization from transfusions. 2008. http://www.emedicine.com/med/topic107.htm. Accessed October 24, 2008.

  e. Evaluation of patient care
    i. Maintenance of vital signs within normal limits; when the patient moves from lying to sitting or standing, change in pulse and blood pressure of no more than 20 points
    ii. Patient urine output exceeding 30 ml/hr
    iii. Near equality in patient's 24-hour intake and output
    iv. Stability of patient's weight
 5. **Fatigue**
  a. Description of problem
    i. Potential for activity intolerance related to disease or the treatment of disease
    ii. Clinical findings include reports of fatigue, weakness, malaise, inability to sleep, and inability to concentrate; changes in vital signs with activity
  b. Goals of care
    i. Vital signs within normal limits for the patient
    ii. Patient's ability to accomplish the activities of daily living without tachycardia or hypotension
    iii. Patient's report of a reduction in fatigue
    iv. Patient's ability to concentrate and socialize normally
  c. Collaborating professionals on health care team
    i. Nurse
    ii. Pharmacist
    iii. Physician
    iv. Psychologist
  d. Interventions: See Table 7-14
  e. Evaluation of patient care
    i. Pulse increase of no more than 20 beats/min with nonaerobic activity and return to baseline within 5 minutes of stopping the activity
    ii. Patient's statement that the level of fatigue experienced in performing the activities of daily living is manageable

■ **TABLE 7-14**
■ ■ **Fatigue Intervention Activity Bundle**

Root cause	**Energy expenditure/energy resource variant:** Chronic neutropenia and thrombocytopenia, chemotherapy, radiation therapy, and side effects contribute to patient expressions of weariness and lack of ability to perform independent functions.
Interventions for fatigue	1. Determine the patient's or family's and/or significant other's perception of the causes of fatigue.
	2. Assess and manage treatable contributing factors (pain, emotional distress, sleep disturbances, anemia, hypoxia, organ dysfunction, infection, and fluid and electrolyte imbalances).
	3. Provide a diet high in vitamin C for stress.
	4. When feasible, provide aromas of cooking (bread or cookies baking, soup) to stimulate appetite and motivate the patient to expend the energy required to walk to the kitchen, as possible.
	5. Encourage scheduled aerobic exercise to combat cancer fatigue.
	6. Cluster care and limit the number of interruptions during scheduled rest periods.
	7. Provide stress management and a calm environment to promote relaxation.
	8. Make distractions (music, games, videos, books, magazines, humor, socialization) available.
	9. Establish an on-site or on-unit library to make learning resources available to technical personnel.
	10. Assess the energy needed for an activity and gauge expenditure of the patient's energy resources.
	11. Schedule activities at times of peak energy in order to conserve energy for priority activities.
	12. Reassure the patient that treatment-related fatigue does not directly indicate disease progression.
	13. See Interventions to Protect Against and Detect Infection in Table 7-9.
	14. See Interventions to Prevent and Detect Dehydration in Table 7-11.
	15. See Interventions to Prevent and Detect Hypoxia in Table 7-10.
	16. See Interventions to Prevent Hemorrhage in Table 7-10.

From Schneider S. Interventions for clients with hematologic problems. In: Ignatavicius DD, Workman ML, eds. *Medical-Surgical Nursing: Critical Thinking for Collaborative Care.* 4th ed. Philadelphia, PA: Saunders; 2002.

SPECIFIC PATIENT HEALTH PROBLEMS

Anemia

1. **Pathophysiology**
   a. Anemia is a reduction in the number of RBCs, the quantity of hemoglobin, or the volume of RBCs. Because the main function of RBCs is oxygenation, anemia results in varying degrees of hypoxia. The body compensates for anemia by increasing cardiac output and respiratory rate; by redistributing blood to sustain blood supply to the brain and heart through a reduction in blood supply to the skin, gut, and kidneys; and by increasing the kidney's production of erythropoietin to stimulate erythropoiesis.
   b. Acute blood loss, such as with arterial rupture, dramatically changes the body's hemodynamic status and necessitates emergency intervention. With chronic blood loss occurring over weeks or months, such as in slow gastrointestinal bleeding or menorrhagia, the body has time to compensate, and thus the symptoms of chronic blood loss may be more insidious. Patients with chronic anemia may be admitted to the progressive care unit, where anemia can complicate other medical conditions that do necessitate treatment in a progressive care setting.
2. **Etiology and risk factors**
   a. Inadequate RBC production
      i.   Aplastic anemia
      ii. Chronic inflammatory disease (e.g., rheumatoid arthritis, chronic osteomyelitis)

      iii. End-stage renal disease

      iv. Bone marrow infiltration with malignant cells

      v. Current or recent treatment with antineoplastic chemotherapy

      vi. History of radiation therapy to bones where blood cells are made (i.e., vertebrae, ribs, skull, pelvis, femur, or humerus)

      vii. Bone marrow transplantation

      viii. Dietary deficiencies, particularly in iron, cobalamin (B_{12}), or folate

      ix. Certain drugs (e.g., zidovudine)

  b. Increased RBC destruction

      i. Immune mediated

        (a) Autoimmune hemolytic anemia

        (b) Cytotoxic hypersensitivity reaction (e.g., drug-induced)

      ii. RBC membrane defects (e.g., hereditary spherocytosis)

      iii. Hemoglobin defects

        (a) Sickle cell anemia is an autosomal recessive genetic disorder found primarily in persons of African descent that results from substitution of the amino acid valine for glutamic acid at position 6 of the β-globin protein; this substitution leads to the production of defective hemoglobin, hemoglobin S (HbS). The deoxygenation of HbS leads to distortion of the RBC into the classic sickle cell shape.

        (b) The major consequence of the sickle cell shape is that RBCs are less able to deform and thus obstruct the microcirculation. Sickle-shaped RBCs have a life span of 10 to 20 days (vs. 120 for nonsickled RBCs) and hemolyze rapidly.

        (c) Clinical manifestations of sickle cell anemia are commonly divided into vaso-occlusive, hematologic, and infectious crises.

          (1) Vaso-occlusive crisis occurs when the microcirculation is occluded by sickled RBCs, which causes ischemic injury to the organ perfused; pain is the most frequent complaint.

          (2) Hematologic crisis is manifested by sudden exacerbation of anemia with a corresponding drop in hemoglobin level.

          (3) Infectious crisis is due to a compromised immune system that is susceptible to common infectious agents such as *Haemophilus influenzae, Streptococcus pneumoniae, Mycoplasma pneumoniae, Salmonella typhimurium, S. aureus,* and *Escherichia coli.*

        (d) Treatment for patients with sickle cell anemia includes rest, hydration, supplemental oxygen, analgesia, antibiotic therapy, and blood transfusion as needed.

      iv. Mechanical (e.g., trauma from prosthetic heart valves)

  c. Major blood loss

3. Signs and symptoms

  a. Symptoms: Fatigue; dyspnea, especially with exertion; shortness of breath; possible bone pain if the bone marrow is infiltrated with malignant cells; altered mental status (e.g., dizziness, especially when changing position from lying down to sitting or standing; inability to concentrate; confusion)

  b. Signs: Pallor, possibly jaundice; possible hepatosplenomegaly with liver disease and some types of malignant disease, tenderness of the liver and spleen with palpation and percussion; tachycardia, hypotension, and orthostatic changes in vital signs

4. Diagnostic study findings

  a. Laboratory

      i. Urine: Can test positive for blood

      ii. Stool: Can test positive for blood

      iii. Blood

        (a) Hemoglobin level of less than 7 g/dl, hematocrit (HCT) of less than 21%

        (b) Other findings vary with the cause of anemia and can include increased reticulocyte count, decreased serum iron level, increased or decreased total iron-binding capacity, decreased ferritin level, increased indirect bilirubin level, positive Coombs' test result.

  b. Radiologic: Gastrointestinal series may be obtained to detect the source of bleeding

c. Biopsy: Bone marrow biopsy may be performed to evaluate bone marrow production of RBCs or detect the presence of bone marrow infiltration with malignant cells

d. Endoscopy: To detect the source of bleeding

5. **Goals of care**
   a. Adequate gas exchange
   b. Absence of dehydration due to bleeding
   c. Tolerable level of fatigue

6. **Collaborating professionals on health care team**
   a. Nurse
   b. Blood bank specialist
   c. Pharmacist
   d. Physician

7. **Management of patient care**
   a. Anticipated patient trajectory: Patients with anemia can have an acute event related to loss of RBCs due to hemorrhage or a chronic disorder related to inadequate production of RBCs and/or hemoglobin. Throughout their course of recovery and discharge, patients with anemia may be expected to have needs in the following areas:
      i. Positioning: High Fowler's position for shortness of breath
      ii. Nutrition: Diet or feeding supplement with iron, vitamin B_{12}, and folate may need to be considered
      iii. Pharmacology: Patient may need education on taking oral iron preparations with food to prevent peptic ulcers and on treating constipation as a primary side effect
      iv. Treatment: Invasive treatment with whole blood or packed RBCs
   b. Potential complications
      i. Shortness of breath
         (a) Mechanism: Due to diminished oxygen-carrying capacity
         (b) Management: Place the patient in a position of comfort to ease the work of breathing; oxygen administration and transfusion of packed RBCs may be required
      ii. Weakness and fatigue
         (a) Mechanism: Inadequate circulating hemoglobin decreases oxygen availability to cells, creating decreased energy stores in the body
         (b) Management: Conserve the patient's energy by assisting with nutrition and the activities of daily living, passive range-of-motion exercises; consider providing supplemental oxygen if the patient is out of bed to a chair or is ambulating

8. **Evaluation of patient care**
   a. Absence of dyspnea
   b. Pink skin color, skin warm to the touch
   c. Heart rate of 60 to 100 beats/min
   d. Hemoglobin level higher than 7 g/dl, HCT higher than 21%

Thrombocytopenia

1. **Pathophysiology: The number of platelets available to assist with coagulation is inadequate, which puts the patient at increased risk of hemorrhage. Thrombocytopenia is usually defined as platelets fewer than 140,000/mm³.**

2. **Etiology and risk factors**
   a. Decreased platelet production
      i. Bone marrow infiltration with malignant cells (e.g., leukemia, multiple myeloma, malignant metastases)
      ii. Current or recent treatment with antineoplastic agents
      iii. History of radiation therapy to the bones in which blood cells are made
      iv. Bone marrow aplasia
   b. Increased platelet destruction
      i. Disseminated intravascular coagulation (DIC): DIC is a hypercoagulable disorder that can be caused by cancer or infection. The normal coagulation cascade is overstimulated resulting in simultaneous thrombosis and hemorrhage. DIC is always secondary to another pathologic process.

     ii. Antibody mediated
         (a) Immune thrombocytopenic purpura (ITP)
            (1) Agents known to induce ITP include sulfonamides, thiazide diuretics, chlorpropamide, quinidine, and gold.
            (2) Patients with HIV infection are at increased risk for development of ITP.
         (b) Heparin-induced thrombocytopenia (HIT) and thrombosis (see Hypercoagulable Disorders)
         (c) Alloimmunization after multiple platelet transfusions
     iii. Thrombotic thrombocytopenic purpura (TTP) or hemolytic uremic syndrome (HUS)
     iv. Sepsis
  c. Sequestration of platelets in the spleen (e.g., with liver disease and portal hypertension)
  d. Massive transfusion of RBCs over a short period of time, which can lead to a dilutional thrombocytopenia

3. Signs and symptoms
  a. Symptom: Unexplained bleeding
  b. Signs: Pallor, petechiae, purpura, ecchymoses; oozing of blood from venipuncture sites, conjunctival bleeding; bleeding from the oropharynx, gastrointestinal tract, or genitourinary tract and splenomegaly may be present

4. Diagnostic study findings
  a. Laboratory
     i. Urine: Can test positive for blood
     ii. Stool: Can test positive for blood
     iii. Blood
         (a) Platelet count is lower than $50,000/mm^3$.
         (b) Both hemoglobin level and HCT are usually decreased as a result of blood loss.
  b. Radiologic: Spleen ultrasonography or liver-spleen scan to determine the size of the spleen
  c. Bone marrow biopsy to determine whether adequate numbers of platelets are being made in the bone marrow

5. Goals of care
  a. Absence of hemorrhage
  b. Prevention of injury

6. Collaborating professionals on health care team
  a. Nurse
  b. Blood bank specialist
  c. Pharmacist
  d. Physician

7. Management of patient care
  a. Anticipated patient trajectory: Children with thrombocytopenia usually have symptoms after a viral infection, and the disorder resolves spontaneously in 90% of cases. Adult ITP and ATP are not as well understood; only 10% to 20% of adult patients have a spontaneous remission. Patients may be expected to have needs in the following areas:
     i. Positioning: Handle with care because of ease of bruising
     ii. Transport: May need supplies for spontaneous nose bleeding or oral bleeding; inform team members of risk for bruising
     iii. Discharge planning: Patient and family may need education about home environmental risks for injury that may precipitate spontaneous bleeding, need to seek health care for monitoring of platelet counts or if bleeding occurs, and effects of steroid therapy
  b. Potential complications
     i. Bleeding
         (a) Mechanism: Platelet count lower than $50,000/mm^3$
         (b) Management: Treatment for ITP can include administration of steroids, IV administration of immunoglobulin, platelet transfusion, splenectomy, and immunosuppressive therapy

8. Evaluation of patient care
  a. Absence of clinical or spontaneous bleeding

    b. Platelet count above 50,000/mm³

    c. Absence of bruising related to injury

Hypercoagulable Disorders

1. **Pathophysiology**
    a. Hypercoagulable disorders occur when the normal mechanisms of hemostasis involving platelets and clotting factors are disrupted, which results in uncontrolled or inappropriate clotting. Paradoxically, a secondary bleeding disorder develops in many of these patients when their reserves of platelets and clotting factors are depleted.
    b. Venous thromboses result from activation of the coagulation cascade caused by venous stasis, ischemia, or infarction. Arterial emboli result when a venous thrombus breaks away from its site of origin and migrates into the arterial vascular system. Pulmonary embolus, myocardial infarction, and thrombotic cerebrovascular accidents can be caused by arterial emboli. Patients are often admitted to progressive care and critical care units for hemodynamic and neurologic support as well as for thrombolytic therapy with streptokinase, urokinase, or tissue plasminogen activator. Anticoagulation therapy puts these patients at risk for bleeding, although they have an underlying hypercoagulable disorder.
    c. TTP appears to be an exaggerated immunologic response to vessel injury that results in extensive thrombus formation and decreased blood flow to the affected site. These patients are critically ill; fever, thrombocytopenia, hemolytic anemia, renal impairment, and neurologic symptoms develop. HUS appears to be a variant of TTP that is seen more commonly in children. Patients with HUS tend to have more severe renal impairment, but fewer neurologic signs and symptoms, than do patients with TTP.
    d. DIC is another hypercoagulable disorder.
    e. HIT is a form of thrombocytopenia caused by an immune reaction to heparin that occurs 5 to 14 days after the initiation of heparin therapy. A decrease in platelet count occurring before 5 days of heparin therapy is usually a transient condition called nonautoimmune heparin-associated thrombocytopenia (formerly called type I HIT).
2. **Etiology and risk factors**
    a. Changes in blood flow (e.g., deep vein thrombosis)
    b. Changes in circulating blood coagulation factors (e.g., TTP, HIT)
    c. Changes in the vessel wall
3. **Signs and symptoms**
    a. Symptoms: Tenderness or pain with palpation
    b. Signs: Unexplained bleeding, sudden painful swelling of one extremity, and other signs may be present, depending on the organ system involved; temperature exceeding 101° F (38.3° C), petechiae, purpura, ecchymoses, hematomas; circumference of one extremity different from that of the other corresponding extremity; changes in vital signs; with an arterial thrombosis, decreased blood flow in one extremity may be detected by Doppler ultrasonography
4. **Diagnostic study findings**
    a. Laboratory
        i. With venous stasis, laboratory values may be normal until anticoagulation therapy begins.
        ii. With TTP, RBC levels are decreased; reticulocyte count, bilirubin level, and lactate dehydrogenase levels are increased; fragmented RBCs are seen on peripheral smear.
        iii. With HIT, platelet count is less than 50,000/mm³ or a sudden drop from patient's baseline by 30% to 50% after initiation of heparin therapy.
    b. Radiologic: Angiography or venography can indicate vessel blockage
5. **Goals of care**
    a. Prevention of ischemic injury
    b. Prevention of dehydration
    c. Absence of hemorrhage
    d. Restoration of homeostatic coagulation
6. **Collaborating professionals on health care team**
    a. Transfusion specialist
    b. Blood bank specialist

    c. Pharmacist

    d. Nurse

    e. Physician

7. **Management of patient care**

    a. If HIT is suspected, stop all exposure to heparin including unfractionated and low–molecular-weight heparin, flushes, and heparin-coated devices. Initiate therapy with alternative, nonheparin anticoagulant. Assess for complications (e.g., lower limbs for deep venous thrombosis).

    b. Anticipated patient trajectory: Full recovery from the complications of hypercoagulopathies, such as deep venous thrombosis, polycythemia, and temporary hyperviscosity of blood, can reasonably be expected when the patient is given early thrombolytic therapy combined with watchful collaborative care. Hypercoagulable disorders complicated by comorbidities, poor response to thrombolytics or collaborative care, and septicemia, however, may lead to loss of limbs because of ischemia or life-threatening DIC. Patients may be expected to have needs in the following areas:

        i. Positioning: Care in handling the patient because of the ease of bruising and propensity to create an embolus

        ii. Skin care: Prevention of complications of immobility and prolonged bed rest, which could lead to tissue alterations and ischemia

        iii. Pain management: Patient-controlled analgesia for deep venous thrombosis, joint swelling

        iv. Treatments: Thrombolytic therapy and potential blood product administration

    c. Potential complications

        i. Bleeding

            (a) Mechanism: Platelet count lower than 50,000/mm^3

            (b) Management: Clotting factor replacement and platelet transfusion, administration of antithrombolytics

8. **Evaluation of patient care**

    a. Absence of clinical or spontaneous bleeding

    b. Platelet count higher than 50,000/mm^3

    c. Absence of bruising related to injury

    d. Pain management

Neutropenia

1. **Pathophysiology**

    a. Occurs when the total number of neutrophils is abnormally low and puts the patient at increased risk of infection. The longer the patient is neutropenic, the greater the chance of infection. Patients are often admitted to critical care units with a diagnosis such as sepsis or acute leukemia that is complicated by neutropenia.

    b. The most common sites of infection seen in neutropenic patients are the lung (pneumonia), blood (septicemia), skin, urinary tract, and gastrointestinal tract (mucositis, esophagitis, perirectal lesions). The major infectious gram-negative bacilli include *Klebsiella pneumoniae* and *E. coli*. The major infectious gram-positive cocci include *S. aureus, Enterococcus,* and *Staphylococcus epidermidis*. Because affected patients do not have adequate numbers of WBCs to mount an immunologic response, the classic signs of infection may be absent. Fever may be the only sign of infection.

2. **Etiology and risk factors**

    a. Decreased neutrophil production

        i. Bone marrow infiltration with malignant cells

        ii. Recent history of antineoplastic chemotherapy, especially if high-dose chemotherapy was administered as part of bone marrow transplantation

        iii. Any history of radiation therapy to bones in which blood cells are made

        iv. Use of certain drugs (e.g., zidovudine, clozapine)

        v. Autoimmune disorder (e.g., systemic lupus erythematosus, rheumatoid arthritis)

    b. Increased neutrophil use: Overwhelming sepsis

3. **Signs and symptoms**

  a. Symptoms: Malaise; reports of fever, chills, and night sweats; sore throat; dyspnea; shortness of breath; abdominal pain, sinus pain, headache; confusion; pain with swallowing, urination, or defecation
  b. Signs: Cough, diarrhea, temperature exceeding 101° F (38.3° C), loss of integrity of skin and mucous membranes (especially at IV and central venous catheter sites), lymphadenopathy, tachycardia, hypotension, crackles, and rhonchi
4. **Diagnostic study findings**
  a. Laboratory: ANC lower than 500/μl
  b. Radiologic: Findings are usually noncontributory to the diagnosis of neutropenia, but studies may be indicated to identify the source of infection secondary to neutropenia
  c. Bone marrow biopsy
5. **Goals of care: Absence of infection**
6. **Collaborating professionals on health care team**
  a. Nurse
  b. Blood bank specialist
  c. Pharmacist
  d. Physician
7. **Management of patient care**
  a. Anticipated patient trajectory: Mortality rate is 18% to 40% in the first 48 hours for patients with an ANC lower than 500/μl. The goal of therapy is to support the patient until his or her own WBCs are available to fight infection.
  b. Potential complications
    i. Infection resulting in febrile episodes
      (a) Mechanism: Low WBC availability decreases the ability to fight infection
      (b) Management: Protect the patient from sources of community or nosocomial infection, institute neutropenic precautions (see Table 7-9)
8. **Evaluation of patient care: Protection successful in avoiding infectious processes**

Organ Transplant and Rejection

1. **Pathophysiology**
  a. When tissue from one person is transplanted into another person, the immune system of the recipient can recognize the transplanted tissue, or allograft, as foreign. Rejections occur through various mechanisms:
    i. Type III, Arthus-type hypersensitivity reaction in the blood vessels of the graft immediately after transplantation
    ii. Cytotoxic T lymphocytes (T_C) can directly attack the allograft, which results in acute transplant rejection and occurs within days of the transplantation.
    iii. B lymphocytes can make antibodies against the allograft; these activate the complement pathways and attract platelets. Fibrin accumulates on the transplanted tissue, causing ischemia. In this way the allograft is slowly rejected over many months to years.
  b. Human leukocyte antigen matching of donor to recipient before transplantation is an attempt to choose a donor whose antigens match the recipient's as closely as possible so that the recipient's immune system is not triggered to attack the allograft after the transplantation procedure.
  c. Allogeneic BMT is fundamentally different from solid organ transplantation. In allogeneic BMT, the immune system itself is being transplanted into a new host. Therefore, it may attack any tissue in the new host, resulting in graft-versus-host disease (GVHD). Because GVHD is usually a limited (albeit serious) problem, the majority of patients undergoing allogeneic BMT can eventually discontinue immunosuppressive therapy. In patients receiving solid organ transplants, the host's own immune system attacks the donated organ, so recipients must receive lifelong immunosuppressive therapy.
2. **Etiology and risk factors: Activation of the immune response against transplanted tissue**
3. **Signs and symptoms**
  a. Symptoms: Malaise, poor appetite, myalgia, tenderness of the allograft
  b. Signs: Swelling of the allograft, temperature exceeding 101° F (38.3° C)

4. **Diagnostic study findings: Specific to the organ transplanted**
5. **Goals of care**
   a. Nonproliferation of immunocompetent cells
   b. Suppression of the activity of helper T cells (T_H) and T_C cells
   c. Engraftment of donor tissue or organ
6. **Collaborating professionals on health care team**
   a. Nurse
   b. Blood bank specialist
   c. Pharmacist
   d. Physician
   e. Transplant surgery team
7. **Management of patient care**
   a. Anticipated patient trajectory: Hyperacute rejection and graft failure can occur immediately after transplantation; acute rejection can occur weeks to months later; chronic rejection can progress over a period of several years
   b. Potential complications
      i. Proliferation of immunocompetent cells
         (a) Mechanism: Antigens on transplanted tissue cells are immediately recognized as nonself, and rejection of donor tissue occurs
         (b) Management: Immunosuppression (see Immunosuppression section)
8. **Evaluation of patient care**
   a. Immunosuppression
   b. Engraftment of donor tissue or organ

Immunosuppression

1. **Pathophysiology**
   a. Immunosuppression occurs when some defect in the immunologic system puts the patient at increased risk for infection. The longer the patient is immunosuppressed, the greater the risk of infection. Neutropenia is one form of immunosuppression (see Neutropenia). Although there are primary forms of immune dysfunction, patients are more often admitted to critical care units with immunosuppression as a complication of an underlying disease.
   b. Various drugs prescribed to suppress one part of the immune system have untoward effects on other parts of the hematologic and immunologic systems. After organ transplantation, various drugs are used to suppress the immune system and prevent transplant rejection. These drugs act primarily on B cells and T cells and suppress not only the immunologic response to the allograft but also the patient's ability to fight bacteria, viruses, fungi, and parasites.
2. **Etiology and risk factors**
   a. Immunosuppressive agents
   b. Genetic (e.g., severe combined immunodeficiency disease)
   c. Decreased neutrophil production (see Neutropenia)
   d. HIV infection (see HIV Infection)
3. **Signs and symptoms: See Neutropenia**
4. **Diagnostic study findings: Laboratory cultures give positive results for unusual or opportunistic organisms (e.g., *Pneumocystis carinii*)**
5. **Goals of care: See Neutropenia and Table 7-9**
6. **Collaborating professionals on health care team: See Neutropenia**
7. **Management of patient care: See Neutropenia and Table 7-9**
8. **Evaluation of patient care: See Neutropenia and Table 7-9**

HIV Infection

1. **Pathophysiology**
   a. HIV type 1, previously known as human T-lymphotropic virus type 3 (HTLV-3), is a retrovirus that infects cells expressing CD4 on their cell membranes, primarily T_H lymphocytes and macrophages. The HIV copies its RNA into the host cell's DNA and then remains

quiescent until the host cell is activated to mount an immunologic response. Activation of the host CD4 cells also initiates replication and production of the HIV RNA, which is released into the circulation. This newly made HIV then infects other cells expressing CD4.

b. Disease course

    i. The initial stage of HIV infection lasts 4 to 8 weeks. High levels of virus are in the blood. The patient experiences generalized flulike symptoms.

    ii. The virus then enters a latent stage in which it is inactive in infected, resting CD4 cells, replicating only when the host cell is activated for an immune response. Levels of virus are high in the lymph nodes, where CD4 cells reside, but low in the blood. T_C cells, which express CD8 and so are not infected by HIV, and B cells attempt to destroy the CD4 cells harboring the virus. However, the T_C cells and B cells are crippled without adequate T_H support. This latent stage lasts on the average between 2 and 12 years, during which time the patient is asymptomatic. During this time, the number of CD4 cells declines.

    iii. During the third stage of HIV infection, the patient begins to have opportunistic infections. Levels of CD4 cells are usually below $500/mm^3$ and declining, whereas levels of virus in the blood are increasing. This stage can last 2 to 3 years.

    iv. Once the CD4 cell levels drop below $200/mm^3$, the patient is considered to have AIDS. Virus levels in the blood are high. This stage ends in death, usually within 1 year.

2. Etiology and risk factors: HIV is transmitted via intimate sexual contact, contaminated needles or contaminated blood products, from mother to fetus, and from mother to breast-feeding infant

3. Signs and symptoms

  a. Symptoms and history: Fatigue, night sweats, sore throat, dyspnea, shortness of breath, pain, history of frequent infections, social history of IV drug abuse with shared needles, history of unprotected sexual contact with persons possibly infected with HIV, history of blood transfusion

  b. Signs: Weight loss, diarrhea, temperature exceeding 101° F (38.3° C), loss of integrity of skin and mucous membranes, possible cachexia, possible lymphadenopathy, tachycardia, hypotension, crackles, and rhonchi

4. Diagnostic study findings

  a. Laboratory

    i. Western blot test result that is positive for HIV (*Note:* Enzyme-linked immunosorbent assay [ELISA] is a less expensive screening test for HIV antibody. If the ELISA result is positive, a Western blot test should be performed to confirm the findings, because false-positive results do occur with ELISA.)

    ii. CD4 lymphocyte counts that are lower than $500/mm^3$

    iii. Nonreactive results on skin test panel

    iv. Infection with unusual or opportunistic organisms (e.g., *P. carinii*)

  b. Radiologic: Infiltrates on chest radiograph

5. Goals of care

  a. Education about prevention of the spread of HIV infection

  b. Maintenance of universal precautions

  c. Containment of associated opportunistic diseases

  d. Ability of the patient to express fear, grief, and social isolation

6. Collaborating disciplines

  a. Nurse

  b. Chaplain

  c. Social worker

  d. Physician

  e. Pharmacist

  f. Psychiatrist

7. Management of patient care

  a. Anticipated patient trajectory: The time from initial HIV infection to the development of AIDS ranges from months to years depending on demographic characteristics, lifestyle, and interventional factors. Progression to death accelerates with the development of multiple opportunistic infections. Throughout their course of clinical care and discharge, patients may be expected to have needs in the following areas:

  i. Nutrition: Avoid fatty foods if chronic diarrhea is present, avoid fruits with peels, maintain good hydration, maintain high protein consumption, encourage consumption of foods that the patient likes, assess for oral lesions and hygiene

  ii. Infection control: Education of the patient and the family or significant others may be key in decreasing the spread of infection by sexual contact, IV needle use, and maternal-child transmission; health care workers must use universal precautions

  iii. Pharmacology: Education for the patient and the family or significant others may be warranted to describe antiretroviral therapy, prophylactic treatment for opportunistic infections, and use of hematopoiesis-stimulating factors

  iv. Psychosocial issues: There is no cure for HIV infection or AIDS; therefore, individual coping ability should be explored

  v. Ethical issues: Presence of HIV infection or AIDS raises the concern of intentional spread of infection

 b. Potential complications

  i. AIDS dementia complex

   (a) Mechanism: HIV invasion of the central nervous system, which occurs in 70% of cases

   (b) Management: Initiation of fall precautions and support for cognitive, motor, or behavioral impairment

  ii. Opportunistic infections

   (a) Mechanism: Suppression of immune responses resulting from infection with HIV

   (b) Management: Antiretroviral therapy with zidovudine, didanosine (ddI, Videx), zalcitabine (ddC, Hivid), or stavudine (d4T, Zerit); prophylactic antibiotic therapy with TMP-SMX, aerosolized pentamidine (Pentam), and/or other agents; antiretroviral therapy with agents with HIV-1 protease inhibitors such as saquinavir (Invirase), indinavir (Crixivan), nelfinavir (Viracept), and/or ritonavir (Norvir)

 8. Evaluation of patient management

  a. Controlled infective state

  b. Ability of the patient to express fears, anxiety, and grief

  c. Low number and severity of opportunistic infections

REFERENCES AND BIBLIOGRAPHY

Physiologic Anatomy

Guyton AC, Hall JE. *Textbook of Medical Physiology*. 11th ed. Philadelphia, PA: Saunders; 2006.

McCance KL, Huether SE. *Pathophysiology: The Biologic Basis for Disease in Adults and Children*. 5th ed. St Louis, MO: Mosby; 2006.

McMahon TJ, Exton Stone A, Bonaventura J, et al. Functional coupling of oxygen binding and vasoactivity in S-nitrosohemoglobin. *J Biol Chem*. 2000;275:16738-16745.

★ Metcalf D. Cellular hematopoiesis in the twentieth century. *Semin Hematol*. 1999;36(4 suppl 7):5-12.

Murphy KM, Travers P, Walport M. *Janeway's Immunobiology*. 7th ed. New York, NY: Garland; 2007.

Porth CM. *Pathophysiology: Concepts of Altered Health Status*. 6th ed. Philadelphia, PA: Lippincott Williams & Wilkins; 2002.

Patient Assessment

Deglin JH, Vallerand AH. *Davis Drug Guide for Nurses*. 11th ed. Philadelphia, PA: FA Davis; 2009.

Hankins J, Lonsway RAW, Hedrick D, et al. *Infusion Therapy in Clinical Practice*. 2nd ed. St Louis, MO: Saunders; 2001.

Ignatavicius DD, Workman ML, eds. *Medical-Surgical Nursing: Critical Thinking for Collaborative Care*. 5th ed. Philadelphia, PA: Saunders; 2006.

Pagana KD, Pagana TJ. *Mosby's Diagnostic and Laboratory Test Reference*. 6th ed. St Louis, MO: Mosby; 2003.

Van Leeuwen AM, Kranpitz TR, Smith L. *Davis's Comprehensive Handbook of Laboratory and Diagnostic Tests With Nursing Implications*. 2nd ed. Philadelphia, PA: FA Davis; 2006.

Wilson BA, Shannon MT, Stang CL. *Nurse's Drug Guide*. Upper Saddle River, NJ: Prentice Hall; 2004.

Specific Patient Health Problems
Anemia

Coyer SM, Lash AA. Pathophysiology of anemia and nursing care implications. *Medsurg Nurs.* 2008;17(2):77-83.

Herrington JD, Davidson SL, Tomita DK, et al. Utilization of darbepoetin alfa and epoetin alfa for chemotherapy-induced anemia. *Am J Health Syst Pharm.* 2005;62(1):54-62.

Mickle J, Reinke D. A review of anemia management in the oncology setting: a focus on implementing standing orders. *Clin J Oncol Nurs.* 2007;11(4): 534-539, 590-594.

Pearl RG, Pohlman A. Understanding and managing anemia in critically ill patients. *Crit Care Nurse.* 2002;(Suppl):1-16.

Powars DR, Chan LS, Hiti A, et al. Outcome of sickle cell anemia: a 4-decade observational study of 1056 patients. *Medicine.* 2005;84(6):363-376.

Shermock KM, Horn E, Rice TL. Erythropoietic agents for anemia of critical illness. *Am J Health Syst Pharm.* 2008;65(6):540-546.

Sobrero A, Puglisi F, Guglielmi A, et al. Fatigue: a main component of anemia symptomatology. *Semin Oncol.* 2001;28(2 suppl 8):15-18.

Spence RK. Medical and economic impact of anemia in hospitalized patients. *Am J Health Syst Pharm.* 2007;64(16 Suppl 11):S3-S10.

★ Volberding P. Consensus statement: anemia in HIV infection: current trends, treatment options, and practice strategies. *Clin Ther.* 2000;22(9):1004-1020.

Thrombocytopenia

Ansani NT. Heparin-induced thrombocytopenia and thrombosis: A review of pharmacologic therapy. *J Pharm Technol.* 2001;17(5):189-197.

Argatroban is a new option for patients with heparin-induced thrombocytopenia. *Drugs Ther Perspect.* 2001;17(19):1-4.

Cantrell SW, Ward KS, Van Wicklin SA. Translating research on venous thromboembolism into practice. *AORN J.* 2007;86(4):590-602.

Efird LE, Kockler DR. Fondaparinux for thromboembolic treatment and prophylaxis of heparin-induced thrombocytopenia. *Ann Pharmacother.* 2006;40:1383-1387.

Fukuyama SN, Itano J. Thrombocytopenia secondary to myelosuppression. *Am J Nurs.* 1999;(Suppl):5-8, 34-36.

Krimmel T, Brant JM. Test your knowledge. Disseminated intravascular coagulation. *Clin J Oncol Nurs.* 2003;7(4):479-481.

Mayer B. Hematologic disorders and oncologic emergencies. In: Urden LD, Stacy KM, Lough ME, eds. *Thelan's Critical Care Nursing.* 5th ed. St Louis, MO: Mosby; 2006.

Nguyen TN, Gal P, Ransom JL, et al. Lepirudin use in a neonate with heparin-induced thrombocytopenia. *Ann Pharmacother.* 2003;37(2):229-233.

Reardon JE Jr, Marques MB. Evaluation of thrombocytopenia. *Lab Med.* 2006;37(4):248-250.

Schneider M. Thrombotic microangiopathy (TTP and HUS): advances in differentiation and diagnosis. *Clin Lab Sci.* 2007;20(4):216-220.

Hypercoagulable Disorders

Cooney MF. Heparin-induced thrombocytopenia: advances in diagnosis and treatment. *Crit Care Nurse.* 2006;26(6):30-37.

Dickey TL. The hypercoagulable state as a risk factor for venous thromboembolism, part I. *J Am Acad Physician Assist.* 2002;15(11):28-30, 32, 35.

Gardner J. Factor V Leiden with deep venous thrombosis. *Clin Lab Sci.* 2003;16(1):6-9.

Mayer B. Hematologic disorders and oncologic emergencies. In: Urden LD, Stacy KM, Lough ME, eds. *Thelan's Critical Care Nursing.* 5th ed. St Louis, MO: Mosby; 2006.

Meissner MH, Chandler WL, Elliott JS. Venous thromboembolism in trauma: a local manifestation of systemic hypercoagulability? *J Trauma Injury Infect Crit Care.* 2003;54(2):224-231.

Mulroy JF, De Jong MJ. Syndromes of hypercoagulability: protein C and protein S deficiencies in acutely ill adults. *Am J Nurs.* 2003;103(5):64KK, 64MM, 64OO.

Neufeld EJ. Coagulation disorders and treatment strategies. *Hematol Oncol Clin North Am.* 1998;12(6):ix-x, 1141-1144.

Selleng K, Warkentin TE, Greinacher A. Heparin-induced thrombocytopenia in intensive care patients. *Crit Care Med.* 2007;35(4):1165-1176.

Spero JA. Venous thromboembolism and hypercoagulability. *Top Emerg Med.* 2000;22(3):9-22.

Subar M. Clinical evaluation of hypercoagulable states. *Clin Geriatr Med.* 2001;17(1):57-70.

Swanson JM. Heparin-induced thrombocytopenia: a general review. *J Infusion.* 2007;30(4):232-240.

Todisco M, Casaccia P, Rossi N. Severe bleeding symptoms in refractory idiopathic thrombocytopenic purpura: a case successfully treated with melatonin. *Am J Ther.* 2003;10(2):135-136.

van Cott EM, Laposata M. Your lab focus: overview. Algorithms for hypercoagulation testing. *Lab Med.* 2003;34(3):216-220, 222.

Warkentin TE, Greinacher A, Koster A, Lincoff AM. American College of Chest Physicians. Treatment and prevention of heparin-induced thrombocytopenia: American College of Chest Physicians Evidence-Based Clinical Practice Guidelines (8th Edition). *Chest.* 2008.133(6 Suppl):340S-380S.

Neutropenia

Bow EJ. Management of the febrile neutropenic cancer patient: lessons from 40 years of study. *Clin Microbiol Infect.* 2005;11(suppl 5):24-29.

Corey L, Boeckh M. Persistent fever in patients with neutropenia. *N Engl J Med.* 2002;346(4):222-224.

Kannangara S. Management of febrile neutropenia. *Community Oncol.* 2006;3(9):585-591.

Klastersky J, Paesmans M, Rubenstein EB, et al. The Multinational Association for Supportive Care in

Cancer Risk Index: a multinational scoring system for identifying low-risk febrile neutropenic cancer patients. *J Clin Oncol*. 2000;18(16):3038-3051.

Langan RC, Bordelon PC. Initial management of the febrile cancer patient with neutropenia. *Fam Pract Recertif*. 2007;29(7):30-34.

Mutnick AH, Kirby JT, Jones RN. CANCER Resistance Surveillance Program: initial results from hematology-oncology centers in North America. *Ann Pharmacother*. 2003;37(1):47-56.

Reigle BS, Dienger MJ. Sepsis and treatment-induced immunosuppression in the patient with cancer: tables/charts. *Crit Care Nurs Clin North Am*. 2003;15(1):109-118.

Santolaya ME, Alvarez AM, Becker A, et al. Prospective, multicenter evaluation of risk factors associated with invasive bacterial infection in children with cancer, neutropenia, and fever. *J Clin Oncol*. 2001;19(14):3415-3421.

Segal BH, Freifeld AG. Antibacterial prophylaxis in patients with neutropenia. *J Natl Compr Cancer Netw JNCCN*. 2007;5(2):235-242.

Soni S, Radel E. Neutropenia: striking a balance between caution and alarm. *Contemp Pediatr*. 2002;19(8):77-78, 82-85.

Wilson BJ. Dietary recommendations for neutropenic patients. *Semin Oncol Nurs*. 2002;18(1):44-49.

Transplant Rejection

Bahruth AJ. What every patient should know … pre-transplantation and posttransplantation. *Crit Care Nurs Q*. 2004;27(1):31-60.

Hartley C. Organ donation and transplantation. In: Urden LD, Stacy KM, Lough ME, eds. *Thelan's Critical Care Nursing*. St Louis, MO: Mosby; 2006.

Hoffman FM, Nelson BJ, Drangstveit MB, et al. Caring for transplant recipients in a nontransplant setting. *Crit Care Nurse*. 2006;26(2):53-66, 68-74.

Mancini MC, Cush EM, Launius BK, et al. The management of immunosuppression: the art and the science. *Crit Care Nurs Q*. 2004;27(1):61-64.

Sayegh MH, Carpenter CB. Transplantation 50 years later–progress, challenges, and promises. *N Engl J Med*. 2004;351(26):2761-2766.

Shafer TJ, Wagner D, Chessare J, et al. Organ donation breakthrough collaborative: increasing organ donation through system redesign. *Crit Care Nurse*. 2006;26(2):33-42, 44-49.

Immunosuppression

Cohen SM. Current immunosuppression in liver transplantation. *Am J Ther*. 2002;9(2):119-125.

Hartley C. Organ donation and transplantation. In: Urden LD, Stacy KM, Lough ME, eds. *Thelan's Critical Care Nursing* (5th ed). St Louis, MO: Mosby; 2006.

Huizinga R. Update in immunosuppression. *Nephrol Nurs J*. 2002;29(3):261-267.

Immunosuppressive therapies: an overview. *Dis Manag Digest*. 2000;4(5):2-3, 14-15.

Mancini MC, Cush EM, Launius BK, et al. The management of immunosuppression: the art and the science. *Crit Care Nurs Q*. 2004;27(1):61-64.

Nseir S, Di Pompeo C, Diarra M. Relationship between immunosuppression and intensive care unit–acquired multidrug-resistant bacteria: a case-control study. *Crit Care Med*. 2007;35(5):1318-1323.

Reigle BS, Dienger MJ. Sepsis and treatment-induced immunosuppression in the patient with cancer. *Crit Care Nurs Clin North Am*. 2003;15(1):109-118.

HIV Infection

Abel E, Painter L. Factors that influence adherence to HIV medications: Perceptions of women and health care providers. *J Assoc Nurses AIDS Care*. 2003;14(4):61-69.

Covington LW. Update on antiviral agents for HIV and AIDS. *Nurs Clin North Am*. 2005;40(1):149-165.

Drug resistance guide being pondered by CDC: as HIV drug resistance rises, surveillance needed. *AIDS Alert*. 2003;18(11):146-147.

Ferri RS, Adinolfi A, Orsi AJ, et al. Treatment of anemia in patients with HIV infection, part 2: Guidelines for management of anemia. *J Assoc Nurses AIDS Care*. 2002;13(1):50-59.

Goldschmidt RH, Dong BJ. Treatment of AIDS and HIV-related conditions: 2001. *J Am Board Fam Pract*. 2001;14(4):283-309.

Mitchell B. Clinical update. A background and critical analysis of the treatment of pneumocystis carinii pneumonia (PCP) in HIV/AIDS. *Aust Nurs J*. 2007;14(9):20-23.

Orsega S. Treatment of adult HIV infection: antiretroviral update and overview. *J Nurse Pract*. 2007;3(9):612-624.

The Gastrointestinal System

SYSTEMWIDE ELEMENTS

Physiologic Anatomy

1. **Upper gastrointestinal (GI) tract (Figure 8-1)**
   a. Mouth and accessory organs
      i. Lips, gums and teeth, and inner structures of the cheeks, tongue, hard and soft palate, and salivary glands
      ii. Chewing prepares food by softening and moving it around, mixing it with saliva, and forming a bolus.
      iii. Skeletal muscles for chewing are coordinated by cranial nerves V, VII, IX, X, XI, XII.
      iv. Saliva aids in swallowing; approximately 570 ml/day of saliva is secreted. Submandibular, parotid, and sublingual salivary glands along with minor salivary glands in the oral mucosa secrete mixed saliva, which is 99% water and 1% solids, and includes electrolytes and organic protein molecules.
   b. Pharynx
      i. Extends from the cricoid cartilage to the level of the sixth cervical vertebra
      ii. Swallowing receptors are stimulated by the autonomic nervous system when a food bolus moves toward the back of the mouth. The motor impulses to swallow are transmitted via cranial nerves V, IX, X, and XII.
   c. Esophagus
      i. Transports food from the mouth to the stomach and prevents retrograde movement of the stomach contents
      ii. Collapsible tube about 25 cm long that lies posterior to the trachea and the heart
         (a) Begins at the level of the sixth cervical vertebra and extends through the mediastinum and diaphragm to the level of the first thoracic vertebra, where it attaches to the stomach below the level of the diaphragm
         (b) Upper portion of the esophagus is striated skeletal muscle, which is gradually replaced by smooth muscle so that the lower third of the esophagus is totally smooth muscle.
         (c) Motor and sensory impulses for swallowing and food passage derive from the vagus nerve. Lower esophagus also innervated by splanchnic and sympathetic neurons. Food moves by the strong muscular contraction of peristalsis and by gravity. In the absence of gravity, nutrients transported by muscular contractions.
         (d) Sphincters: Hypopharyngeal (proximal) prevents air from entering the esophagus during inspiration; gastroesophageal (distal) prevents gastric reflux into the esophagus

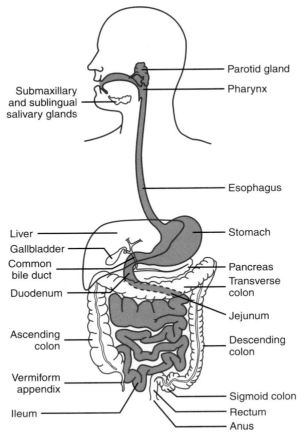

FIGURE 8-1 ■ Digestive tract of the human being. (From Westfall UE, Heitkemper M. Gastrointestinal physiology. In: Clochesy JM, Breu C, Cardin S, et al, eds. *Critical Care Nursing.* 2nd ed. Philadelphia, PA: Saunders; 1996:979.)

    iii. Blood supply
        (a) Arterial supply: Celiac trunk includes the gastric, pyloric, right, and left gastro-epiploic arteries
        (b) Venous drainage: Splanchnic bed drains the entire GI tract; gastric vein drains the stomach and esophagus
        (c) Direct drainage into the azygos and hemiazygos veins of the mediastinum; all of these then drain into the portal vein

  d. Stomach
    i.   Food storage reservoir and site of the start of the digestive process. Normal capacity is 1000 to 1500 ml but can hold up to 6000 ml.
    ii.   Layers of the stomach and intestinal wall (Figure 8-2)
        (a) Mucosa: Cells produce mucus that lubricates and protects the inner surface. These cells are replaced every 4 to 5 days. This layer receives the majority of the blood supply of the stomach.
           (1) Epithelium: Contains the gastric, cardiac, fundic, and pyloric glands
              a) Gastric cells: Contain microvilli that monitor intragastric pH
              b) Cardiac glands: Secrete alkaline mucus, a lubricant that continually bathes and protects the epithelial lining from autodigestion
              c) Fundic glands
                  1) Chief cells: Secrete pepsinogen, an inactive form of pepsin, in response to food ingestion; in its active form, pepsin digests proteins
                  2) Parietal cells: Secrete hydrochloric acid, which lowers pH and kills bacteria, and intrinsic factor, a glycoprotein necessary for vitamin B_{12} absorption

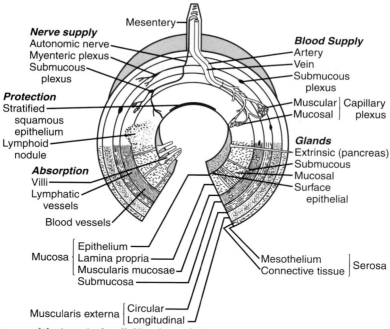

FIGURE 8-2 ■ Layers of the intestinal wall. Histology of the gastrointestinal tract, stomach through large intestine. (From Kinney MR, Dunbar S, Brooks-Brunn J, et al, eds. *AACN's Clinical Reference for Critical Care Nursing.* St Louis, MO: Mosby; 1998:982.)

  (2) Lamina propria: Contains lymphocytes; site of gut immunologic response
  (3) Muscularis mucosae: Contains thin smooth muscle layer
 (b) Submucosa: Contains connective tissue and elastic fibers, blood vessels, nerves, lymphatic vessels, and structures responsible for secreting digestive enzymes
 (c) Circular and longitudinal smooth muscle layers: Continue the modification of food into a liquid consistency and move it along the GI tract. Movements are tonic and rhythmic, occurring every 20 seconds. Electrical activity is constantly present in the smooth muscle layers.
 (d) Serosa: Outermost layer
 iii. Gastric hormones
 (a) Gastrin
  (1) Hormone secreted in response to distention of antrum or fundus by food
  (2) Stimulates secretion of hydrochloric acid by the parietal cells and secretion of pepsin by chief cells
  (3) Increases gastric blood flow
 (b) Histamine: Hormone secreted by mast cells in the presence of food that is critical to the regulation of gastric acid secretions
  (1) Stimulates gastric acid and pepsin secretion
  (2) Initiates contraction of the gallbladder
  (3) Relaxes sphincter of Oddi
  (4) Increases GI motility
 iv. Gastric secretion
 (a) Approximately 1500 to 3000 ml is secreted daily and mixes with food entering the stomach.
 (b) Phases of gastric secretion are as follows:
  (1) Cephalic phase: Fibers of the vagus nerve stimulate the stomach to secrete gastrin (from the antrum) and hydrochloric acid
  (2) Gastric phase: Vasovagal reflexes stimulate the parasympathetic system to increase the secretion of gastrin

   v. Gastric emptying
- (a) Is proportional to the volume of material in the stomach
- (b) Depends on the character of the ingested material: Liquids, digestible solids, fats, indigestible solids
- (c) Factors accelerating gastric emptying: Large volume of liquids; anger; insulin
- (d) Factors inhibiting gastric emptying: Fat, protein, starch, sadness, duodenal hormones
- (e) Vomiting
  - (1) Coordinated by the vomiting center in the medulla in response to afferent impulses from various regions of the body
  - (2) Stimuli that induce vomiting: Tactile stimulation to the back of the throat, increased intracranial pressure (ICP), intense pain, dizziness, anxiety
  - (3) May be preceded by autonomic nervous system discharge: Sweating, increased heart rate, increased salivation, nausea, muscular force by the diaphragm and abdomen

  vi. Blood supply
- (a) Arterial: Celiac artery flows into the right gastric artery, left gastric artery, gastroduodenal artery, and finally into the right gastroepiploic artery; the splenic artery flows into the left gastroepiploic artery
- (b) Venous drainage: Splanchnic bed drains the entire GI tract, the gastric vein drains the stomach and esophagus; both vessels drain into the portal vein

 vii. Innervation
- (a) Intrinsic nervous system (intramural neurons) within the wall of the GI tract is independent of central nervous system controls.
  - (1) Myenteric (Auerbach's) plexus: Located between the circular and longitudinal muscles; stimulation increases muscle tone, contractions, velocity, and excitation of the digestive tract
  - (2) Submucosal (Meissner's) plexus: Located between the circular and submucosal layers; influences secretions of the digestive tract; contains secretomotor and enteric vasodilator neurons
- (b) Extrinsic system: Via the central nervous system, parasympathetic system, and sympathetic system
  - (1) Parasympathetic: Fibers arise from the medulla and spinal segments (i.e., vagus nerves)
    - a) Cranial segments: Transmission via the vagus nerve; innervate the stomach, pancreas, and first half of the small intestine
    - b) Sacral segments: Innervate the distal half of the large intestine, sigmoid, rectum, and anus
    - c) Enhances function of the intrinsic nervous system and the secretion of acetylcholine
    - d) Increases glandular secretion and muscle tone; decreases sphincter tone
  - (2) Sympathetic: Motor and sensory fibers arise from the thoracic and lumbar segments; distribution is via the sympathetic ganglia (i.e., celiac plexus)
    - a) Fibers run alongside blood vessels and secrete norepinephrine.
    - b) Inhibit GI activity by acting on smooth muscle

2. Middle GI tract: Small intestine
  a. Approximately 5 m long; extends from the pylorus to the ileocecal valve
  b. Consists of three divisions: Duodenum, jejunum, ileum
  c. Primary function: Absorption of nutrients
  d. Layers of the intestinal wall (see Figure 8-2)
-   **i.** Mucosa: Innermost layer; receives the majority of the blood supply; the predominant site of nutrient absorption
  - (a) Epithelium: Covered with villi and microvilli that increase the surface area of the small intestine several hundred times; contain glands, crypts of Lieberkühn (intestinal glands) that secrete approximately 2 L of fluid every 24 hours and goblet cells that secrete mucus

(b) Lamina propria: Contains lymphocytes; site of gut immunologic responsiveness
(c) Muscularis mucosae: Contains thin smooth muscle
  ii. Submucosa: Contains loose connective tissue and elastic fibers, blood vessels, lymphatic vessels, and nerves
  iii. Muscularis: Muscle layer; function is involuntary and involved in motility
  iv. Serosa: Outermost layer; protects and suspends intestine within the abdominal cavity
e. Peristalsis: Propulsive movements that move the intestinal contents toward the anus. Approximately 3 to 5 hours is necessary for passage through the entire small intestine.
f. Blood supply
  i. Arterial: Derived from the celiac artery (first portion of the duodenum) and the superior mesenteric arteries (remainder of the duodenum, jejunum, ileum, cecum)
  ii. Venous drainage: Splanchnic bed drains the entire GI tract
    (a) Superior mesenteric vein: Drains the small intestine and the ascending and transverse colon
    (b) Inferior mesenteric vein: Drains the sigmoid colon and rectum
g. Innervation: Same as for stomach
h. Small intestine digestive enzymes not secreted, but integral components of the mucosa
  i. Bile and pancreatic enzymes are secreted into the duodenum.
  ii. In the jejunum and the ileum, food is digested and absorbed.
  iii. Up to 3000 ml/day of digestive enzymes (e.g., lipase, amylase, maltase, and lactase)
  iv. pH is approximately 7.0.
i. Intestinal hormones
  i. Secretin: Secreted by the mucosa of the duodenum in response to acidic gastric juice from the stomach and to alcohol ingestion
    (a) Augments the action of cholecystokinin (CCK)
    (b) Stimulates release of the alkaline component of pancreatic juice and the secretion of water
    (c) Increases the bile secretion rate
    (d) Decreases the motility of most of the GI tract
  ii. CCK: Secreted by the mucosa of the jejunum in response to the presence of fat, protein, and acidic contents in the intestine
    (a) Increases contractility and emptying of the gallbladder and blocks the increased gastric motility caused by gastrin
    (b) Stimulates secretion of pancreatic digestive enzymes, bicarbonate, and insulin
  iii. Gastric inhibitory peptide (GIP): Secreted by the mucosa of the upper portion of the small intestine in response to the presence of carbohydrates and fat in the intestine; inhibits gastric acid secretion and motility, slowing the rate of gastric emptying
  iv. Vasoactive intestinal peptide: Secreted throughout the gut in response to acidic gastric juice in the duodenum
    (a) Main effects are similar to those of secretin.
    (b) Stimulates the secretion of intestinal juices to decrease the acidity of chyme and inhibits gastric secretion
  v. Somatostatin: Secreted throughout the intestine in response to vagal stimulation, ingestion of food, and release of CCK, GIP, glucagon, and secretin
    (a) Inhibits the secretion of saliva, gastric acid, pepsin, intrinsic factor, and pancreatic enzymes
    (b) Inhibits gastric motility, gallbladder contraction, intestinal motility, and blood flow to the liver and intestine
    (c) Inhibits the secretion of insulin and growth hormone
  vi. Serotonin: Secreted throughout the intestine in response to vagal stimulation, increased luminal pressure, and the presence of acid or fat in the duodenum; inhibits gastric acid secretion and mucin production
j. Functions: Almost all absorption occurs in the small intestine via four mechanisms: Active transport, passive diffusion, facilitated diffusion, and nonionic transport

     i.   Vitamin absorption: Occurs primarily in the intestine by passive diffusion, except for the fat-soluble vitamins, which require bile salts for absorption, and vitamin B_{12}, which requires intrinsic factor

    ii.   Water absorption: Approximately 8 L of water per day is absorbed by the small intestine

   iii.   Electrolyte absorption: Most occurs in the proximal small intestine

   iv.   Iron absorption: Absorbed in the ferrous form in the duodenum

      (a) Facilitated by ascorbic acid

      (b) Increases in states of iron deficiency

    v.   Carbohydrate absorption: Complex carbohydrates are broken down into monosaccharides or basic sugars (fructose, glucose, galactose) by specific enzymes (e.g., amylase, maltase)

    vi.   Protein absorption: Protein is broken down into amino acids and small peptides; essential amino acids are lysine, phenylalanine, isoleucine, valine, methionine, leucine, threonine, and tryptophan

   vii.   Fat absorption

3. Lower GI tract

   a. Colon

      i.   Approximately 6.5 cm in diameter and 1.5 m long; extends from terminal ileum at the ileocecal valve to the rectum

     ii.   Ileocecal valve: Prevents return of feces from the cecum into the ileum

   b. Divisions of the colon

      i.   Cecum: Blind pouch to which the appendix is attached; about 2.5 cm from the ileocecal valve

     ii.   Ascending colon: Extends from the cecum to the lower border of the liver, where it forms the right hepatic flexure

    iii.   Transverse colon: Crosses the upper half of the abdominal cavity, curving downward at the lower end of the spleen at the left colonic (splenic) flexure anterior to the small intestine

    iv.   Descending colon: Extends from the splenic flexure to the sigmoid colon

     v.   Sigmoid colon: S-shaped curve extending from the descending colon to the rectum

    vi.   Rectum: Extends from the sigmoid colon to the anus

   c. Layers of the large intestine wall (see Figure 8-2): No villi and no secretion of digestive enzymes. Layers similar to those of the middle GI tract with exceptions:

      i.   Epithelial surface contains cells that absorb water and electrolytes.

     ii.   Crypts covered by epithelial cells that produce mucus

   d. Blood supply (Figure 8-3)

      i.   Arterial supply

        (a) Superior mesenteric artery supplies the ascending colon and part of the transverse colon.

        (b) Inferior mesenteric artery feeds the transverse colon, sigmoid colon, and upper rectum.

        (c) Hypogastric arteries give rise to the middle and inferior rectal and hemorrhoidal arteries.

        (d) Rectal arteries, which arise from the internal iliac arteries, supply the distal rectum.

     ii.   Venous drainage

        (a) Superior mesenteric vein drains the ascending colon and part of the transverse colon.

        (b) Inferior mesenteric vein drains the transverse colon, sigmoid colon, and rectum.

        (c) Internal iliac vein

   e. Colonic functions

      i.   Absorption of water and electrolytes: Approximately 500 ml of chyme (the byproduct of digestion) enters the colon per day and, of this, 400 ml of water and electrolytes is reabsorbed

     ii.   Breakdown of cellulose by enteric bacteria

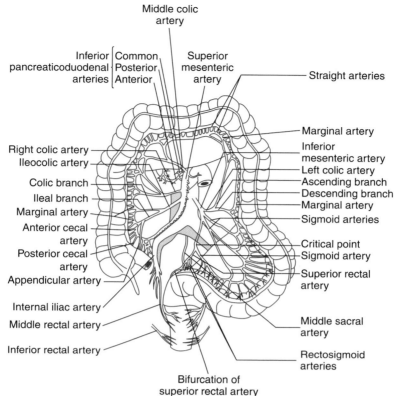

FIGURE 8-3 ■ Arterial and venous blood supplies to the primary and accessory organs of the alimentary canal. (From Ruppert SD, Englert DM. Patients with gastrointestinal bleeding. In: Clochesy JM, Breau C, Cardin S, et al, eds. *Critical Care Nursing.* 2nd ed. Philadelphia, PA: Saunders; 1996:1028.)

      iii. Synthesis of vitamins (folic acid, vitamin K, riboflavin, nicotinic acid) by enteric bacteria

      iv. Storage of fecal mass until it can be expelled from the body

          (a) Takes approximately 18 hours from the time food enters the colon until the intestinal contents reach the distal portion of the colon

          (b) Time from ingestion of food to defecation of the residue may be 24 hours or longer

      v. Motility

          (a) Peristalsis: Propulsive movements that push GI contents toward the anus

          (b) Haustral churning: The major type of movement in the colon

          (c) Factors that enhance motility: Bacterial enterotoxins, viral infections of the gut, regional enteritis, ulcerative colitis, increased bile salts, osmotic overload, laxatives

          (d) Factors that inhibit motility: Low-bulk diet, parenteral nutrition, bed rest, dehydration, ileus, fasting, drugs

          (e) Poor motility causes more absorption, and the development of hard feces in the transverse colon causes constipation.

          (f) Aging causes a reduction in peristalsis and decreased GI motility throughout the GI system.

  f. Innervation: Same as for the stomach and small intestine

  g. Gut defenses

      i. The gut encounters a variety of potentially harmful substances daily; these can include natural toxins in food, insecticides, preservatives, chemical waste products, and airborne particulate matter that is swallowed.

      ii. Mechanisms exist within the GI tract to protect the integrity of the gut and thus the individual.

    iii. Fluid and cellular layers are as follows:
- **(a)** Aqueous layer: Stationary layer immediately adjacent to the microvillus border of the enterocytes; consists of acids, digestive enzymes, and bacteria depending on the location in GI lumen
- **(b)** Mucosal barrier: Physical and chemical barriers that protect the wall of the gut from harmful substances. Surfaces of the stomach, intestine, biliary and pancreatic ducts, and gallbladder have cells that synthesize and release mucus.
- **(c)** Epithelial cells: Tight junctions between cells regulated by hormones and cytokines make them relatively impervious to large molecules and bacteria; rapid proliferation of cells minimizes the adherence of flora. The level of permeability varies within the various segments of the GI tract.
- **(d)** Mucus-bicarbonate barrier: Forms a layer of alkalinity between the epithelium and luminal acids that neutralizes the pH and protects against surface shear

    iv. Motility: Prevents bacteria in the distal small intestine from migrating proximally into the sterile parts of the upper GI system
- **(a)** Stomach
  - **(1)** Expulsion of toxic substances as a result of stimulation of the vomiting center in the medulla
  - **(2)** Barrier against the reflux of duodenal contents back into the stomach
- **(b)** Colon: Moves pathogens and potential carcinogens out of the body

    v. Gut immunity: Necessary because the gut is a reservoir of potentially pathogenic bacteria
- **(a)** B lymphocytes that bear surface immunoglobulin A (IgA) or synthesize secretory IgA that prevents antigens from binding to mucous cells
- **(b)** Macrophages in the lamina propria
  - **(1)** Gut-associated lymphoid tissue in the submucosa (lamina propria or Peyer's patches) of the GI tract
  - **(2)** Glutamine is the primary fuel of the gut and maintains the gut mucosal barrier.

    vi. Gastric acid: Intragastric pH below 4.0 is essential
- **(a)** Protects the stomach from ingested bacteria and other harmful substances
- **(b)** Prevents bacteria from entering the intestine

    vii. Commensal bacteria: Natural gut flora are stable and protective in a healthy person by competing with pathogenic species for nutrients and attachment sites and produce inhibitory substances against pathogenic species
- **(a)** Stomach, duodenum, and jejunum are sterile.
- **(b)** Ileum contains aerobic and anaerobic bacteria: dietary intake is a major factor in determining intestinal flora.
- **(c)** Large intestine contains large numbers of aerobic and anaerobic bacteria and smaller numbers of yeast and fungi.

    viii. Impaired gut barrier function facilitates bacterial translocation, which is the egress of bacteria and/or their toxins across the mucosal barrier and into the lymphatic vessels and portal circulation.

4. Accessory organs of digestion (Figure 8-4)
  a. Liver
    i. Largest solid organ, weighing approximately 3 lb (1500 g), located in the right upper quadrant, beneath the diaphragm
    ii. Consists of three lobes divided into eight independent segments, each of which has its own vascular inflow, outflow, and biliary drainage. Because of this division into self-contained units, each can be resected without damaging those remaining.
- **(a)** Right lobe: Anterior (segments V and VIII) and posterior (segments VI and VII)
- **(b)** Left lobe: Medial (segment IV) and lateral (segments II and III); the left lobe extends across the midline into the left upper quadrant
- **(c)** Caudate lobe (segment I)

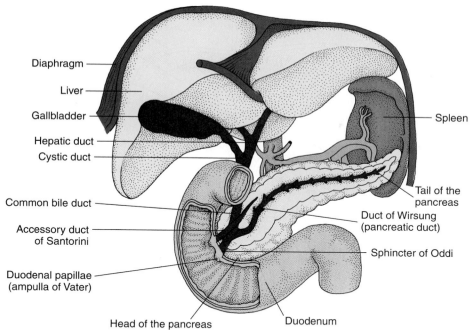

FIGURE 8-4 ■ Anatomy of the liver and biliary tract. (From Westfall UE, Heitkemper M. Gastrointestinal physiology. In: Clochesy JM, Breau C, Cardin S, et al, eds. *Critical Care Nursing*. 2nd ed. Philadelphia, PA: Saunders; 1996:992.)

  iii. Microscopically the liver consists of functional units called lobules composed of portal triads in which the bile ducts, hepatocytes, and artery are located. The portal triads are then bounded by sinusoids and a central vein. A cross section of a classic lobule or acinus is hexagonal.
  iv. Blood supply (Figure 8-5): Derived from both a vein and an artery
   (a) 25% of cardiac output flows through the liver per minute.
   (b) Portal vein (after draining the mesenteric veins and pancreatic and splenic veins) and hepatic artery (off the aorta via the celiac trunk) enter the liver at the porta hepatis or hilum (a horizontal fissure in the liver, containing blood and lymph vessels, nerves, and the hepatic ducts).
   (c) 75% is supplied by the portal vein; each segment receives a branch of the portal vein, and 25% is supplied by the hepatic artery.
   (d) Small branches of each of these vessels enter the acinus at the portal triad (an area in the liver consisting of the portal vein, branches of the hepatic artery, and tributaries to the bile duct).
   (e) Functionally, the liver can be divided into three zones, based on oxygen supply. Zone 1 encircles the portal tracts where the oxygenated blood from hepatic arteries enters. Zone 3 is located around the central veins, where oxygenation is poor. Zone 2 is located in between.
   (f) Blood from both the portal vein and the hepatic artery mixes together in the hepatic sinusoids and then flows through the sinusoids to the hepatic venules (zone 3) through the central veins, branches of the hepatic vein.
   (g) Sinusoids
    (1) Found between plates (layers) of hepatocytes; have a porous lining with fenestrations that allows nutrients in the blood plasma to wash freely over exposed surfaces (the spaces of Disse)
    (2) Sinusoidal lining consists of endothelial cells, Kupffer cells, perisinusoidal fat-storing cells, and pit cells.
   (h) Venous drainage: Begins in the central veins in the center of the lobules; central veins empty into the hepatic veins, which empty into the inferior vena cava

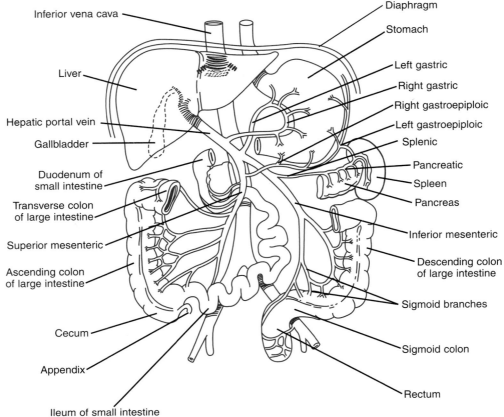

FIGURE 8-5 ■ Hepatic portal circulation. (From Totora GJ, Anagnostakos NP. *Principles of Anatomy and Physiology.* 4th ed. New York, NY: Harper & Row; 1984:510.)

    v.   Biliary duct system for draining bile
- (a) Begins at the sinusoidal level as bile canaliculi, which branch into ductules, intralobular bile ducts, and larger intrahepatic ducts
- (b) Intrahepatic ducts come together at the porta hepatis to form the common hepatic duct, which becomes the common bile duct after joining with the cystic duct, and drains into the duodenum.

   vi. Physiology: The liver is a metabolically complex organ with interrelated digestive, metabolic, exocrine, hematologic, and excretory functions. The many functions it performs are interwoven; each lobe is an independent functional unit, so that up to 80% of the liver can be destroyed and it will regenerate.
- (a) Digestive functions: Plays a role in the synthesis, metabolism, and transport of carbohydrates, fats, and proteins
    - (1) Carbohydrates: Maintains normal serum glucose levels by
        - a) Glycogen storage: Approximately 900 kcal of glycogen reserves are stored in the adult liver
        - b) Glycogenesis: Conversion of excess carbohydrates to glycogen for storage in the liver as a metabolic reserve
        - c) Glycogenolysis: Conversion of large stores of glycogen in muscles and liver to glucose
        - d) Gluconeogenesis: Manufacture of glucose from noncarbohydrate substrate (fat, fatty acids, glycerol, amino acids)
    - (2) Fats
        - a) Bile secretion for fat digestion plays a role in fat and lipid synthesis, metabolism, and transport.

        b) Principal site of synthesis and degradation of lipids (cholesterol, phospholipids, lipoprotein): Produces approximately 1000 mg of cholesterol per day

        c) Exogenous lipoprotein metabolism

        d) Endogenous lipoprotein metabolism: Major lipoprotein synthesized by the liver is very low-density lipoprotein (VLDL); one third of VLDL remnants are converted to low-density lipoprotein (LDL)

           1) Direct removal of VLDL remnants

           2) Removal of 75% of LDL remnants by LDL receptors in the liver

        e) Conversion of excess carbohydrate to triglyceride, which is stored as adipose tissue

        f) Conversion of triglyceride to glycerol and fatty acids for energy

        g) Storage of triglyceride and fat-soluble vitamins (A, D, E, and K)

        h) Storage of fats, cholesterol, proteins, vitamin B_{12}, and minerals

     (3) Protein

        a) Production of plasma proteins (albumin, prealbumin, transferrin, clotting factors, haptoglobin, ceruloplasmin, α_1-antitrypsin, complement, α-fetoprotein)

        b) Deamination: Metabolism of amino acids

        c) Transamination: Conversion of amino acids to ammonia, conversion of ammonia to urea for urinary excretion

  (b) Endocrine functions: Metabolism of glucocorticoids, mineralocorticoids, hormones

  (c) Exocrine functions

     (1) Excretion of bile pigment

     (2) Excretion of cholesterol

     (3) Urea synthesis

     (4) Detoxification of drugs and foreign substances

  (d) Hematologic functions: Synthesis of bilirubin, coagulation factors

  (e) Excretory functions

     (1) Detoxifies and eliminates drugs, hormones, and toxic substances

     (2) Produces and secretes 600 to 1000 ml/day of bile

     (3) Stores vitamin B_{12}, copper, and iron

     (4) Filters blood via Kupffer cells (macrophages) that reside in the liver sinusoids

b. Gallbladder: Pear-shaped saclike organ that serves as a reservoir for bile

   i. Attached to the inferior surface of the liver in the area that divides the right and left lobes (gallbladder fossa)

   ii. Approximately 7 to 10 cm long; holds and concentrates approximately 30 ml of bile

   iii. Blood supply: Arterial blood supply is from the cystic artery; venous drainage is via a network of small veins

   iv. Innervation: Splanchnic nerve, right branch of the vagus nerve

   v. Cystic duct: Attaches the gallbladder to the common hepatic duct

    (a) Union of the cystic duct and the common hepatic duct forms the common bile duct.

    (b) Common bile duct either joins the pancreatic duct outside the duodenum or forms a common channel through the duodenal wall at the ampulla of Vater.

    (c) Intraduodenal segment of the common bile duct and the ampulla is the sphincter of Oddi.

   vi. Presence of CCK in the blood (in response to chyme in the duodenum)

    (a) Facilitates delivery of bile to the duodenum

    (b) Contracts the gallbladder

    (c) Relaxes the sphincter of Oddi

   vii. Bile is composed of water, bile salts, and bile pigments.

    (a) Bile salts are responsible for the absorption and emulsification of fat and fat-soluble vitamins.

     (b) Bile pigments are high in cholesterol and phospholipids; give feces a brown color.

     (c) Bilirubin is the major bile pigment; it is a breakdown product of hemoglobin metabolism from senescent red blood cells.

     (d) Serum bilirubin

       (1) Total: Indirect bilirubin plus direct bilirubin; when total bilirubin level is elevated and the cause is unknown, indirect and direct bilirubin fractions can be measured

       (2) Indirect (unconjugated): Bilirubin bound to albumin before it binds to glucuronic acid; fat soluble. Causes of elevation of indirect bilirubin concentration in serum include the following:

         a) Any hemolytic process (e.g., ABO mismatch in blood transfusion, β-hemolytic streptococcal infection)

         b) Gilbert's syndrome, a common disorder characterized by a mild, chronic fluctuating increase in the level of unconjugated bilirubin

         c) Inherited deficiency of bilirubin, which results in variations of the Crigler-Najjar syndrome

         d) Diffuse hepatocellular necrosis

       (3) Direct (conjugated): Bilirubin bound to glucuronic acid, water soluble; concentration elevates with biliary tract obstruction (except cystic duct), diffuse biliary tract damage, acute cellular rejection after liver transplantation. Causes of elevation of direct bilirubin concentration in serum include the following:

         a) Bile duct obstruction (e.g., stones, tumor, biliary stricture after liver transplantation)

         b) Cholecystitis

         c) Necrosis of the bile duct (e.g., hepatic artery thrombosis)

         d) Autoimmune diseases of biliary stasis (e.g., primary biliary cirrhosis, primary sclerosing cholangitis)

         e) Inherited disorders of conjugated bilirubin excretion (e.g., Dubin-Johnson syndrome, Rotor's syndrome)

c. Pancreas: Soft, flattened gland with a lobular structure but without an external capsule

  i.   12 to 20 cm long, located in the retroperitoneal area

  ii.   Head lies in the C-shaped curve of the duodenum at the level of the body of L2.

  iii. Body extends horizontally behind the stomach.

  iv. Tail is contiguous with the spleen, lying between the two layers of the peritoneum that form the lienorenal ligament at the level of the body of L1.

  v.   Blood supply

     (a) Arterial blood supplies from the celiac axis, which divides into the common hepatic, splenic, and left gastric arteries and the superior mesenteric artery

     (b) Venous drainage via the portal vein, which is formed by the joining together of the superior mesenteric and splenic veins

  vi. Innervation

     (a) Sympathetic efferent innervations via the greater, lesser, and least splanchnic nerves have an inhibitory function.

     (b) Parasympathetic innervation via the vagal nerves, which stimulate exocrine secretion

  vii. Duct of Wirsung: Main pancreatic duct whose terminal end, the sphincter of Oddi in the ampulla of Vater, empties into the duodenum; shares the sphincter of Oddi with the common bile duct

  viii. Duct of Santorini: Accessory pancreatic duct (present in 40% to 70% of persons) that lies anterior and opens into the second part of the duodenum proximal to the duct of Wirsung

  ix. Pancreatic secretions: Consist of aqueous and enzymatic components

     (a) Aqueous component

       (1) Approximately 1 L of fluid per day is secreted.

(2) Ductule cells secrete water and bicarbonate.
    (b) Enzymatic component
       (1) Acinar cells (part of the exocrine function of the pancreas) secrete the pancreatic enzymes.
       (2) Amylase (for digestion of starches) and lipase (for digestion of fats) are secreted as active enzymes.
       (3) Pancreatic proteases are secreted as inactive precursors and are converted to active enzymes in the lumen of the small intestine (for digestion of proteins).
   x. Food in the intestine stimulates the secretion of enzymes. Changes in the proportions of various nutrients in the diet result in changes in the proportions of enzymes in the pancreatic secretions. Adaptation of the pancreatic secretions is accomplished by hormones that operate at the level of gene expression:
      (a) GIP and secretin increase the expression of the lipase gene.
      (b) CCK increases the expression of the protease genes.
      (c) In individuals with diabetes, insulin regulates the expression of the amylase gene; however, how amylase expression is normally regulated in individuals without diabetes is unknown.
      (d) Certain conditions decrease pancreatic secretion: pancreatitis, cystic fibrosis, tumors, and protein deficiency.
   xi. Endocrine cells found in the islets of Langerhans
      (a) Alpha cells secrete glucagon, which is responsible for glycogenolysis and gluconeogenesis.
      (b) Beta cells secrete insulin, which facilitates the use of glucose by tissues.
      (c) Delta cells secrete somatostatin, which inhibits the secretion of insulin, glucagon, and growth hormone.
      (d) Polypeptide cells are associated with the hypermotility of the GI tract and diarrhea.

Patient Assessment

1. **Nursing history**
   a. Patient health history
      i. Chief complaint
      ii. History of present illness
      iii. Past medical conditions (e.g., neurologic conditions, cirrhosis, diabetes), eating disorders, or communicable diseases (e.g., viral hepatitis, jaundice)
      iv. Surgical history (e.g., appendectomy, gastric bypass)
      v. Allergies
         (a) Food allergies, intolerances (e.g., lactase deficiency causes lactose intolerance)
         (b) Drug allergies
      vi. Pain: Location, duration, character, severity, alleviating and aggravating factors, relationship to changes in eating, bowel habits, or position
      vii. Oral health status: Teeth, gums, tongue, pharynx
      viii. Nausea or vomiting: Duration, alleviating and aggravating factors, description of vomitus (undigested food, unrecognizable digested product, blood—bright red or resembling coffee grounds), timing, and relationship to pain
      ix. Loss of appetite (loss of desire or interest in food), duration, association with other symptoms
      x. Dysphagia: Difficulty in swallowing, types of foods and/or liquids causing difficulty
      xi. Heartburn (dyspepsia, reflux): Duration, alleviating and aggravating factors
      xii. Fecal elimination: Diarrhea or constipation, color of stools, presence of blood (black, maroon, or bright red color); clay-colored stool—absence of bile pigment as a result of biliary obstruction or advanced cirrhosis
      xiii. Urinary elimination: Color of urine; dark (tea-colored) urine—acute hepatocellular necrosis or severe biliary obstruction

      xiv. Fatigue, weakness
      xv. Easy bruising or bleeding
      xvi. Fever, night sweats
      xvii. Muscle wasting, atrophy: Wasting of the muscle over the temporal bones in the face or the thenar muscle of the thumb
      xviii. Weight loss or weight gain, obesity
      xix. Eating disorders
   b. Family history
      i. Carcinoma, liver disease, pancreatitis, peptic ulcer disease
      ii. Diabetes mellitus, anemia, tuberculosis
      iii. Inflammatory bowel disease: Crohn's disease, ulcerative colitis
      iv. Obesity
   c. Social history
      i. Substance abuse: Tobacco use, alcohol use, drug use
      ii. Sexual history: Heterosexual, homosexual relationships; involvement with prostitutes
      iii. Place of birth, travel history
      iv. History of tattoos, piercings
   d. Medication history (all medications evaluated but specifically herbal supplements, vitamins, anabolic steroids, motility agents, antacids, histamine or proton pump inhibitors, anticholinergics, antibiotics, antidiarrheals, laxatives, enemas, narcotics, sedatives, barbiturates, stimulants, antihypertensives, diuretics, anticoagulants, analgesics, nonsteroidal, steroids, chemotherapy agents)
2. Nursing examination of patient
   a. Physical examination data
      i. Inspection
         (a) Anatomic landmarks are used to locate and describe normal and abnormal assessment findings.
           (1) Xiphoid process, subcostal margins, costovertebral angle
           (2) Abdominal quadrants (Figure 8-6), midline of abdomen
           (3) Umbilicus, rectus abdominis muscle
           (4) Anterior superior iliac spine, symphysis pubis, inguinal ligament
           (5) Flanks
         (b) General appearance: Physical signs of altered nutritional status (e.g., cachexia, obesity)

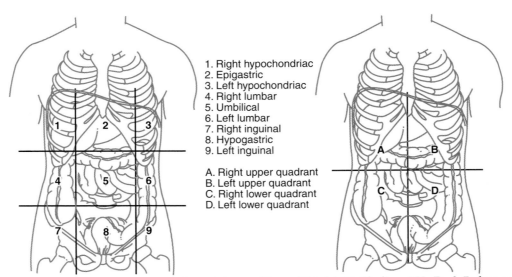

1. Right hypochondriac
2. Epigastric
3. Left hypochondriac
4. Right lumbar
5. Umbilical
6. Left lumbar
7. Right inguinal
8. Hypogastric
9. Left inguinal

A. Right upper quadrant
B. Left upper quadrant
C. Right lower quadrant
D. Left lower quadrant

FIGURE 8-6 ▪ Regions and quadrants of the abdomen. (From Wright JE, Shelton BK. *Desk Reference for Critical Care Nursing.* Boston, MA: Jones & Bartlett; 1993:854.)

    (c) Oral cavity: Gingivitis, lesions (e.g., herpes simplex, *Candida albicans,* leukopla-kia), ability to swallow, presence of odors (e.g., ketones, fetor, alcohol)

    (d) Abdominal profile: Evaluate with the patient lying supine on the examination table or bed

      (1) Symmetry, size (girth), and contour of the abdomen from the costal margins to the symphysis pubis (flat, rounded, scaphoid, protuberant)

        a) Abdominal distention can be due to fluid, fat, flatus, fetus, feces, malig-nancies, nonmalignant tumors.

        b) Asymmetry can be due to these causes as well as to obstructions, cysts, or scoliosis.

      (2) Condition of umbilicus (protruding; nodular; inverted; with calculus, ecchy-moses, or drainage)

      (3) Caput medusae: Engorged abdominal veins around the umbilicus are seen in patients with portal hypertension or obstruction of the superior or inferior vena cava

      (4) Collateral vessels that come to the skin surface and traverse the abdomen: Seen in obesity and ascites

      (5) Masses, visible peristalsis or pulsations

      (6) Striae, ecchymoses, hematomas, scars, wounds, stomas, hernias, engorged veins, diastasis recti, fistulas, tubes, or drains

      (7) Spider angiomas: Found above the umbilicus on the anterior and posterior thorax, head, neck, and arms

      (8) Jaundice: Evident in skin and sclerae

  ii. Auscultation: Performed in all quadrants before percussion and palpation to note location and characteristics of bowel and other sounds

    (a) Normal bowel sounds: Low-pitched, continuous gurgles heard in abdominal quadrants

    (b) Abnormal bowel sounds

      (1) Factors related to hypoactive or absent sounds: Peritonitis, paralytic ileus, anesthesia, inflammation, electrolyte imbalance, gastric or intra-abdominal bleeding, pneumonia, both mechanical and nonmechanical obstruction

      (2) Factors related to hyperactive sounds: Hyperkalemia, gastroenteritis, gastric or esophageal bleeding, diarrhea, laxative use, mechanical obstruction

    (c) Bruit: Denotes increased turbulence or significant dilatation

      (1) Aortic bruit can be heard 2 to 3 cm above the umbilicus in the epigastric area and denotes partial aortic occlusion.

      (2) Hepatic bruit can be heard over the liver and may indicate primary liver can-cer, alcoholic hepatitis, or vascular liver metastases.

      (3) Renal artery bruit can be heard to the left and/or right of midline in the epi-gastric areas in renal artery stenosis.

      (4) Iliac artery bruit can be heard in the left and/or right inguinal areas.

      (5) Venous hum or murmur heard over the liver denotes liver disease such as alcoholic hepatitis, hemangiomas, or dilated periumbilical circulation.

      (6) Friction rub over the spleen denotes inflammation or infarction of the spleen.

      (7) Peritoneal friction rub indicates peritoneal irritation.

      (8) Hepatic friction rub over the liver can be heard in cases of abscess and vari-ous types of hepatitis (e.g., syphilitic).

  iii. Percussion

    (a) Percussion notes or tones

      (1) Tympany is noted when percussing air-filled organs such as the stomach.

      (2) Resonance is noted when striking air-filled lungs.

      (3) Dullness is noted over solid organs such as the liver or spleen.

    (b) Percussion to evaluate the sizes of the liver and spleen

      (1) Liver size can be estimated by percussing from the right clavicle straight down the right midclavicular line to detect changes in percussion tones.

a) Beginning at the midclavicular line below the umbilicus, percuss for the lower edge of the liver. Over the bowel, the percussion tone is tympanic and transitions to dull, which denotes the lower edge of the liver.

b) At the level of the fifth intercostal space, percuss downward. The percussion tone transitions from the resonance of the lung tissue to dull, which denotes the upper edge of the liver.

c) Distance between the upper and lower edges of the liver at the midclavicular line is normally about 12 cm. A span of greater than 12 cm or less than 6 cm is abnormal. Gas in the colon, pregnancy, or tumors can impair accurate assessment of the liver span.

(2) Spleen can be percussed (dull tones) only if grossly enlarged (e.g., portal hypertension) at the left midclavicular line below the left costal margin. To determine the presence of masses or abnormal fluid (ascites) and air collections:

a) Collections can be confirmed by shifting dullness (fluid remains dependent with changes in position).

b) Fluid waves can be elicited by placing the hands on either side of the abdomen, then tapping one hand against the abdomen and feeling the wave transmitted to the opposite hand.

c) Difference between fluid and fat can be determined by placing the hands on either side of the abdomen, having an assistant place his or her hand on the midline, and then pressing downward with one hand. Transmission of fat waves will be halted by the center hand, whereas fluid waves will continue toward the opposite hand.

iv. Palpation

(a) Light and deep palpation are done to determine the tone of the abdominal wall (relaxed, tense, rigid), areas of tenderness or pain, and the presence and characteristics of masses. Light palpation is done before deep palpation to determine areas of tenderness or resistance (guarding); observe the patient's face for nonverbal signs of discomfort.

(b) Visceral tenderness: Dull, poorly localized (e.g., bowel obstruction)

(c) Somatic tenderness: Sharp, well localized (e.g., late appendicitis, capsular stretching of the swollen liver)

(d) Rebound tenderness: Occurs when palpation is suddenly withdrawn; associated with peritonitis

(e) Contralateral tenderness: Tenderness on the side opposite palpation (e.g., early appendicitis)

(f) Referred tenderness: Tenderness in an area distant from the source (e.g., right shoulder blade pain referred from the gallbladder)

(g) Murphy's sign: Severe right upper quadrant tenderness elicited on deep palpation under the right costal margin, exacerbated by deep inspiration and associated with cholecystitis

(h) To determine liver size: Palpate at the patient's right side

(1) Right flank area is supported with the left hand, and the fingertips of the right hand are slid under the right costal margin, using firm pressure.

(2) Fingertips are advanced as the patient inhales deeply, and the liver edge moves 1 to 3 cm downward.

(3) Fingertips are held steady as the patient exhales and inhales again, and the smooth (normal) edge of the liver may be felt moving past the fingertips.

(4) The liver is not normally palpated more than 1 to 2 cm below the right costal margin (in cases of alcoholic liver disease or fatty liver disease, the liver may be enlarged with the margins projecting down into the abdomen 4 to 5 cm).

(i) To determine spleen size: Palpate from the patient's right side

(1) Left flank area is supported with the right hand, and the fingertips of the left hand are slid under the left costal margin, using firm pressure.

(2) Fingertips are advanced as the patient inhales deeply, and the spleen edge moves 1 to 3 cm downward.

(3) Fingertips are held steady as the patient exhales and inhales again, and the smooth (normal) edge of the spleen may be felt moving past the fingertips.

(4) The spleen is not normally palpable, except in cases of enlargement or inferior displacement.

b. Monitoring data

   i. Heart rate, blood pressure, intake and output

   ii. Daily weights, calorie counts, or dietary intake notations

   iii. Estimation of metabolic expenditures

3. **Appraisal of patient characteristics: Patients in progressive care units with acute GI problems have conditions that vary in complexity. During their hospitalization their clinical status may move along the continuum of care from improvement to deterioration in a nonlinear fashion. This potential for gradual or abrupt changes in clinical condition with possibly life-altering effects creates barriers in the ability to monitor life-sustaining functions with precision. Clinical attributes of patients with acute GI disorders that the nurse needs to assess include the following:**

a. Resiliency

   i. Level 1—*Minimally resilient:* A 92-year-old woman with a history of aortic valve replacement and dementia who presents with lower GI bleeding and anemia after doubling daily aspirin dose for 2 months

   ii. Level 3—*Moderately resilient:* A 68-year-old male accountant 3 days after a ruptured appendix and repair in whom signs of sepsis and acute renal failure develop

   iii. Level 5—*Highly resilient:* A 16-year-old male high school student with blunt abdominal trauma after a motor vehicle accident. He was wearing a seatbelt, and the vehicle air bags deployed.

b. Vulnerability

   i. Level 1—*Highly vulnerable:* A 45-year-old woman with a diagnosis of cirrhosis and spontaneous bacterial peritonitis who has an esophageal variceal hemorrhage during hospitalization

   ii. Level 3—*Moderately vulnerable:* A 56-year-old attorney with acute pancreatitis, high fever, and positive blood culture results

   iii. Level 5—*Minimally vulnerable:* A 24-year-old Chinese man with acute hepatitis B viremia

c. Stability

   i. Level 1—*Minimally stable:* An 84-year-old man, with do not resuscitate orders, with a recent history of surgical aortic aneurysm repair who came to the emergency department with bowel ischemia

   ii. Level 3—*Moderately stable:* A 62-year-old newly retired man with colon cancer who is undergoing chemotherapy after tumor resection

   iii. Level 5—*Highly stable:* A 45-year-old homemaker who has undergone a cholecystectomy for gallstones and had no prior health problems

d. Complexity

   i. Level 1—*Highly complex:* A 36-year-old grocery store clerk with cirrhosis and newly diagnosed liver cancer who is listed for liver transplantation shortly after separating from his wife and moving back in with his parents

   ii. Level 3—*Moderately complex:* An 18-year-old man who had abdominal trauma in a motor vehicle accident that killed his girlfriend

   iii. Level 5—*Minimally complex:* A 34-year-old married mechanic after small bowel resection for Crohn's disease

e. Resource availability

   i. Level 1—*Few resources:* An illiterate 78-year-old widower with no children who has a small bowel obstruction due to cancer and has minimal income, has no transportation, and cannot afford his medications or insurance copayment

   ii. Level 3—*Moderate resources:* A 48-year-old field worker with cirrhosis with decompensations of encephalopathy and ascites who has a 17-year-old son. He has medical and Supplemental Security Income disability benefits that will cover the cost of medications.

   iii. Level 5—*Many resources:* A 58-year-old college professor, who is married with three grown children who live locally and who has chronic hepatitis C cirrhosis

f. Participation in care

   i. Level 1—*No participation:* A 51-year-old migrant field worker with no known family in the United States who has encephalopathy from fulminant liver failure due to exposure to agricultural chemicals

   ii. Level 3—*Moderate level of participation:* A 68-year-old widow being discharged after upper GI bleeding from a peptic ulcer. She underwent gastric resection, and her primary caregiver will be her daughter.

   iii. Level 5—*Full participation:* A 25-year-old secretary with a mild episode of pancreatitis, recovering without complications and planning her follow-up care with her husband and a good family friend who is a nurse

g. Participation in decision making

   i. Level 1—*No participation:* A 98-year-old woman with Alzheimer's disease who has no family and who has been in a motor vehicle accident with severe abdominal injuries, renal failure, and sepsis

   ii. Level 3—*Moderate level of participation:* A 45-year-old businessman, married with two young children, who has esophageal cancer and is undergoing esophageal resection followed by chemotherapy. The patient and his wife are overwhelmed by the changes in their lives and unsure of what the treatment options and posthospitalization issues are.

   iii. Level 5—*Full participation:* A 34-year-old tennis coach with severe gastroenteritis that resolved after 2 days in the hospital who is planning to continue his recovery using vacation time

h. Predictability

   i. Level 1—*Not predictable:* A 43-year-old health food store manager in whom jaundice, elevated liver enzyme levels, and encephalopathy suddenly develop and who has no prior history or risk factors for liver disease

   ii. Level 3—*Moderately predictable:* A 34-year-old Vietnamese general manager with jaundice, abnormal liver test results, malaise, and hepatosplenomegaly after returning from a trip to South America

   iii. Level 5—*Highly predictable:* A 40-year-old store manager who recently underwent liver transplantation and is progressing well toward discharge

4. Diagnostic studies

  a. Laboratory

   i. Complete blood cell count (CBC)

   ii. Serum electrolyte, glucose, blood urea nitrogen (BUN), creatinine, calcium, magnesium, ammonia, and cholesterol levels

   iii. Liver function tests: Total protein, albumin, serum alanine aminotransferase (ALT; formerly serum glutamate pyruvate transaminase [SGPT]), aspartate aminotransferase (AST; formerly serum glutamic-oxaloacetic transaminase [SGOT]), alkaline phosphatase, lactate dehydrogenase, γ-glutamyl transferase (GGT) levels

   iv. Serum bilirubin level: Total, indirect, direct

   v. Ceruloplasmin level

   vi. Serum amylase, lipase, cholinesterase levels

   vii. Prothrombin time (PT), international normalized ratio (INR)

   viii. Level of α-fetoprotein, a tumor marker used to diagnose liver cancer; level of carbohydrate antigen 19-9 (CA 19-9), a tumor marker used for the diagnosis of pancreatic or hepatobiliary cancer

   ix. Carcinoembryonic antigen level

   x. Levels of smooth muscle antibody (SMA), antimitochondrial antibody (AMA), antinuclear antibody (ANA), antineutrophil cytoplasmic antibody (ANCA), and anti–liver-kidney microsomal antibody (anti-LKM antibody), an assay used to diagnose autoimmune disorders

xi. Fasting lipid levels

xii. Hepatitis serologic testing (hepatitis A, B, C)

xiii. Blood cultures (if an infectious process is suspected or with new onset of ascites or abdominal pain)

xiv. Urine: Amylase, lipase, and bilirubin levels; culture and sensitivity testing; urinalysis; microalbumin level

xv. Nutritional parameters
   (a) Total iron-binding capacity, serum iron level, ferritin level
   (b) Serum transferrin, prealbumin, retinol-binding protein levels
   (c) 24-hour urine urea nitrogen, creatinine, sodium levels

xvi. Stool: Occult blood, fat, protein, ova and parasites, cultures

b. Radiologic

   i. Abdominal flat-plate radiography: To visualize the position, size, and structure of the abdominal contents, truncal skeleton, and soft tissues of the abdominal wall. Dilated bowel loops, free air, fluid accumulations, and intramural bowel gas can be identified on plain radiographic films.

   ii. Upper GI series: Contrast is used to visualize the position, contours, and size of the entire upper GI tract (especially the stomach and duodenum); to detect ulcers, tumors, strictures, and obstructions. Barium swallow is used to examine swallowing, motility, and emptying in the esophagus.

   iii. Small bowel follow-through: To visualize the small bowel from the ligament of Treitz to the ileocecal valve to detect ulcers, tumors, diverticula, polyps, and inflammatory bowel disease

   iv. Lower GI series: Barium enema is used to visualize the position, contours, and size of the entire lower GI tract; to detect ulcers, tumors, strictures, obstructions, polyps, inflammatory bowel disease, and diverticula; and to evaluate melena after inconclusive upper GI series

   v. Esophagogastroduodenoscopy (EGD) or upper endoscopy: Visualization and photography of the esophagus, stomach, and proximal duodenum by means of an endoscope
   (a) To detect obstruction, strictures, ulcers, or tumors
   (b) To evaluate melena, hematemesis, heme-positive nasogastric drainage, dysphagia, odynophagia, dyspepsia, nausea, vomiting, or unexplained abdominal pain
   (c) To perform biopsy and obtain brush cytology and culture specimens; to place stents; to remove foreign bodies; to place feeding tubes; or to control bleeding

   vi. Flexible sigmoidoscopy: Visualization and photography of the rectum, sigmoid colon, and descending colon up to 65 cm by means of a flexible sigmoidoscope or colonoscope
   (a) To detect inflammatory disease, tumors, obstruction, strictures, and polyps
   (b) To evaluate unexplained chronic diarrhea or pain, lower GI bleeding
   (c) To perform biopsy, obtain specimens for brush cytology studies, perform polypectomy, and obtain culture specimens; to remove foreign bodies; and to control bleeding

   vii. Colonoscopy: Visualization and photography of the colon from the rectum to the ileocecal valve by means of a colonoscope
   (a) To detect polyps, strictures, obstruction, tumors, or inflammatory disease
   (b) To evaluate lower GI bleeding, unexplained chronic abdominal pain, unexplained iron-deficiency anemia, or changes in bowel patterns
   (c) To perform biopsy, obtain specimens for brush cytology studies, perform polypectomy, and obtain culture specimens; to remove foreign bodies; and to control bleeding

   viii. Endoscopic retrograde cholangiopancreatography (ERCP): Visualization and photography of the biliary and/or pancreatic ducts by means of a flexible (fiberoptic) endoscope
   (a) To detect tumors, bile duct stones, obstruction, and pancreatitis

        (b) To evaluate jaundice, elevated levels on liver tests, and chronic unexplained abdominal pain

        (c) To perform biopsy and obtain specimens for brush cytology studies and cultures; to place stents; or to remove stones

    ix. Angiography: Selective catheterization of the visceral arterial system and portal venous system, to reveal vessel sizes, patency, and flow rates of the vessels as well as the direction of the blood flow

    x. Cholangiography: Radiopaque dye is used to enhance the radiograph and allow visualization of the gallbladder and bile ducts

    xi. Computed tomography (CT) of the abdomen: Can be done with or without intravenous, oral, or rectal contrast

        (a) To visualize the gallbladder, liver, pancreas, spleen, loops of the small and large intestine, extrahepatic bile ducts, and portal vein

        (b) To determine the presence of vascular problems, infection, tumors, and pancreatic pseudocyst

        (c) Use of contrast-enhanced images allows for improved visualization of tumors, vascularity of masses, and differences within bowel loops.

    xii. Positron emission tomography (PET): Use of radioisotopes (carbon, oxygen, nitrogen, and fluorine, and some metals such as copper and gallium and their decay products) to reveal physiologic function, not anatomic structure. It is used to evaluate for colorectal, liver, pancreatic, and neuroendocrine diseases.

    xiii. Magnetic resonance imaging (MRI)

        (a) Same applications as CT with a greater potential for tissue characterization and a greater ability to diagnose and characterize diffuse liver and pancreatic disease

        (b) Can also detect arterial and venous blood flow, vessel patency, bile ducts, and the presence of strictures within the ducts

        (c) Less effective than CT for evaluating disorders of the bowel because the movement of the intestine degrades MRI images

    xiv. Ultrasonography of the abdomen: To visualize the sizes and echotextures of the gallbladder, liver, pancreas, and spleen; to determine the presence or absence of disease (fatty infiltration, cirrhosis), the cause of masses (cysts, abscesses, tumors), and the presence of foreign bodies (gallstones); to evaluate the bile ducts and accumulation of fluids; and to determine the direction of blood flow, the development of collateral vessels, and vessel patency

    xv. Capsule endoscopy: Swallowable wireless miniature camera to visualize the gastrointestinal mucosa

  c. Other testing

    i. Biopsy: Needle or forceps aspiration of tissue from the esophagus, stomach, duodenum, colon, rectum, or liver or soft tissues masses for histologic analysis

    ii. Abdominal paracentesis: Withdrawal of peritoneal fluid for diagnostic purposes or symptomatic relief by means of a large-bore needle

    iii. Peritoneoscopy (laparoscopy): Examination of the structures and organs within the abdominal cavity by means of a laparoscope

    iv. Gastric lavage: Insertion of a gastric tube through the nose or mouth to examine the gastric contents or secretions for occult blood or pH

    v. Schilling's test: Vitamin B_{12} absorption test to determine whether vitamin B_{12} absorption is defective and if the cause is intrinsic factor deficiency. Oral radioactively labeled vitamin B_{12} and intrinsic factor, and intramuscular nonradioactive vitamin B_{12} are administered, and 24- to 48-hour urine excretion is measured.

Patient Care

1. Inability to establish or maintain a patent airway

  a. Description of problem: With acute hemorrhage or encephalopathy there may be an inability to maintain the airway because of altered levels of consciousness or possible aspiration due to vomiting. Clinical findings may include altered rate and depth of respirations, decreased oxygen saturation, dyspnea or tachypnea, and cyanosis.

    b. Goals of care: Reestablish and maintain a patent airway and transfer to a higher level of care

    c. Collaborating professionals on health care team: Physician, nurse, anesthesiologist, respiratory therapist, radiologist

    d. Interventions: See Chapter 2

    e. Evaluation of patient care: Patent airway and no signs of aspiration

2. **Fluid volume deficit**

    a. Description of problem: Associated with hemorrhage, GI fluid and blood losses, third-spacing, or sepsis. Clinical findings may include the following:

        i. Anxiety or diminished mental status

        ii. Tachycardia and decreased pulse pressure

        iii. Orthostatic hypotension progressing to profound hypotension

        iv. Oliguria, anuria

        v. Decreased hemoglobin level, hematocrit, and platelet count; increased INR; hematemesis or melena

        vi. Elevated BUN, creatinine, lactate levels

        vii. Metabolic acidosis

    b. Goals of care: Restore normal circulating fluid volume

    c. Collaborating professionals on health care team: Physician, nurse, laboratory technician, pharmacist, blood bank personnel

    d. Interventions: See Chapters 3 and 5

    e. Evaluation of patient care: Restoration of adequate circulating volume as evidenced by vital signs, serum electrolyte and lactate levels, urine output, and oxygen delivery

3. **Electrolyte and/or acid-base imbalances**

    a. Description of problem: May be related to hemorrhage, GI losses, third-spacing, sepsis, or renal failure (see Chapters 2 and 5 for specific clinical findings)

    b. Goals of care: Restore and maintain electrolyte balance and normalize pH

    c. Collaborating professionals on health care team: Physician, nurse, pharmacist, laboratory technician, respiratory therapist

    d. Interventions: See Chapters 2 and 5

    e. Evaluation of patient care: Maintenance of normal values for serum electrolytes, lactate, and arterial blood gases

4. **Impaired nutrition**

    a. Description of problem: May be associated with inadequate intake, anorexia (intake less than body requirements) due to nausea, vomiting, diarrhea, reduced absorption, or increased metabolic needs

    b. Goals of care: Ensure that minimum daily requirements for both calories and nutrients are met

    c. Collaborating professionals on health care team: Physician, dietitian, total parenteral nutrition team, pharmacist

    d. Interventions

        i. Perform accurate monitoring and recording of patient weight; monitoring of intake and output, including calorie count.

        ii. Assess bowel sounds and for signs of malabsorption or obstruction.

        iii. Complete a comprehensive nutritional assessment, including increases in energy requirements.

        iv. Administer oral and/or parenteral nutritional support, and monitor the patency of feeding tubes if used.

        v. Monitor for complications of central venous catheters if used.

        vi. Monitor patient response to and tolerance of the nutritional regimen (e.g., electrolyte balance, hydration, hypoglycemia, or hyperglycemia).

    e. Evaluation of patient care

        i. Meeting of the nutrient and caloric needs of the body as evidenced by lean muscle weight gain

        ii. Enhancement of immune response

        iii. Minimization of negative nitrogen balance

SPECIFIC PATIENT HEALTH PROBLEMS

Acute Abdomen

1. **Pathophysiology: Condition of complex etiology characterized by the sudden onset of abdominal pain, associated with inflammation of the peritoneal cavity and usually necessitating emergency surgical intervention**
2. **Etiology and risk factors**
    a. Perforated or ruptured viscus (esophagus, stomach, liver, pancreas, gallbladder, bile duct, bowel, appendix, or diverticulum) caused by erosion, technical error during surgery or other procedure, foreign body, trauma, or infection
    b. Perforated or ruptured blood vessel as in peptic ulcer disease, abdominal aortic aneurysm, tumor, or trauma
    c. Bowel ischemia: Decrease in blood flow or tissue perfusion that can be acute or chronic, occlusive or nonocclusive
        i.   Arterial occlusion (embolus or thrombus)
        ii. Venous occlusion (hypercoagulable state, trauma)
        iii. Nonocclusive (cardiopulmonary bypass, vasoconstrictive medication, dehydration, shock, or congestive heart failure)
    d. Bowel obstruction: Blockage of the forward flow of intestinal contents
        i.   Classification: Acute, subacute, chronic, or intermittent (only acute obstruction leads to infarction or strangulation)
        ii. Extent: Partial, complete
        iii. Location
            (a) Intrinsic: Originates within the lumen of the intestine
            (b) Extrinsic: Originates outside the lumen of the intestine
        iv. Effects on the intestine
            (a) Simple: Does not occlude blood supply
            (b) Strangulated: Occludes blood supply
            (c) Closed loop: Obstruction at each end of an intestinal segment
        v.   Causal factors
            (a) Mechanical (gallstones, tumor, impactions, foreign bodies, inflammatory bowel diseases, adhesions, volvulus, intussusception)
            (b) Functional (paralytic ileus after abdominal surgery or caused by electrolyte imbalances, peritonitis, spinal fractures, megacolon, ischemia, pancreatitis)
            (c) Infection (abscess, sepsis)
            (d) Extra-abdominal cause (cirrhosis, altered host response)
3. **Signs and symptoms**
    a. Persistent severe abdominal pain, referred pain
    b. Nausea, vomiting, reflux, or anorexia
    c. Alteration in bowel patterns
    d. Abdominal distention; hyperactive or hypoactive bowel sounds
    e. Guarding of the abdomen, rebound tenderness
    f. Fever, pallor, tachypnea
    g. Dehydration
    h. Evidence of blunt or penetrating trauma
    i. Fecal odor of gastric drainage
4. **Diagnostic study findings: Differential diagnosis is complex**
    a. Laboratory
        i.   Elevated white blood cell (WBC) count with a shift to the left: Elevated segmented neutrophil and basophil counts, increased numbers of bands (immature neutrophils)
        ii. Elevated alkaline phosphatase level
        iii. Findings consistent with a diagnosis of pancreatitis; elevated serum amylase, lipase levels
        iv. Findings consistent with hemorrhage
        v.   Arterial blood gas levels: Metabolic acidosis

vi. Blood and body fluid culture results positive for infectious organisms
   b. Radiologic
      i. Abdominal flat-plate radiography: Alteration in the position, size, or structure of abdominal contents; free air or free fluid in the abdomen
      ii. Abdominal ultrasonography: Masses (cysts, abscesses, tumors), foreign bodies (gallstones), infarction
      iii. Cholangiography: Cholangitis
      iv. ERCP: Biliary or pancreatic stones, obstruction of ducts
      v. Arteriography: Bleeding, infarction
      vi. Abdominal CT or MRI: Vascular problems, infection, masses, or pancreatic pseudocyst
   c. EGD: Bleeding from peptic ulcer, esophageal tear
   d. Flexible sigmoidoscopy or colonoscopy: Lower GI ulceration, perforation, bleeding, abscess, ischemia
   e. Abdominal paracentesis: Blood, bile, pus, urine, or feces in abdominal cavity
   f. Peritoneoscopy (laparoscopy): Bleeding, perforation, rupture, abscess, ischemia
5. **Goals of care**
   a. Restore hemodynamic equilibrium and fluid balance.
   b. Restore electrolyte balances.
   c. Restore optimal GI function.
   d. Minimize other organ dysfunction and damage.
   e. Provide pain relief.
   f. Eliminate any infectious process.
6. **Collaborating professionals on health care team: Physician, nurse, dietitian, respiratory therapist, pharmacist, radiologist or technician, consultant (e.g., hepatologist, infectious disease specialist)**
7. **Management of patient care**
   a. Anticipated patient trajectory: Patients with an acute abdomen can differ greatly in their clinical course and status at discharge, depending on factors such as age and preexisting conditions. Throughout their course of recovery and discharge, patients with an acute abdomen may be expected to have needs in the following areas:
      i. Positioning: As the patient's condition and comfort dictate
      ii. Skin care: Postoperative wound care and pressure relief are required, because the patient is susceptible to skin breakdown from diarrhea, fistula formation, wound drainage, dehydration, hypotension, and malnutrition
      iii. Pain management: Hypotension makes pain management more complex; however, dosage reduction and nonpharmacologic techniques may be effective. Frequent reassessment and gradual titration of medication required. (See discussion of pain in Chapters 4 and 10.)
      iv. Nutrition: Nutritional needs will be increased because of increased metabolic needs. There will have been a reduction in intake before surgery because of the acute condition. After surgery the reduction in intake will continue in the face of increased metabolic demands of surgery, fever, wound healing, and complications such as infection. Cause of the condition and the caloric requirements will determine how these metabolic needs are met (enteral or parenteral route).
      v. Infection control: Patients with blunt or penetrating trauma, infection, or pancreatitis will have an increased risk of infectious complications resulting from the ruptured viscus or translocation of bacteria. Vigilance is required to identify signs and symptoms of an infectious process early and initiate treatment promptly.
      vi. Transport: Patient will undergo a variety of diagnostic tests and procedures, which will require that the patient be maintained in a mobile environment. Monitoring of various tubes, drains, and catheters is required in addition to monitoring of vital signs.
      vii. Discharge planning: Patient may need assistance at home for dressings, intravenous antibiotics, wound care, parenteral or enteral nutrition. Physical therapy may also be required.

       viii. Pharmacology: Patients will be receiving a complex variety of medications after surgery (antibiotics, insulin, narcotics, anxiolytics, vasopressors, inotropic agents, proton pump inhibitors, diuretics, cathartics)

       ix. Psychosocial issues: Due to the acute nature of the illness, the family may be unprepared for role changes and financial issues. There may be significant alteration in body image and/or resumption of prior roles in the family.

       x. Treatments: After surgery the patient can receive noninvasive treatments (motility agents) as well as invasive treatments (additional surgery)

       xi. Ethical issues: Living will, durable power of attorney for health care, refusal of treatment, consent for treatment

  b. Potential complications

     i. Sepsis

       (a) Mechanism: Translocation of bacteria through the lumen of an ischemic GI tract, abscess, invasive monitoring lines

       (b) Management: See Chapter 9

     ii. Myocardial infarction

       (a) Mechanism: Myocardial ischemia resulting from reduced preload

       (b) Management: See Chapter 3

     iii. Dehydration

       (a) Mechanism: Hemorrhage, third-spacing, nausea, vomiting, diarrhea, intraoperative losses

       (b) Management: See Chapter 5

     iv. Renal insufficiency

       (a) Mechanism: Reduction in mean arterial pressure, infection, hypotension, nephrotoxic drugs, hepatorenal syndrome

       (b) Management: See Chapter 5

     v. Fistula formation or abscesses

       (a) Mechanism: Pancreatic enzymes or perforation of bowel

       (b) Management

         (1) Wound care to minimize fluid collections and abscesses

         (2) Administration of antibiotics to prevent or minimize complications

8. Evaluation of patient care

  a. Hemodynamic stability

  b. Fluid, electrolyte, nitrogen, and acid-base balance

  c. Freedom from pain

  d. Absence of infection

  e. Absence of complications

Acute (Fulminant) Liver Failure

1. Pathophysiology

  a. Clinical syndrome defined as the development of hepatic encephalopathy within 8 weeks of symptoms or within 2 weeks of the onset of jaundice

  b. Occurs in individuals with a history of normal liver function and is characterized by massive hepatocellular necrosis as evidenced by a raised serum ALT level; prolonged coagulation and hypoglycemia can also occur

  c. Except in cases of acute fulminant liver failure caused by acetaminophen toxicosis, the mortality rate is 80% to 100% without liver transplantation.

2. Etiology and risk factors

  a. Viral hepatitis: Acute hepatitis A and B

  b. Autoimmune hepatitis

  c. Acetaminophen toxicosis: Liver failure from intentional overdose and unintentional therapeutic misadventure has a better prognosis than that resulting from other causes

  d. Hepatotoxic drugs or substances

  e. Mushroom poisoning (e.g., owing to *Amanita phalloides*, *Amanita verna*, and *Amanita venosa*; *Galerina autumnalis*, *Galerina marginata*, and *Galerina venenata*; *Gyromitra* species)

  f. Viral infections: Herpesvirus family, especially in immunocompromised patients

g. Acute Wilson's disease, acute Budd-Chiari syndrome

h. Veno-occlusive disease and graft-versus-host disease after bone marrow transplantation

i. Reye's syndrome

3. **Signs and symptoms**

a. Prodromal symptoms (vague, flulike symptoms), fever

b. Jaundice

c. Hyperventilation, respiratory alkalosis

d. Hepatic encephalopathy (confusion): Rapid progression to hepatic coma

e. Profound coagulopathy and hypoglycemia

f. Hepatorenal syndrome

g. Sepsis, metabolic acidosis

h. Intracranial hypertension

i. Hyperdynamic circulation

j. Systolic ejection murmur

k. Eventual cardiovascular collapse

l. Liver is enlarged during the acute inflammatory stage, then becomes atrophied as hepato-cellular necrosis progresses.

4. **Diagnostic study findings**

a. Laboratory

   i. Increased levels of AST, ALT, and, to a lesser degree, alkaline phosphatase and GGT. Severe elevations followed by a progression back to normal that may be misinterpreted as improvement in the patient's status but is not a favorable sign if it occurs in the setting of increasing PT, INR, and bilirubin levels; indicates near-complete hepatocellular necrosis.

   ii. Increased serum bilirubin, creatinine, BUN levels

   iii. Prolonged PT and INR

   iv. Levels of factors V and VII less than 20% of normal (poor prognostic sign)

   v. Decreased serum glucose level, hemoglobin level, and hematocrit

   vi. Increased serum lactate level, serum ammonia level, and WBC count

   vii. Positive results on cultures of body fluids

   viii. Positive results on hepatitis serologic testing or tests for autoimmune markers depending on cause

   ix. Positive urine toxicology screen results

   x. Positive stool guaiac test results

b. Radiologic

   i. Chest radiograph: Bilateral infiltrates or evidence of aspiration pneumonitis

   ii. CT scan of the head: Normal until very late in the process

   iii. Cerebral perfusion scan may show decreased or absent flow late in the process; performed before liver transplantation to rule out brain death.

c. Pressure measurement

   i. Increased ICP, increased mean arterial pressure, normal cerebral perfusion pressure (early signs)

   ii. Increased ICP, normal or decreased mean arterial pressure, decreased cerebral perfusion pressure (late signs)

5. **Goals of care**

a. Optimize liver function.

b. Stabilize for liver transplantation if appropriate.

c. Monitor and treat complications.

6. **Collaborating professionals on health care team: Physician, nurse, pharmacist, laboratory technician, respiratory therapist, consultant**

7. **Management of patient care**

a. Anticipated patient trajectory: Very unstable with long recovery. Liver transplantation may be necessary when progression of liver failure continues; this requires either a graft from a living donor or a cadaveric liver. Patients may be expected to have needs in the following areas:

   i. Positioning: Head of bed raised 30 degrees for treatment of increased ICP

ii. Skin care: Itching can be severe with the onset of jaundice; scratching is unconscious, which results in excoriations; in patients with prolonged coagulation times, this can result in hematoma formation

iii. Pain management: Difficult because of liver failure. Pain is rare because encephalopathy inhibits the reception of transmitted pain impulses. Consultation with a hepatologist necessary if pain medication required.

iv. Nutrition: Metabolic rate can be increased; fluid balance is a problem with renal failure. Special enteral and parenteral solutions required because of liver and renal dysfunction.

v. Infection control: Immobility, altered level of consciousness, invasive lines, and depressed immune system result in increased risk of infection

vi. Transport: Monitor for changes in ICP; mobile environment increases the risk of infection

vii. Discharge planning: Recovery is long, and the patient and family will need assistance with home care, rehabilitation, medications, office visits

viii. Pharmacology: Patient will be taking a complex regimen of medications, and alternative choices (shorter-acting drugs or drugs with shorter half-lives) and dosing patterns (every 12 hours instead of every 6 or 8 hours) will be required because of liver dysfunction

ix. Psychosocial issues: Acuity of the situation will have a profound impact on the family and increase stress

x. Treatments
   (a) Noninvasive: Medications
   (b) Invasive: Surgery, endoscopy with esophageal variceal ligation or sclerosis, colonoscopy with cauterization, angiography with embolization

xi. Ethical issues: Cause of the liver disease can affect the potential for liver transplantation and may lead to a discussion regarding end-of-life issues

b. Potential complications
   i. Infection or sepsis
      (a) Mechanism: Depressed immune system and breaks in the skin barrier due to monitoring needs; altered level of consciousness and risk of aspiration
      (b) Management: See Chapter 9
   ii. Brainstem herniation (most common cause of death in fulminant liver failure) or intracranial hemorrhage
      (a) Mechanism: Increased coagulation times increase the risk of intracranial bleeding and pulmonary hemorrhage; increased risk of hypoxia, which increases the risk of cerebral edema
      (b) Management: See Chapter 4
   iii. Renal failure
      (a) Mechanism: Progression of liver failure may lead to renal failure (hepatorenal syndrome)
      (b) Management: See Chapter 5
   iv. Respiratory failure
      (a) Mechanism: Pulmonary edema, hemorrhage, pneumonia, altered mental status
      (b) Management: See Chapter 2
   v. Liver transplantation
      (a) Treatment option for fulminant liver failure and end-stage liver disease, and certain cases of hepatoma
      (b) Liver disease may recur in the transplanted liver.
      (c) Currently approximately 20,000 patients need liver transplantation; however, only about 6000 are done per year.
         (1) Cadaveric (deceased) donor
            a) Donor is declared brain dead.
            b) Either entire liver or split liver can be used.
            c) Donor and recipient are matched by blood group, age, size.

(2) Living donor
   a) Donor provides 60% of his or her liver.
   b) Donor is between the ages of 21 and 45 years in most cases.
   c) Recipient is usually in healthier condition than those receiving cadaveric organs because of the ability to transplant earlier in the disease course.
   d) During the early postoperative period the patient requires monitoring for primary nonfunction of the new liver, monitoring for improvement in mentation and levels of coagulation factors, and monitoring for infection.

8. **Evaluation of patient care: Normalization of liver functions, neurologic function, renal function, and vital signs**

Chronic Liver Failure: Decompensated Cirrhosis

1. **Pathophysiology**
   a. Cirrhosis is a chronic and usually slowly progressive disease of the liver involving the diffuse formation of connective tissue (fibrosis), nodular regeneration of the liver after necrosis, and chronic inflammation.
   b. Changes are often irreversible.
   c. Once the diagnosis of cirrhosis has been made, there is generally a 5- to 10-year period before decompensation.

2. **Etiology and risk factors**
   a. Alcoholism (Laënnec's cirrhosis): Development of cirrhosis preceded by a reversible stage of alcoholic hepatitis
   b. Postnecrotic cirrhosis
      i.   Viral hepatitis (chronic active hepatitis B, C, F, or G)
      ii.   Drug or toxin induced (prescription drugs, herbs, heavy metals)
      iii. Autoimmune hepatitis
   c. Autoimmune diseases of biliary stasis (primary biliary cirrhosis, primary sclerosing cholangitis)
   d. Inborn errors of liver metabolism: Wilson's disease (copper metabolism), hemochromatosis (iron metabolism), α_1-antitrypsin deficiency
   e. Nonalcoholic fatty liver disease, associated with obesity, hyperlipidemia, protein-calorie malnutrition, diabetes mellitus, chronic corticosteroid use, jejunoileal bypass, short bowel syndrome
   f. Hepatic vein thrombosis (Budd-Chiari syndrome)
   g. Right-sided heart failure: Cardiac cirrhosis

3. **Signs and symptoms**
   a. Fatigue, alteration in sleep pattern: Insomnia, day-night reversal
   b. Pruritus
   c. Muscle wasting, weight loss
   d. Abdominal distention with ascites
   e. Anemia, hematomas, ecchymoses
   f. Clay-colored stools
   g. Fetor hepaticus: Musty breath, poor dentition
   h. Altered mental status, asterixis
   i. Visible stigmata of liver disease: Jaundice, temporal and upper body muscle wasting, parotid enlargement, spider angiomas, palmar erythema, leukonychia, possible clubbing of the fingers, testicular atrophy, gynecomastia in males, striae, the development of abdominal wall collaterals, caput medusae
   j. Umbilical hernia, incisional hernia, splenomegaly
   k. Hyperdynamic circulation: Increased heart rate, systolic ejection murmur
   l. Possible decrease in lung sounds in the bases because of pleural effusions
   m. Hepatic bruit (hepatoma or alcoholic hepatitis superimposed on cirrhosis)

4. **Diagnostic study findings**
   a. Laboratory: Depend on the cause and stage of disease

    i. ALT, AST, alkaline phosphatase, GGT levels: Not usually markedly elevated in advanced cirrhosis but depend on the cause of the liver disease

    ii. Bilirubin level: Elevated in advanced cirrhosis except in diseases of biliary stasis, in which it is elevated early in the disease

    iii. PT, INR: Prolonged PT and increased INR; the most sensitive index of synthetic liver function in a readily available laboratory test

    iv. Platelet count: May be decreased because of splenomegaly

    v. Blood ammonia level: May be elevated (may be affected by a variety of factors not related to liver disease)

    vi. Hemoglobin level, hematocrit: Decreased

    vii. BUN, creatinine levels: Decreased until hepatorenal syndrome occurs

    viii. Serum sodium level: Decreased (at times critically)

    ix. Hepatitis serologic findings: Variable

    x. Ascitic fluid: WBC increased absolute neutrophil count, culture results positive for a specific organism

  b. Radiologic

    i. CT: Liver volume decreased, spleen volume increased, possible presence of ascites or tumor

    ii. MRI, magnetic resonance venography, magnetic resonance arteriography, magnetic resonance cholangiopancreatography: To evaluate organs, vessels, bile ducts for abnormalities (portal vein thrombosis, liver cancer)

    iii. Abdominal ultrasonography: To determine liver and spleen sizes, portal vein patency, presence of hepatoma, bile duct dilatation, presence of small amounts of ascites

  c. ERCP: May show dilated bile ducts or beading (narrowing) of ducts

  d. Upper GI endoscopy: Reveals esophageal, gastric, and/or duodenal varices

  e. Abdominal paracentesis if ascites present: To test fluid for infection (important)

  f. Liver biopsy: For staging of inflammation and fibrosis

5. Goals of care

  a. Optimize remaining liver function.

  b. Stabilize decompensations.

6. Collaborating professionals on health care team: Physician, nurse, dietitian, laboratory technician, physical therapist, consultant (hepatologist, gastroenterologist, surgeon)

7. Management of patient care

  a. Anticipated patient trajectory: Patient with chronic liver failure may plateau before decompensation then deteriorate rapidly. Patients may be expected to have needs in the following areas:

    i. Positioning: Development of orthostatic hypotension dictates the need for slow, deliberate movements to prevent dizziness and falls. Patient with encephalopathy may not be able to coordinate thoughts and movements.

    ii. Skin care: Skin will be very dry, and there will be an increase in bruising due to reduction of the platelet count and levels of coagulation factors

    iii. Pain management: See Acute (Fulminant) Liver Failure

    iv. Nutrition: Ascites may cause early satiety; low zinc levels in liver disease may result in diminished taste or metallic taste; severe muscle wasting and malnutrition develop

    v. Infection control: Depressed immune system increases the risk of infection; presence of ascites creates the risk of peritonitis

    vi. Transport: Mobile environment increases the risk of infection; ascites creates the risk for spontaneous bacterial peritonitis

    vii. Discharge planning: Recovery periods are short, and rehospitalization can be frequent as the patient decompensates. Family and patient will need assistance with home care, rehabilitation, medications, office visits.

    viii. Pharmacology: Patient will be taking a complex regimen of medications, and alternative choices (shorter-acting drugs or drugs with shorter half-lives) and dosing patterns (every 12 hours instead of every 6 or 8 hours) will be required because of liver dysfunction

ix. Psychosocial issues: Chronicity of the situation will have a profound impact on the family unit and increase stress. Depression can occur in both the patient and primary caregiver.

x. Treatments

(a) Noninvasive: Medications

(b) Invasive: Surgery, endoscopy with esophageal variceal ligation or sclerosis, colonoscopy with cauterization, angiography with embolization

xi. Ethical issues: Lack of available organs and prolonged hospitalizations increase the risk of sepsis, which prevents transplantation and leads to discussions of withdrawal of life support

b. Potential complications

i. Portal hypertension

(a) Mechanism

(1) Increased hydrostatic pressure (higher than 10 mm Hg) within the portal venous system as a result of disruption of the normal liver architecture, which increases the resistance to blood flow into and out of the liver (25% of the cardiac output per minute)

(2) Development of esophageal varices and gastroesophageal variceal bleeding

(3) Splenomegaly: Increased size and congestion of the spleen as a result of portal hypertension, with backward venous congestion via the splenic vein, which results in pancytopenia (anemia, leukopenia, thrombocytopenia)

(b) Management

(1) Restriction on the amount of weight to be lifted (no more than 40 lb)

(2) Frequent monitoring for consequential cytopenia

(3) Use of β-blockers or scheduled endoscopic treatments

(4) Sarfeh shunts may be used for refractory bleeding.

(5) Transjugular intrahepatic portosystemic stents may be used for refractory bleeding.

ii. Ascites

(a) Mechanism: Caused by transudation of fluid from the liver surface as a result of portal and lymphatic hypertension and increased membrane permeability, which lead to increased hydrostatic pressure and decreased oncotic pressure in the portal venous system, characterized by a rise in hepatic sinusoidal pressure, excess hepatic lymph, and hypoalbuminemia

(b) Management

(1) Low-sodium diet, use of diuretics

(2) Accurate intake and output measurements

(3) Monitoring for refractory conditions (increasing ascites with increasing creatinine level)

(4) Transjugular intrahepatic portosystemic stents may be used for refractory ascites.

iii. Spontaneous bacterial peritonitis

(a) Mechanism: Result of the translocation of bacteria from GI lumens to the ascitic fluid

(b) Management

(1) Paracentesis to verify primary versus secondary peritonitis

(2) Administration of antibiotics

(3) Adjustment of diuretic therapy

iv. Malnutrition

(a) Mechanism: Reduced caloric intake, reduced synthesis of albumin by the liver, increased caloric needs

(b) Management

(1) Nutritional supplements

(2) Enteral feedings

(3) Parenteral nutrition

v.   Hepatic encephalopathy
   (a) Mechanism
      (1) Neuropsychiatric syndrome that develops when nitrogenous and other potentially toxic compounds arising from gut flora accumulate as a result of impaired transformation and elimination
      (2) Four grades of alteration of mentation (Table 8-1)

■ **TABLE 8-1**
■ ■ **Clinical Assessment of Hepatic Encephalopathy**

	Grade I	Grade II	Grade III	Grade IV
Level of consciousness	Awake	Decreased, but opens eyes spontaneously	Somnolent to semistuporous but arousable to verbal and painful stimuli; does not open eyes spontaneously	Comatose; no response to pain
Orientation	Total orientation with trivial lack of awareness then progression to disorientation	Minimal disorientation to time and place progressing to severe confusion	Complete disorientation when aroused	Coma
Intellectual functions	Mental clouding; slowness in answering questions; impaired handwriting; subtle changes in intellectual function; impaired performance on addition takes; decrease in psychometric test scores	Amnesia for past events; impaired performance on subtraction tasks; decrease in psychometric test scores	Inability to perform computations	Coma
Behavior	Forgetfulness, restlessness, irritability, untidiness, apathy, disobedience	Subtle personality changes, inappropriate behavior, decreased inhibitions	Lethargy; bizarre behavior (e.g., unprovoked rage)	Coma
Mood	Euphoria, anxiety, depression, crying	Lethargy or apathy, paranoia	Increased apathy	Coma
Neuromuscular function	Muscular incoordination, tremors, yawning, insomnia	Hypoactive reflexes, asterixis, ataxia, slurred speech	Inability to cooperate; nystagmus and Babinski's sign	Coma

HEPATIC ENCEPHALOPATHY TYPES
A. Encephalopathy associated with acute liver failure
B. Encephalopathy associated with portal-systemic bypass and/or intrinsic hepatocellular disease
C. Encephalopathy associated with cirrhosis and portal hypertension or portal systemic shunts
   Subcategory of type C
      Episodic hepatic encephalopathy subdivisions: Precipitated, spontaneous, recurrent
      Persistent hepatic encephalopathy subdivisions: Mild, severe, treatment dependent
      Minimal hepatic encephalopathy

From Ferenci P, Lockwood A, Mullen K, et al. Hepatic encephalopathy—definition, nomenclature, diagnosis, and quantification: final report of the working party at the 11th World Congresses of Gastroenterology, Vienna 1998. *Hepatology*. 2002;35:716-721.

(b) Management
(1) Neurologic monitoring for altered level of consciousness (see Chapter 4)
(2) Administration of lactulose to enhance GI motility
(3) Maintenance of airway
vi. Pulmonary complications
(a) Mechanism: Variety of pulmonary conditions develop as a result of hypoxemia, increased intrapulmonary vascular shunting, and changes in intrapleural and intra-abdominal pressures; for example, pleural effusions, hepatopulmonary syndrome (pulmonary capillary vasodilation and intrapulmonary shunts)
(b) Management: See Chapter 2
vii. Hepatorenal syndrome
(a) Mechanism: "Functional" form of acute renal failure that occurs in patients with advanced end-stage liver disease, resulting from decreased effective circulating plasma volume and the release of mediators of vasoconstriction, which cause diversion of renal blood flow
(b) Management: See Chapter 5
viii. Infection or sepsis
(a) Mechanism: Depressed immune system and breaks in the skin barrier due to monitoring needs; altered level of consciousness and risk of aspiration
(b) Management: See Chapter 9
8. **Evaluation of patient care: Optimization of liver function, neurologic function, vital signs, renal function**

Acute Pancreatitis

1. **Pathophysiology**
   a. Overview: Inflammation of the pancreas results when activated pancreatic proteases digest pancreatic tissue itself. Pancreatic secretions build up, and trypsin accumulates and activates the other pancreatic proteases. Normal defense mechanisms are overwhelmed, which results in pancreatic tissue autodigestion.
   b. Classification of pancreatitis
      i. Acute pancreatitis: Single episode characterized by abdominal pain and elevated levels of enzymes (amylase, lipase) with inflammation of the pancreas, which returns to normal after resolution of the episode
         (a) 80% of cases are related to biliary stones or alcohol use.
         (b) Mild pancreatitis does not have other organ damage or complications, and recovery is uneventful. Severe pancreatitis is characterized by impaired pancreatic function and systemic complications; recovery prone to complications.
      ii. Recurrent chronic pancreatitis: Progressive destruction of the acinar cells as a result of persistent inflammation
         (a) Classification of chronic pancreatitis: Lithogenic (chronic calcifying stones), obstructive, inflammatory, or fibrotic
         (b) Cause can be alcohol use, malnutrition, or idiopathic causes.
   c. Regardless of the initiating mechanism, acinar cell injury occurs with activation of pancreatic proenzymes to their active forms, which results in autodigestion of the pancreas.
   d. Three processes contribute to the initiation of pancreatitis.
      i. Obstruction of the pancreatic duct
      ii. Pancreatic ischemia
      iii. Premature activation of zymogens (inactive digestive enzymes), leading to premature release of active pancreatic enzymes, which begin autodigestion of the pancreas
         (a) Release of cytokines (platelet-activating factor, tumor necrosis factor, interleukin-1), which damage the pancreas
         (b) Release of kinins, which create capillary wall permeability
         (c) Pancreatic and peripancreatic edema with loss of up to 6 L of fluid into the interstitial space

(d) Release and activation of systemic inflammatory mediators (cytokines), including complement, kinins, histamine, prostaglandin, clotting factors; results in systemic effects, including systemic inflammatory response syndrome (SIRS)

(e) End results include increased vascular permeability, vasodilation, vascular stasis, and microthrombosis, with significant effects on other organ systems.

   e. Forms of acute pancreatitis

     i. Mild, edematous (interstitial pancreatitis): Accounts for 95% of cases; mortality rate is 5%; edematous pancreas with minimal or no necrotic damage; gross architecture is preserved

     ii. Severe, hemorrhagic (necrotizing pancreatitis): Accounts for 5% of cases; mortality rate is 50%

     iii. Extensive peripancreatic tissue necrosis and hemorrhage. There is necrosis of fat throughout the abdomen. Retroperitoneal hemorrhage caused by tissue necrosis or erosion of a pseudocyst into the vascular structure, vascular inflammation, and thrombus may occur.

2. Etiology and risk factors

   a. Alcoholism

   b. Obstruction of the pancreatic ducts

     i. Gallstones (biliary, pancreatic)

     ii. Structural abnormalities (duodenum-ampulla, bile ducts, pancreatic duct)

     iii. Tumor

     iv. Inflammation, infection

     v. Edema

   c. Complication of abdominal surgery or diagnostic procedure (e.g., ERCP)

   d. Abdominal trauma: Blunt or penetrating

   e. Drug toxicity: Cyclosporine, corticosteroids, azathioprine, thiazides, sulfonamides, tetracycline, estrogens

   f. Familial hyperlipidemia

   g. Chronic hyperparathyroidism, hypercalcemia

   h. Infection: *Mycoplasma, Streptococcus, Salmonella,* Paramyxovirus (mumps), cytomegalovirus, echovirus, Epstein-Barr virus, coxsackievirus, hepatitis virus

   i. Shock

3. Signs and symptoms

   a. Vary from a mild, almost asymptomatic case to a fulminant condition of massive pancreatic necrosis

   b. Abdominal pain manifested in 95% of cases

     i. Epigastric or right upper quadrant pain that is knifelike and twisting in nature; begins suddenly and reaches the apex quickly; may radiate to all abdominal quadrants and the lumbar area; associated with nausea and vomiting, low-grade fever

     ii. Diminished bowel sounds, tenderness on palpation

   c. Visceral tenderness

     i. Initial tenderness that is diffuse, caused by capsular distention and release of kinins

     ii. May cause the patient to double over, with a facial expression of pain, nausea, vomiting, pallor, diaphoresis

   d. Somatic tenderness: Extrapancreatic involvement (peritoneal, retroperitoneal)

     i. Sharp, well localized, yet can be diffuse

     ii. Accompanied by nausea, vomiting, rigid abdomen, rebound tenderness

     iii. Standard dosages of analgesics may be ineffective for pain relief.

   e. Low-grade fever

   f. Diaphoresis

   g. Anorexia, vomiting, diarrhea

   h. Dehydration

   i. Abdominal distention

   j. Jaundice; dark, foamy urine

   k. Steatorrhea: Bulky, pale, foul-smelling stools

   l. Cullen's sign: Bluish discoloration of the periumbilical area

m. Turner's sign: Bluish discoloration of the flanks

n. Peritoneal lavage reveals blood in the peritoneal cavity ("beef broth" tap).

o. Hypoactive or absent bowel sounds

p. Rebound tenderness

4. **Diagnostic study findings**

   a. Laboratory

   i.   Elevated serum amylase level that peaks between 4 and 24 hours after the onset of pancreatitis and returns to normal within 4 days; the degree of elevation does not necessarily correlate with the severity of the illness. Not a sensitive test unless done early after the onset of signs and symptoms.

   ii.   Elevated serum lipase level: Stays elevated longer than does serum amylase level

   iii. Elevated urine amylase and lipase levels: In patients with good renal function, these are better indexes of pancreatic damage than are serum levels

   iv.   Decreased serum ionized calcium level (less than 2.0 mg/dl): Calcium binds to areas of fat necrosis

   v.   Intermittently elevated serum glucose level: Indicates beta-cell involvement

   vi.   Presence of C-reactive protein

   vii. Increased trypsin level

   viii. Elevated WBC count and serum bilirubin, BUN, triglyceride levels

   ix.   Elevated serum AST, ALT, lactate dehydrogenase, alkaline phosphatase levels

   x.   Decreased albumin level

   xi.   Elevated or decreased hematocrit

   b. Radiologic

   i.   Abdominal plain film: Presence of dilated duodenum (sentinel loop) or transverse colon

   ii.   CT: Evidence of pancreatic inflammation, pseudocyst, abscess, obstruction of the pancreatic duct, peripancreatic and retroperitoneal necrosis

   iii. MRI: Similar to CT in identifying inflammation; also identifies areas of poor perfusion and debris in fluid collections

   iv.   Ultrasonography: Evidence of diffuse pancreatic enlargement, pseudocyst, or abscess, or presence of gallstones, bile duct dilatation

   c. ERCP: Not accurate for the diagnosis of acute pancreatitis but can provide evidence of biliary or pancreatic stones. Early ERCP with sphincterotomy and stone extraction may ameliorate the course of biliary pancreatitis.

5. **Goals of care**

   a. Optimize pancreatic function.

   b. Minimize complications.

6. **Collaborating professionals on health care team: Physician, nurse, dietitian, laboratory technician, physical therapist, consultant (gastroenterologist, surgeon), pain management team**

7. **Management of patient care**

   a. Anticipated patient trajectory: May be variable, with improvements, plateaus, decompensations, then rapid deterioration. Relapses may occur after weeks of improvements. Patients may be expected to have needs in the following areas:

   i.   Positioning: For patient comfort

   ii.   Skin care: Prevention of excoriation due to fistula drainage; keep clean and dry

   iii. Pain management: Essential, as there can be severe pain affecting multiple other organ systems. Consultation with a pain management team is necessary, because certain narcotics will affect the pancreatic sphincters.

   iv.   Nutrition: Patient will need to be on nothing-by-mouth (NPO) status initially, sometimes for weeks, which necessitates the use of total parenteral nutrition (TPN) or lower elemental enteral feedings. Enteral feeding is safe and cost-effective and is associated with fewer septic and metabolic complications.

   v.   Infection control: Depressed immune system increases the risk of infection. Pain may lead to shallow respirations and atelectasis or pneumonia. Pleural effusions may become infected.

     vi. Transport: Frequent diagnostic testing increases the risk of infection and catheter dislodgment

     vii. Discharge planning: Recovery periods are prolonged, and rehospitalizations occur; patient will need assistance with home care, rehabilitation, medications, frequent office visits

     viii. Pharmacology: Patient will be taking a complex regimen of medications, and alternative drug choices and dosing patterns will be necessary because of the potential for liver and kidney dysfunction

     ix. Psychosocial issues: Chronicity of the illness will increase the stress on the family unit. Depression may occur in both the patient and primary caregiver.

     x. Treatments
        (a) Noninvasive: Medications
        (b) Invasive: Surgery

     xi. Ethical issues: Need for ongoing care with the use of multiple resources over very long periods, withdrawal of life support due to inability to prevent or resolve multiple organ failure

  b. Potential complications

     i. Local complications: Wound infections and skin breakdown in the area of wounds, incisions, and fistulas
        (a) Mechanism: Pancreatic enzymes autodigest body tissues they contact, which leads to fistula formation, and increased skin breakdown
        (b) Management
            (1) Keep skin clean and dry.
            (2) Use ostomy bags or drains to minimize drainage contact with skin.

     ii. Hypovolemia
        (a) Mechanism: Massive third-spacing of fluids may result in fluid collections, necrosis, pseudocysts, abscesses, fistulas, intestinal obstruction
        (b) Management: See Chapter 5

     iii. SIRS and sepsis
        (a) Mechanism: Can develop when peripancreatic or ascitic fluid collections become infected and spread through areas of necrosis
        (b) Management: See Chapter 9

     iv. Multiple organ dysfunction syndrome (MODS)
        (a) Mechanism: Result of sepsis in the setting of an abscess or necrotizing pancreatitis
        (b) Management: See Chapter 9

     v. Adult respiratory distress syndrome (ARDS)
        (a) Mechanism: Respiratory failure in the setting of sepsis, which leads to increased $\dot{V}/\dot{Q}$ mismatch, decreased compliance
        (b) Management: See Chapter 2

     vi. Acute renal tubular necrosis, acute renal failure
        (a) Mechanism: Hypotension, inadequate preload, use of nephrotoxic antibiotics, vasoconstriction from vasoactive medications
        (b) Management: See Chapter 5

     vii. Disseminated intravascular coagulation
        (a) Mechanism: Due to sepsis, hypotension, elevated cytokine levels
        (b) Management: See Chapter 7

     viii. Pain
        (a) Mechanism: Pancreatitis is usually described by patients as the worse pain they have ever had. This can be due to gallstones or to the inflammation of the tissues where autodigestion is occurring.
        (b) Management (see also the discussion of pain in Chapters 4 and 10): Administration of analgesics and use of nonpharmacologic pain treatments (distraction, imagery)

8. Evaluation of patient care

  a. Normalization of pancreatic functions, vital signs, digestive function

  b. Relief of pain

Gastrointestinal Bleeding

1. **Pathophysiology**
   a. Peptic ulcer disease
      i. Both duodenal and gastric ulcers are classified as peptic ulcers. The mucosal lining of the stomach and duodenum is digested by pepsin and acid, which causes ulcerations, due to either an imbalance between acid and pepsin production or the loss of the protective factors of bicarbonate, mucus, and cell renewal in the affected mucosa.
      ii. In duodenal ulcers there is an oversecretion of acid. In gastric ulcers there is a reduction in the gastric mucosal barrier caused by decreased mucosal blood flow, altered cellular renewal, reduction in mucus secretion, bacterial infection, or damaging agents.
      iii. Infection with *Helicobacter pylori,* a bacterium, contributes to the development of gastric ulcers; a high incidence of colonization with *H. pylori* is found in people with gastric ulcers.
   b. Variceal bleeding: Esophageal varices develop in 50% of patients with alcoholic cirrhosis within 2 years of their diagnosis. Esophageal variceal hemorrhage accounts for one third of deaths in patients with cirrhosis and portal hypertension. The mortality rate is 30% to 50% for each episode of bleeding.
      i. Portal circulation is high flow (approximately 1100 ml/min) with low pressure (about 7 mm Hg); an increase in resistance (either intrahepatic or extrahepatic) to blood flow in this system results in portal hypertension.
      ii. Spontaneous rupture and bleeding occur when the portosystemic gradient is higher than 12 mm Hg, which causes the formation of varices in collateral venous channels between the portal and systemic circulation.
      iii. Varices in the distal esophagus and at the esophagogastric junction are the most prone to bleeding; however, varices can also form in the peritoneum, retroperitoneum, and throughout the GI tract, including the rectum (Figure 8-7).

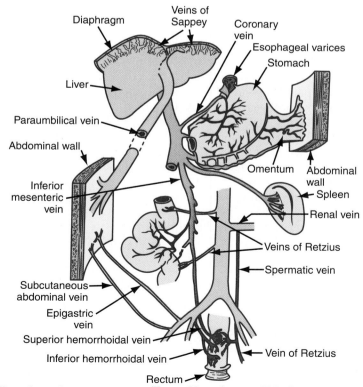

FIGURE 8-7 ■ Collateral circulation in the liver. (From Krumberger JM. Gastrointestinal disorders. In: Kinney MR, Packa DR, Dunbar SB, eds. *AACN's Clinical Reference for Critical-care Nursing.* St Louis, MO: Mosby; 1993:1149.)

    c. Other causes of upper GI bleeding

        i. Mallory-Weiss syndrome: Tear in the mucosa or submucosa at the gastroesophageal junction. Tear is usually longitudinal, caused by forceful or prolonged vomiting; 75% of cases occur in males with a history of excessive alcohol ingestion or salicylate use.

        ii. Esophagitis

        iii. Stress ulcers (gastric, duodenal): Extremely common in critically ill patients; associated with sepsis, shock, burns, trauma, acute head injuries, renal failure, hepatic failure, ARDS, mechanical ventilation, and major operative procedures; characterized by mucosal ischemia that leads to alterations that result in the loss of protective functions

    d. Causes of lower GI bleeding

        i. Crohn's disease: Less common, usually due to deep ulceration in the colon

        ii. Ulcerative colitis: Can cause exsanguination due to diffuse ulceration

        iii. Colitis resulting from ischemia, radiation, chemotherapy

        iv. Diverticula: Most common cause of acute massive colonic blood loss

        v. Intestinal polyps: Intermittent or occult bleeding

        vi. Angiodysplasia (arteriovenous malformation of the mucosa): Common cause of chronic or intermittent low-grade bleeding in aged patients

        vii. Hemorrhoids

2. Etiology and risk factors

    a. Gastric ulcers associated with decreased tissue resistance; three to four times more common in men; associated with malignancy; may lead to nonhealing ulcer in stomach

    b. Duodenal ulcers associated with increased hydrochloric acid level

        i. Most frequent sites are the pylorus and the first portion of the duodenum.

        ii. Can occur at any age; common among young adults

        iii. Seem to have a seasonal trend, with higher incidence in the spring and fall

        iv. Pharmacologic agents may play a role: Salicylates, indomethacin, phenylbutazone, nonsteroidal anti-inflammatory drugs (NSAIDs), corticosteroids, antineoplastic agents, vasopressors, reserpine

        v. Caffeine use, alcohol abuse, cigarette smoking

        vi. Familial tendency

    c. Variceal bleeding is associated with portal hypertension.

        i. Prehepatic (presinusoidal) factors in which the wedge hepatic venous pressure is less than the portal pressure: Portal vein thrombosis due to the presence of cirrhosis, hepatoma, umbilical vein catheterization in infancy, or hypercoagulable state

        ii. Intrahepatic (sinusoidal) factors in which the wedge hepatic venous pressure is increased and equals the portal pressure: Postnecrotic cirrhosis (e.g., chronic active hepatitis and cirrhosis), alcoholic cirrhosis

        iii. Posthepatic (postsinusoidal) factors in which the site of obstruction to flow is distal to the sinusoids: Hepatic vein thrombosis (e.g., Budd-Chiari syndrome), veno-occlusive disease after bone marrow transplantation

        iv. Diseases causing portal hypertension: Splenomegaly or splenic vein thrombosis not due to liver disease; fulminant hepatitis; cirrhosis of various causes; metastatic carcinoma; diseases of the hepatic venules, veins, or inferior vena cava; cardiac diseases

3. Signs and symptoms

    a. Ulcers

        i. Epigastric pain with bleeding: Heartburn; with duodenal ulcers, pain is relieved by food; pain stops when bleeding begins

        ii. Nausea, vomiting

        iii. Hematemesis (blood is bright red or resembles coffee grounds)

        iv. Melena

        v. Weight loss

        vi. Abdominal tenderness, guarding

        vii. Hyperactive bowel sounds

        viii. Orthostatic hypotension

        ix. Narrow pulse pressure

    b. Esophageal varices

        i. Sudden onset of hematemesis (may be projectile): Coffee-ground vomitus or bright red blood

        ii. Coagulopathy: Prolonged PT, increased INR, decreased platelet count

        iii. Hyperdynamic circulation: Increased cardiac output, decreased systemic vascular resistance, systolic ejection murmur

        iv. Hemodynamic changes: Decreased pulse pressure, orthostatic hypotension, tachycardia

        v. Increased minute ventilation

        vi. Lethargy, malaise

        vii. Pale skin and/or mucous membranes

4. Diagnostic study findings

    a. Laboratory

        i. Hemoglobin level, hematocrit: Decreased; true extent of blood loss may not be immediately apparent

        ii. BUN level: May be elevated

        iii. PT, INR: Prolonged PT, increased INR

        iv. Albumin: May be decreased

        v. Platelet count: May be decreased in cirrhosis

        vi. Blood tests or stomach biopsy: To detect colonization by *H. pylori*

        vii. Guaiac testing of nasogastric drainage and stool for occult blood

    b. Radiologic

        i. Upright chest radiography or upright and lateral abdominal radiography: Shows free air under the diaphragm with perforated, bleeding ulcers

        ii. Upper GI series: To localize an ulcer

        iii. Selective mesenteric angiography: To localize the site of bleeding when endoscopy cannot be performed

        iv. Upper GI endoscopy: To reveal the location of an ulcer, rule out other causes of bleeding

            (a) Differential diagnosis for variceal bleeding is complex and includes peptic ulcer disease, gastritis, Mallory-Weiss tear of the esophagus, and Boerhaave's syndrome, among others.

            (b) Definitive identification is made by endoscopic examination of the esophagus, stomach, and duodenum and/or colonoscopy.

            (c) During endoscopy it is possible to grade and classify esophageal, gastric, and/or duodenal varices according to size, location, and risk factors.

        v. Superior mesenteric artery arteriography: To measure hepatic vein pressure gradient and to image the portal and hepatic venous systems

        vi. Angiography: To evaluate blood flow, identify the source of bleeding; can be used to embolize a vessel

        vii. CT: To document cirrhosis, identify the presence of collateral circulation, and rule out hepatoma

        viii. Doppler ultrasonography: To evaluate patency of and flow in the portal vein and hepatic veins

    c. Nasogastric intubation: To obtain gastric aspirate

5. Goals of care

    a. Minimize blood loss; replenish losses.

    b. Optimize hemodynamic status.

    c. Restore circulating blood volume.

    d. Provide pain relief.

6. Collaborating professionals on health care team: Physician, nurse, dietitian, laboratory technician, consultant (gastroenterologist, surgeon)

7. Management of patient care

    a. Anticipated patient trajectory: Once bleeding is halted, rapid stabilization is possible. If it is difficult to halt the hemorrhage, then the patient course is more problematic. Patients may be expected to have needs in the following areas:

i. Positioning: Head of the bed raised to prevent aspiration; the patient may need to lie on the side to minimize the risk of aspiration

ii. Skin care: Prevention of breakdown due to lower GI bleeding or decreased skin perfusion; keep clean and dry

iii. Pain management: Gastric ulcer pain may be sharp or dull and may worsen with food consumption. Proton pump inhibitors and pain medication may reduce the discomfort as the ulcer heals. Aspirin and other NSAIDs should be avoided because they may worsen the condition. Pain management is individualized depending on comorbidities (encephalopathy, renal failure).

iv. Nutrition: Patient will need to be on NPO status because of bleeding; depending on the duration and cause; the use of TPN or lower elemental enteral feedings may be necessary

v. Infection control: Depressed immune system increases the risk of infection if surgery is performed; risk of aspiration is significant

vi. Transport: A significant amount of the treatment can be done at the bedside, which will minimize the need for transport

vii. Discharge planning: Recovery periods may be either short or prolonged, depending on the cause of the bleeding and comorbidities; this may be a new diagnosis requiring increased patient and family education

viii. Pharmacology: Patients will be taking few medications unless infection ensues. Most medications will be related to treatment of the primary cause of the bleeding and prevention of complications. If shock is prolonged, dosing will need to be altered for liver or kidney dysfunction.

ix. Psychosocial issues: Acute nature of the situation will have a profound impact on the family unit and increase stress

x. Treatments
   (a) Noninvasive: Medications
   (b) Invasive: Surgery, variceal ligation or cautery via endoscopy, cautery via colonoscopy, embolization via angiography

xi. Ethical issues: Blood replacement (against some religious views), advance directives

b. Potential complications
   i. Hypovolemia
      (a) Mechanism: Can occur as a result of massive third-spacing of fluids or hemorrhage
      (b) Management
         (1) Third-spacing: Rapid replacement of fluids
         (2) Hemorrhaging: Administration of blood products, use of a Minnesota tube
         (3) Either third-spacing or hemorrhaging: Use of vasoactive medications; accurate and rapid recording of intake and output
         (4) GI surgery for gastric ulcers or refractory variceal bleeding
   ii. Aspiration
      (a) Mechanism: Vomiting of blood or GI contents, hypotension, or encephalopathy prevents the ability to protect the airway and can result in aspiration, which may lead to bacterial pneumonia
      (b) Management: See Chapter 2
   iii. Acute renal tubular necrosis, acute renal failure
      (a) Mechanism: Prolonged hypotension, use of vasoactive medications or nephrotoxic antibiotics
      (b) Management: See Chapter 5

8. **Evaluation of patient care**
   a. Normalization of GI functions, neurologic function, vital signs, and renal function
   b. Cessation or control of GI bleeding

Hepatitis

1. **Pathophysiology: Acute inflammation of the entire liver, characterized on biopsy specimens by centrilobular necrosis and infiltration of the portal tracts by leukocytes. May be a multisystem infection involving many organs: Regional lymphadenopathy, splenomegaly,**

ulceration of the GI tract, acute pancreatitis, myocarditis, **serum sickness, vasculitis, and nephritis.**

2. **Etiology and risk factors**
   a. Causes may be viral, drug related, or autoimmune.
   b. Less acute forms can produce subacute hepatic necrosis or cholestatic liver disease, or can silently progress to cirrhosis.
   c. Multiple viruses cause hepatitis in humans.
      i. Hepatitis A virus infection (formerly called infectious hepatitis)
         (a) RNA virus infection that occurs sporadically or endemically
         (b) Fecal-oral transmission; can also be transmitted by ingestion of raw or under-cooked shellfish contaminated by sewage dumped into the ocean
         (c) Usually self-limiting
      ii. Hepatitis B virus infection (formerly called serum hepatitis)
         (a) In infected individuals, DNA virus is present in all body secretions.
         (b) Transmission
            (1) Mother-to-neonate vertical transmission
            (2) Homosexual and heterosexual transmission
            (3) Parenteral transmission (intravenous drug abuse, transfusion of blood or blood products, hemodialysis, exposure to contaminated equipment, body piercings, razors)
         (c) Associated with hepatitis delta virus (hepatitis D virus, an RNA virus), a small RNA particle that is unable to replicate on its own but is capable of infection when in the presence of hepatitis B virus (hepatitis B surface antigen needed)
      iii. Hepatitis C virus infection (formerly called non-A, non-B hepatitis)
         (a) RNA virus
         (b) Transmission
            (1) Parenteral transmission (intravenous drug abuse, nasal cocaine use, transfusion of blood or blood products, hemodialysis, body piercings, razors, toothbrush sharing, acupuncture, health care exposure)
            (2) Sexual and maternal: Low frequency of transmission to neonate (5% to 12% risk of vertical transmission)
            (3) Accounts for more than 90% of posttransfusion hepatitis
      iv. Hepatitis D virus infection
         (a) Single-stranded RNA virus
         (b) Worldwide distribution
         (c) Requires presence of hepatitis B virus to establish infection
         (d) Transmitted parenterally and as a coinfection with hepatitis B; may lead to fulminant hepatitis
      v. Hepatitis E virus infection
         (a) RNA virus
         (b) Epidemiology and clinical course similar to those of hepatitis A
         (c) Most prevalent among young adults
      vi. All viruses in the herpesvirus family (herpes simplex, cytomegalovirus, Epstein-Barr virus, varicella-zoster virus)
   d. Autoimmune hepatitis
      i. Idiopathic hepatitis characterized by chronic inflammation and plasma cells in liver tissue, autoantibodies, and increased serum globulin levels
      ii. Predominance in women aged 30 to 45 years
      iii. Associated with four antibodies: ANA, anti–smooth muscle antibodies (ASMA), ANCA, anti-LKM
   e. Drug-related hepatitis
      i. Form of drug allergy in which the immune response is directed toward the liver cells, causing necrosis that affects a particular region of the liver lobule (e.g., acetaminophen causes centrilobular necrosis)
      ii. Severe reaction produces diffuse necrosis and/or cholestasis.
      iii. Prognosis is variable.

  f. Categories (or types) of hepatitis
   i. Acute hepatitis: Acute onset of inflammation, usually self-limiting
   ii. Acute fulminant hepatitis
   iii. Asymptomatic carrier state (viral hepatitis)
    (a) Infected person is unable to clear hepatitis antigen because of ineffective cellular immunity.
    (b) Carrier is able to transmit hepatitis to others but suffers no liver damage.
   iv. Chronic hepatitis
    (a) Hepatitis antigen, chronic liver inflammation, and viral replication persist for at least 6 months.
    (b) Progressive liver damage may develop into cirrhosis.
3. Signs and symptoms
  a. Anicteric (not jaundiced) cases: Usually asymptomatic except for flulike symptoms; occasionally hepatomegaly, splenomegaly, and lymphadenopathy may occur
  b. Icteric cases (small proportion of cases)
   i. Prodromal period associated with not feeling well: Malaise, fatigue
   ii. Subsidence of symptoms with the onset of jaundice
   iii. Among smokers and drinkers, loss of the desire to smoke or drink
   iv. Dark urine, followed by lightening of the urine
   v. Fever, nausea, vomiting, diarrhea
   vi. Hepatomegaly, splenomegaly
4. Diagnostic study findings
  a. Laboratory
   i. Increased WBC count, serum total bilirubin level
   ii. Increased levels of ALT, AST, and, to a lesser degree, alkaline phosphatase and GGT
   iii. Positive results on hepatitis serologic testing (Table 8-2)
   iv. Presence of autoimmune markers: ANA, ASMA, ANCA, anti-LKM
  b. Radiologic: Ultrasonography may show hepatomegaly or splenomegaly, or give normal results
5. Goals of care
  a. Minimize symptoms.
  b. Optimize liver function and functional status.
  c. Restore physical and mental energy.
6. Collaborating professionals on health care team: Physician, nurse, dietitian, laboratory technician, consultant (hepatologist)
7. Management of patient care
  a. Anticipated patient trajectory: Can be a slow recovery with symptomatic irritations; however, some will progress to fulminant liver failure or cirrhosis. Patients may be expected to have needs in the following areas:
   i. Skin care: Prevention of breakdown due to pruritus caused by deposition of bile salts, dryness, itching
   ii. Pain management: Avoid acetaminophen as well as aspirin and other NSAIDs in severe cases of hepatitis
   iii. Nutrition: If disease is severe, nutritional supplements may be required
   iv. Discharge planning: Recovery periods occur after prolonged illness without relapse. If the disease is fulminant, the hospital course may vary from long hospitalization to liver transplantation.
   v. Pharmacology: Caution required with medications because of decreased liver function and possible renal impairment
   vi. Psychosocial issues: In the acute or chronic state, the psychosocial issues may involve body image and intimacy issues (fear of transmission); however, the acute nature of fulminant hepatitis will have a profound impact on the family unit and increase stress. If this is a new condition, there may be significant educational needs and complex treatment decisions.
   vii. Treatments: Medications, transplantation
   viii. Ethical issues: Social stigma related to disease etiology

■ **TABLE 8-2**
■ ■ **Serologic Testing for Viral Hepatitis**

Serologic Test	Description and Purpose
HEPATITIS A VIRUS (HAV)	
HAV total antibody	Presence in serum confers lifelong immunity
HAV IgM	Level rises early during infection (detectable at 3-4 wk after exposure and just before liver test values become elevated); indicates acute infection; returns to normal in approximately 8 wk
HAV IgG	Level rises slowly during infection (detectable at 6-12 wk after exposure and persists for more than 10 yr after infection)
HEPATITIS B VIRUS (HBV)	
HBsAg	HBV *surface* antigen; most commonly used marker for HBV infection; detectable within 30 days of exposure and persists up to 3 mo after jaundice appears unless a carrier state develops, in which case it will persist longer; presence in serum (seropositivity) indicates active HBV infection
Anti-HBs	Antibody to HBsAg; presence in serum (seropositivity) indicates HBV immunity due to HBV infection or vaccination; detectable 4-12 wk after HBsAg disappears
HBeAg	HBV *e* antigen; found only in sera positive for HBsAg; presence in serum (seropositivity) indicates high titer of HBV (extensive viral replication) and increased infectiousness (ongoing viral replication); detectable 4-6 wk after exposure; persistence of this marker in blood predicts development of chronic HBV infection
HBcAg	HBV *core* antigen; not detectable in serum, detectable only in hepatocytes
Anti-HBc (total)	Antibody to HBcAg; detectable 3-12 wk after exposure during what is referred to as the "window phase" (after HBsAg disappears but before antibody to HBsAg appears)
HBV DNA	HBV DNA detected by process of nucleic acid hybridization
PCR for HBV DNA	Test detects polymerase-containing virions; PCR process amplifies DNA in blood so that it is easily detected; very sensitive test
HEPATITIS C VIRUS (HCV)	
HCVAb	Antibody to HCV; presence in serum (seropositivity) is diagnostic for chronic infection only; absence (seronegativity) does not exclude the diagnosis of HCV infection; false-positive results may occur
HCV RNA	HCV RNA detected by process of nucleic acid hybridization; presence in serum is diagnostic of viremia in acute or chronic HCV hepatitis; test also used to monitor response to interferon-α therapy
HCV genotype	Test identifies six different genotypes and several subtypes of the virus; used to determine appropriate treatment options and durations
PCR for HCV RNA	Detects polymerase-containing virions; PCR process amplifies RNA in blood so that it is easily detected; very sensitive test
bDNA	Quantitative test of HCV RNA for determining amount of virus; research assay not yet licensed by the Food and Drug Administration
HEPATITIS D VIRUS (HDV; HEPATITIS DELTA VIRUS)	
HDAg (total)	HDV antigen; detectable only concurrently with HBV infection
HDV IgM	Level rises early in infection; if persistent, may indicate chronic infection
HDV IgG	Level rises slowly during infection; persists for life
HDVAb	Antibody to HDV; detectable only concurrently with HBV infection
HDV RNA	Detected by process of nucleic acid hybridization
HEPATITIS E VIRUS (HEV)	
PCR for HEV RNA	Detects polymerase-containing virions; PCR process amplifies RNA in blood so that it is easily detected; very sensitive test

From Pagana KD, Pagana TM. *Mosby's Manual of Diagnostic and Laboratory Tests.* 2nd ed. St Louis, MO: Mosby; 2002.
IgG, Immunoglobulin G; *IgM,* immunoglobulin M; *PCR,* polymerase chain reaction test.

   b. Potential complications
       i. Cirrhosis (see Chronic Liver Failure)
       ii. Ascites (see Chronic Liver Failure)
       iii. Encephalopathy (see prior coverage and Chapter 4)
       iv. Increased ICP (see Chapter 4)
       v. Liver failure (see Acute [Fulminant] Liver Failure)
       vi. Infection or sepsis (see Chapter 9)
       vii. Renal failure (see Chapter 4)
       viii. Liver cancer (see prior coverage)
       ix. Malnutrition (see prior coverage)
8. Evaluation of patient care
   a. Normalization of liver function, neurologic function, vital signs, renal function
   b. Increased mental and physical energy

Inflammatory Bowel Disease

1. Pathophysiology
   a. Crohn's disease
       i. Chronic transmural inflammation of the digestive tract that can involve one or more areas of any portion of the GI tract from the mouth to the anus
       ii. Ileum, colon, perianal area most common sites of inflammation
       iii. Extraintestinal organs may be affected.
       iv. Incurable condition associated with relapses and remissions
       v. Inflammation begins in the intestinal mucosa and spreads inward and outward to involve the mucosa and serosa. Bowel becomes congested, thickened, and rigid, with adhesions. Edema and thickening of the muscularis mucosae may narrow the lumen of the involved colon.
       vi. Fistulas, abscesses, and perforation may occur.
   b. Ulcerative colitis
       i. Idiopathic inflammation involving the mucosa of the colon
       ii. Inflammation is continuous and circumferential; begins in the rectum and progresses proximally toward the cecum.
       iii. Inflammation begins at the base of the crypts of Lieberkühn; small erosions form and coalesce into ulcers, followed by abscess formation, necrosis, and ragged ulcerations of the mucosa.
2. Etiology and risk factors
   a. Crohn's disease
       i. Cigarette smoking, NSAID use
       ii. Exact etiology unknown; possible causes include bacterial, viral, allergic, autoimmune, and hereditary factors
       iii. Prevalence equal in men and women; most common age at onset is 10 to 30 years
       iv. Other concurrent autoimmune disorders common
       v. Familial predisposition
       vi. Increased suppressor T-cell activity and alterations in IgA production
   b. Ulcerative colitis
       i. Etiology unknown: Genetic, infectious, and immunologic factors suspected
       ii. Other concurrent autoimmune disorders common
       iii. Prevalence higher among women, especially those of Jewish descent; onset usually between 10 and 40 years of age
3. Signs and symptoms
   a. Crohn's disease
       i. Pain: Initially, a constant right-sided pain that mimics appendicitis; later, crampy abdominal pain most often associated with eating
       ii. Meals omitted to avoid pain; weight loss, malnutrition, cachexia
       iii. Nausea and vomiting, watery diarrhea, steatorrhea, anal excoriation or fistula
       iv. Arthralgias, malaise, fever
       v. Aphthous ulcers of the lips and mouth

      vi. Vitamin B_{12} deficiency (when the ileum is involved)

      vii. Metabolic bone disease

  b. Ulcerative colitis

      i. Sensation of rectal urgency

      ii. Crampy abdominal pain and tenderness, hypertympanic abdomen

      iii. Bloody, purulent, watery diarrhea: Up to 30 stools per day

      iv. Weight loss, cachexia, orthostasis

      v. Vomiting, dehydration, fever

      vi. Extracolonic manifestations such as anemia, arthritis, hepatic dysfunction

4. Diagnostic study findings

  a. Crohn's disease

      i. Laboratory

         (a) Decreased hemoglobin level, hematocrit, potassium level, serum albumin level

         (b) Increased WBC count, alkaline phosphatase level

         (c) Occult blood in stool

      ii. Radiologic: "String sign" (irregular narrowing of the distal ileum) on abdominal radiograph

      iii. Sigmoidoscopy: Inflammation of the intestinal mucosa and surrounding musculature, as well as longitudinal and transverse ulcers (cobblestoning) and stenosis of the intestinal lumen

      iv. Colonoscopy: To determine the extent of disease

      v. Rectal biopsy: Inflammation of the intestinal mucosa and surrounding musculature

  b. Ulcerative colitis

      i. Laboratory

         (a) Decreased hemoglobin level, hematocrit, potassium level, serum albumin level

         (b) Increased WBC count, alkaline phosphatase level

         (c) Occult blood in stool

      ii. Radiologic: Abdominal radiograph reveals crypt abscess, mucosal ulcerations, dilated loops of bowel

      iii. Proctosigmoidoscopy: Shows diffuse erythema, mucosal inflammation, loss of vascular network, mucosal bleeding

5. Goals of care

  a. Crohn's disease

      i. Optimize GI function.

      ii. Restore and maintain nutritional status.

      iii. Relieve symptoms.

  b. Ulcerative colitis

      i. Minimize complications.

      ii. Restore and maintain nutritional status.

      iii. Optimize colon function.

6. Collaborating professionals on health care team: Physician, nurse, dietitian, laboratory technician, consultant (gastroenterologist, surgeon)

7. Management of patient care (for both Crohn's disease and ulcerative colitis)

  a. Anticipated patient trajectory: These are chronic condition with exacerbations. Patients may be expected to have needs in the following areas:

      i. Positioning: Position of comfort; usually the head of the bed is raised

      ii. Skin care: Prevention of breakdown due to diarrhea; keep clean and dry

      iii. Pain management: Will be individualized; antidiarrheal agents and anticholinergics to ease cramping

      iv. Nutrition: Each patient will have variations in nutritional intake; high-fiber, low-sugar diet and adjustment for food allergies such as milk or yeast allergies

      v. Infection control: Perforation or ulceration risk

      vi. Discharge planning: Chronicity of these conditions may result in frequent rehospitalizations for exacerbations

      vii. Pharmacology: Patients will be taking a variety of medications to control symptoms, such as antidiarrheal agents, anticholinergics, vitamin supplements

      viii. Psychosocial issues: Chronic nature of these diseases and their impact on the patient's social structure may lead to isolation and may significantly affect the family unit and increase stress

      ix. Ethical issues: Advance directives

  b. Potential complications

      i. Crohn's disease

        (a) Acute complications

          (1) Toxic megacolon (loss of contractility and massive dilatation of colon)

          (2) GI hemorrhage

          (3) Perforation of the ileum

          (4) Bowel obstruction

        (b) Chronic complications

          (1) Rheumatoid arthritis

          (2) Sclerosing cholangitis

          (3) Urinary calculi

          (4) Iron-deficiency anemia

      ii. Ulcerative colitis

        (a) Toxic megacolon: Associated with fulminant disease

        (b) Friable colon

        (c) Increased risk of colon cancer

        (d) SIRS and sepsis: Can develop if the colon perforates

      iii. Management

        (a) Crohn's disease

          (1) Monitor for infections or peritonitis.

          (2) Check the stool for pus, blood.

          (3) Keep an accurate record of intake and output to optimize nutritional status.

          (4) Optimize bowel function; minimize episodes of diarrhea, abdominal pain.

          (5) Administer medications as ordered.

        (b) Ulcerative colitis

          (1) Monitor for exacerbation of symptoms.

          (2) Keep accurate intake and output measurements.

          (3) Monitor electrolyte, hemoglobin levels.

          (4) Optimize nutritional status.

          (5) Administer medications as ordered.

8. Evaluation of patient care: Optimization of GI functions

REFERENCES AND BIBLIOGRAPHY

Physiologic Anatomy

Blumberg RS, Stenson WF. The immune system and gastrointestinal inflammation. In: Yamada T, ed. *Textbook of Gastroenterology*. Vol 1. 4th ed. Philadelphia, PA: Lippincott Williams & Wilkins; 2003.

Furness JB, Clerc N, Vogalis F, et al. The enteric nervous system and its extrinsic connections. In: Yamada T, ed. *Textbook of Gastroenterology*. Vol 1. 4th ed. Philadelphia, PA: Lippincott Williams & Wilkins; 2003.

McCance KL, Huether SE. *Pathophysiology: The Biologic Basis for Disease in Adults and Children*. 5th ed. St Louis, MO: Mosby; 2005.

Stacy KM. Gastrointestinal anatomy and physiology. In: Urden LD, Stacy KM, Lough ME, eds. *Thelan's Critical Care Nursing*. 5th ed. St Louis, MO: Mosby; 2006.

Patient Assessment

Nakamura T, Terano A. Capsule endoscopy: past, present, and future. *J Gastroenterol*. 2008;43(2): 93-99.

Stacy KM. Gastrointestinal clinical assessment and diagnostic procedures. In: Urden LD, Stacy KM, Lough ME, eds. *Thelan's Critical Care Nursing*. 5th ed. St Louis, MO:, Mosby; 2006.

Acute Abdomen

Chan FK, Leung WK. Peptic ulcer disease. *Lancet*. 2002;360:933-942.

Johnson LR. Secretion. In: Johnson LR, ed. *Essential Medical Physiology*. 3rd ed. Amsterdam, The Netherlands: Academic Press; 2003.

Langell JT, Mulvihill SJ. Gastrointestinal perforation and the acute abdomen. *Med Clin North Am*. 2008;92(3):599-625.

Miller SK, Alpert PT. Assessment and differential diagnosis of abdominal pain. *Nurse Pract.* 2006;31(7):38-47.

Acute (Fulminant) Liver Failure

Blei AT. Portal hypertension and its complications. *Curr Opin Gastroenterol.* 2007;23(3):275-282.

Bureau C, Garcia-Pagan JC, Otal P, et al. Improved clinical outcome using polytetrafluoroethylene-coated stents for TIPS: results of a randomized study. *Gastroenterology.* 2004;126(2):469-475.

Ferenci P, Lockwood A, Mullen K, et al. Hepatic encephalopathy—definition, nomenclature, diagnosis, and quantification: final report of the working party at the 11th World Congresses of Gastroenterology, Vienna 1998. *Hepatology.* 2002;35:716-721.

Garcia-Tsao G. Portal hypertension. *Curr Opin Gastroenterol.* 2006;22(3):254-262.

Hayes PC, Simpson KJ. Approach to the patient with fulminant (acute) liver failure. In: Yamada T, ed. *Textbook of Gastroenterology.* Vol 2. 4th ed. Philadelphia, PA: Lippincott Williams & Wilkins; 2003.

Jones DE. Pathogenesis of primary biliary cirrhosis. *Postgrad Med J.* 2008;84(987):23-33.

Qureshi W, Adler DG, Davila R, et al. ASGE guideline: the role of endoscopy in the management of variceal hemorrhage. *Gastrointest Endosc.* 2005;62(5):651-655.

Sargent S. Hepatic nursing. Pathophysiology and management of hepatic encephalopathy. *Br J Nurs.* 2007;16(6):335-339.

Schuppan D, Afdhal NH. Liver cirrhosis. *Lancet.* 2008;371(9615):838-851.

Chronic Liver Failure: Decompensated Cirrhosis

Bureau C, Garcia-Pagan JC, Otal P, et al. Improved clinical outcome using polytetrafluoroethylene-coated stents for TIPS: results of a randomized study. *Gastroenterology.* 2004;126(2):469-475.

Dib N, Oberti F, Cales P. Current management of the complications of portal hypertension: variceal bleeding and ascites. *CMAJ.* 2006;174(10):1433-1443.

Dove LM, Wright TL. Chronic viral hepatitis. In: Friedman LS, Keefe EB, eds. *Handbook of Liver Disease.* Philadelphia, PA: Elsevier; 2002.

Ferenci P, Lockwood A, Mullen K, et al. Hepatic encephalopathy—definition, nomenclature, diagnosis, and quantification: final report of the working party at the 11th World Congresses of Gastroenterology, Vienna 1998. *Hepatology.* 2002;35:716-721.

Heidelbaugh JJ, Bruderly M. Cirrhosis and chronic liver failure: part I. Diagnosis and evaluation. *Am Fam Physician.* 2006;74(5):756-762.

Heidelbaugh JJ, Bruderly M. Cirrhosis and chronic liver failure: part II. Complications and treatment. *Am Fam Physician.* 2006;74(5):767-776.

Qureshi W, Adler DG, Davila R, et al. ASGE guideline: the role of endoscopy in the management of variceal hemorrhage. *Gastrointest Endosc.* 2005;62(5):651-655.

Tripathi D, Redhead D. Transjugular intrahepatic portosystemic stent-shunt: technical factors and new developments. *Eur J Gastroenterol.* 2006;18(11):1127-1133.

Acute Pancreatitis

Carroll JK, Herrick B, Gipson T, Lee SP. Acute pancreatitis: diagnosis, prognosis, and treatment. *Am Fam Physician.* 2007;75(10):1513-1520.

Cothren C, Burch JM. Acute pancreatitis. In: Harken AH, Moore EE, eds. *Abernathy's Surgical Secrets: Questions and Answers Reveal the Secrets to Successful Surgery.* 5th ed. Philadelphia, PA: Hanley & Belfus; 2004.

Gourgiotis S, Germanos S, Ridolfini MP, et al. Surgical management of chronic pancreatitis. *Hepatobiliary Pancreat Dis Int.* 2007;6(2):121-133.

Holcomb SS. Stopping the destruction of acute pancreatitis. *Nursing.* 2007;37(6):42-48.

Hughes E. Understanding the care of patients with acute pancreatitis. *Nursing Standard.* 2003;18:45.

Johnson LR. Secretion. In: Johnson LR, ed. *Essential Medical Physiology.* 3rd ed. Amsterdam, The Netherlands: Academic Press; 2003.

McClave S, Chang WK, Dhaliwal R, Heyland DK, et al. Nutrition support in acute pancreatitis: a systematic review of the literature. *JPEN J Parenter Enteral Nutr.* 2006;30(2):143-156.

Owyang C. Chronic pancreatitis. In: Yamada T, ed. *Textbook of Gastroenterology.* Vol 1. 4th ed. Philadelphia, PA: Lippincott Williams & Wilkins; 2003.

Gastrointestinal Bleeding

Barba K, Fitzgerald P, Wood S. Managing peptic ulcer disease. *Nursing2007.* 2007;37(7):56hn1-56hn4.

Dib N, Oberti F, Cales P. Current management of the complications of portal hypertension: variceal bleeding and ascites. *CMAJ.* 2006;174(10):1433-1443.

Elta GH. Approach to the patient with gross gastrointestinal bleeding. In: Yamada T, ed. *Textbook of Gastroenterology.* Vol 2. 4th ed. Philadelphia, PA: Lippincott Williams & Wilkins; 2003.

Krumberger J. How to manage an acute upper GI bleed. *RN.* 2005;68(3):34-39.

Martins NB, Wassef W. Upper gastrointestinal bleeding. *Curr Opin Gastroenterol.* 2006;22(6):612-619.

Spirt MJ, Stanley S. Update on stress prophylaxis in critically ill patients. *Critical Care Nurse.* 2006;26(1):18.

Hepatitis

Czaja AJ. Autoimmune hepatitis. In: Friedman LS, Keefe EB, eds. *Handbook of Liver Disease.* Philadelphia, PA: Elsevier Science; 2002.

Dove LM, Wright TL. Chronic viral hepatitis. In: Friedman LS, Keefe EB, eds. *Handbook of Liver Disease.* Philadelphia, PA: Elsevier Science; 2002.

Wilson TR. The ABCs of hepatitis. *Nurse Pract.* 2005;30(6):12-15.

Inflammatory Bowel Disease

Marrero F, Qadeer MA, Lashner BA. Severe complications of inflammatory bowel disease. *Med Clin North Am.* 2008;92(3):671-686.

Nightingale A. Diagnosis and management of inflammatory bowel disease. *Nurse Prescribing.* 2007;5(7):289-296.

Stenson WF, Korzenik J. Inflammatory bowel disease. In: Yamada T, ed. *Textbook of Gastroenterology.* Vol 1. 4th ed. Philadelphia, PA: Lippincott Williams & Wilkins; 2003.

Shock, Systemic Inflammatory Response Syndrome, and Sepsis

SYSTEMWIDE ELEMENTS

Physiologic Anatomy

1. **Definitions***
   a. *Shock*: A life-threatening, complex process of ineffective tissue perfusion that results in cellular, metabolic, and hemodynamic alterations. The imbalance between oxygen supply and demand causes inadequate peripheral tissue perfusion, impaired cellular function, and impaired organ perfusion. If not detected and promptly treated, shock can lead to organ system failure and death. Early identification of shock can dramatically reduce mortality. The five types of shock are cardiogenic, hypovolemic, anaphylactic, neurogenic, and septic shock (see Chapter 3).
   b. *Systemic inflammatory response syndrome (SIRS)*: Systemic inflammatory response to a variety of severe clinical insults (such as pancreatitis, ischemia or reperfusion, multiple trauma and tissue injury, hemorrhagic shock, and immune-mediated organ injury) in the absence of infection (Figure 9-1). Response is manifested by two or more of the following conditions:
      i. Temperature above 100.4° F (38° C) or below 96.8° F (36° C)
      ii. Heart rate above 90 beats/min
      iii. Respiratory rate above 20 breaths/min or arterial partial pressure of carbon dioxide ($Paco_2$) below 32 mm Hg
      iv. White blood cell (WBC) count above 12,000/mm³ or below 4000/mm³, or more than 10% immature (band) forms
   c. *Infection*: Microbial phenomenon characterized by an inflammatory response to the presence of microorganisms or the invasion of normally sterile host tissue by organisms
   d. *Bacteremia*: Presence of viable bacteria in the blood
   e. *Sepsis*: A documented infection with at least two of the four SIRS criteria
      i. In 2002, the PIRO model was developed as a tool to diagnose and track the progression of sepsis
         (a) *P*: Predisposition for individual patients to respond to infection in different ways
         (b) *I*: Infection
         (c) *R*: Response to inflammation
         (d) *O*: Organ dysfunction

---

*Accepted definitions by Bone, Balk, Cerra, and colleagues (1992) with modifications made by the Society of Critical Care Medicine in 2002.

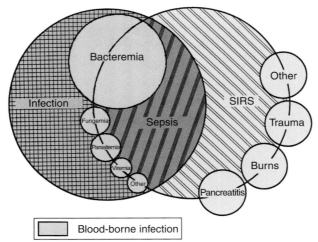

FIGURE 9-1 ■ Interrelationship between systemic inflammatory response syndrome (*SIRS*), sepsis, and infection. (From Bone RC, Balk RA, Cerra FB, et al. Definitions for sepsis and organ failure and guidelines for the use of innovative therapies in sepsis. *Chest.* 1992;101:1645.)

  ii.   In an effort to improve patient outcomes with sepsis, important initiatives have been developed to promote early awareness, detection, and treatment of severe sepsis. In 2008, the Society of Critical Care Medicine consensus group updated the set of clinical guidelines for early identification and management of sepsis. The Surviving Sepsis Campaign recommendations form the basis for a group of time-sensitive interventions called "sepsis bundles." Those caring for patients in non–intensive care unit (ICU) settings can have significant impact to improve survival rates by recognizing sepsis early.

  iii.   Early signs of sepsis include the following:
    (a) Systolic blood pressure (BP) less than 90 mm Hg
    (b) Mean arterial pressure less than 65 mm Hg
    (c) Decrease in systolic BP of more than 40 mm Hg
    (d) Decrease in urine output

  f. *Severe sepsis*: Sepsis associated with organ dysfunction of one or more organ systems, hypoperfusion, or hypotension. Associated signs and symptoms include chills, tachypnea, unexplained alterations in mental status, tachycardia, altered WBC count, decreased platelet count, elevated numbers of immature neutrophils, decreased skin perfusion, decreased urine output, skin mottling, poor capillary refill, hypoglycemia, and petechiae.

  g. *Septic shock*: Sepsis-induced state with hypotension (systolic BP less than 90 mm Hg or a reduction of 40 mm Hg from baseline) despite adequate volume resuscitation along with perfusion abnormalities that may include, but are not limited to, lactic acidosis, oliguria, and acute alterations in mental status. Frequently, patients have cardiovascular system failure as evidenced by hypotension and reduced perfusion to vital organs. Patients receiving inotropic or vasopressor agents may not be hypotensive at the time that perfusion abnormalities are measured.

  h. *Multiple organ dysfunction syndrome (MODS)*: Presence of progressive physiologic dysfunction in two or more organ systems after an acute threat to systemic homeostasis. Patients with a medical and surgical history, with special emphasis on sepsis, shock, trauma, recent surgical procedures, recent infections, and preexisting organ compromise, may exhibit early signs of tachycardia and hypotension.

2. **Epidemiology**
  a. Sepsis is the tenth leading cause of death in the United States.
    i.   Sepsis is the leading cause of death in ICUs.
    ii.   Sepsis develops in more than 750,000 people annually, with 2000 new cases per day in the United States.
    iii. Septic shock develops in approximately 40% of patients with sepsis.
    iv.   More than 1 million cases are expected by 2010.

    b. Mortality rates in the United States: Approximately 225,000 people die each year of either septic shock or bacteremia
        i. Sepsis carries a mortality rate of 20%.
        ii. Severe sepsis and septic shock carry a mortality rate of 30% to 60%.
    c. Health care costs of severe sepsis exceed $17 billion annually.

3. Influences of gender on the response to sepsis: Gender-based differences exist in the response to infection and sepsis
    a. Females: Estrogen may enhance immune function to the extent of inducing autoimmune disease
        i. Estrogen provides a protective effect in the presence of sepsis.
        ii. Monocytes produce more interleukin-1, cause chemotaxis and phagocytosis.
    b. Males: Testosterone suppresses immune function, placing males at risk for worse outcomes; androgens depress the immune response
    c. Once sepsis or septic shock develops, there is no difference in the mortality rate between males and females.

4. Cellular pathophysiology
    a. Many experts agree that, before the development of SIRS, a physiologic insult occurs. The insult may take the form of an infection, traumatic injury, surgical incision, burn injury, or pancreatitis. The initial physiologic response to the insult is the development of a proinflammatory state characterized by the expression of multiple mediators in an effort to limit damage from the insult (Figure 9-2).
    b. Gram-positive bacteria are responsible for approximately 50% of infections resulting in sepsis; gram-negative bacteria account for approximately 25%; 15% of the infections are due to a mix of gram-positive and gram-negative organisms; fungal pathogens account for 5% to 10% of the infections.
    c. When phagocytic cells destroy bacteria, a cascade of events follows. Sequence of events varies depending on whether gram-negative or gram-positive organisms are involved.

5. Etiology and risk factors
    a. Most common sites of origin of bacteremia and sepsis
        i. Respiratory tract
        ii. Intra-abdominal and pelvic sites
        iii. Urinary tract
        iv. Skin
        v. Intravascular catheters

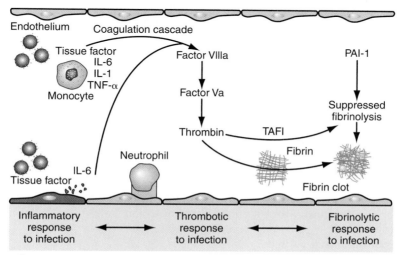

FIGURE 9-2 ■ Inflammation, coagulation, and impaired fibrinolysis in severe sepsis. *IL,* Interleukin; *PAI,* plasminogen activator inhibitor; *TAFI,* thrombin activatable fibrinolysis inhibitor; *TNF,* tumor necrosis factor. (From Ahrens T, Vollman K. Severe sepsis management: are we doing enough? *Crit Care Nurse.* 2003;23[5 suppl]:2-16.)

    b. Most common organisms in hospitalized patients: Gram-negative aerobes

        i. *Escherichia coli*

        ii. *Klebsiella* and *Citrobacter* species

        iii. *Pseudomonas aeruginosa*

    c. Other gram-negative aerobes: *Enterobacter* and *Proteus*

    d. Infections with gram-positive organisms are becoming more common because these organisms are associated with use of intravascular catheters and invasive devices. Most common aerobic organisms are the following:

        i. *Staphylococcus aureus*

        ii. Coagulase-negative staphylococci

        iii. *Streptococcus pyogenes*

        iv. *Streptococcus pneumoniae*

        v. Less common organisms

            (a) Methicillin-resistant *S. aureus*

            (b) Oxacillin-resistant *S. aureus*

            (c) Vancomycin-resistant enterococci

    e. Other organisms

        i. Viruses, protozoa, parasites

        ii. Fungi, such as *Candida albicans*

        iii. Anaerobic organisms: *Clostridium, Bacteroides fragilis*

    f. Predisposing factors for the development of bacteremia or sepsis

        i. Extremes of age: Elderly and very young

        ii. Granulocytopenia

        iii. Prior antimicrobial therapy

        iv. Severe burn injury, recent trauma, recent surgical procedures, and invasive procedures

        v. Functional asplenia

        vi. Immunosuppression: Infection with human immunodeficiency virus (HIV), chemotherapy, corticosteroids, and bone marrow suppression

        vii. Malnutrition and total parenteral nutrition

        viii. Alcohol use and abuse; abuse of other drugs

Patient Assessment

1. Nursing history

    a. Patient health history: Suspect sepsis when known or suspected infection and two or more systems of SIRS. Significant medical and surgical history, with a review of all major systems and the identification of recent invasive procedures and recent travel history.

        i. History of chronic disease (diabetes mellitus; alcoholism; and liver, heart, and renal failure) places the patient at risk.

        ii. Acute illness: Trauma, burns, cholelithiasis, intestinal obstruction, pancreatitis, appendicitis, peritonitis, diverticulitis

        iii. Wounds

    b. Family health history: Chronic disease or infections

    c. Social history: Significant others, ability of the patient and significant others to manage stress, financial obligations of the patient and significant others, and parenting responsibilities of the patient

    d. Medication history, especially medications with immunosuppressive properties (chemotherapeutic drugs, corticosteroids) and antibiotics

    e. Nutritional history, with a special focus on the causes of primary malnutrition (anorexia nervosa, alcohol abuse) and secondary malnutrition (iatrogenic malnutrition, surgical malnutrition)

2. Nursing examination of patient

    a. Physical examination data

        i. Inspection: Clinical presentation may vary, depending on the patient's underlying health and organ function

(a) Acute distress with anxiety, restlessness, confusion, and disorientation progressing to unresponsiveness

(b) Flushed, warm, dry skin or pale, cold, mottled skin (particularly in the elderly), decreased capillary refill; shaking chills and shivering in some patients

(c) Tachypnea and dyspnea

(d) Decreased urinary output; significant edema or positive fluid balance

(e) Petechiae, purpura

ii. Palpation

(a) Tachycardia with rapid, weak, and thready peripheral pulses. Initially, pulses may be bounding and rapid with a hyperdynamic state.

(b) Warm skin (elderly may present with cool skin rather than hyperthermia)

(c) Abdominal distention

iii. Percussion: Dullness over areas of consolidation

iv. Auscultation

(a) Pulmonary crackles from interstitial pulmonary edema; wheezing without a history of bronchospastic airway disease

(b) Hypotension, narrowed or widened pulse pressure

(c) Absence of bowel sounds; may progress to paralytic ileus

b. Monitoring data

i. Core temperature: Above 100.4° F (38° C) or below 96.8° F (36° C)

ii. Heart rate above 90 beats/min

iii. Respiratory rate: Higher than 30 breaths/min

iv. BP: Below 90 mm Hg systolic or fall in systolic BP of more than 40 mm Hg

3. Appraisal of patient characteristics: During hospitalization, any patient is at risk for the development of an infection that can lead to sepsis. Although the signs can be subtle, early identification, treatment, and transfer to a higher level of care are paramount to increased survival rates. The potential for gradual or abrupt changes in clinical condition with possibly life-threatening effects creates challenges. This requires the progressive care nurse to prevent infections, carefully monitor, and recognize populations at risk. Clinical attributes of patients that the nurse needs to assess include the following:

a. Resiliency

i. Level 1—*Minimally resilient:* A 84-year-old woman with hemorrhagic stroke, hemiparalysis, and left lower lobe pneumonia

ii. Level 3—*Moderately resilient:* A 68-year-old male accountant 3 days postoperative after a ruptured appendix and repair, in whom signs of sepsis and acute renal failure develop

iii. Level 5—*Highly resilient:* A 16-year-old male high school student 7 days postoperative after a ruptured appendix and repair

b. Vulnerability

i. Level 1—*Highly vulnerable:* A 57-year-old woman in whom lupus and bacterial pneumonia are diagnosed and who refuses intravenous (IV) antibiotic therapy

ii. Level 3—*Moderately vulnerable:* A 56-year-old attorney with acute pancreatitis, high fever, and positive blood culture results

iii. Level 5—*Minimally vulnerable:* A 24-year-old woman with sinusitis

c. Stability

i. Level 1—*Minimally stable:* A 92-year-old malnourished woman with multiple open wounds in whom a fever, tachycardia, leukocytosis, and minimal urine output develop

ii. Level 3—*Moderately stable:* A 66-year-old man with testicular cancer who is undergoing chemotherapy and who has redness developing around his peripherally inserted central catheter

iii. Level 5—*Highly stable:* A 38-year-old college professor who has mitral valve prolapse and requires prophylactic antibiotics before dental procedures

d. Complexity
   i.   Level 1—*Highly complex:* A 68-year old man who undergoes hemodialysis three times a week, is being evicted from his home, and has an arteriovenous graft that is swollen and red
   ii. Level 3—*Moderately complex:* A 52-year-old migrant worker with newly diagnosed esophageal varices who aspirates and is hyperglycemic and tachypneic
   iii. Level 5—*Minimally complex:* A 21-year-old college student with a diagnosis of mononucleosis
e. Resource availability
   i.   Level 1—*Few resources:* A 88-year-old widower with no nearby relatives who requires a revision of his total knee replacement that has a related infection. He lives in a rural area and is unable to obtain transportation for his antibiotic therapy treatments.
   ii. Level 3—*Moderate resources:* A 48-year-old self-employed carpenter who underwent a cardiac catheterization and has a diagnosis of cardiomyopathy. He does not have health insurance, and his sister is a registered nurse.
   iii. Level 5—*Many resources:* A 58-year-old who has pancreatitis and who is married with two grown children who live locally
f. Participation in care
   i.   Level 1—*No participation:* A 91-year-old widower without children who has a postoperative infection and requires complex dressing changes on discharge
   ii. Level 3—*Moderate level of participation:* A 62-year-old man being discharged after removal of a pacemaker around which infection had developed. His wife will assist in administering IV antibiotics via his peripherally inserted central catheter.
   iii. Level 5—*Full participation:* A 21-year-old nursing student who has a tonsillectomy during semester break
g. Participation in decision making
   i.   Level 1—*No participation:* A 88-year-old man with dementia who has been in a motor vehicle accident and in whom renal failure, pneumonia, and sepsis develop
   ii. Level 3—*Moderate level of participation:* A 34-year-old women, newly divorced with four young children at home, who is admitted with necrotizing fasciitis requiring emergent surgery
   iii. Level 5—*Full participation:* A 47-year-old teacher who has a mastoidectomy after recurrent ear infections and plans to recuperate during school break
h. Predictability
   i.   Level 1—*Not predictable:* A 73-year-old in whom hypotension, tachycardia, and reduced mental alertness develop. He had an endotracheal tube inserted and was receiving mechanical ventilation before being transferred from ICU last week after exacerbation of chronic obstructive pulmonary disease
   ii. Level 3—*Moderately predictable:* A 44-year-old physician with fever, chills, and malaise after returning from a cruise to South America
   iii. Level 5—*Highly predictable:* A 58-year-old manager who recently underwent carotid endarterectomy and is being discharged

4. **Diagnostic studies**
   a. Laboratory
      i.   Arterial blood gas levels
           (a) Respiratory alkalosis with $Paco_2$ below 32 mm Hg attempting to compensate for metabolic acidosis, with pH below 7.35 and decreased HCO_3
           (b) Late: Respiratory acidosis with $Paco_2$ above 45 mm Hg
           (c) Oxygen saturation by pulse oximetry above 92%
      ii. Complete blood cell count and differential: Either increased (>12,000/mm^3) or decreased (<4000/mm^3) or above 10% immature (band) forms
      iii. Serum glucose levels: Elevated from the stress response
      iv. Blood cultures and antibiotic sensitivities
           (a) Identification of causative organisms; blood culture results are positive in only 50% of patients with sepsis for uncertain reasons (bacteremia may be intermittent)
           (b) Urine, sputum, and wound cultures to correlate with blood cultures

    v. Elevated blood urea nitrogen and creatinine levels

    vi. Coagulation studies: May show elevations in prothrombin time and partial thrombo-plastin time; decreased fibrinogen level and increased level of fibrin split products

    vii. Decreased platelet levels

    viii. Decreased C-reactive protein and elevated procalcitonin levels

    ix. Elevated serum enzyme levels, indicating liver or cardiac impairment

Patient Care

1. **Infection and exaggerated inflammatory process**
   a. Description of problem
      i. Exaggerated or "malignant" inflammation
      ii. Inadequate primary defenses (broken skin, traumatized tissues) and secondary defenses (immunosuppression), invasive procedures, and/or malnutrition
      iii. Defining characteristics: See definition of SIRS
   b. Goals of care
      i. WBC count is 4000 to 12,000/mm^3.
      ii. Temperature is 96.8° to 100.4° F (36° to 38° C).
      iii. Heart rate is 60 to 100 beats/min.
      iv. Respiratory rate is 12 to 20 breaths/min.
   c. Collaborating professionals on health care team: Registered nurse, medical/surgical attending physician, respiratory therapist, pharmacist, dietitian, infectious disease specialist, pastoral counselor
   d. Interventions
      i. Administer antimicrobial agents on time.
      ii. Monitor antibiotic levels, particularly aminoglycoside levels, for renal and ototoxic effects.
      iii. Monitor for reaction to antibiotics.
         (a) Superinfection: Infection with organisms such as *C. albicans* is usually controlled by normal body flora
         (b) Allergy: Rash and anaphylactic shock
         (c) Resistance: Reemergence of symptoms of fever, purulence, and increased WBC count
      iv. Monitor compliance with unit infection control protocols, as recommended by the Centers for Disease Control and Prevention.
         (a) Hand washing, hospital personnel and visitors
         (b) Dressing changes
         (c) Wound isolation
         (d) Management of indwelling devices
         (e) Use of maximum barrier precautions and aseptic technique during catheter insertions
         (f) Diagnosis of infection
         (g) Removal of foci of infection
      v. Provide twice-a-day teeth brushing and oral cleansing every 2 hours, and maintain 30-degree head of bed if patient is unable to handle secretions.
      vi. Assist with treatments to limit the nidus of infection.
         (a) Removal of necrotic tissue
         (b) Débridement of burned tissue
         (c) Drainage of abscesses
      vii. Stabilize fractures promptly to limit tissue damage and inflammation.
      viii. Maintain strong rapport with the family and provide frequent updates and education, because the course of this disease is often unpredictable.
   e. Evaluation of patient care
      i. No clinical manifestations of SIRS are evident.
      ii. Culture and sensitivity test results are negative.
2. **Maldistribution of blood flow (renal, cerebral, cardiopulmonary, gastrointestinal, peripheral)**
   a. Description of problem

      i.   Hyperdynamic state: The usual presentation

      ii.   Subsequent development of hypovolemia

      iii. Increase in lactic acid levels

      iv. Inability of the tissues to use oxygen

      v.   Decreased urine output

      vi. Diminished bowel sounds and/or paralytic ileus

      vii. Excessive microvascular coagulation and impaired fibrinolysis

      viii. Decreased systemic vascular resistance as evidenced by hypotension (systolic BP below 90 mm Hg)

      ix. Changes in the sensorium (restlessness, anxiety, and disorientation progressing to unresponsiveness)

b. Goals of care

      i.   Oxygen delivery and consumption are normal or supranormal.

      ii.   Urine output is at least 1 ml/kg/hr.

      iii. Restore mean arterial pressure to 60–65 mm Hg.

      iv. Bowel sounds are present, and there is no abdominal distention.

      v.   Sensorium is clear; the patient is oriented to time, place, and person.

c. Collaborating professionals on health care team: Initiate transfer to higher level of care if sepsis is suspected

d. Interventions

      i.   Monitor screening parameters for early identification of sepsis.

      ii.   Administer supplemental oxygen.

      iii. Be prepared to administer fluid resuscitation bolus volumes of 20 ml/kg while waiting to transfer to higher level of care.

          (a) Type of fluid may be either crystalloid or colloid to restore circulating volume.

      iv. Be prepared to administer vasoactive medications as needed if fluid resuscitation fails to maintain BP and organ perfusion.

      v.   Monitor for symptoms of diminished visceral perfusion.

          (a) Decreased or absent bowel sounds

          (b) Elevated serum amylase level

          (c) Decreased platelet count

      vi. Avoid Trendelenburg's position, which may impair gas exchange and decrease cerebral perfusion.

      vii. Maximize oxygen delivery and utilization; minimize oxygen demand.

          (a) Control hyperthermia.

             (1) Use tepid baths or a cooling blanket.

             (2) Prevent chills and shivering.

             (3) Remove extra blankets.

             (4) Use antipyretic agents other than aspirin to reduce fever.

      viii. Limit patient activity; maintain a restful environment; provide uninterrupted rest; maintain family visitations as appropriate.

      ix. Manage pain, anxiety, and restlessness with medications and nursing interventions.

e. Evaluation of patient care

      i.   Vital signs are within normal limits.

      ii.   Peripheral pulses are present and equal bilaterally.

      iii. Urine output is at least 1 ml/kg/hr.

      iv. Sensorium is clear.

3. Impaired oxygenation and ventilation: See Chapter 2

4. Altered thermoregulation

  a. Description of problem

      i.   Related to the body's response to infection and the inflammatory process

      ii.   Core temperature below 96.8° F (36° C) or above 100.4° F (38° C)

      iii. Flushed, warm skin or pale, cool skin

      iv. Increased or decreased metabolic rate

    b. Goals of care

        i. Core temperature is between 96.8° and 100.4° F (36° and 38° C).

        ii. Skin is warm and dry.

    c. Collaborating professionals on health care team: See Infection and Exaggerated Inflammatory Process

    d. Interventions

        i. Monitor core temperature hourly.

        ii. After the source of increased or decreased temperature is identified, maintain normothermia by the use of antipyretic medication as prescribed; avoid aspirin products.

        iii. Use tepid baths or a cooling blanket to reduce hyperthermia.

            (a) Monitor core temperature at all times to reduce the risk of hypothermia.

            (b) Do not decrease temperature too rapidly, because this may lead to shaking chills.

            (c) Reposition frequently, and check for tissue breakdown if a cooling blanket is used.

        iv. Use warming blankets and a warmed ambient temperature to manage hypothermia.

    e. Evaluation of patient care: Normothermia is achieved

5. Catabolic state resulting in malnutrition

    a. Description of problem

        i. Increased body temperature

        ii. Increased body metabolism

        iii. Decreased intake of nutrients

        iv. Loss of body weight

    b. Goals of care

        i. Stable body weight is as appropriate for gender and body frame.

        ii. Nitrogen balance is positive.

        iii. Muscle mass is adequate.

    c. Collaborating professionals on health care team: See Infection and Exaggerated Inflammatory Process

    d. Interventions: See Chapter 8

        i. Initiate enteral feedings within 48 hours to limit gastrointestinal microbial translocation.

        ii. Establish caloric requirements based on body size and degree of hypermetabolism; 20 to 25 kcal/kg/day is average.

        iii. Maintain glucose level at 80 to 110 mg/dl because hyperglycemia is associated with a poor prognosis.

        iv. Provide family/significant others with distinct goals for nutritional support.

    e. Evaluation of patient care

        i. Serum albumin level is above 3.5 g/dl.

        ii. Body weight is within 2 kg of normal.

        iii. There is no evidence of electrolyte or vitamin imbalances.

Anaphylactic Hypersensitivity Reactions

1. Pathophysiology

    a. There are four types of hypersensitivity reaction, classified according to the time between the exposure and the reaction, the immune mechanism involved, and the site of the reaction.

        i. Type I immediate hypersensitivity reactions are mediated by immunoglobulin E (IgE) in reaction to common allergens such as dust, pollen, animal dander, insect sting, some foods, and various drugs. These reactions can be local, resulting in local swelling and discomfort, or systemic, resulting in anaphylaxis and possibly in death if not recognized and treated promptly.

        ii. Type II immediate hypersensitivity reactions are mediated by antibody and complement. These reactions can occur with a mismatched blood transfusion or as a response to various drugs.

        iii. Type III immediate hypersensitivity reactions result in tissue damage caused by precipitation of antigen-antibody immune complexes. These reactions can occur with serum sickness or in response to various drugs.

      iv. Type IV delayed hypersensitivity reactions result from migration of immune cells to the site of exposure days after the exposure to the antigen. These reactions can occur in contact dermatitis, measles rash, or tuberculin skin testing or in response to various drugs. Transplanted graft rejection is a type IV hypersensitivity reaction.

    b. After a first, sensitizing exposure to a specific allergen, such as an insect sting, in which abnormally large amounts of IgE antibodies are made, subsequent exposures to the same allergen trigger an exaggerated antibody reaction. When the patient comes in contact with the antigen a second time, IgE triggers the release of histamine, heparin, and other cytokines from mast cells, causing bronchiole constriction, peripheral vasoconstriction, and increased vascular permeability, which quickly progress to airway obstruction, pulmonary edema, peripheral edema, hypovolemia, hypotension, shock, and circulatory collapse.

2. Etiology and risk factors
    a. Drugs (e.g., penicillin, local anesthetics, vaccines, contrast dye)
    b. Insect stings
    c. Foods (e.g., shellfish, milk, eggs, fish, wheat)

3. Signs and symptoms
    a. Symptoms: Apprehension, dyspnea, restlessness
    b. Signs: Urticaria, facial edema, tachypnea, stridor, cyanosis, tachycardia, hypotension, wheezing

4. Diagnostic study findings: Usually noncontributory to the diagnosis of anaphylaxis

5. Goals of care
    a. Patent airway, maintenance of breathing and circulation
    b. Absence of hypovolemia due to shock
    c. Stable hemodynamic state

6. Collaborating professionals on health care team
    a. Nurse
    b. Pharmacist
    c. Physician
    d. Respiratory therapist

7. Management of patient care
    a. Anticipated patient trajectory: Patients experiencing an anaphylactic hypersensitivity or anaphylactoid event differ in their clinical course depending on age, medical history, number of prior exposures, and the extent of prior reactions. Throughout their course of recovery, airway and circulatory compromise or collapse may threaten life. Mild hypersensitivity reactions with localized symptoms can be prevented from becoming acute if pharmacologic management is immediate. Patients may be expected to have needs in the following areas:
        i. Positioning: Use a chin lift in the supine position or high Fowler's position to provide a patent airway
        ii. Transport: Maintain a patent airway, circulatory support, and cervical neck traction until the patient is hemodynamically stable
        iii. Discharge planning: Patient education may be required to reinforce the importance of wearing a MedicAlert bracelet, the home use of epinephrine, the need to contact health care personnel immediately at the onset of a hypersensitivity reaction, and the importance of avoiding allergens
    b. Potential complications
        i. Cardiopulmonary arrest
            (a) Mechanism: Antibody response to allergen results in vasodilation and bronchoconstriction
            (b) Management: Cardiopulmonary resuscitation, administration of corticosteroids (IV Solu-Cortef or Solu-Medrol) and histamine blockers (diphenhydramine [Benadryl], 25 to 50 mg; epinephrine, 0.2 to 0.5 ml subcutaneously or 0.5 ml of 1:1000 IV)
        ii. Respiratory compromise
            (a) Mechanism: Histamine release creates interstitial edema and potential bronchoconstriction resulting in pulmonary edema
            (b) Management: Administration of corticosteroids, histamine blockers, and supplemental oxygen

8. **Evaluation of patient care**
   a. Patent airway with uncompromised breathing
   b. Absence of circulatory collapse or compromise
   c. Controlled local clinical manifestations, such as hives or urticaria

---

REFERENCES AND BIBLIOGRAPHY

Sepsis, Systemic Inflammatory Response Syndrome, and Septic Shock

Ahrens T, Tuggle D. Surviving severe sepsis: early recognition and treatment. *Crit Care Nurse.* 2004;Oct(suppl):2-15.

★ Balk RA. Severe sepsis and septic shock: definitions, epidemiology, and clinical manifestations. *Crit Care Clin.* 2000;16:179-192.

Beery TA. Sex differences in infection and sepsis. *Crit Care Nurs Clin North Am.* 2003;15:55-62.

Bochud P, Calandra T. Pathogenesis of sepsis: new concepts and implications for future treatment. *BMJ.* 2003;326:262-266.

★ Bone RC, Balk RA, Cerra FB, et al. Definitions for sepsis and organ failure and guidelines for the use of innovative therapies in sepsis. *Chest.* 1992;101:1644-1655.

Dellinger RP, Carlet JM, Masur H, et al. Surviving Sepsis Campaign guidelines for management of severe sepsis and septic shock. *Crit Care Med.* 2004;32:858-872.

Dellinger RP, Levy MM, Carlet JM. Surviving Sepsis Campaign: international guidelines for management of severe sepsis and septic shock. *Crit Care Med.* 2008;36(1):296-327.

Ely ES, Kleinpell R, Goyette RE. Advances in the understanding of clinical manifestations and therapy of severe sepsis: an update for critical care nurses. *Am J Crit Care.* 2003;12:120-135.

Felblinger DM. Malnutrition, infection, and sepsis in acute and chronic illness. *Crit Care Nurs Clin North Am.* 2003;15:71-78.

Filbin MR, Stapczinski JS. Shock, septic. Medscape website. Emedicine. http://www.medscape.com/files/emedicine/topic533.htm. Accessed June 30, 2008.

Garretson S, Malberti S. Understanding hypovolaemic, cardiogenic and septic shock. *Nurs Stand.* 2007;21(50):46-55, 58, 60.

Giuliano KK. Physiological monitoring for critically ill patients: testing a predictive model for the early detection of sepsis. *Am J Crit Care.* 2007;16(2):122-131.

Griffiths RD. Nutrition support in critically ill septic patients. *Curr Opin Clin Nutr Metab Care.* 2003;6:203-210.

Guven H, Altintop L, Baydin A, et al. Diagnostic value of procalcitonin levels as an early indicator of sepsis. *Am J Emerg Med.* 2002;20:202-206.

Holzinger U, Feldbacher M, Bachlechner A. Improvement of glucose control in the intensive care unit: an interdisciplinary collaboration study. *Am J Crit Care.* 2008;17(2):150-156.

Institute for Healthcare Improvement. IHI contributing to bold international campaign to dramatically reduce mortality from sepsis. http://www.ihi.org/IHI/Topics/CriticalCare/Sepsis/ImprovementStories/HIContributingto Bold International Campaign to Dramatically Reduce Mortality from Sepsis.htm. Published 2005. Accessed June 30, 2008.

Kleinpell RM. Advances in treating patients with severe sepsis: role of drotrecogin alfa (activated). *Crit Care Nurse.* 2003;23:16-29.

Kleinpell RM. Recognizing and treating five shock states. http://www.nurse.com/ce/course.html?CCID-3723. Published 2007. Accessed June 30, 2008.

Kleinpell RM. The role of the critical care nurse in the assessment and management of the patient with severe sepsis. *Crit Care Nurs Clin North Am.* 2003;1:27-34.

Kleinpell RM. Working out the complexities of severe sepsis. *Nurse Pract.* 2005;30(4):43-44, 46-48.

Kleinpell RM, Graves BT, Ackerman M. Incidence, pathogenesis, and management of sepsis: an overview. *AACN Clinical Issues.* 2006;17:385-393.

Kumar A, Roberts D, Wood KE, et al. Duration of hypotension before initiation of effective antimicrobial therapy is the critical determinant of survival in human septic shock. *Crit Care Med.* 2006;34:1589-1596.

Levy MM, Fink MP, Marshall JC, et al. 2001 SCCM/ESICM/ACCP/ATS/SIS International Sepsis Definitions Conference. *Crit Care Med.* 2003;31:1250-1256.

Martin GS, Mannino DM, Eaton S, et al. The epidemiology of sepsis in the United States from 1979 through 2000. *N Engl J Med.* 2003;348:1546-1554.

Mathiak G, Neville LF, Grass G. Targeting the coagulation cascade in sepsis: did we find the "magic bullet"? *Crit Care Med.* 2003;31:310-311.

Munford RS. Severe sepsis and septic shock. Harrison's Practice website. http://www.harrisonspractice.com/practice/ub/view/Harrison's_Principles_of_Internal_Medicine/Severe_Sepsis_and_Septic_Shock. Accessed June 30, 2008.

O'Grady NP, Alexander M, Dellinger E, et al. Guidelines for the prevention of intravascular catheter-related infections. Centers for Disease Control and Prevention. *MMWR Recomm Rep.* 2002;51:1-29.

Patel BM, Chittock DR, Russell JA, et al. Beneficial effects of short-term vasopressin infusion during severe septic shock. *Anesthesiology.* 2002;96: 576-582.

Pearl RG, Pohlman A. Understanding and managing anemia in critically ill patients. *Crit Care Nurse.* 2002;Dec(suppl):1-16.

Raising the bar with bundles. Treating patients with an all-or-nothing standard. *Joint Commission Perspectives on Patient Safety.* 2006;6(4):5-6.

Rivers E, Nguyen B, Havstad S, et al. Early goal-directed therapy in the treatment of severe sepsis and septic shock. *N Engl J Med.* 2002;345:1368-1377.

Rivers EP, Coba V, Whitmill M. Early goal-directed therapy in severe sepsis and septic shock: a contemporary review of the literature. *Curr Opin Anesthesiol.* 2008;21(2):128-140.

Robson WP. The Sepsis Six: helping patients to survive sepsis. *Br J Nurs.* 2008;17(1):16-21.

Shafazand S, Weinacker AB. Blood cultures in the critical care unit: improving utilization and yield. *Chest.* 2002;132:1727-1736.

Sommers MS. The cellular basis of septic shock. *Crit Care Nurs Clin North Am.* 2003;15:13-25.

★ Task Force of the American College of Critical Care Medicine, Society of Critical Care Medicine. Practice parameters for hemodynamic support of sepsis in adult patients. *Crit Care Med.* 1999;27:639-660.

Townsend S, Dellinger RP, Levy MM, Ramsay G. *Implementing the Surviving Sepsis Campaign.* Des Plaines, IL: Society of Critical Care Medicine; 2005.

Anaphylactic Hypersensitivity Reactions

Brown SG. The pathophysiology of shock in anaphylaxis. *Immunol Allergy Clin North Am.* 2007;27(2):165-175.

Carlson B. Shock. In: Urden LD, Stacy KM, Lough ME, eds. *Thelan's Critical Care Nursing.* 5th ed. St Louis, MO: Mosby; 2006.

Clark S, Camargo CA Jr. Epidemiology of anaphylaxis. *Immunol Allergy Clin North Am.* 2007;27(2):145-163.

Golden DBK. What is anaphylaxis? *Curr Opin Allergy Clin Immunol.* 2007;7(4):331-336.

Griffiths M. Emergency treatment of anaphylaxis: implications for nurses. *Prim Health Care.* 2008;18(2):14-15.

Jevon P. Severe allergic reaction: management of anaphylaxis in hospital. *Br J Nurs.* 2008;17(2): 104-108.

Ogawa Y, Grant JA. Mediators of anaphylaxis. *Immunol Allergy Clin North Am.* 2007;27(2):249-260.

CHAPTER 10

Psychosocial Aspects of Progressive Care

Psychosocial Considerations

1. **Scope of progressive care nursing practice**
   a. "The scope of practice for nursing care of the acutely and critically ill patients of all ages encompasses the dynamic interaction of the acutely and critically ill patient and his or her family, the nurse and environment of care" (Figure 10-1).
   b. Needs or characteristics of the patient and family influence and drive the characteristics or competencies of the critical care nurse.
   c. Challenges of meeting psychosocial needs
      i. Other conflicting priorities such as addressing the physiologic instability of the patient may preclude or inhibit nurses from meeting the psychosocial needs of the patient and family.
      ii. Psychosocial needs often involve family members (an aspect unique to psychosocial needs in contrast to physiologic needs); for example, issues such as grief and loss, and powerlessness may pertain more to the family than to the patient in some situations (e.g., brain-dead patient).
      iii. Value systems in critical care units often emphasize performing nursing tasks over attending to the psychosocial needs of the patient and family.
      iv. Meeting psychosocial needs demands a coordinated, multidisciplinary approach to care.
      v. Critical care environment is often a barrier to effectively meeting psychosocial needs.
      vi. Growing evidence supports an interrelationship between psychosocial and physiologic problems (e.g., stress and immunity).
   d. Patient
      i. Progressive care patients share some common, predictable psychosocial needs (e.g., the need for reassurance and support).
      ii. Specific patient psychosocial needs vary depending on patient and family characteristics and the patient's status on the health-to-illness continuum.
      iii. The more compromised the patient, the more complex the patient's needs.
      iv. Progressive care patients' psychosocial needs are based on patient characteristics, including resiliency, vulnerability, stability, complexity, resource availability, participation in care and decision making, and the predictability of the illness
      v. Patient characteristics and needs influence family members' needs and psychosocial issues.

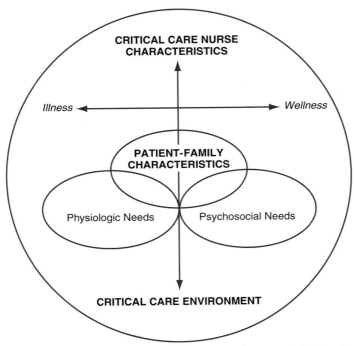

FIGURE 10-1 ■ Complexity of the psychosocial needs of critically ill patients and their families.

e. Family
  i. Definition of *family*
    (a) Traditional: A group of two or more people who reside together and who are related by birth, marriage, or adoption
    (b) Contemporary: A group of people who love and care for each other
    (c) As the patient defines it
  ii. Families of high-acuity patients share a variety of predictable psychosocial needs.
  iii. Specific psychosocial needs of family members vary depending on patient characteristics, family characteristics, and the patient's status on the health-to-illness continuum (e.g., cultural diversity issues).
  iv. Predictable needs of family members of progressive care patients include the following:
    (a) To obtain information
    (b) To receive support and reassurance
    (c) To be with the patient
    (d) To participate in preparation for home care
f. Progressive care nurse
  i. Progressive care nurse characteristics influence the extent to which patient and family psychosocial needs are met.
  ii. Continuum of nursing characteristics includes clinical judgment, advocacy and moral agency, caring practices, collaboration, systems thinking, response to diversity, clinical inquiry, and facilitation of learning.
g. Progressive care team
  i. Members of the progressive care team include the nurse, physician, respiratory therapist, social worker, clergy, physical therapist, occupational and speech therapist, discharge planners, case managers, and others as needed.
  ii. Psychosocial needs of the patient and family are met through the collaborative efforts of a multidisciplinary team; each member brings a unique perspective and specific expertise to the shared plan of care and patient goals.
h. Progressive care environment (interaction among elements—hence complexity)
i. Location of the progressive care patients

i. For progressive care patients and families the actual location may vary on the basis of institutional criteria.

ii. The use of AACN's Synergy Model for Patient Care is an effective tool that will assist in defining the progressive care patient needs. As in critical care, the geographic domain of progressive care is expanding.

iii. Care provided to progressive care patients is not limited by geography but is based on the needs and required interventions of the patient.

iv. Specific progressive care units (PCUs) can be identified; patients requiring progressive care nursing can be located throughout the hospital.

v. Progressive care can be very specialized, with care focused on a specific system such as cardiac, or more generalized, as in the care of patients with multisystem problems

vi. Physical environment: Noise, lights, lack of privacy, odors, drafts, and hot or cold rooms are sources of environmental stress and an important consideration for patient who has relocated to progressive care from a critical care unit

2. **Common elements**
   a. Life cycle
      i. Patients and family members come to PCUs at all phases of the life cycle.
      ii. Growth and development of the patient and family members influence psychosocial needs, response to illness, and behaviors (e.g., body image changes may present serious psychologic stressors to young adults).
      iii. Erikson's eight stages of the life cycle: See Table 10-1

TABLE 10-1
Erikson's Eight Stages of the Life Cycle

Stage*	Developmental Tasks	Approach
ACQUISITION OF HOPE		
Trust versus mistrust (0-2 yr)	Incorporative stage by oral, tactual, and visual senses Needs are met; sense of trust of self and others develops. Mother figure important	Provide oral gratification. Provide soft touch, cuddling. Use gentle voice. Provide safe, warm environment. Physical and emotional safety: Enable mother to stay with patient. Supply special toys and blanket. Be a consistent care provider.
ACQUISITION OF WILL		
Autonomy versus shame (2-3 yr)	Muscle system maturation Coordination of holding on and letting go Beginning of autonomous will Self-control without loss of self-esteem Illness may be seen as shameful and/or dirty or bad.	Use gentle firmness and reassurance by word and act. Talk to patient before performing procedures. Enhance self-esteem. Foster autonomy and self-reliance. Take time to explain in simple terms; use touch and gentle words.
ACQUISITION OF PURPOSE		

Initiative versus guilt (3-6 yr)	Becomes part of family relationships:
	    I am a person, but what kind of person?
	    Identifies with parents
	Social circles widen; makes friends.
	Has enough language skills to understand and *misunderstand*
	Imagination increases to point of frightening self.
	Child psychomotor skills, mental curiosity, social nature intrude on how child thinks.
	Curious about sexuality Early sense of responsibility and conscience
		Satisfy curiosity with simple and practical information.
		Provide comfort when patient has bad dreams (loss of life, limb).
		Dispel fantasies; encourage questions. Answer within patient's understanding.
		Make patient a partner in treatment, within patient's limits.
		Enable family to visit or stay with patient.
		Be a consistent provider.

Continued

▨ **TABLE 10-1**
▨ ▪ **Erikson's Eight Stages of the Life Cycle—Cont'd**

Stage*	Developmental Tasks	Approach
ACQUISITION OF COMPETENCE		
Industry versus inferiority (6-12 yr)	Active period of socialization Period of learning: *I am what I learn* Balance between *what I want to do* and *what I am told to do* If child is too rigid, develops overly strict sense of duty, which restricts socialization and creativity Needs to work and learn to feel good about self Wants to be recognized by doing things well Needs time for self and others	Respect patient's need for privacy. Provide balance of social time and alone time. Let patient help with care. Teach about what is going on around area. Use gentle firmness. Engage in conversation about school activities, sports, classes, hobbies. Engage in active listening. Recognize importance of respect and dignity. Recognize importance of friends' communicating and visiting.
ACQUISITION OF FIDELITY		
Identity versus role confusion (13-20 yr)	Searches for self, *new self emerging*, with physical growth and development of secondary sex characteristics Takes very seriously how he or she thinks others see him or her, in comparison with what he or she feels about self Needs to incorporate new changes and old roles and skills into a person that fits with image of today Identity equals how he or she thinks others see him or her. Identity diffusion is confusion between what person thinks others see and what person believes about self.	Use name of patient. Recognize that peers are important and have a powerful influence on patient's identity. Foster decision making by patient within safety parameters. Encourage patient to believe that he or she is part of the treatment process. Encourage patient to talk about plans and dreams, what he or she wants to do. Recognize importance of personal grooming. Focus on strengths. Provide information to patient. Make patient's input part of treatment process.
ACQUISITION OF LOVE		
Intimacy versus isolation (21-45 yr)	Increased importance of human closeness Work and study for life's role Interpersonal intimacy with another adult Endless talking aboout what one feels, what others seem to feel, expectations and hopes If intimacy not accomplished, will isolate self and lack spontaneity	Recognize importance of patient's family. Allow involvement of significant others. Encourage patient to talk about plans of life, what he or she does and hopes to accomplish. Make patient's input part of treatment planning. Share information, involve family. Talk about children, work, hobbies. Communicate openly and honestly about patient's condition.
ACQUISITION OF CARE		
Generativity versus stagnation (45-65 yr)	Individuals combine their personalities and energies in producing fulfilling relationships, possibly common offspring, creativity, job fulfillment. Believes in self; enhanced self-esteem and self-concept allows for closeness of relationships When unable to develop relationships, become self-absorbed or withdrawn	Show respect and concern. Recognize patient's need to be involved in treatment along with significant others. Provide information to patient and family. Engage in information sharing. Even if patient is unconscious, talk to him or her. Explain what is happening.

■ **TABLE 10-1**
■ ■ **Erikson's Eight Stages of the Life Cycle—Cont'd**

Stage*	Developmental Tasks	Approach
ACQUISITION OF WISDOM		
Ego integrity versus despair (≥65 yr)	Acceptance of one's own life as significant and others' as important Feels responsible for own life, *I accept what I am* > (responsible for own life), life has dignity and love Emotional integration provides the strength to deal with life as it is *right now*.	Treat with respect and dignity. Address as Mr./Mrs./Ms. or by title. Involve patient in treatment planning. Encourage expressions of life experiences. Recognize that significant others are very important in the decision-making process. Provide control of pain to enhance dignity and *clarity of mind*.

* Ages are approximate and should be considered only as a guide

   b. Needs of the patient
      i. Maslow categorized needs in terms of a hierarchy.
         (a) Physiologic requirements
         (b) Safety and security
         (c) Love and sense of belonging
         (d) Self-esteem
         (e) Self-actualization
      ii. Basic needs must be satisfied before higher-level needs can be met.
      iii. Needs change throughout the life cycle.
      iv. Illness may require refocusing on the achievement of basic needs.
   c. Family issues
      i. Family system theories
         (a) Derived from general system theory—a method of viewing systems that are composed of related parts that interact together as a whole
         (b) Can be used by progressive care nurses to understand family cultural patterns and dynamics, including communication patterns, power, economics, and interaction. Also help give insight into dysfunctional family relationships.
      ii. Family systems
         (a) Groups of individuals bonded together by their interests
         (b) Community whose members nurture and support one another
         (c) Members have a set of rules, roles, power structure, forms of communication, and styles of problem solving that allow tasks to be accomplished effectively.
         (d) Illness alters rules, roles, power, and so on, in the family, which creates stress and the need for adaptation to a new environment and situation.
         (e) Influenced by cultural factors, spiritual support
      iii. Caregiver issues
         (a) Caregivers, including family members and nursing staff, are exposed to environmental stressors; may lead to role strain.
         (b) Can lead to exhaustion if not recognized and managed effectively
   d. Environmental considerations along the continuum of care
      i. The environment can directly affect the ability to meet a patient's needs, including the need for rest and sleep (e.g., lack of doors on patient rooms, fluorescent overbed lighting).
      ii. Staff awareness and behaviors also can have a profound effect on modifying environmental influences that affect the patient.
      iii. Other factors are the progressive care nurse's ability to understand the stress experienced by the patient as he or she moves from one environment to another, and the patient's ability to cope with change.
      iv. The progressive care environment provides for additional privacy and should be conducive to accommodating the patient's normal rest patterns.

■ **BOX 10-1**
■ **STRATEGIES FOR CREATING A HEALING ENVIRONMENT**

- Provide the patient with reassurance that the patient is being closely watched and that you are available to meet the patient's needs.
- Create a personalized space for the patient, keep the patient's personal items (such as eyeglasses) within reach, and display cherished items (such as family pictures).
- Ensure privacy and dignity (e.g., close curtains and doors and talk quietly during sensitive conversations).
- Provide information about caregivers (e.g., write the names of nurses and other caregivers on a dry-erase board in the room).
- Use dimmers to adjust the brightness of lights.
- Adjust the curtains to block out bright lights.
- Provide natural light and outside views when possible.
- Use incandescent lighting if possible.
- Decrease sensory deprivation by allowing family visitation, surrounding the patient with familiar items, providing radio or television, etc., according to the patient's desires.
- Use music therapy, which provides comforting background noise and helps manage stress, anxiety, and pain.

    v. Patients received on the PCU from the critical care unit may have experienced some form of delirium. Ouimet et al found in their study that delirium developed in 31.8% of intensive care unit (ICU) patients who had a mean APACHE score of 16.5 or greater.

    vi. Strategies for creating a healing environment: See Box 10-1

  e. Stress

    i. Definition: Condition that exists in an organism when it encounters stimuli

    ii. Illness is a stressful situation. Directed interventions by the nurse can lessen stress and/or the impact of stress on the patient and family. Nursing presence and the anticipation of patient needs have been reported to be associated with less stressful critical care experiences

    iii. Selye identified two types of stress.

      (a) Eustress: Condition that exists in an organism when it meets with nonthreatening stimuli

      (b) Distress: Condition that exists in an organism when it meets with noxious stimuli

    iv. Common psychologic stressors for acutely ill patients and their families

      (a) Powerlessness (lack of control)

      (b) Sleep deprivation

      (c) Grief and loss

      (d) Sensory overload or deprivation

      (e) Pain

      (f) Posttraumatic stress disorder

    v. Response to stress

      (a) Noxious psychosocial stimuli can overwhelm the body's compensatory ability to maintain homeostasis and can elicit a stress response.

      (b) Major neural response to a stressful stimulus is activation of the sympathetic nervous system.

      (c) Relationship between psychologic stress and health: Psychoneuroimmunologic research has identified a relationship between stress and immune function (i.e., an increased stress response is associated with decreased immunity)

Patient and Family Psychosocial Assessment

1. **Nursing history**

  a. Patient history

    i. Identify preexisting psychiatric, psychologic, and social problems.

    ii. Identify preillness coping mechanisms.

    iii. Identify sources of support (e.g., family, friends, spiritual support, pets).

    iv. Identify patient proxy, living will, durable power of attorney, and so on.

    b. Family history: Family assessment data obtained on admission or as soon as possible
        i.   Health care proxy or family spokesperson
        ii.   Contact information (e.g., home and cell phone numbers, pager numbers)
        iii. Diversity issues (culture, language, etc.) that affect the patient and family
        iv. Coping strategies
        v.   Family caregivers
        vi. Support systems (family, friends, church group, other spiritual support)
        viii. Family concerns regarding this hospitalization
        ix. Best time for family to visit the patient
        x.   Preferred method of meeting and communicating with PCU team members (e.g., participation in scheduled PCU rounds, scheduled evening meetings, phone calls)

2. **Nursing examination of patient**
    a. Physical examination
    b. Cognitive assessment (e.g., ability to concentrate, level of judgment, presence of confusion)
    c. Behavioral assessment (sleep patterns, level of agitation, interaction with family and staff)
    d. Review of findings from other diagnostic studies (e.g., computed tomographic [CT] scan, electroencephalogram [EEG])
    e. Assessment of episode of delirium/disorientation and coping along the critical care continuum of care environment

3. **Appraisal of patient characteristics: Almost all patients with an acute illness experience some psychosocial issues during the course of their illness. However, each patient and family are unique and bring a unique set of characteristics to the care situation. Examples of characteristics of patients and family that the nurse needs to assess include the following: The AACN Progressive Care Task Force has described the synergy of the progressive care patient as moderately stable with less complexity, requires moderate resources, and requires intermittent nursing vigilance; or stable with a high potential for becoming unstable and requires increased intensity of care and vigilance. Characteristics of progressive care patients include a decreased risk of a life-threatening event, a decreased need for invasive monitoring, increased stability, and an increased ability to participate in their care**
    a. Resiliency
        i.   Level 1—*Minimally resilient:* A 47-year-old man who is admitted for observation after a suicide attempt of ingestion of half a bottle of aspirin
        ii.   Level 3—*Moderately resilient:* A 23-year-old man with a 9-year history of "problem drinking," stabilized and transferred from the critical care unit to progressive care after chest trauma suffered in an alcohol-related automobile accident and being prepared for transfer to a military hospital where he will receive extended treatment for alcohol abuse
        iii. Level 5—*Highly resilient:* A healthy 21-year-old female college student with a 3.9 grade point average who comes to the emergency department exhibiting multiple abrasions and unruly, belligerent, and delirious behavior after attending her first "spring break-out celebration," which included drinking and some drug experimentation
    b. Vulnerability
        i.   Level 1—*Highly vulnerable:* An 84-year-old woman who is living alone, has developed signs and symptoms of dementia and severe depression, and has forgotten to eat or drink for several days
        ii.   Level 3—*Moderately vulnerable:* An extremely overweight 37-year-old woman who admits to feeling "even more depressed" after her unsuccessful suicide attempt and numerous diets, pills, and diet plans that have not worked. Her primary physician relates that she does not meet the criteria for surgical treatment of morbid obesity.
        iii. Level 5—*Minimally vulnerable:* A 44-year-old single father, admitted for monitoring overnight subsequent to an automobile crash in which he was cited for aggressive driving, who relates that since his recent divorce he occasionally has had episodes when his anger quickly escalates to violent behaviors. He fears "taking it out" on his two sons.
    c. Stability
        i.   Level 1—*Minimally stable:* A 65-year-old woman who is transferred from the critical care unit after experiencing acute respiratory distress syndrome after the ingestion of

an alkali solution during an attempted suicide. She has been extubated for 2 days and is alert but nonresponsive to all attempts to engage in conversation.

ii. Level 3—*Moderately stable:* A 50-year-old man with a history of drinking four beers a day who is admitted to the PCU for an initial episode of gastrointestinal bleeding resulting from a duodenal ulcer. He is receiving benzodiazepines to prevent delirium tremens from acute alcohol withdrawal.

iii. Level 5—*Highly stable:* A 25-year-old woman is admitted to the PCU from the emergency department, to which she was brought by friends who could not wake her after a night of heavy drinking. She is now awake and alert.

d. Complexity

i. Level 1—*Highly complex:* An 89-year-old man who has liver failure resulting from the ingestion of 200 acetaminophen tablets after the death of his wife and who is transferred to the PCU from the critical care unit. He has multiple medical problems, including terminal lung cancer. He stated in his suicide note that he "is tired" and wants to be with his wife. He now has a "do not resuscitate" order.

ii. Level 3—*Moderately complex:* A 60-year-old patient with amyotrophic lateral sclerosis who has just been transferred from the critical care unit after an episode of acute respiratory failure. The patient has already stated he does not desire mechanical ventilation to prolong life. The family is supportive of the patient's wishes but does not want the patient to suffer or be left alone.

iii. Level 5—*Minimally complex:* A 50-year-old woman in the PCU for the management of gastrointestinal bleeding resulting from nonsteroidal anti-inflammatory drug use, who has delirium after receiving sedatives

e. Resource availability

i. Level 1—*Few resources:* A homeless woman who is admitted for observation from the emergency department after an attempt at suicide by slicing her wrist. She has no identification, and she refuses to talk with the staff.

ii. Level 3—*Moderate resources:* An 83-year-old woman who is admitted from a local nursing home to the PCU with possible urosepsis. The patient's family has been paying out of pocket for the nursing home but says "the money is almost gone."

iii. Level 5—*Many resources:* A 60-year-old male computer executive who has delirium tremens 4 days after undergoing elective hip surgery. His family is very supportive and confident the patient would be concerned if he realized how his drinking (three to four glasses of wine per day) had affected him. The patient has excellent insurance coverage for both inpatient care and outpatient substance abuse treatment.

f. Participation in care

i. Level 1—*No participation:* An 85-year-old male patient who underwent a complicated aortic aneurysm repair 4 days earlier and transferred from the ICU today. The patient has a 10-year history of dementia and is now having delirium. The ICU had experienced a great deal of difficulty with mobilizing the patient. He is restless and uncooperative.

ii. Level 3—*Moderate level of participation:* A 37-year-old man who has a diagnosis of cardiomyopathy and will undergo tests to be placed on a transplant list. Running has been his life, and he is listless and depressed.

iii. Level 5—*Full participation:* A. 70-year-old man who is admitted to the PCU after colectomy and small bowel resection. He asks the nurse for more pain medication so that he can "sit up more and take some deep breaths" as his preoperative instructions directed.

g. Participation in decision making

i. Level 1—*No participation:* A 65-year-old female patient whose daughter faints after she is told that her mother has inoperable metastasis of lung cancer. The mother is requesting the daughter's participation in the decision regarding chemotherapy. The daughter is crying and does not want to discuss it.

ii. Level 3—*Moderate level of participation:* A 67-year-old man who requires a tracheostomy for long-term airway management after a suicide attempt and whose wife requests multiple consultations from other pulmonary services

       iii.   Level 5—*Full participation:* A 65-year-old patient with cancer and chronic pain who has asked to have do not resuscitate orders and to be "allowed to die with dignity"

  h. Predictability

       i.   Level 1—*Not predictable:* A 75-year-old woman with ovarian cancer who is admitted after ingesting 10 capsules of acetaminophen to "stop the pain"

       ii.   Level 3—*Moderately predictable:* A 60-year-old patent with acute upper respiratory tract congestion and asthma who has delirium resulting from a combination of hypoxemia and electrolyte imbalances

       iii.   Level 5—*Highly predictable:* A 20-year-old patient who is admitted with altered consciousness after drinking at a college fraternity party

4. **Diagnostic studies**

  a. Laboratory studies

  b. EEG

  c. Cerebral blood flow studies

Psychosocial Care Issues

1. **Interdependence—Many of the psychosocial issues and concerns of the acutely ill patient are interdependent. For example, inadequately managed pain may lead to feelings of powerlessness, anxiety, and depression that, in turn, heighten the patient's perception of pain (Figure 10-2).**

2. **Powerlessness**

  a. Description of problem

       i.   Perceived lack of control over the outcome of a specific situation. The ability of an event to engender a sense of powerlessness is influenced by the individual's self-esteem and self-concept and where the individual is in the life cycle.

       ii.   Progressive care patients have experienced loss of their ability to control even the most basic of functions, including the ability to communicate, to breathe on their own, and to control bladder and bowel function. Depending on the philosophy and organization of the critical care environment, they may experience loss in the ability to participate in decision making about their own health care and future.

       iii.   Progressive care patients who have been transferred from the critical care unit may be skeptical regarding their progress toward recovery.

       iv.   Progressive care patients may question the ability of the progressive care nurse to care for their acute illness needs.

       v.   Patients may fear being alone.

  b. Goals of care

       i.   Patient communicates needs and wishes verbally or nonverbally.

       ii.   Patient (and family as appropriate) participates in decision making regarding the plan of care.

       iii.   Patient and family members do not demonstrate signs of dysfunction associated with powerlessness, such as the following:

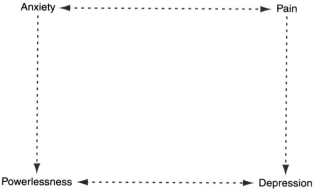

FIGURE 10-2 ■ Relationship between psychosocial needs and problems during a critical illness.

  (a) Withdrawal
  (b) Aggressive behavior
  (c) Demanding behavior
  (d) Excessive repetition of the same questions
  (e) Placing of unrealistic demands on the staff
  (f) Blaming of the staff for the patient's condition
   iv. Patient participates in decision making regarding daily care activities (e.g., timing of bath, sleep, visiting hours).
 c. Collaborating professionals on health care team
   i. Nurse
   ii. Physician
   iii. Respiratory therapist
   iv. Physical therapist
   v. Social worker
   vi. Clergy
   vii. Case manager
 d. Interventions
   i. Promote patient-nurse communication.
  (a) Methods of communication should be based on patient preferences and abilities.
  (b) Utilize available interpreter services for non-English-speaking patients and family members.
  (c) Enlist help from family members and volunteers in the communication process.
   ii. Involve the patient and family in the care-planning process and decision making.
  (a) Ask the patient (or health care proxy) what level of involvement he or she would like in the care-planning process.
  (b) Encourage the patient and family members to keep a record of questions and concerns.
  (c) Provide the patient, proxy, or a family member with daily (or more frequent) updates regarding the patient's status and care plan.
   iii. Encourage the patient and family members to meet with spiritual support persons if they would find this helpful.
   iv. Prepare the patient for procedures: explain what will be happening, when it will happen, and how the patient will be affected.
 e. Evaluation of patient care: Patient and family are active participants in care planning and delivery (to the extent possible)
3. Sleep deprivation
 a. Patients who have transitioned from the critical care environment may have experienced a decrease in the amount, consistency, and/or quality of sleep that occurs in a 24-hour period. Sleep fragmentation occurs when the patient fails to complete a 90-minute average sleep cycle that includes both rapid eye movement and non–rapid eye movement sleep.
   i. Circadian rhythm refers to the 24-hour cycle that is linked to light/dark phases.
   ii. Biologic functions such as heart rate, metabolic rate, breathing rate, and temperature are affected by the circadian cycle.
   iii. Imbalance in the secretion of melatonin can result in a wide range of sleep disorders.
 b. Goals of care
   i. Work with patient to restore a normal sleeping pattern.
   ii. Patient states that he or she feels rested.
   iii. Patient does not demonstrate signs and symptoms of sleep deprivation, including the following:
  (a) Altered mental status (e.g., confusion, delusions)
  (b) Decreased alertness

       (c) Irritability
       (d) Aggressive behavior
       (e) Restlessness
       (f) Anxiety
       (g) Exhaustion

  c. Collaborating professionals on health care team
     i. Nurse
     ii. Physician
     iii. Pharmacist
     iv. Respiratory therapist

  d. Interventions
     i. Prepare patient's environment to optimize normal sleep time rest.
     ii. Monitor the room temperature.
     iii. Help patient to remain physically active during normal waking hours.
     iv. Decrease the noise level to promote sleep.
     v. Decrease overhead lighting to promote sleep.
     vi. Provide adequate pain relief.
     vii. Teach the patient and family relaxation techniques to promote rest and sleep.
     viii. Administer pharmacologic agents as needed to promote sleep (e.g., melatonin, benzodiazepines, diphenhydramine). Note: Long-term use of benzodiazepines can abolish stage IV sleep.
     ix. Consult with a pharmacist regarding the best drug choices for promoting sleep, particularly for high-risk populations such as the elderly.
     x. Allow individualized family visitation that promotes sleep patterns.

  e. Evaluation of patient care
     i. Patient's signs and symptoms of sleep deprivation are resolved.
     ii. Patient states that he or she feels rested.

4. Grief and loss
  a. Description of problem: The grief reaction is the emotional response to a loss in which something valued is changed or altered so that it no longer has its previously valued traits
     i. Grief can be experienced during an acute or a critical illness by both the patient and family members.
     ii. Grief may result from loss (or potential loss) of health, body image, role, and financial security.
     iii. Degree of grief experienced is related to the meaning of the loss to the individual, the adequacy of coping responses, and the availability of support systems.
     iv. Expressions of grief have wide variation and are culturally determined.

  b. Goals of care
     i. Patient and family express feelings of grief and loss (if they choose).
     ii. Patient and family are able to state the prognosis and current plan of care.

  c. Collaborating professionals on health care team
     i. Nurse
     ii. Clergy
     iii. Social worker
     iv. Physician

  d. Interventions
     i. Appreciate cultural variation in expressions of grief.
     ii. Allow the patient and family members to express grief in their own way.
     iii. Provide privacy for family members and patients.
     iv. Provide ongoing, honest information to the patient and family regarding the patient's illness and expected recovery.
     v. Provide the patient and family with teaching regarding the normal grief response.

  e. Evaluation of patient care: Patient and family express grief in a culturally appropriate way

5. Sensory overload or deprivation: See Box 10-1

SPECIFIC PATIENT HEALTH PROBLEMS

Anxiety

1. Definition: According to the American Psychiatric Association, *anxiety* is the apprehensive anticipation of future danger or misfortune accompanied by a feeling of dysphoria or somatic symptoms of tension. Focus of anticipated danger may be internal or external.
2. Etiology and risk factors: Results from multiple sources in the PCU, including the following:
   a. Unstable physiologic status (e.g., hypoxemia with shortness of breath)
   b. Pain
   c. Fear of the unknown
   d. Procedures
   e. Separation from family and support system
   f. Underlying psychiatric disorder (including panic disorders, phobias, and posttraumatic stress disorder)
   g. Fear or change in security associated with change in status or move from critical care into progressive care
      i. Lack of having nurse close by
      ii. Removal of perceived life-saving equipment
      iii. Decrease in the visibility of nurse or staff
3. Signs and symptoms: See Box 10-2
4. Diagnostic study findings
   a. When behavioral manifestations of anxiety are present, possible physiologic causes (e.g., hypoxemia, hypoglycemia) must be ruled out.
   b. Toxicologic screen: To assess for possible drug-induced anxiety
   c. Mental Status Examination: Findings may be abnormal with severe anxiety
5. Collaborative diagnoses of patient needs: Minimize anxiety for the patient and family by preparing them for potentially anxiety-producing situations
6. Goals of care
   a. Patient does not demonstrate signs or symptoms of anxiety (e.g., no tachypnea, tachycardia, muscle tension).
   b. Patient communicates that he or she is not anxious.
7. Management of patient care
   a. Anticipated patient trajectory: With reassurance, support, and pharmacologic therapy as needed, anxiety can be minimized
      i. Treatments
         (a) Nonpharmacologic
            (1) Reassure the patient and give explanations about the patient's condition and treatment plan.
            (2) Ask the patient to discuss fears and worries.
            (3) Assure the patient that adequate sedation and pain medication will be provided during painful procedures.
            (4) Assure the patient and family that the patient will be monitored and observed frequently.
            (5) Allow family members to stay with the patient as much as possible to provide support.
            (6) Use music therapy.
            (7) Use pet therapy if available.
            (8) Establish hourly rounding to reassure the patient.
         (b) Pharmacologic
            (1) Benzodiazepines
            (2) Sedatives and hypnotics
            (3) Pain medication (as needed)

■ **BOX 10-2**
■ **CLINICAL MANIFESTATIONS OF ANXIETY**

COGNITIVE
- Apprehension
- Difficulty concentrating
- Hypervigilance
- Impaired judgment
- Self-consciousness
- Worry

BEHAVIORAL
- Easy fatigue
- Fidgeting
- Refusal of medical treatment
- Restlessness
- Sleep disturbances
- Unrealistic demands for attention

PHYSIOLOGIC
CARDIAC
- Chest pain
- Dysrhythmias
- Increased blood pressure
- Palpitations
- Tachycardia

RESPIRATORY
- Choking sensation
- Shortness of breath
- Tachypnea

NEUROMUSCULAR
- Dilated pupils
- Dizziness
- Light-headedness
- Muscle and motor tension
- Tremors

GASTROINTESTINAL
- Anorexia
- Nausea
- Vomiting

GENITOURINARY
- Frequency
- Urgency

   ii.   Discharge planning
      (a) Teach the patient and family methods of anxiety reduction (e.g., imagery, distraction).
      (b) Patient may require follow-up (psychiatric and/or social services) for unresolved anxiety issues.
      (c) Patient may require follow-up teaching regarding pharmacologic and nonpharmacologic interventions to treat anxiety.

Pain

1. **Description**
   a. *Pain* is an individual, subjective, and complex biopsychosocial process whose existence cannot be proved or disproved. Unrelieved pain is a major psychologic and physiologic stressor for patients.
   b. **McCaffery states that p**ain is "whatever the person says it is, existing whenever he says it does"
   c. **Mersky describes p**ain as "an unpleasant sensory and emotional experience".
      i.   Amount of tissue damage is not the only predictor of when and how pain is experienced.
      ii. Other factors influence the response to the cognitive integration of pain (e.g., age, gender, culture, beliefs, mood, previous pain experiences, current diagnosis and situation, amount of perceived control over the situation).
      iii. Negative impact of pain on one's quality of life can include suffering, fear, anxiety, depression, and hopelessness
2. **Etiology and risk factors**
   a. Acute conditions
      i.   Surgical events (e.g., incisions; presence of drains, tubes, orthopedic hardware)
      ii. Traumatic injuries (e.g., fractures, lacerations)

        iii. Medical conditions (e.g., pancreatitis, ulcerative colitis, migraine headache)

        iv. Psychologic conditions (e.g., anxiety), which can increase pain perception, prolong the pain experience, and lower the pain threshold

   b. Procedures (e.g., turning; suctioning; placement or removal of catheters, tubes, or drains; paracentesis)

   c. Immobility

   d. Preexisting chronic pain conditions

        i. Musculoskeletal conditions (e.g., arthritis, low back pain, fibromyalgia)

        ii. Other conditions (e.g., cancer, stroke, diabetic neuropathy)

   e. Pain can also be perceived without the current presence of a physiologically unpleasant stimulus.

3. **Signs and symptoms**

   a. See Chapter 4 for physiologic aspects of pain

   b. Most reliable indicator of pain is the patient's self-report

   c. Other important points related to manifestations of pain include the following:

        i. Patients in pain often demonstrate one or more behavioral signs or indicators of pain intensity (see Table 4-22).

        ii. When patients are unable to respond or self-report pain, behavioral indicators may be used. Because of the individuality of pain expression, these indicators may be absent despite the presence of severe pain, which may cause clinicians to conclude erroneously that pain is not present.

        iii. When conditions known to be painful exist, assume that pain is present and proceed with appropriate treatment.

        iv. Several barriers and misconceptions about pain hinder effective pain management (Table 10-2), including the clinician's personal values and beliefs, and confusion about addiction, tolerance, and physical dependence with regard to pain medications. See Table 10-3 for distinctions in these terms as they relate to pain and opioid use.

   d. Practitioners must accept and respond to patient reports of pain.

   e. Decrease in or elimination of a pain behavior after an analgesia intervention can indicate a reduction in pain and reflect an ongoing need for analgesia.

   f. The Capp/Rogers National Pain Care Policy Act of 2007 (HR 2994) provides support to address the barriers that people in pain often face.

        i. Improving pain care research

        ii. Education on pain care

        iii. Training in pain management

        iv. Improving access to pain care

4. **Diagnostic study findings**

   a. **Puntillo states that** "pain is described by the person experiencing it; it doesn't have to be diagnosed any other way."

   b. Diagnostic studies may supplement, but should not replace, a comprehensive physical examination and history.

   c. Diagnostic studies can help to accurately identify the causes for pain; however, the absence of positive study findings should not be used to deny the existence of pain.

   d. While diagnostic studies are in progress, treatment of pain should be initiated. It is rarely justified to defer analgesia until a diagnosis is made.

5. **Goals of care**

   a. Pain, including procedural pain, is consistently controlled at or below the patient's stated comfort level (e.g., a pain score of 2 to 3 on a scale of 0 to 10).

   b. In a patient unable to provide a self-report of pain, there is a marked decrease or absence of pain behaviors after pharmacologic intervention.

   c. Patient demonstrates a decrease in anxiety and other psychologic effects of unrelieved pain.

   d. Patient is able to comfortably perform or participate in activities necessary for recovery.

   e. Patient has increased periods of uninterrupted sleep.

   f. Medication adverse effects are avoided or managed.

   g. Length of hospital stay is not extended because of poorly managed pain.

   h. Patient is satisfied with pain management.

■ **TABLE 10-2**
■ ■ **Barriers to Pain Management in the Critically Ill Patient**

Barrier	Comment
Pain management often is not a priority because of life-threatening illness or other physiologic conditions.	Patients have the right to effective pain management, and every effort should be made to include analgesia in the treatment plan.
Cultural beliefs about pain (e.g., pain builds character, pain is a sign of weakness or a form of punishment) may affect pain management.	Provide education about harmful effects of pain, benefits of effective pain management, and need to report the effectiveness of pain management.
Lack of knowledge about the process of pain (see Chapter 4)	Meaning and expression of pain vary among patients.
• Individuality of a patient's pain response	Self-report is the single most reliable indicator of pain (patient is the authority on his or her pain, not you).
• Failure to accept a patient's self-report of pain	Pain is not an acceptable consequence of surgery or trauma.
• Harmful effects of pain	Unrelieved pain can lead to life-threatening complications, delayed healing, increased length of hospital stay, and development of future pain issues.
Lack of knowledge about pharmacology of opioids (see Chapter 4)	Respiratory depression is preventable in most cases by slow opioid titration and decrease of dosage when increased sedation occurs.
• Exaggerated fear of opioid-induced adverse effects, especially respiratory depression	
• Ignorance of onset, peak, duration of action, equianalgesia	Physicians often underprescribe opioids, and nurses often administer the lowest prescribed dose, which contributes to the undertreatment of pain.
Exaggerated fears related to addiction (see Table 10-3)	When opioids are used for pain relief, the addiction rate is less than 1%.
• Fear of creating addiction or causing relapse in a patient with a history of addiction	Patients with chronic pain often are knowledgeable about which analgesics and dosages they need to relieve their pain. This is not always a sign of addiction.
• Fear of being lied to about the severity of pain in order to obtain drugs to support an existing addiction	
Inability to communicate (see Chapter 4)	Use translators as indicated.
• Language barrier or aphasia	Assume pain is present on basis of physical findings (e.g., trauma, surgery, procedures), and treat with analgesics.
• Mechanical ventilation	
• Use of neuromuscular blocking agents, sedatives	
• Other conditions (e.g., delirium, coma)	
Noisy and chaotic critical care environment	Sleep deprivation, anxiety, and lack of control can negatively affect the patient's perception of, response to, and tolerance of pain.

6. **Management of patient care**
   a. The Joint Commission's 2008 standards were developed in collaboration with the University of Wisconsin–Madison Medical School. The standards include the following:
      i. "Patients have the right to pain management" (RI.2.160).
      ii. "When pain is identified, the patient is assessed and treated by the hospital or referred for treatment" (PC.8.10).
   b. Anticipated patient trajectory
      i. Assessment
         (a) Perform thorough history taking (including a pain history), physical examination, and pain assessment.
         (b) Identify the underlying cause whenever possible.
         (c) Identify any previously effective methods of coping with and relieving pain.
      ii. Treatments
         (a) Nonpharmacologic methods

■ **TABLE 10-3**
■ ■ **Definitions Related to the Use of Opioids in the Treatment of Pain**

Term	Definition	Comment
Addiction	Chronic, neurobiologic disease Persistent pattern of compulsive and dysfunctional opioid use characterized by an impaired control over drug use, continued use despite harm, use for effect other than pain relief, and craving	When opioids are used for pain relief, the incidence of addiction is less than 1%. Patients with addictive disease are at high risk for undertreatment of pain and have the right to receive quality pain management. Be prepared to titrate opioids and benzodiazepines to dosages higher than usual on basis of assessment findings (e.g., pain, side effects, mood).
Physical dependence	Physiologic state of reliance on an opioid, evidenced by withdrawal symptoms if the opioid is abruptly stopped or an opioid antagonist is given Does not, in and of itself, imply addiction	Signs and symptoms of withdrawal include lacrimation, rhinorrhea, pupil dilation, yawning, tremor, gooseflesh, insomnia, diarrhea, vomiting, irritability, elevated blood pressure, muscle cramps, dysphoria.
Tolerance	State of adaptation characterized by the need for increasing or more frequent doses of medication to maintain an effect Does not, in and of itself, imply addiction	Tolerance occurs to both the analgesic and adverse effects of opioids (except constipation).
Pain tolerance	Point at which an increasing intensity of a stimulus is felt as painful	Individual, influenced by many factors (e.g., endorphin levels)
Pain threshold	Duration or intensity of pain that a person is willing to endure	Individual, influenced by many factors (e.g., energy level, past pain experiences)

Data and definitions compiled from American Academy of Pain Medicine, American Pain Society, American Society of Addiction Medicine. *Consensus Document: Definitions Related to the Use of Opioids for the Treatment of Pain.* Glenview, IL: American Academy of Pain Medicine; 2001; http://www.asam.org/ppol/paindef.htm; American Society of Pain Management Nurses. *ASPMN Position Statement: Pain Management in Patients With Addictive Disease.* Pensacola, FL: American Society of Pain Management Nurses; 2002; and McCaffery M, Pasero C. *Pain: Clinical Manual.* 2nd ed. St Louis, MO: Mosby; 1999.

       (1) May be used to supplement, but not replace, analgesic medications. Table 10-4 provides an overview of these therapies.
       (2) There is a lack of conclusive scientific evidence to support the efficacy of their use for pain management.
           a) Results are unpredictable.
           b) Many do not relieve pain; some may only make pain more tolerable for brief intervals.
           c) Patients must be willing and physically and mentally able to try them.
       (3) No universally accepted categorizations or definitions of these methods exist. Broad categories include the following:
           a) Cutaneous stimulation and physical modalities
           b) Cognitive and behavioral modalities
           c) Complementary and alternative medicine
       (4) Use of these methods in the progressive care patient is limited because of the severity of the patient's illness and other demands on the nurse's time.
     (b) Pharmacologic methods (see also Chapter 4)
       (1) Analgesics are the mainstay of treatment for acute and cancer pain and some chronic noncancer pain.
       (2) Three classes of analgesic are nonopioids, opioids, and coanalgesics (adjuvants).

■ **TABLE 10-4**
■ ■ **Nonpharmacologic Approaches to Pain Management in the Critically Ill Patient***

Examples	Indications	Presumed Mechanism of Pain Reduction	Comments
CUTANEOUS STIMULATION†			
Superficial heat • Hot packs • Hot water bottles • Heating pads • Chemical gel packs	Joint and muscle pain, spasm, and stiffness, as from surgery Trauma Arthritis Acute low back pain	Activation of large myelinated primary afferent fibers may modify response of spinal cord to noxious stimuli.	May apply at pain site or distal, proximal, or contralateral to pain Avoid both heat and cold over radiation-therapy sites.
Superficial cold • Ice packs • Towels soaked in ice water • Gel packs	Itching Heat preferred for thrombophlebitis Cold preferred for acute trauma and migraine pain; avoid in peripheral vascular disease	May decrease muscle spasm, sensitivity to pain Heat may increase elastic properties of muscles. Cold may cause local numbing.	Skin must be protected to avoid tissue damage. Cold often more effective and long-lasting than heat
Massage	Stress, anxiety Muscle tension, spasm, pain Immobility	May inhibit transmission of painful stimuli Relaxes muscles	May be acceptable form of touch to convey care and concern Family can be involved.
TENS	Acute surgical, musculoskeletal, neuropathic pain	May inhibit transmission of painful stimuli	Avoid if patient has on-demand pacemaker
Vibration	Muscle, joint and neuropathic pain Avoid in thrombophlebitis, headaches.	Paresthesia or numbness over site	May change pain from sharp to dull Can be substituted for TENS
PHYSICAL†			
Mobilization Range-of-motion exercises Physical therapy Repositioning	Prolonged immobility and decreased function	Relieves muscle tension Keeps joints and ligaments flexible	Helps decrease loss of function, strength
Immobilization	Some postoperative conditions, fractures	Relieves muscle tension Keeps joints and ligaments flexible	Maintains joints in position of maximum function
COGNITIVE-BEHAVIORAL			
Distraction Television Reading Visiting Imagery Music, singing Humor	Mild to moderate pain of brief duration, such as procedural pain	In general, thought to interfere with neural perception of pain in the brain Refocuses or directs attention away from painful stimuli	Pain awareness may be increased after distraction, so patient may need analgesia to rest.
Relaxation • Deep or rhythmic breathing • Progressive muscle relaxation • Imagery • Massage • Music • Repetition of word or phrase	Muscle tension Anxiety, stress Acute or chronic pain	May be related to reduction in muscle tension, distress, and anxiety	May not "look" like patient is in pain Teach and use as coping skill for stress reduction. Dim light and noise reduction promote relaxation.

Continued

■ **TABLE 10-4**
■ ■ **Nonpharmacologic Approaches to Pain Management in the Critically Ill Patient*—Cont'd**

Examples	Indications	Presumed Mechanism of Pain Reduction	Comments
Education • Pain-management concepts	Any pain condition Throughout shift	Reduces stress, anxiety Increases sense of control	Teach patient, family, significant other.
CAM MODALITIES			
Prayer Meditation Biofeedback Hypnosis Aromatherapy Yoga Therapeutic touch Reflexology Acupuncture Herbs Vitamins	Mainly chronic pain conditions Same methods for acute pain, such as prayer or massage	Promote balance, harmony, and healing by interaction of mind, body, and spirit.	Overlap exists between CAM and other nonpharmacologic approaches.

* In most clinical situations, these approaches should be used in addition to analgesics.
† Physician order may be required.
TENS, Transcutaneous electrical nerve stimulation; *CAM*, complementary and alternative medicine.

    iii. Discharge planning: Patient and family teaching regarding the following:
        (a) Appropriate use of pain scales or other methods to be used to assess pain
        (b) Effective pain management concepts and options (e.g., pain medications and the difference between addiction, physical dependence, and tolerance)
        (c) Pain management as an important part of patient care
        (d) Responsibility of the patient to report ineffective pain relief and concerns regarding the pain management plan
    iv. Useful pain management resources: See pain section in the reference list

Delirium (Acute Confusional State)

1. **Definition:** Clinical state associated with a disturbance of consciousness that is accompanied by a change in cognition that cannot be accounted for by a preexisting or evolving dementia. Delirium develops over a short time (hours to days) and fluctuates during the course of a day. Delirium is often a temporary condition.
2. **Etiology and risk factors**
    a. Incidence (rates)
        i. 50% of the critically ill experience delirium
        ii. 80% of terminally ill develop delirium near death
    b. Delirium due to a general medical condition
        i. Hypoxia
        ii. Hypercapnia
        iii. Metabolic acidosis
        iv. Heart, kidney, liver failure
        v. Hyperthyroidism or hypothyroidism
        vi. Hyperparathyroidism
        vii. Cerebrovascular accident, transient ischemic attack
        viii. Concussion
        ix. Postictal state
        x. Electrolyte imbalances (hyperkalemia, hypokalemia)
        xi. Hyperglycemia or hypoglycemia
        xii. Alcohol or drug withdrawal

        xiii. Infection

        xiv. Pain

    c. Substance-induced delirium (due to a medication, toxin exposure, drug abuse)

        i. Anesthetics (emergence delirium)

        ii. Analgesics

        iii. Sedatives (e.g., benzodiazepines)

        iv. Antiemetics

        v. Cardiac medications (e.g., antihypertensives, digoxin)

        vi. Steroids

        vii. Anticholinergics

        viii. Delirium due to multiple causes

        ix. Other (i.e., not able to be specified)

3. Signs and symptoms

    a. Cognitive

        i. Diminished attention span

        ii. Reduced ability to focus

        iii. Disorientation to person, place, time

        iv. Confusion over daily events

        v. Hallucinations (visual are more common)

        vi. Abnormal results on a Mental Status Examination (i.e., Folstein Mini-Mental State Examination)

    b. Behavioral: May vary markedly from patient to patient

        i. Excessive restlessness

        ii. Sluggishness and lethargy

        iii. Inappropriate behavior

        iv. Irritability

        v. Picking or groping at bed linens, gown

        vi. Attempting to get out of bed (when unsafe)

        vii. Crying out, screaming, moaning, muttering

        viii. Personality changes

        ix. Changes in affect

    c. Physiologic

        i. Tremors (alcohol withdrawal)

        ii. Seizures (alcohol withdrawal)

4. Diagnostic study findings: Dependent on the underlying problem (e.g., may have abnormal electrolyte levels, CT scan results)

5. Collaborative diagnoses of patient needs

    a. Assess for possible factors that could contribute to delirium.

    b. Decrease the use of medications that could contribute to delirium.

6. Goals of care

    a. Patient is oriented to person, time, and place.

    b. Patient does not demonstrate signs or symptoms of anxiety, fear, and confusion.

    c. Patient responds to simple, concrete questions.

7. Management of patient care

    a. Anticipated patient trajectory: With treatment of the underlying cause of delirium, the problem can be managed and eliminated

        i. Treatments

            (a) Nonpharmacologic

                (1) Assess for delirium (e.g., Confusion Assessment Method–ICU)

                (2) Provide for adequate rest and sleep.

                (3) Review medication list with the physician, and discontinue suspect medications.

                (4) Monitor and manage electrolyte and acid-base disorders.

                (5) Consult a psychiatrist if delirium does not resolve with standard management.

                (6) Use restraints only as needed for patient safety.

(7) Explain to family members the nature of delirium and why it occurs. Stress the temporary nature of the condition in hospitalized patients.

(8) Give family members updates on patient management and progress (e.g., findings related to the underlying cause of the delirium).

(9) Reassure the family that the patient is not in control or responsible for his or her behaviors.

(b) Pharmacologic: Avoid additional drugs unless needed for patient, family, or staff safety

(1) There are currently no drugs with Food and Drug Administration (FDA) approval for the treatment of delirium.

(2) Antipsychotic (e.g., haloperidol) is recommended by the American Psychiatric Association and the Society of Critical Care Medicine.

(3) Benzodiazepine (in combination with an antipsychotic). Note: Benzodiazepines may worsen delirium, especially in the elderly. Use the smallest dosage possible.

(4) Few evidence-based protocols are available; for an example see http://www.icudelirium.org/delirium/training-pages/DeliriumProto%2001_30_07.pdf

  ii. Discharge planning

   (a) No specific needs anticipated related to delirium

   (b) May require follow-up with primary care provider

Depression

1. Definition: Mood state characterized by feeling of sadness, lowered self-esteem, and pessimistic thinking and guilt. Depressive episodes and depressive disorders are psychiatric diagnoses given to patients based on specific criteria (e.g., etiology, length of depression).

2. Etiology and risk factors

 a. According to the APA, the incidence in the medically ill ranges from 6% to 72%.

 b. Causes of depression include the following:

  i. Psychodynamic

   (a) Illness progression

   (b) Fear and anxiety regarding the illness and the outcome of the illness

   (c) Illness-related regimen

   (d) Reaction to loss and deprivation

   (e) Partial or complete loss of self-esteem

  ii. Cognitive: Patient's beliefs (thoughts such as "It's all my fault") may lead to depression

  iii. Biochemical

   (a) Neurotransmitter imbalance

   (b) Thyroid dysfunction

   (c) Hypocalcemia or hypercalcemia

   (d) Medications (e.g., antihypertensives, thiazides, spironolactone, β-blockers, digoxin [at toxic levels], steroids, benzodiazepines, cocaine withdrawal, alcohol)

  iv. Social

   (a) Lack of social support

   (b) Abandonment or isolation

  v. Other

   (a) Lack of sleep

   (b) Chronic or acute unmanaged pain

3. Signs and symptoms

 a. Cognitive

  i. Decreased ability to concentrate

  ii. Difficulty making decisions

 b. Behavioral

  i. Psychomotor agitation

  ii. Abnormal sleep patterns

  iii. Apparent sadness (tears, furrowed brow, downturned corners of the mouth, lack of eye contact)

      iv. Fatigue

      v. Recurrent thoughts of death

4. Diagnostic study findings

  a. Diagnosis based on history and clinical examination (i.e., cognitive and behavioral changes)

  b. Diagnostic test results may be abnormal if there is an underlying physiologic problem contributing to the depression (e.g., digoxin toxicosis)

  c. Mini-Mental State Examination to rule out delirium (delirium may be confused with depression)

  d. EEG: Sleep EEG abnormalities may be present in up to 90% of inpatients during a major depressive episode

5. Collaborative diagnoses of patient needs

  a. Allow the patient to participate in goal setting with the ICU team.

  b. Treat manageable symptoms such as pain and anxiety that may contribute to depression.

  c. Review the plan of care with the patient, and stress areas of improvement as appropriate.

  d. Allow the patient control over the environment as much as possible.

  e. Assist the patient in understanding the biochemical nature of depression (when appropriate).

6. Goals of care

  a. Patient verbalizes concerns about his or her medical condition, treatment plan, and so on, that led to feelings of depression.

  b. Patient is able to describe the presumed cause and management of depression for his or her particular situation.

  c. Patient is able to describe his or her role in the plan of care.

  d. Patient sets realistic goals with the health care team regarding the plan of care.

7. Management of patient care

  a. Anticipated patient trajectory: With counseling, ongoing support from family and friends, and, when indicated, pharmacologic therapy, patients with depression can resume and maintain normal lives

      i. Treatments

         (a) Nonpharmacologic

            (1) Assist in performing a differential diagnosis: Grief reaction, mood disorder, organic brain syndrome, delirium, dementia, metabolic conditions presenting as depression (e.g., hypercapnia, metabolic acidosis, uremia).

            (2) Discuss the treatment plan and progress with the patient—engage the patient in care planning as appropriate.

            (3) Discuss concerns over possible or actual depressed state.

            (4) Acknowledge that a depressed mood can be normal during or after a serious illness.

            (5) Provide a mechanism to increase social support (family support, social services).

            (6) Attend to any suicidal ideation (is the patient a threat to self or others?).

            (7) Secure a psychiatric referral as appropriate.

         (b) Pharmacologic: Antidepressants (e.g., tricyclics, selective serotonin reuptake inhibitors)

      ii. Discharge planning

         (a) Provide information to the patient and family about depression and available treatments.

         (b) Discuss pharmacologic therapy, including mode of action, benefits, and side effects.

         (c) Patient may require follow-up evaluation and teaching on pharmacologic and nonpharmacologic treatments for depression.

         (d) The FDA notified health care professionals that all makers of antidepressant medications require warning that there may be an increase in suicidal thinking in young adults 18 to 24 years of age during the first 1 to 2 months of treatment

Alcohol Withdrawal

1. **Definition: Presence of a characteristic withdrawal syndrome that develops after the cessation of (or reduction in) heavy and prolonged alcohol use**
2. **Etiology and risk factors: Abrupt cessation of alcohol use in persons with a physical dependence**
3. **Signs and symptoms (12 to 48 hours after cessation of alcohol intake): Withdrawal syndrome includes two or more symptoms of autonomic hyperactivity (e.g., sweating, pulse >100 beats/min, insomnia, agitation)**
   a. Mild to moderate dependency
      i.   Agitation
      ii. Anxiety
      iii. Tremors
      iv. Nausea and vomiting
      v.   Weakness
      vi. Diaphoresis
      vii. Hallucinations
   b. Delirium tremens (48 to 72 hours after cessation of alcohol intake)
      i.   Anxiety attacks
      ii.   Sleeplessness
      iii. Disorientation
      iv.   Confusion
      v.   Cognitive impairment
      vi.   Delirium
      vii. Tachycardia
      viii. Fever
      ix.   Grand mal seizure
4. **Diagnostic study findings**
   a. Blood alcohol level: Elevated on admission
   b. Liver function studies: Values may be elevated
   c. Clinical Institute Withdrawal Assessment for Alcohol (CIWA-Ar) or Clinical Institute Withdrawal Assessment for Alcohol DSM-IV version (CIWA-AD) to quantify the severity of withdrawal and guide collaborative diagnoses of patient needs
5. **Goals of care**
   a. Patient does not demonstrate signs or symptoms of withdrawal (e.g., seizures, agitation, irritability) that affect patient, family, and staff safety.
   b. Patient states negative effects of alcohol on body systems (e.g., liver failure).
6. **Management of patient care**
   a. Anticipated patient trajectory: With aggressive pharmacologic and nonpharmacologic management, patients undergoing acute alcohol withdrawal should recover without incident. Life-long counseling and support (e.g., Alcoholics Anonymous) is needed for patients with an alcohol addiction.
      i. Treatments
         (a) Nonpharmacologic
             (1) Protect the patient, family, and staff from harm (e.g., use padded bed rails).
             (2) Use a nonthreatening, supportive manner with the patient.
             (3) Engage the patient in short, directed conversations.
             (4) Decrease stimulation that could precipitate aggressive or violent behaviors.
         (b) Pharmacologic
             (1) Administer medications to a patient who is at risk for withdrawal or who demonstrates withdrawal behaviors.
             (2) Benzodiazepines (give based on results of CIWA-Ar or Severity Assessment Scale)
             (3) Adjunctive pharmacologic treatment (e.g., thiamine, folate, multivitamins)
             (4) Mayo-Smith, Beecher, Fischer, et al found in a meta-analysis that sedative-hypnotic agents are more effective than neuroleptic agents in reducing duration of delirium and mortality.

    ii. Discharge planning
       (a) Patient referral to Alcoholics Anonymous for current and future management
       (b) Referral of family members to Al-Anon or Alateen
   iii. Ethical issues: Staff may have ethical issues or conflicts caring for patients whose health problems they perceive to be "self-inflicted"

Aggression and Violence

1. **Definition:** *Aggression* is forceful physical or verbal behavior that may or may not cause harm to others. *Violence* is the ultimate maladaptive coping response and is the acting out of aggression that results in injury to others or destruction of property.
2. **Etiology and risk factors:** Violence in the progressive care setting may be triggered by the accumulation of stress in patients or family members who have feelings of desperation and who lack coping skills and/or resources to resolve a situation by other means. Aggression and violence can be present with the following:
   a. Personality disorders
   b. Organic illness
   c. Psychiatric illness
   d. Substance abuse or withdrawal
3. **Signs and symptoms**
   a. Cognitive
     i. Inability to think clearly and rationally
     ii. Paranoia
   b. Behavioral
     i. Anger, yelling, use of profanity
     ii. Agitation
     iii. Pacing (family member)
     iv. Verbal threats
     v. Striking, pushing, kicking of staff
   c. Physiologic
     i. Tachycardia
     ii. Tachypnea
     iii. Increased blood pressure
     iv. Increased muscle tension
4. **Diagnostic study findings**
   a. Mental Status Examination: To help rule out organic brain disease
   b. Laboratory tests: To rule out metabolic problems
   c. Drug screens: May reveal toxic drug levels, high blood alcohol levels
5. **Collaborative diagnoses of patient needs**
   a. Protect patient, family, and staff from injury.
   b. Provide the patient and family members with support and information early in the PCU stay.
   c. Attend to aggressive behavior rapidly and definitively.
   d. Be proactive in using appropriate resources (e.g., social services, security).
6. **Goals of care: Patient does not demonstrate aggressive or violent behaviors toward self or others**
7. **Management of patient care**
   a. Anticipated patient trajectory: With ongoing support and counseling, patients exhibiting aggressive and/or violent behaviors have the potential to modify these behaviors and live normal lives
     i. Treatments
       (a) Nonpharmacologic
         (1) Review medication list and discontinue suspect medications.
         (2) Identify and remove other possible causes or stimuli that precipitate aggressive or violent behaviors (e.g., argumentative, challenging family members).
         (3) Involve social service personnel early in the patient's stay, particularly in high-risk situations (e.g., known alcohol abuse in family members).
         (4) Patient issues

a) Verbal, chemical, and physical restraints may be required to relieve symptoms and maintain safety.
b) Use of physical restraints requires a plan and explanation of their use to the patient and family, daily renewal of the restraint order, close monitoring, and use of alternative methods of restraint as appropriate.
(5) Patient and family member issues
a) Speak in a calm, soft, noncondescending manner.
b) Allow the patient and family member to ventilate verbally without interruption.
c) Focus on the particular incident at hand.
d) Place clear limits on what will and will not be tolerated—outline the consequences of aggressive or violent behavior.
e) Do not attempt to educate the patient and family about aggression and violence during the aggressive or violent episode.
f) Obtain psychiatric consultation as needed.
(b) Pharmacologic
(1) Anxiolytics
(2) Neuroleptics (i.e., haloperidol)
ii. Discharge planning
(a) Discuss strategies for avoiding aggression or violence in the future.
(b) Post-ICU support and psychiatric follow-up may be required.
(c) Refer the individual to anger management classes.

Suicide

1. **Definition: A *suicide attempt* is the actual implementation of a self-injurious act with the express purpose of ending one's life. Patients coming to a critical care setting have often been unsuccessful in their suicide attempt and are admitted for actual or potential medical problems (e.g., respiratory depression, liver failure following acetaminophen overdose). A patient who has attempted suicide may be admitted to the ICU to determine whether the person meets the criteria for brain death.**
2. **Etiology and risk factors**
   a. Self-destructive behaviors resulting from a perceived, overwhelming threat to oneself
   b. Important differential diagnoses include the following:
      i. Unintentional drug overdose or other injury (i.e., gunshot) related to altered mental status, cognitive impairment, or physical handicap (visual impairment)
      ii. Elder or spousal abuse
3. **Signs and symptoms: May vary markedly depending on the type and extent of the injury present and the time that has elapsed since the injury**
   a. Cognitive and behavioral
      i. Altered level of consciousness and orientation
      ii. Severe anxiety (if conscious)
      iii. Severe depression (if conscious)
      iv. Marked disorientation or confusion
   b. Physiologic (related to the agent used in the suicide attempt, the extent of injury, and the time that has elapsed)
      i. Drug overdose
         (a) Tachycardia (amphetamines)
         (b) Bradycardia (digitalis)
         (c) Tachypnea (salicylates)
         (d) Bradypnea (barbiturates, opiates)
         (e) Dilated pupils (amphetamines)
         (f) Constricted pupils (opiates)
      ii. Trauma (gunshot wounds, stabbing, auto "accident")
         (a) Cardiovascular involvement: Hypotension, shock
         (b) Pulmonary involvement: Pneumothorax, lung contusions
4. **Diagnostic study findings**

a. Related to the method of attempted suicide
   i. Elevated liver enzyme levels: Acetaminophen overdose
   ii. Abnormal CT scan results: Gunshot wound to the head
   iii. Abnormal arterial blood gas levels
      (a) Metabolic acidosis: Salicylate, methanol overdose
      (b) Respiratory acidosis: Barbiturate, benzodiazepine, and/or opiate overdose
      (c) Respiratory alkalosis: Lower doses of salicylates
   iv. Electrolyte abnormalities: Hyperkalemia with digitalis overdose
   v. Abnormal coagulation results (increased international normalized ratio and prothrombin time): Warfarin overdose
   vi. Hypoglycemia: Insulin overdose
   vii. Drug screens: Urine and blood

5. **Collaborative diagnoses of patient needs**
  a. Provide a safe environment for the patient, family, and staff.
  b. Demonstrate trust, respect, and acceptance of the patient.

6. **Goals of care**
  a. Patient discusses suicidal thoughts with health care team.
  b. Patient verbalizes the need for help.
  c. Patient verbalizes needs and concerns.
  d. Patient verbalizes positive feelings about self.
  e. Patient verbalizes desire to recover.
  f. Patient is future oriented.

7. **Management of patient care (see Box 10-3 for more information related to the nursing care of the suicidal patient)**
  a. Anticipated patient trajectory: Outcomes for patients who have attempted suicide vary significantly depending on the mechanism and extent of injury. Many suicidal patients can live normal lives if they receive counseling and support.
   i. Treatments (will be specific to the mechanism of injury)
      (a) Institute specific treatment related to toxin ingestion, wounds (e.g., gastric lavage for drug overdose when indicated). Consult the poison control center or POISINDEX System (Thomson Micromedex) when relevant.
      (b) Assess the patient's risk for future suicide attempts.
      (c) If the patient is at continued risk for a suicide attempt, provide for protection from injury (e.g., constant observation, restraints). See The Joint Commission standards for the use of physical restraints (http://www.jointcommission.org).
      (d) Once the patient's condition has stabilized, allow for opportunities to discuss the attempted suicide and the patient's feelings (e.g., hopelessness, anger, shame, sadness) in a private setting.
      (e) Obtain a mental health consultation (patient's private psychiatrist, staff psychiatrist, or advanced practice nurse).

▨ BOX 10-3
▨ CHARACTERISTICS OF SUICIDAL PATIENTS

- The acute crisis period or high-lethality time is of short duration; it can be counted in hours or days.
- Suicidal patients are usually ambivalent about dying. At the same time that they plan suicide, they have fantasies of rescue.
- People who commit suicide may have talked about it or may not have talked about it.
- Suicidal persons usually give clues about their intentions.
- Suicidal behavior has no racial, social, religious, cultural, or economic boundaries.
- Suicide has no characteristic genetic qualities; however, its incidence is higher in families in which there have been previous suicides.
- Suicidal behavior does not necessarily mean that the person is mentally ill; in some cases, suicide is viewed as a logical last step by someone who is overwhelmed by stress.
- Most important, directly asking a person about suicidal intent will not cause suicide.

        (f) Facilitate visits from the patient/family support system (friends, clergy).

        (g) Allow family members to verbalize their feelings and concerns related to the suicide or attempted suicide.

    ii. Discharge planning

        (a) Varies depending on patient factors (e.g., physical and psychologic state) and family and social support systems

        (b) Provide information on a 24-hour suicide prevention hotline.

        (c) Provide phone numbers and websites for illness-specific support services (e.g., http://www.americanheart.org;http://www.cancer.org;http://www.nationalmssociety.org).

    iii. Ethical issues: Attempted assisted suicide by the patient and family in cases of terminal disease or unbearable chronic condition (see Chapter 1)

Dying Process and Death

1. **Description: Process of dying in the critical care setting can take many forms. Patient may die suddenly as a result of the injury or condition, after a protracted illness, after the withdrawal of life support, or as a result of brain death.**
   a. Care of patients and family members during or after the dying process is heavily influenced by the circumstances surrounding the patient's death.
   b. Kübler-Ross (1969) described five psychologic stages of the dying process (Table 10-5).
      i. Denial or isolation
      ii. Anger, rage, envy, resentment
      iii. Bargaining
      iv. Depression
      v. Acceptance
2. **Signs and symptoms**
   a. Clinical death: Cardiopulmonary arrest
   b. Brain death: Lack of brainstem function
      i. Loss of spontaneous respiratory effort (i.e., failed apnea test)
      ii. Loss of cough and/or gag reflex
      iii. Loss of oculocephalic reflex (doll's eyes phenomenon is seen)
      iv. Loss of caloric response following instillation of ice water against the tympanic membrane
3. **Diagnostic study findings: Most commonly used in the diagnosis of brain death. Studies include EEG, cerebral blood flow studies.**
4. **Collaborative diagnoses of patient needs**
   a. Ensure that the patient does not experience discomfort (pain, shortness of breath, etc.) or anxiety during the dying process.
   b. Ensure that family members' needs to be with the patient, receive reassurance and support, and have hope for a peaceful death are met.
5. **Goals of care**
   a. Patient and family members openly discuss fears and concerns regarding the dying process.
   b. Patient rates pain as within the goal range (determined by the patient).
   c. Patient does not complain of shortness of breath.
   d. Brain death: Family members recognize the brain-dead patient as legally dead and do not confuse brain death with a vegetative state
6. **Management of patient care (see Table 10-5 for more information on caring for the dying patient)**
   a. Anticipated patient trajectory: A peaceful death, in the manner desired by the patient and family, is the expected outcome
      i. Treatments
         (a) Nonpharmacologic
            (1) Ensure that do-not-resuscitate orders are written when appropriate.
            (2) Allow the patient and family members to discuss fears and concerns regarding the dying process.
            (3) Allow the patient and family members time to be alone (if desired).
            (4) Use nonpharmacologic methods of pain relief (see Pain).

■ **TABLE 10-5**
■ ■ **Kübler-Ross Stages of Grieving and Suggested Nursing Interventions**

Stage of Grieving	Nursing Interventions
Denial	Because denial operates protectively in a person on the verge of crisis, it is important for the nurse to respond to dying patients by • Listening to find out their perceptions of their situation • Showing acceptance whenever they are found to be in the dying process • Not encouraging false beliefs • Attempting to understand why they are behaving as they are
Anger	Allow patients to express their feelings to you and to ask, "Why me?" Remember, you need not attempt to answer that unanswerable question. • The anger that patients are expressing is not directed at you personally but, rather, toward what you represent (continued life) and toward their own painful situation.
Bargaining	Find out what kind of help patients need to complete their unfinished business. • Try to make time just to be with dying persons and to listen.
Depression	Avoid interrupting the grieving process. • Support patients in their grief. • Share your feelings of sadness appropriately, if you feel sad.
Acceptance	During this stage, the issue of letting go of a dying person arises. Show your support by • Not deserting the patient or family • Respecting their acceptance of death • Assisting the family with letting go of someone whom they love by listening and by intervening in areas in which family members feel they need help Other interventions for comfort and dignity include • Adequate medication for control of pain • Frequent mouth care • Positioning for comfort • Allowing family members to visit more frequently when the patient desires closer contact with loved ones • Supporting the family's involvement in providing comfort measures for the dying person

(5) Determine cultural preferences related to the dying process and postmortem care.

(6) Assist the dying person and his or her family members to validate their feelings (e.g., anger, pain).

(7) Acknowledge the grieving that accompanies the dying process.

(8) Help the patient and family to prepare for the dying process by describing possible symptoms and how they can be treated.

(9) Explain the role of pain medication—to relieve pain versus hasten dying.

(10) Determine the patient's and family's desires for spiritual support and assist in obtaining support (notify clergy, etc.).

(11) Assist with the withdrawal of life support (e.g., extubation); use guidelines for the withdrawal process (http://www.americanheart.org).

(12) Allow family members to be present if they choose.

(13) Provide for patient comfort (e.g., mouth care, positioning, suctioning).

      (b) Pharmacologic

          (1) Pain medication

          (2) Sedatives

          (3) Oxygen therapy

          (4) Diuretics and other agents as needed for patient comfort

    ii. Discharge planning: Bereavement support services for the family after the patient's death

REFERENCES AND BIBLIOGRAPHY

Psychosocial—General References

American Association of Critical-Care Nurses. *The Synergy Model of Certified Practice*. Aliso Viejo, CA: American Association of Critical-Care Nurses; 2003.

American Association of Critical-Care Nurses. *Progressive Care Fact Sheet*, 2003. http://www.aacn.org/WD/Practice/Content/progressivecarefactsheet.pcms?menu=Practice. Retrieved 11/04/2008.

American Psychiatric Association. *Diagnostic and Statistical Manual of Mental Disorders (DSM-IV-TR)*. 4th ed., text rev. Washington, DC: American Psychiatric Association; 2000.

★ Bell L, ed. *Standards for Acute and Critical Care Nursing Practice*. Aliso Viejo, CA: American Association of Critical-Care Nurses; 2008.

Biondi M, Kotzalidis GD. Human psychoneuroimmunology today. *J Clin Lab Anal*. 1990;4:22-38.

Caine RM. Psychological influences in critical care: perspectives from psychoneuroimmunology. *Crit Care Nurse*. 2003;23(2):60-70.

Caine RM, Ter-Bagdasarian L. Early identification and management of critical incident stress. *Crit Care Nurse*. 2003;23(1):59-65.

Carlson VR, Mroz I. Barriers to effective patient care. In: Grenvik A, Ayres SM, Holbrook PR, et al, eds. *Textbook of Critical Care*. 4th ed. Philadelphia, PA: Saunders; 2000.

Curley MAQ. Patient-nurse synergy: optimizing patients' outcome. *Am J Crit Care*. 1998;7:64-72.

★ Erikson E. *Childhood and Society*. 2nd ed. New York, NY: WW Norton; 1963.

★ Erikson E. *Identity, Youth and Crisis*. New York, NY: WW Norton; 1968.

★ Fortinash KM, Holoday-Worret PA. *Psychiatric Nursing Care Plans*. 3rd ed. St Louis, MO: Mosby; 1999.

★ Grumet GW. Pandemonium in the modern hospital. *N Engl J Med*. 1993;328:433-437.

Hardin SR, Kaplow R, eds. *Synergy for Clinical Excellence: The AACN Synergy Model for Patient Care*. Boston, MA: Jones and Bartlett; 2005.

★ Holland C, Cason CL, Prater LR. Patient's recollections of critical care. *Dimens Crit Care Nurs*. 1997;16:132-141.

Jastremski CA, Harvey M. Making changes to improve the intensive care unit experience for patients and their families. *New Horiz*. 1998; 6(1):99-109.

Keltner NL, Schwecke LH, Bostrom CE. *Psychiatric Nursing*. 4th ed. St Louis, MO: Mosby; 2003.

Maslow AH. *Toward a Psychology of Being*. Princeton, NJ: Van Nostrand; 1968.

Mullen JE. The synergy model in practice: the synergy model as a framework for nursing rounds. *Crit Care Nurse*. 2002;22:66-68.

★ Pettigrew J. Intensive nursing care: the ministry of presence. *Crit Care Clin North Am*. 1990;2: 503-508.

Pope DS. Music, noise, and the human voice in the nurse-patient environment. *Image*. 1995;27:291-295.

★ Satir V. *Conjoint Family Therapy*. Palo Alto, CA: Science & Behavior Books; 1967.

Schrader KA. Stress and immunity after traumatic injury: the mind-body link. *AACN Clinical Issues*. 1996;3:351-358.

Seligmann J. Variation on a theme. *Newsweek*. 1990;114:38.

★ Selye H. *Stress Without Distress*. Philadelphia, PA: Lippincott; 1974.

Solomon GF. Psychoneuroimmunology: interactions between the central nervous system and immune system. *J Neurosci Res*. 1987;18:1-9.

Topf M, Bookman M, Armand D. Effects of critical care unit noise on the subjective quality of sleep. *J Adv Nurs*. 1996;24:545-551.

Urban N. Patient and family responses to the critical care environment. In: Kinney MR, Dunbar SB, Brooks-Brunn J, et al, eds. *AACN Clinical Reference for Critical-care Nursing*. 4th ed. St Louis, MO: Mosby; 1998.

US Bureau of the Census. Uses for questions on the Census 2000 forms. http://census.gov/dmd/www/content.htm.

Patient Care

Andrews M, Boyle J. *Transcultural Concepts in Nursing*. 4th ed. Philadelphia, PA: Lippincott Williams & Wilkins; 2003.

Arbour R. Sedation and pain management in critically ill adults. *Crit Care Nurse*. 2000;20(5):39-56.

Beers MH, Berkow R. *The Merck Manual of Diagnosis and Therapy*. 17th ed. Whitehouse Station, NJ: Merck; 1999.

Carpenito-Moyet LJ. *Nursing Diagnosis: Application to Clinical Practice*. 10th ed. Philadelphia, PA: Lippincott Williams & Wilkins; 2004.

Chlan L, Tracy MF. Music therapy in critical care: indications and guidelines for intervention. *Crit Care Nurse*. 1999;19(3):35-41.

Cullen L, Titler M, Drahozal R. Protocols for practice: family and pet visitation in the critical care unit. *Crit Care Nurse*. 1999;19(3):84-87.

Gawlinski A, Hamwi D, eds. Acute care nurse practitioner: clinical curriculum and certification review. Philadelphia, PA: Saunders; 1999.

Gerdner LA, Buckwalter KC. Music therapy. In: Bulechek GM, McCloskey JC, eds. *Nursing Interventions: Effective Nursing Treatments*. 3rd ed. Philadelphia, PA: Saunders; 1999.

Giuliano KK, Bloniasz E, Bell J. Implementation of a pet visitation program in critical care. *Crit Care Nurse*. 1999;19(3):43-50.

Henneman EA, Cardin S. Family-centered critical care: a practical approach for making it happen. *Crit Care Nurse.* 2002;22(6):12-19.

★ Leske JS. Needs of relatives of critically ill patients: a follow-up. *Heart Lung.* 1986;15:189-193.

Stuart GW, Sundeen S. *Principles and Practice of Psychiatric Nursing.* 6th ed. St Louis, MO: Mosby; 2002.

Tullmann DF, Dracup K. Creating a healing environment for elders: complimentary and alternative therapies. *AACN Clinical Issues.* 2000;11:34-50.

Anxiety

Bally K, Campbell D, Chesnick K, et al. Effects of patient-controlled music therapy during coronary angiography on procedural pain and anxiety distress syndrome. *Crit Care Nurse.* 2003;23(2):50-51.

Keegan L. Alternative and complementary modalities for managing stress and anxiety. *Crit Care Nurse.* 2000;20:93-96.

Simon NM, Pollack MH, Labbate LA, et al. Recognition and treatment of anxiety in the intensive care unit patient. In: Irwin RS, Rippe JM, eds. *Intensive Care Medicine.* 5th ed. Philadelphia, PA: Lippincott; 2003.

Wong HLC, Lopez-Nahas V, Molassiotis A. Effect of music therapy on anxiety in ventilator dependent patients. *Heart Lung.* 2001;30:376-387.

Pain

★ Acute Pain Management Guideline Panel. *Acute Pain Management in Adults: Operative Procedures, Quick Reference Guide for Clinicians No 1.* Rockville, MD: Agency for Health Care Policy and Research, Public Health Service, US Department of Health and Human Services; 1992. AHCPR Pub No 92-0019.

American Academy of Pain Medicine, American Pain Society, American Society of Addiction Medicine.*Consensus Document: Definitions Related to the Use of Opioids for the Treatment of Pain.* Glenview, IL: American Academy of Pain Medicine; 2001. http://www.asam.org/Definitions Related to the Use of Opioidsin Pain Treatment.html.

American Geriatrics Society. The management of pain in older persons: AGS panel on chronic pain in older persons. *J Am Geriatr Soc.* 1998;46(5):635-651.

American Pain Society. *Principles of Analgesic Use in the Treatment of Acute Pain and Cancer Pain.* 5th ed. Glenview, IL: American Pain Society; 2003.

American Society of Pain Management Nurses. *ASPMN Position Statement: Pain Management in Patients With Addictive Disease.* Pensacola, FL: American Society of Pain Management Nurses; 2002.

Ardery G, Herr K, Titler M, et al. Assessing and managing acute pain in older adults: a research base to guide practice. *Medsurg Nurs.* 2003;12(1):7-18.

Cullen L, Greiner J, Titler MG. Pain management in the culture of critical care. *Crit Care Nurs Clin North Am.* 2001;13(2):151-166.

Dalton JA, Coyne P. Cognitive-behavioral therapy: tailored to the individual. *Nurs Clin North Am.* 2003;38(3):465-476.

Graf C, Puntillo K. Pain in the older adult in the intensive care unit. *Crit Care Clin.* 2003;19(4):749-770.

Hamill-Ruth RJ, Marohn ML. Evaluation of pain in the critically ill patient. *Crit Care Clin.* 1999;15(1):35-54.

Jacobi J, Fraser GL, Coursin BD, et al. Clinical practice guidelines for the sustained use of sedatives and analgesics in the critically ill adult. *Crit Care Med.* 2002;30(1):119-141.

Joint Commission. *Comprehensive Accreditation Manual for Hospitals (CAMH): The Official Handbook.* Oakbrook Terrace, IL: The Joint Commission; 2008.

Kanner R, ed. *Pain Management Secrets.* 2nd ed. Philadelphia, PA: Hanley & Belfus; 2003.

Koestler AJ, Doleys DM. The psychology of pain. In: Tollison CD, Satterthwaite JR, Tollison JW, eds. *Practical Pain Management.* Philadelphia, PA: Lippincott Williams & Wilkins; 2002.

Lang JD Jr. Pain: a prelude. *Crit Care Clin.* 1999;15(1):1-16.

Loeser JC, Butler SH, Chapman CR, et al, eds. *Bonica's Management of Pain.* 3rd ed. Baltimore, MD: Lippincott Williams & Wilkins; 2001.

★ McCaffery M. *Nursing Practice Theories Related to Cognition, Bodily Pain, and Man-Environment Interactions.* Los Angeles, CA: University of California at Los Angeles Student's Store; 1968.

McCaffery M, Pasero C. *Pain: Clinical Manual.* 2nd ed. St Louis, MO: Mosby; 1999.

Mersky H. Classification of chronic pain: description of chronic pain syndromes and definitions of pain terms. *Pain.* 1979;3(suppl):S217.

Munden J, Eggenberger T, Goldberg KE, et al. eds. Pain management made incredibly easy. Philadelphia, PA: Lippincott Williams & Wilkins; 2003.

National Pharmaceutical Council, Inc. *Pain: Current Understanding of Assessment, Management, and Treatments.* Reston, VA: National Pharmaceutical Council, Inc.; 2001.

Pace S, Burke T. Intravenous morphine for early pain relief in patients with acute abdominal pain. *Acad Emerg Med.* 1996;3(12):1086-1092.

Pasero C. Pain in the critically ill patient. *J Perianesth Nurs.* 2003;18(6):422-425.

Puntillo K. Pain: assessment, treatment and the coming thunder. Interview by Michael Villaire. *Crit Care Nurse.* 1995;15(6):75-81.

Puntillo KA, Morris AB, Thompson CL, et al. Pain behaviors observed during six common procedures: results from Thunder Project II. *Crit Care Med.* 2004;32(2):421-427.

Puntillo KA, White C, Morris AB, et al. Patients' perceptions and responses to procedural pain:

results from Thunder Project II. *Am J Crit Care.* 2001;10(4):238-251.

Rakel B, Barr JO. Physical modalities in chronic pain management. *Nurs Clin North Am.* 2003;38(3):477-494.

Snyder M, Wieland J. Complementary and alternative therapies: what is their place in the management of chronic pain? *Nurs Clin North Am.* 2003;38(3):495-508.

St. Marie B, ed. *ASPMN: Core Curriculum for Pain Management Nursing.* Philadelphia, PA: Saunders; 2002.

Titler MG, Rakel BA. Nonpharmacologic treatment of pain. *Crit Care Nurs Clin North Am.* 2001;13(2):221-232.

Websites

Agency for Healthcare Research and Quality. http://www.ahrq.gov.

American Academy of Pain Management. http://www.aapainmanage.org.

American Academy of Pain Medicine. http://www.painmed.org.

American Pain Society. http://www.ampainsoc.org.

American Society for Pain Management Nursing. http://www.aspmn.org.

American Society of PeriAnesthesia Nurses. http://www.aspan.org.

American Society of Regional Anesthesia and Pain Medicine. http://www.asra.com.

International Association for the Study of Pain. http://www.iasp-pain.org.

Medscape. http://www.medscape.com.

Oncology Nursing Society. http://www.ons.org.

Pain/Palliative Care Resource Center. http://www.cityofhope.org/prc/.

The Joint Commission. http://www.jointcommission.org.

Delirium (Acute Confusional State)

Burns SM. Delirium during emergence from anesthesia: a case study. *Crit Care Nurse.* 2003;23(1):66-69.

Inouye SK, van Dyck CH, Alessi CA, et al. Clarifying confusion: the confusion assessment method. *Ann Intern Med.* 1990;112:941-948.

Ouimet S, Kavanagh BP, Gottfried SB, Skrobik Y. Incidence risk factors and consequences of ICU delirium. *Intensive Care Med.* 2007;33:66-73.

Truman B, Ely EW. Monitoring delirium in critically ill patients: using the confusion assessment method for the intensive care unit. *Crit Care Nurse.* 2003;23(2):25-36.

Depression

American Psychiatric Association. *Diagnostic and Statistical Manual of Mental Disorders (DSM-IV-TR).* 4th ed., text rev. Washington, DC: American Psychiatric Association; 2000.

Food and Drug Administration Alert. http://www.fda.gov/medwatch/safety/2007/safety07.htm#Antidepressant.

Alcohol Withdrawal

Mayo-Smith MF, Beecher LH, Fischer TL, et al. Management of alcohol withdrawal delirium. An evidence-based practice guideline. *Arch Intern Med.* 2004;164(13):1405-1412.

Schumacher L. Identifying patients "at risk" for alcoholic withdrawal syndrome and a treatment protocol. *J Neurosci Nurs.* 2000;32:158-163.

★ Sellers EM, Sullivan JT, Somer G. Characterization of DSM-III-R criteria for uncomplicated alcohol withdrawal provides an empirical basis for DSM-IV. *Arch Gen Psychiatry.* 1991;48:442-447.

Sommers MS, Dyehouse JM, Howe SR, et al. Nurse, I only had a couple of beers: validity of self-reported drinking before serious vehicular injury. *Am J Crit Care.* 2002;11:106-114.

★ Sullivan JT, Sykora K, Schneiderman J, et al. Assessment of alcohol withdrawal: the revised Clinical Institute Withdrawal Assessment for Alcohol scale (CIWA-Ar). *Br J Addict.* 1989;84: 1353-1357.

Website

Alcoholics Anonymous. http://www.aa.org.

Suicide

Cummins RO. *Advanced Cardiac Life Support Provider Manual.* Dallas, TX: American Heart Association; 2001.

Simons M. Patient contracting. In: Bulechek GM, McCloskey JC, eds. *Nursing Interventions: Effective Nursing Treatments.* 3rd ed. Philadelphia, PA: Saunders; 1999.

Website

American Association of Poison Control Centers. http://www.aapcc.org.

Dying Process and Death

Chapple HS. Changing the game in the intensive care unit: letting nature take its course. *Crit Care Nurse.* 1999;19(3):25-34.

Cummins RO. *Advanced Cardiac Life Support Provider Manual.* Dallas, TX: American Heart Association; 2001.

★ Kübler-Ross E. *On Death and Dying.* New York, NY: Macmillan; 1969.

Myers TA, Eichhorn DJ, Guzzetta CE, et al. Family presence during invasive procedures and resuscitation: the experience of family members, nurses, and physicians. *Am J Nurs.* 2000;100:32-42.

Websites

American Cancer Society. http://www.cancer.org.

American Heart Association. http://www.americanheart.org.

The ICU Delirium and Cognitive Impairment Study Group. http://www.icudelirium.org/delirium/training-pages/DeliriumProto%2001_30_07.pdf.

Index

Page numbers followed by b indicate box(es); f, figure(s); t, table(s).